Man against Disease

Arthur G. Clegg, B.Sc., F.I.Biol.
Sometime Principal Lecturer in Biological Science,
City of Sheffield College of Education.

P. Catherine Clegg, B.Sc., Ph.D., M.B., Ch.B.
Sometime Lecturer in Physiology, University of Sheffield.

 Heinemann Educational Books
London

Heinemann Educational Books Ltd
22 Bedford Square, London WC1B 3HH

London   Edinburgh   Melbourne   Auckland
Singapore   Kuala Lumpur   New Delhi
Ibadan   Nairobi   Johannesburg
Exeter (NH)   Kingston

ISBN 0 435 60170 9
© A. G. Clegg and P. C. Clegg 1973
First published 1973
Reprinted 1975, 1977, 1980, 1982
Reprinted 1987

Filmset and printed in Great Britain by
BAS Printers Limited, Over Wallop, Hampshire

Bound by Hunter & Foulis Limited, Edinburgh

Man
against
Disease

Preface

Over the last few years we have been increasingly aware of the need by non-medical students, for a comprehensive account of human health and its disorders. Students of Health Education, Hygiene, Domestic Science, Pharmacy, Human Biology, Zoology, and Social Studies, and teachers of these subjects in Universities, Colleges and schools often experience difficulty in finding 'medical-background' literature which is appropriate to their needs. This book has been written in an attempt to fulfil these needs, by bringing together material from a wide range of sources. It is hoped that pupils in schools (Human Biology and Hygiene, Domestic Science, Biology and ROSLA courses) will also find it useful, as a reference book.

The subjects dealt with in this book range beyond those normally dealt with in conventional courses in Human Biology and Hygiene and it has been somewhat difficult to formulate an appropriate title. We hope that the title chosen, *Man against Disease*, will convey the spirit of the book, which deals not only with the enemies outside, but also those within man.

1973   A.G.C. and P.C.C.

Acknowledgements

Many people have assisted us in the preparation of this book, in allowing us to visit abattoirs, dairies, sewage farms, water works, museums etc., and by allowing us to use their illustrations. Each illustration in the text carries its own acknowledgement but we would especially like to record our appreciation of the generosity of the World Health Organization and the Wellcome Museum of Medical Science, London.

The colour plates following page 72 are reproduced by kind permission of Dr A. M. Ramsay, Dr R. T. D. Emond, and William Heinemann Medical Books Ltd.

By the same authors

Biology of the Mammal, Heinemann Medical Books.

Introduction to mechanisms of hormone action, Heinemann Medical Books.

Hormones, Cells, and Organisms, Heinemann Educational Books.

For David and Jonathan

Contents

COLOURED PLATES SHOWING
SYMPTOMS OF SOME COMMON
DISEASES
[Following page 72]

1. The germ theory of disease

Introduction

DURING the long history of mankind, man's views on the causes of disease have undergone radical changes. At the time of the New Testament disease was looked upon as the result of possession by devils which could be driven out by religious faith, or by magic and charms. Some still hold this view. At other times men have thought that the breathing of foul vapours or 'miasmas' was the cause of disease. This was a popular belief in the mid-nineteenth century when industrial cities lay under a nauseating stench of rotting garbage and human excreta. There were large dunghills in the towns and cities where faeces accumulated until carted away by farmers for use as manure. Where a river ran through the town or city then the sewers—if there were any—discharged their untreated contents directly into the water. But it was not the stench of garbage and faeces which caused such diseases as cholera and typhoid which were so common at these times. It was the presence of germs (minute living organisms, invisible to the naked eye) which could readily spread from a diseased to a healthy person in the overcrowded, unsanitary conditions of the times when water and food could be readily contaminated by urine and faeces from diseased persons.

The men to whom we owe the greatest debt for our understanding of the nature of infectious diseases are a Frenchman, Louis Pasteur (1822–95) and a German, Robert Koch (1843–1910). Pasteur was, by training, a chemist and although he had no medical training his ideas and discoveries were later to revolutionize medical and veterinary science. His researches extended widely and covered the nature of fermentation, disorders of the process of fermentation, e.g. 'diseases' of wine, diseases of silkworms, the causes of infectious disease in man and ways in which he can be made immune to infectious disease. We are in this chapter considering the germ theory of disease, but it is virtually impossible to isolate Pasteur's contribution to this great discovery from his other work. Although his interests ranged widely there was a natural sequence of ideas in his work, and his studies of fermentation and its disorders seemed to lead quite naturally on to his studies of disease in animals and men.

Pasteur and the germ theory of fermentation

The first researches which gained Pasteur notice from the eminent scientists of his day were on the structure of crystals of organic acids. In recognition of this work he was appointed to the post of Professor of Chemistry at Strasbourg. From Strasbourg he went as Professor of Chemistry at Lille. Here he found himself surrounded by an industry engaged in the production of alcohol from the fermentation of sugar beet. Quite naturally, when one of the local distillers was having problems in the fermentation of his sugar beet he consulted the local Professor of Chemistry. Pasteur went to the distillery and examined the large vats in which the sugar beet was fermenting. The owner, a Monsieur Bigo, told Pasteur that in some of the vats the alcohol became contaminated during the process of fermentation and that the yield of alcohol was poor.

Pasteur examined these 'sick' vats and fished out samples of a grey slimy substance from the beet liquor to take back to his laboratory. He did not forget to take other samples from the healthy foaming vats which were producing satisfactory amounts of alcohol. When Pasteur examined these specimens in his laboratory, he saw under the microscope that the juices from the healthy vats contained tiny yellowish globules, some in bunches or chains and others with tiny buds appearing from their sides. These were yeasts, tiny living micro-organisms which had, in fact, been described earlier by other investigators, such as Cagniard de la Tour in France and by Schwann in Germany.

Pasteur performed a variety of experiments with yeasts and with the process of fermentation. He found, for example, that if the yeasts were killed by boiling then fermentation stopped. To Pasteur these yeasts appeared not as accidental contaminants of the fermentation process but as the actual cause of fermentation. It appeared to him that the process of fermentation, in which sugar is converted to alcohol and other substances, is the *result* of the activity of the living micro-organisms. In 1860 the Academy of Science awarded Pasteur its prize in experimental physiology for his studies in fermentation which had led him to develop the 'germ theory' of fermentation.

However, these studies of normal fermentation did not help Monsieur Bigo and his 'sick' beet vats which were producing contaminated alcohol. When Pasteur examined the slime from the 'sick' vats he found that there were very few yeast organisms. Instead there were minute rods dancing around in the fluid. These rods were much smaller than the yeasts, being only 1/10 000 of a centimetre in length. He found that the liquid from the 'sick' vats which contained fantastic numbers of these tiny rods contained no alcohol. Instead of alcohol the liquid contained lactic acid, the acid which accumulates in souring milk. These tiny rods, he thought, must be the living ferments which are converting sugar into lactic acid, just as yeasts are the living ferments which produce alcohol from sugar.

In order to study these tiny rods further, to see if they really were living organisms, he tried to see if they could multiply. He first took some tiny flecks of slime from the 'sick' vats and placed them in sugar water, but in this solution they did not grow or multiply. So he prepared a richer food for them containing the liquid from boiled yeast, sugar and a little chalk to make the food alkaline. To a bottle of this food he then, from the point of a needle, added a tiny speck from the 'sick' vats. He put the bottle in a warm oven and left it there overnight. The following day the bottle contained many grey specks and a grey fluid at the bottom. When he examined a drop of fluid from the bottle he found that it contained millions of tiny rods. The rods had indeed multiplied and produced lactic acid. He was now able to tell M. Bigo that it was these tiny rods in the beet vats which were the cause of the disorders of fermentation.

These studies showed once and for all that the process of fermentation is due to the activity of living organisms. The product of the fermentation, e.g. alcohol, lactic acid or acetic acid (vinegar) depends on the kind of living micro-organism in the fermenting fluid. Pasteur now turned his attention to fermentation in the wine industry. Here grapejuice is fermented in vats to produce alcohol. No yeast is added to the vats for there are living 'wild' strains of yeasts on the skin of the grapes. There are many kinds of wines—champagnes, burgundies, clarets etc. which result from differences in the kind of grapes used and differences in procedure. Each

kind of wine has its own 'illness'. Champagnes are liable to develop a slimy, 'ropy' sediment, clarets are liable to become turbid, burgundies to become bitter, and so on. Pasteur found when he examined wines under the microscope that they contained various micro-organisms in addition to the wild yeasts from the grape skin. He became convinced that these micro-organisms were the cause of the 'illnesses' of the wines. He first tried to kill these micro-organisms in the wines by using chemicals, but later found that they could be killed by heating the wine to 55 °C. This heat treatment prevented the deterioration of the wine on storage and yet it did not alter the flavour or bouquet (smell) of the wine; it is used to process many different foodstuffs to improve their keeping qualities and increase their safety, and is called pasteurization.

Pasteur destroys the concept of 'spontaneous generation' of life

These early studies by Pasteur showed that fermentation was due to the activity of living micro-organisms and that the process of fermentation could be 'diseased' by the presence of other micro-organisms. His next studies, which were highly controversial at the time, explored the origins of these micro-organisms. Where did they come from? In Pasteur's time scientists held the view that these primitive kinds of life—the micro-organisms—could arise 'spontaneously' from inanimate matter. For example, John Needham (1713–81) took some boiling mutton gravy and placed it in a flask which he then corked. In a few days this gravy was literally teeming with micro-organisms. He believed that he had destroyed all life in the gravy by boiling it so that the micro-organisms which appeared later had come from non-living matter in the gravy—'spontaneous generation' was a fact.

But Pasteur realized that if all life in a nutrient solution was killed by boiling then any life which later appeared had come from the atmosphere. A cork is not a very efficient way of preventing contamination of a solution from the atmosphere. Pasteur placed his nutrient solution in a flask and drew out the neck into a swan's-neck tube (Figure 1.1). He then boiled the liquid in the flask, killing all micro-organisms in the liquid, and driving air out of the neck. As the flask cooled, air was drawn into the flask again but micro-organisms became trapped along the moist walls of the tube so that the liquid in the flask remained sterile—it contained no micro-organisms. If, however, the nutrient

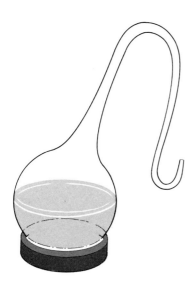

Figure 1.1 Pasteur's swan-neck flask.

solution was shaken to bring it into contact with the upper walls of the flask then the tube rapidly became alive with micro-organisms.

Pasteur and diseases of silkworms

Pasteur went on to study diseases of animals and man. His first study was a disease of silkworms which was ruining the French silk industry. When he arrived in southern France he knew little about silkworms. He was to find that they develop from eggs laid by a moth. After eating a quantity of mulberry leaves the silkworm grows and then spins a cocoon of silk—the raw material for the silk industry. Some of the silk cocoons are allowed to develop into moths which then lay further eggs to provide a supply of more silkworms and cocoons. The disease of the worms which was destroying the silk industry was called pébrine, because the sick worms were covered with tiny pepper-like spots. When he examined the inside of the sick worms he found many tiny globules which were not present in healthy worms. These, he thought, were the cause of the disease. He advised the silk farmers that they should collect the male and female moths in pairs and after the female of each pair had laid her eggs then both parents should be pinned down, their bellies opened and the contents examined for the presence of the tiny globules. If none were found this meant that the eggs would be sound and could be used for

new silkworms in the spring. But the next spring there was disaster, for his prediction did not come true and many worms which hatched from supposedly healthy eggs failed to eat normally and did not spin their cocoons of silk.

These were difficult times, for his studies were being complicated by the presence of two distinct diseases in the silkworms. By careful experiments he was able to show that pébrine was, in fact, a disease caused by a micro-organism which could be spread from one silkworm to another. He found that he could infect healthy worms by allowing them to feed on leaves on which he had smeared crushed-up sick moths. After this meal the worms became covered with pepper-spots and their insides swarmed with tiny globules. The disease could also be transmitted from one generation to the next by infecting worms which were just about to spin a cocoon. These worms spun their cocoons and developed normally into moths, but the moths were loaded with globules and their eggs came to nothing. Pasteur's original mistake in examining moths for the presence of the disease was that he looked only under the skin of the moth's belly for the globules; but it was necessary to grind up the whole animal before it was possible to guarantee that the eggs that it had laid would be free of the disease and produce healthy worms.

Pasteur, Koch and the disease of anthrax

Pasteur had thus been able to show that micro-organisms were responsible for 'diseases' of fermentation and also for the disease of silkworms called pébrine.

In 1877 he provided the then shattering evidence that micro-organisms were the cause of a disease in animals and man. This disease was anthrax, a disease which affects sheep, cattle, horses and goats and sometimes spreads to men handling these animals. In Pasteur's time anthrax was common on farms all over Europe. In sheep and goats it is a rapidly fatal disease in which the blood teems with tiny micro-organisms and death occurs in a matter of hours. The death rate in animals is very high, at 70–100 per cent of affected animals. In man the disease starts in the skin, although it can also attack the lungs or intestine. Local itchiness on the affected skin is followed by the appearance of a small spot which quickly enlarges to form a blood-stained blister surrounded by firm, reddened skin. The patient becomes feverish with headache and aches and pains in the joints.

If the micro-organisms spread from the infected skin into the blood stream, the condition deteriorates and the patient becomes prostrated with a high fever. Before modern methods of treatment the disease had a high mortality, depending on the site at which the organisms were introduced into the skin. Anthrax starting on the neck had a mortality of twenty-four per cent, but if it started on the forehead it had a mortality rate of three per cent. Just as Pasteur was beginning his studies of anthrax a young German physician, Robert Koch, began to study the same problem. In fact, several investigators before Pasteur and Koch had suspected that micro-organisms were the cause of anthrax. They had seen the micro-organisms in the blood of sick animals and had transferred the disease into healthy animals by means of a few drops of infected blood, but their results did not convince the scientists of the day.

capable of producing the disease in animals as was blood taken directly from an animal dying of anthrax. These minute living organisms were the cause of the disease anthrax. They were never found in the blood of a healthy animal.

Koch was able to provide an explanation for the fact that there were some pastures where no sheep could go without contracting anthrax. In some way the micro-organisms could remain dormant on the pastures, even over winter, only

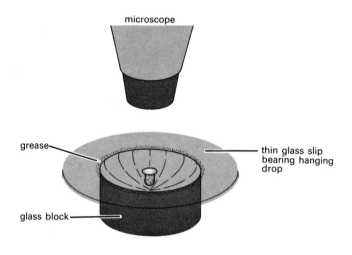

Figure 1.2   Hanging-drop preparation.

Koch's studies anticipated somewhat those of Pasteur. He examined the blood of infected animals and saw the tiny rods of the anthrax bacillus. Koch developed the technique of growing micro-organisms outside the body in serum or on the surface of boiled meat extracts which had been solidified by the addition of gelatine. He was able to sow small pieces of the tissues of sick animals into serum and watch the enormous multiplication of the bacilli. A small drop taken from these cultures and added to further serum produced new generations of bacilli, and after several new sub-cultures were made in this fashion the organisms were just as

later infecting any animals that came to graze on them. This puzzled him because cultures of the rod-like organism which were allowed to dry out for a few days in his laboratory were not then capable of infecting animals. The answer to this problem was provided when he examined cultures of anthrax-producing organisms by means of a special technique. On a clean piece of thin glass which had been heated to destroy all chance micro-organisms, he placed a drop of fluid containing anthrax bacilli. Over this drop he then placed a thick piece of glass containing a concave well scooped out so that the drop would not be touched. He smeared grease around the edge of the thick piece of glass where it touched the thin glass, to prevent the entrance of air or micro-organisms. He turned the apparatus upside down and could observe the drop through the microscope hanging down into the chamber of the thick glass and uncontaminated by micro-organisms from the air (Figure 1.2).

He had kept one of these hanging drop preparations for twenty-four hours, and when he examined the drop under the microscope,

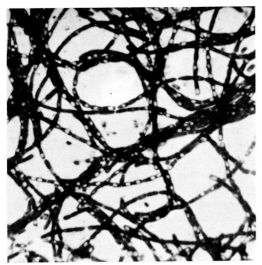

Figure 1.3 Culture of anthrax bacilli with spores. The bacilli tend to stick to one another, end to end, producing long chains. The spores are the clear areas in the bacilli. (*By courtesy of WMMS.*)

instead of finding clearly visible anthrax bacilli he was to find only the faint outlines of the bacilli. Inside each individual bacillus in the thread of bacilli there was a brightly shining oval body (Figure 1.3). He dried this hanging drop and put it away for some weeks. He then took the piece of glass which carried the dried hanging drop and moistened it with serum. As he watched, the glass-like beads transformed again into normal anthrax bacilli. These shining beads were what we call the spores of the microbe, the form in which the anthrax bacillus is resistant to drying, heat and cold, the form in which the bacillus keeps alive in the pastures, even over the winter. The spores which he had prepared by drying the bacilli in air were capable of transformation into bacilli which could infect animals.

It was thus clear that these bacilli were the cause of anthrax in animals. He advised that all animals dying of anthrax should be destroyed at once after they died and if they could not be burned then they should be buried deep in the ground so that the bacilli or their spores could not infect other animals.

Pasteur carried these experiments further. He took the blood of animals dying of anthrax and added it to a nutrient fluid in the laboratory and showed that under these conditions the bacilli multiplied rapidly. He took one drop of infected blood and added it to 50 cm³ of nutrient fluid. After incubation of the fluid he transferred one drop of the nutrient fluid into another 50 cm³ of nutrient fluid. He repeated this process one hundred times in succession so that he had a culture in which the original blood he had added had been so diluted that there was virtually none in the final culture fluid. Only the bacilli could escape the effect of dilution because they were capable of multiplication in the culture fluids. It was obviously the bacilli, and no other component of the original blood, which were the cause of anthrax, for a drop of the hundredth culture could kill an animal as rapidly as a drop of the infected blood.

Pasteur performed many other experiments, the results of which supported this view. For example, he prepared cultures of anthrax bacilli and then he filtered the cultures through membranes which were fine enough to hold back the bacilli. This filtered culture fluid was not infective when it was injected into animals; only the bacilli themselves could produce an infection. The germ theory of human disease was thus firmly established.

Robert Koch was then to provide clear evidence that germs were the cause of two other human diseases, tuberculosis and cholera. The micro-organisms responsible for these diseases were far more difficult to isolate than were anthrax bacilli. Koch had to develop special dyes which could stain the organisms so that they became visible under the microscope. He also put enormous efforts into the task of growing the organisms outside the human body, and succeeded in both of these tasks. He laid down three rules for identifying a particular microbe as a cause of a disease.

1. The microbe must be invariably present in the diseased animal.
2. It must be capable of cultivation outside the body.
3. It must produce the disease when it is injected into a healthy animal.

Pasteur and Koch thus provided the first clear and acceptable evidence for the germ theory of disease. Pasteur made even further contributions by showing that it was possible to modify micro-organisms in such a way that, although they could no longer produce disease when injected into animals, they could make the animal immune to infection by the normal unmodified strain of the micro-organism. After man has suffered from various kinds of infectious disease he develops immunity to a second attack of the disease. Pasteur showed that it was possible to produce this immunity artificially without man having to suffer from the disease. The techniques of producing artificial immunity are the subject of Chapter 6.

2. Disease-causing micro-organisms I Bacteria

BACTERIA are very simple, minute living things consisting of a tiny speck of protoplasm, the basic stuff of all living matter, surrounded by an envelope. In spite of their minute size and simple structure they are true living things and show the four basic signs of life—growth, reproduction, respiration, and assimilation of food.

Structure of bacteria

Shape

Under the microscope individual bacteria are very small creatures of varying shapes and sizes. The shape of bacteria is their only easily visible character and is used as a basis for describing them. Cocci (sing. coccus) are spherical bodies with a diameter of about one micron (1/1000 mm). Some cocci, on division, stick together to form a chain—the streptococci. Other cocci divide irregularly and stick to one another in small bunches; these are the staphylococci. Other cocci are arranged uniformly in pairs—the diplococci (Figure 2.1). Many other bacteria take the form of straight or slightly curved rods. They vary considerably in length from one species to another but they are usually about one micron in diameter. These rod-shaped bacteria are called bacilli and many of them are motile because they carry one or more flagellae (Figure 2.2). There are some curved rods which appear comma-shaped; these are called vibrios such as the organism responsible for cholera. Other bacteria take the form of a long cork-screw shaped rod and these are called spirilla (Figure 2.3). Spirilla, like vibrios, are usually motile. Spirochaetes are much finer flexible filaments twisted into a spiral e.g. *Spirochaeta pallidum* is the organism responsible for syphylis (Figure 2.4).

The microscopic structure of bacteria

Using the ordinary light microscope very little of the detailed structure of bacteria can be seen. The electron microscope, however, can produce much larger magnifications and it has revealed considerable detail of the external and internal structure of bacteria (Figure 2.5). Each bacterial cell is limited by a fairly thick ridged wall which is covered on the outside by a thin film of slime; in some bacteria there is a capsule around the cell wall. Inside the protective cell wall is a delicate cytoplasmic membrane which is enfolded to form a complicated system of tubules which run into the depth of the cell. This enfolded membrane is the 'power house' of the organism. It contains enzymes whose action supplies energy to the cell, including energy for 'pumping' substances into the cell from the outside environment. The cytoplasmic membrane

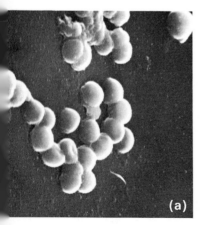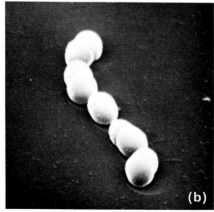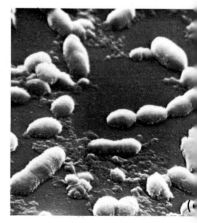

(a)   (b)   (c)

Figure 2.1 Electron micrographs of cocci. (a) *Staphylococcus aureus*, (b) *Streptococcus viridans*, and (c) *Diplococcus pneumoniae*. (*By courtesy of The Upjohn Company.*)

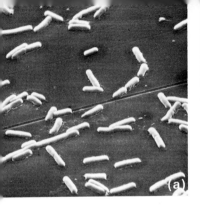
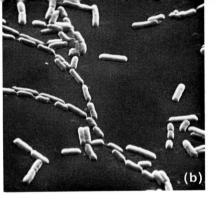
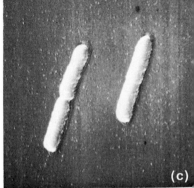

Figure 2.2   Bacilli. (a) *Klebsiella pneumoniae*, (b) *Proteus vulgaris*, and (c) *E. coli*. ((a), (b), and (c) are electron micrographs reproduced by courtesy of The Upjohn Company.) (d) *Salmonella typhimurium*, stained for flagellae. (*By courtesy of the Unilever Research Laboratory.*)

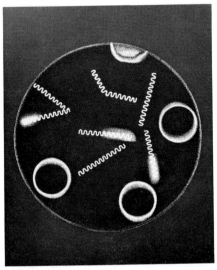

Figure 2.4 (below)   *Spirochaeta pallidum* photographed with the light microscope. (*By courtesy of the WMMS.*)

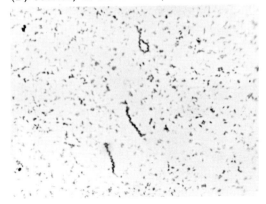

Figure 2.3 (below)   A spirillum. (*By courtesy of the WHO.*)

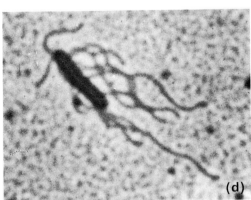

ribosomes — cell
membrane

D.N.A

(a)

slime layer

cell wall

flagellum arising in cytoplasm

capsule   cell wall

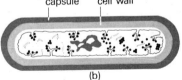

(b)

Figure 2.5 (opposite)   The structure of the bacterial cell as demonstrated by the electron microscope (a) shows a bacterium with flagellae and (b) shows a non-flagellated bacterium having a capsule outside the cell wall.

also manufactures the complex materials that form the cell wall. Inside these two membranes of the cell is the machinery for manufacturing the proteins of the bacterial cell: the nuclear material contains the complex nucleic acid (deoxyribonucleic acid—DNA) which carries 'information', in the form of a chemical code, for all the activities of the cell: the ribosomes (composed of ribonucleic acid and protein) are tiny bodies, about ten to thirty microns in diameter, on which molecules of new protein are manufactured.

Flagellae

Some types of bacteria bear flagellae (Figure 2.2(d)); there is seldom only one and there are usually many, either arising from over the entire surface of the bacterium or concentrated at one or both ends. Each flagellum consists of strands of special protein molecules which can contract, thus enabling the flagellae to move; these contractile flagellae allow the bacterial cell to move, particularly if it is in fluid.

Nuclear material

The use of the electron microscope has revealed a presence of a nucleus in bacterial cells. These are not as complex in structure as are the nuclei of higher plants and animals, and they take the form of a round or oval structure. When the bacterial cell is preparing to divide, a single ring-shaped chromosome appears; this duplicates itself so that each daughter cell comes to

Figure 2.6   Photomicrograph of the cells of *Clostridium botulinum* with spores (phase contrast microscopy). (*By courtesy of The Unilever Research Laboratory.*)

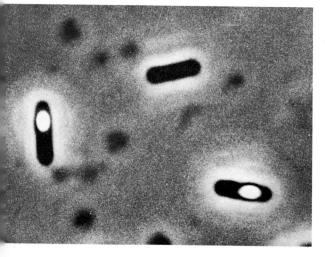

contain a single chromosome. The chromosome carries the gene material—deoxyribonucleic acid (DNA)—which is the information for all the life activities of the bacterial cell.

Spore formation

Some species of bacteria can form very resistant spores (Figure 2.6). Much of the bacterial contents becomes enclosed inside a dense envelope —the endospore. In this form the bacterium may be very resistant to extremes of temperature and to the effects of disinfectants, and it may survive in this form for many years until conditions are suitable for the germination of spores (see also page 4).

Growth and reproduction

All bacteria are unicellular organisms, and growth shows itself by an increase in size of the single cell; since bacteria are only of microscopic dimensions this growth cannot be seen by the human eye. The reproduction of bacteria is mainly by non-sexual means. Only one individual is involved in the process, and undergoes what we call binary fission in which the cell divides into two identical daughter cells. The daughter cells may remain attached to one another, so that chains or bunches of cells are produced. Given optimum conditions of temperature, moisture, oxygen and food supply, bacteria can reproduce indefinitely. Fortunately nature provides efficient checks for indefinite bacterial multiplication. We can readily study bacterial reproduction under optimum conditions in the laboratory. First of all a culture medium is prepared which contains the appropriate organic and mineral substances which are needed for the growth of the particular bacteria in question. To this medium or broth is added a small number of bacteria and the flask containing the broth is then placed in a warm incubator. At intervals a small sample of the broth is removed and the number of bacteria it contains is counted under the microscope. For a few hours after beginning incubation one can observe no increase in the number of bacteria. This is called the lag phase. During this time, however, there is intense metabolic activity in the bacterial cells, which increase greatly in size. After this interval the bacteria begin to divide rapidly, and each cell may undergo division three times in one hour. As each organism and its descendants divide, so the number of bacteria increase in geometric progression, one organism becoming successively 2, 4, 8, 16, 32, 64, 128, 256 . . . and so on. If the logarithm of the number of bacteria in the medium is plotted against time, the result is a straight line. This phase of rapid bacterial division is thus called the logarithmic phase. Sooner or later, however, the medium can support no more bacteria, because of the limited supply of oxygen or nutrients. The multiplication of bacteria now declines to a rate which is sufficient to replace those bacteria which die. This is called the stationary phase of bacterial culture.

Not all species of bacteria, however, need a supply of oxygen. We can divide bacteria into three groups according to their oxygen needs:

1. aerobic bacteria,
2. anaerobic bacteria,
3. facultative bacteria.

Aerobic bacteria must live in an atmosphere or medium which contains oxygen, and if the oxygen supply is reduced then this prevents the bacteria from growing and multiplying. Anaerobic bacteria cannot develop in an atmosphere which contains even traces of free oxygen. Many members of this group cannot, in fact, live in the presence of free oxygen. Although these bacteria cannot live in the presence of free oxygen, they still need this element for their life processes. They obtain oxygen by decomposing organic matter in which the oxygen is locked in complex molecules of carbohydrate, protein and the like. The anaerobes are in fact the putrefying bacteria which are responsible for the decay and destruction of dead animals and plants. Without the activity of this group of micro-organisms, the surface of the earth would be piled high with the corpses of generations of dead animals and plants. The majority of bacteria are, however, facultative in their needs for oxygen; this means that they can live under aerobic or anaerobic conditions, although each species of bacteria has its own preference for either aerobic or anaerobic respiration.

Mutations and bacteria

We have already described the method of asexual bacterial multiplication by the process called binary fission. The daughter cells which result from binary fission have the same genetic structure as the mother cell because each one carries an identical copy of the parent chromosome. Bacterial cells contain probably over a thousand genes in the single chromosome of the cell. Each gene is a short segment of that chemical called DNA which carries the whole or part of the information which determines the character or behaviour of the bacterial cell such as the possession of flagellae, the ability to form spores etc. Before a cell divides, each gene must be copied so that each daughter cell comes to carry the same genetic information as the parent cell. In this process of copying, errors can and do occur, and we call these errors mutations. When a mutation occurs in a dividing bacterial cell, one or other daughter cell will carry a mutant gene which will show itself by some change in the structure or metabolism of the cell. This kind of change in the genetic information occurs in all plant and animal cells. They result in *variation* within a species, and form the raw material for evolution (progressive change) in animals and plants. The *rate* of reproduction in bacteria is, however, so much faster than that of higher plants and animals that a day to man may be a million years to bacteria in terms of opportunity to reproduce and in terms of opportunity to change by means of mutation. Man may have made conquest of many pathogenic bacteria by means of drugs and vaccines, but this conquest has often been of a temporary nature, because he is dealing with a wiley and ever-changing adversary. The use of specific drugs for the treatment of bacterial infections in man was virtually non-existent until 1935 when the first sulphonamide was discovered. The introduction of sulphonamides revolutionized the treatment of many infectious diseases such as gonorrhoea, cerebro-spinal fever (meningococcal meningitis), and pneumonia. During the decade 1935–45 when the sulphonamides were the only anti-bacterial drugs generally available, mutations in the various pathogenic bacteria led to the appearance of strains which were resistant to the action of the sulphonamides. But for the introduction of antibiotics in the 1940s, it is highly likely that by now the sulphonamides would have been almost useless in any infectious disease. Many bacteria are now resistant to the action of the sulphonamides. The change was first seen and progressed most rapidly in the gonococcus—the organism responsible for gonorrhoea. Between 1940 and 1941 70 per cent of patients with gonorrhoea were promptly cured by sulphonamides, but in the period 1944–5 70 per cent failed to respond because of drug resistance by strains of the bacteria. This kind of mutation that alters the responses of bacteria to drugs is of special importance to man. Other types of mutations which have importance for human diseases include those which may affect the virulence of a particular bacterial species.

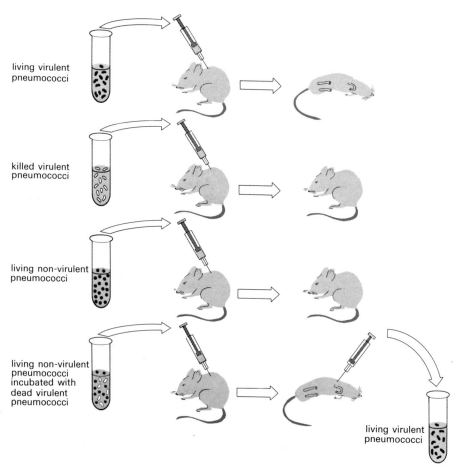

Sexuality in bacteria

We have seen that variation in bacteria can and does arise from mutations which occur in the genetic material during asexual reproduction. However, sexuality also occurs in bacteria, that is the interchange of hereditary characters between two bacterial cells, and this also leads to variation. Studies with the electron microscope have shown that two bacterial cells can fuse together, allowing an interchange of genetic material so that the resulting daughter cells show a combination of hereditary characters.

Bacterial 'transformation'

We have seen two ways in which variation can arise in bacteria. One is by mutation occurring in the genetic material and being transmitted to the offspring of a bacterium during binary fission. Because of the potentially enormous rate of reproduction in bacteria, this kind of mutation can lead to rapid evolution of strains of bacteria possessing new characters. The sexuality of bacteria—the interchange of genetic material between bacterial cells—further contributes to this evolution.

There is another process by which bacteria can exchange new characters, the phenomenon of 'transformation' whereby a packet of genetic information in the form of a fragment of DNA can penetrate into the cell's own genetic apparatus. By this means an entire population of bacteria can, within a few hours, acquire a new character, a rate of evolution which exceeds that of higher organisms by an order of astronomical magnitude.

This phenomenon was first observed as long ago as 1928 when Griffith, a British bacteriologist who was working with bacteria called pneumococci, organisms that are a common cause of pneumonia (Figure 2.7). She found that if she mixed dead pneumococci belonging to a virulent strain with living pneumococci of a normally non-virulent strain and then injected the mixture into mice, the animals rapidly succumbed to a fatal infection. From the bodies

living virulent
pneumococci

killed virulent
pneumococci

living non-virulent
pneumococci

living non-virulent
pneumococci
incubated with
dead virulent
pneumococci

living virulent
pneumococci

Figure 2.7 An illustration of Griffith's work on the transformation of pneumococci.

of these mice she was able to isolate living virulent bacteria. The dead virulent pneumococci had not come to life in the mice but they had somehow 'transformed' the normally harmless strain of pneumococci into lethal microorganisms. We now know that this type of dramatic transformation of the properties of a strain of bacteria appears where a segment of new DNA becomes incorporated into the bacteria cells. Bacteria can acquire additional DNA in several ways. We have seen how this occurs during sexual union of two bacterial cells. A second way whereby a new stretch of DNA can breach the bacterial cell is when the bacteria are attacked by a virus (see also page 28). Just as some bacteria infect and parasitize other organisms, animals and plants, they themselves may be infected and parasitized by viruses. These viruses that parasitize bacteria are called bacteriophages. When a phage attacks the bacteria, it attaches itself to the wall of the bacterial cell and squirts its own DNA into the bacteria. In this act of penetrating the cell wall, it may also introduce fragments of bacterial DNA from the environment which may be incorporated into the DNA of the bacterial cell and so alter the properties of the cell.

There is yet another and important way in which a bacterial cell can be transformed. Some susceptible kinds of bacteria can take up fragments of DNA directly from their environment; presumably this comes from the chromosomes of dead bacterial cells. How this giant molecule crosses the tough cell wall is not known. However some activator, which is a product of the bacteria themselves, appears in the medium in which bacteria are growing and renders them capable of this uptake of fragments of DNA. Whatever the exact mechanism may be that is involved in this kind of interchange of genetic information between populations of bacteria, the process can and does have far-reaching consequences for human disease and for the treatment of infectious disease. One property that can be exchanged between populations of bacteria by 'transformation' is the ability to resist the effects of particular antibiotics and other drugs which are used in the treatment of infections. Thus in one outbreak of dysentery in a mental hospital, the strain of bacteria which was responsible (Shigella species) was found to be resistant to only two drugs (streptomycin and the sulphonamides) at the beginning of the epidemic. Patients were treated with various drugs, and during the course of the epidemic bacteria with eight very different resistance patterns were isolated from patients. We can see what was happening in these patients by isolating a particular drug-resistant strain of Shigella and culturing it with a strain of *Escherichia coli* (normally a very common and harmless commensal of the human bowel flora) which shows no resistance to the drugs that are used in the treatment of dysentery. After twenty-four hours of incubation together, the *E. coli* will acquire the drug resistance from the dysentery bacilli. Furthermore the *E. coli* can transfer this drug resistance to strains of dysentery bacilli previously sensitive to the drugs. Antibiotics may thus produce effects that are both unexpected and unwanted. A particular antibiotic prescribed for a patient with a throat or chest infection may, at the same time as curing the patient of this infection, produce hidden damage in the form of some harmless coliform becoming resistant to the antibiotic; these may later infect dysentery-producing bacteria with the particular drug resistance and thus make treatment of the dysentery more difficult.

The dangers of giving antibiotics to animals

The use of antibiotics in farms or in veterinary practice may at first sight appear to have little relevance for infectious disease in man. Nothing could be further from the truth. In the rearing of various farm animals, antibiotics are commonly used drugs. They may be used to prevent or treat infectious disease in animals but they are also used more widely to promote growth in the animal. How antibiotics increase the growth rate of animals such as pigs and cows is not known, but stimulate growth they do. This practice has led to the development of drug-resistant bacteria in the intestine of animals and these bacteria can and do spread to man. The Swann Report (1969) stresses a dramatic increase in the number of drug-resistant intestinal bacteria in animals. It also shows there is undoubted evidence that these organisms are commonly ingested by man. Feeding antibiotics to animals may be good economics, i.e. the animals grow faster, but they should not be given antibiotics which are used to treat or prevent infections in man.

The culture and identification of bacteria

The early workers with bacteria were plagued by the problem of isolating specific bacteria responsible for a particular disease from all the other kinds of contaminating bacteria present on the skin, in dust, in the air and on laboratory glassware. When they took a sample of blood or pus from a sick patient and tried to culture the bacteria in the laboratory, likely as not their broth cultures would grow scores of different kinds of micro-organisms. Which of these organisms was responsible for the illness and which had come from the air or dust? Robert Koch, the man who discovered the bacteria responsible for diseases such as anthrax, tuberculosis and cholera, was the first worker to provide a solution to this problem. It is said that one day he noticed that half of a boiled potato left on a table in his laboratory had collections of tiny coloured droplets on its surface, some grey, some red, some yellow. Using a fine piece of platinum wire he attacked each coloured drop in turn. The first grey droplet when examined in a drop of water under the microscope, was found to contain thousands of bacteria, each one identical in shape and size to its neighbour. The next droplet from the potato, a yellow one, again contained thousands of identical micro-organisms but these were of a different shape from the organisms in the grey droplet; these organisms were like minute cork-screws which rotated and swarmed about in the water under the microscope. He found that each coloured droplet from the potato was a pure culture of a particular kind of micro-organism. When the potato had been exposed to air, different kinds of micro-organisms had settled on it. Each one multiplied where it landed, producing a small coloured spot which was a pure culture of a particular kind of bacteria.

Following on these observations Koch developed the technique of growing cultures of bacteria on nourishing broths which were stiffened by the addition of gelatine. If a mixture of microbes is spread on to the surface of such a jelly, each microbe multiplies at the place where it settles, and under optimum conditions produces a pure colony of microbes which is not only visible to the naked eye but shows such features as colour, size and shape of colony which are characteristic of the particular species of microbe.

Koch also discovered that some microbes are much more difficult to culture than others, because they are extremely demanding in terms of the nature of the culture medium. After many unsuccessful trials he was able to grow the temperamental tubercle bacillus on a medium containing fresh serum.

Culture media

We can divide media in which bacteria are cultured into two main classes:

1. broths consisting basically of a water extract of meat,
2. solid media which are solidified by the addition of either agar-agar, obtained from seaweed, or gelatine.

When media are solidified by the addition of agar-agar, they melt just below the boiling point of water but do not set again until the temperature is lowered to 42 °C. If it is necessary to enrich the medium for the growth of more delicate micro-organisms then blood or serum can be added to the melted agar at a tempeature that will not harm the additives. Blood-agar is a very useful growth medium for almost all bacteria will grow well on it.

When a sample of biological material, e.g. blood, pus, urine etc., is being examined for the presence of disease-causing bacteria, the first problem which is met is the presence in the material of numerous contaminating bacteria, such as harmless commensals which are unrelated to the disease. The biological material is first sown thinly on a large surface area of a solid medium with the intention of seeding individual bacteria. As these bacteria grow and multiply they produce small colonies of bacteria, visible to the naked eye. Each colony consists of a mass of one species of bacteria. Particular species of bacteria may show special colony characters which help in their identification. Parts of a colony can now be removed and examined under the microscope for special structural and staining qualities that may also help to identify the bacteria. Further specimens of a colony can be removed for culture in other media so that studies can be made of the metabolism of the bacteria, their ability to metabolize various sugars, produce gas or acid and so on. All these may help to identify the bacteria.

During the process of seeding of culture media and during incubation of the culture media under the appropriate conditions (moisture, temperature, presence of various nutrients etc.), strict precautions have to be taken to prevent contamination of the cultures by bacteria in the air, in the breath of the biologist, and by bacteria on glassware and in the culture media. But this is not a practical text and we shall not look in any detail at the special techniques of culturing bacteria.

Using the above techniques it soon became possible to obtain pure cultures of the bacteria responsible for a particular disease in a patient. This may not be an easy task, for certain bacteria require very special culture conditions before they can be persuaded to grow and multiply. Some bacteria such as the *Treponema pallidum*, the organism responsible for syphillis, *cannot* be persuaded to grow outside the body. If we are able to obtain pure cultures of pathogenic bacteria then these can be subjected to further tests. One important and routine study is the microscopic features of the bacteria and their staining properties. Further tests may include the injection of bacteria into laboratory animals to study the virulence of the bacteria: this kind of study may be especially important with bacteria that are responsible for diphtheria or tuberculosis. Some bacteria are so similar in their cultural, staining and metabolic properties that yet other techniques have to be used to distinguish them; these special studies include agglutination reactions with specific sera, but more of these later (page 50).

negative bacteria is stained in the above way, the Gram-positive bacteria stand out as violet-coloured structures; the Gram-negative organisms are colourless and have to be stained with some other contrasting dye such as neutral red. The staining properties of Gram-negative and Gram-positive organisms are due to differences in the composition of their cell walls. The following are the reactions of common commensal or pathogenic bacteria of man to Gram's stain:

Gram-positive	*Gram-negative*
Staphylococci	Neisseria
Streptococci	Salmonellae
Pneumococci	Shigella
Clostridia	Proteus
Yeasts	Vibrio
Moulds	Brucella
	Haemophilus
	Spiroachaetes
	Coliforms

Microscopic examination of bacteria

A study of the staining properties of dried and 'fixed' bacterial cells is a very important step in the identification of bacteria. Bacterial cells which are superficially very similar in their appearance under the microscope may have a very different structure and composition of the cell wall and cytoplasm which can be revealed by the use of appropriate staining reagents. First, thin smears of the bacterial culture are made on clean glass slides. Often a wire with a looped end is used to transfer a small amount of the culture to the slide and the same loop is used to spread out the material into a thin film. Every bacterial culture is regarded as being potentially dangerous and the wire loop is always sterilized in a flame after it has been used. The smear is allowed to dry in air and then 'fixed' by passing it several times through a flame. Fixation partly coagulates the bacterial proteins and causes them to stick to the slide.

Gram's stain is by far the most important stain in bacteriology. Its use divides bacteria into two types, so called Gram-positive and Gram-negative organisms. When Gram-positive organisms are treated with a dye (methyl-violet or gentian violet) followed by iodine, a stain-complex is deposited in the cell wall which cannot be removed by decolourizing agents such as alcohol or acetone. When Gram-negative organisms are similarly treated the dye is washed away by the acetone or alcohol. Thus if a slide bearing a mixture of Gram-positive and Gram-

A second generally used staining test is for the ability of bacteria to hold a dye under acid conditions. Organisms are called acid-fast if they hold a dye in which they have been heated when they are subsequently washed with acid-alcohol. Acid-fast bacteria contain extra lipids in the cell membrane. The tubercle bacillus and other Mycobacteria resist the penetration of ordinary aniline dyes because of their waxy envelope. They are not stained by the Gram stain, but can be stained with a powerful staining solution containing a mordant (fixer) and the penetration of the dye is helped by heat. The stain used consists of basic fuchsin with carbolic acid as a mordant (Ziehl-Neelson's stain). An acid-fast organism is one which will resist de-colourization with 25 per cent sulphuric acid. Certain bacteria of this group—notably the tubercle bacillus, will also resist decolourization by an alcohol-acid mixture, and these bacteria are called 'acid-alcohol-fast'. The distinction is important for identifying the tubercle bacilli from other Mycobacteria which are not pathogens and are 'acid-fast' but not 'acid-alcohol-fast'. In looking at urine for the presence of tubercle bacilli one has to be careful to exclude the acid-fast harmless commensal Mycobacterium called the smegma bacillus (present in the secretions around the opening of the urethra). The smegma bacillus is acid-fast but not acid-alcohol-fast. A variety of other staining techniques may be used to stain spores, capsules, flagellae and spiro-chaetes.

Serological tests

Other laboratory tests can be used to distinguish strains of bacteria which by the normal
cultural and staining properties are identical.
These tests distinguish different proteins in the
various strains and they are best discussed after
we have some understanding of the nature of the
reactions that occur when bacteria and other
micro-organisms are introduced into the animal
body (page 50).

Bacteria. Non-pathogens and pathogens

Harmless bacteria

Bacteria abound in nature. Their total mass on
the earth is vast, at least twenty times the total
mass of *all* animal life. They are present in air,
soil, water. They contaminate every surface and
niche in our homes and even colonize the surface
and parts of the interior of our bodies. A gramme
of fertile soil contains about one hundred million
living bacteria, and the scurf (collections of dead
epidermal cells) on the scalp about five hundred
million bacteria per gramme! The bulk of these
bacteria in the world is far from harmful to man.
Indeed they are essential for the maintenance of
life on this planet (see Chapter 11). Here we are
concerned with the few bacteria that may cause
human disease. It appears that many of the
common disease-producing bacteria have
evolved from bacteria that are harmless commensals of the human body. Many of the pathogenic bacteria are identical in appearance to the
harmless commensals and moreover, when the
pathogenic bacteria do produce disease they
often attack the region of the body which normally carries the harmless commensals which the
pathogenic type so closely resembles.

Let us look then at the flourishing population
of micro-organisms that is harboured by the
normal human body. We will see examples of
bacteria that are normally commensal in their
habits but which, under certain circumstances,
can invade the tissues to cause disease. There
will also be examples of commensals from which
strict pathogens (i.e. those which regularly
cause disease) may have evolved. The micro-
flora and fauna of the human body contain, in
addition to bacteria, fungi, protozoa, an arthropod and at least one virus.

The skin

The skin contains a range of permanent residents, many of which are usually harmless commensals, browsing among the epithelial cells or
living in the various pores that penetrate the
skin—the hair follicles and ducts of sweat glands.
These organisms include a miniature arthropod
(the follicle mite) that lives in and around the
hair follicles and parts of the face. The remaining
organisms include yeasts, bacteria and perhaps
viruses. The fungus responsible for 'athlete's
foot' (page 95) commonly lives as a harmless
species on the cells of the foot and between the
toes; in certain circumstances (page 96) the
fungus proliferates and causes disease. However,
the dominant members of the community on the
skin are bacteria of various types. The skin is
unevenly populated by bacteria and the number
in any one position depends upon various local
factors such as moisture or the presence of
secretions. The densest population occurs on the
face, neck, armpits, and groin. In an adult male
the armpit has a population of over two million
bacteria per square centimetre of epidermis. Of
the bacteria present on the skin, the staphylococcus is important in relation to the production
of disease. Staphylococci can be isolated from
any part of normal human skin and they can be
also isolated from the relatively trivial infections
of skin—pimples and boils. The latter are not
necessarily the same type of staphylococci as
those of normal skin; they are what we call a
different 'strain' of staphylococci and they
probably have evolved from the harmless commensals. There are even more virulent strains
of staphylococci that may invade the tissues of
the body to produce more serious diseases, e.g.
abscesses in bone (osteomyelitis) and in the
breast. Even these virulent staphylococci share
the habits of their commensal ancestors in having
a liking for the skin. Indeed these virulent
staphylococci may colonize the skin (particularly of the nostrils and perineum) and be carried
by apparently healthy individuals. However, if
these individuals work in surgical wards, infant
nurseries, maternity wards and the like, they can
be responsible for epidemics of severe staphylococcal infections.

The mouth and throat

The teeth and the mucous membranes of the
mouth, nose and throat teem with micro-
organisms of many types. Most of the bacteria
are of the round coccus type. The streptococci,
in which the individual cocci are strung together
to form chains, are a member of this group. The
streptococci themselves form a large group of
bacteria, some harmless but others capable of

producing various infections of differing severity. We will be looking at infections caused by pathogenic members of this group of bacteria in other sections of the book (see erysipelas, page 73, tonsillitis and scarlet fever, page 72, rheumatic fever, page 73). The important point here is that the pathogenic members of this group, in appearance at least, are very similar to the harmless commensals that inhabit the entire upper and lower intestinal tract. Another type of bacterium present in the mouth and pharynx is called the pneumococcus. These rather elongated cocci occur in pairs surrounded by a well marked capsule. This is the basic structure of over seventy different types of penumococci that can be distinguished only by means of serological tests (page 50). Many of these pneumococci are carried by normal healthy individuals. They rarely invade the body tissues to cause infection unless the resistance of the host is considerably lowered by other disease processes. Yet other superficially similar pneumococci are not often carried by normal individuals. These pneumococci are commonly responsible for what is called primary pneumonia, that is infection of the normal healthy lung. This term primary distinguishes the pneumonia from secondary pneumonia where the bacterial invaders attack lungs that are already injured by other diseases such as bronchitis.

The streptococci and pneumococci are the Gram-positive bacteria. In the normal healthy mouth and throat there are also representatives of Gram-negative cocci called the Neisseria. Many of the Neisseria are non-pathogenic. One pathogenic representative of this group is worthy of mention—the meningococcus, which is frequently found in the pharynx of healthy people. In overcrowded communities such as armies the number of carriers may be as high as 50 per cent. There are various strains of meningococci which differ in their virulence. Some strains are particularly likely to invade the body, commonly producing an infection of the membranes around the brain, i.e. meningitis. Epidemics of this disease occur in overcrowded communities, although not everyone who harbours a virulent strain of the meningococcus in his pharynx develops meningitis and usually less than one per cent of carriers develop the disease.

There are, of course, other representatives in the micro-flora of the mouth and pharynx, rod-shaped bacteria of various sorts, elongated, spiralled bacteria called spirochaetes, and yeasts.

The stomach and intestine

We can now look at the normal flora of the lower parts of the intestinal tract. In health the stomach is almost sterile for any bacteria that are swallowed are usually quickly killed by the acid contents. Similarly the upper reaches of the small bowel contain few bacteria but these increase in number such that in the colon the bulk of the faecal contents consists of bacteria! In this vast population of micro-organisms there are many different representative forms, streptococci, staphylococci, and many types of rod-shaped forms for which we shall use the old-fashioned term bacilli. In addition there are spirochaetes and yeasts. We will look at two representatives of this vast micro-flora in relation to disease, *Bacillus coli* and a group of anaerobic spore-bearing bacilli of the group called clostridia.

Bacillus coli is not the commonest of bacteria in the bowel and faeces but is much the best known. It grows readily on the simplest of media in the laboratory and was easily grown by the early bacteriologists when they cultured faeces (Figure 2.2 (c)). It was called *Bacillus coli communis*—the common bacillus of the large bowel. Nowadays we know that this supposed single species contains very many different strains. Inside the bowel *B. coli* is usually a harmless intestinal commensal, but outside the bowel it may cause various infections, in particular infections of the kidneys and bladder. However, in the context of our discussion of the evolution of pathogenic bacteria the *B. coli* is important in that it is probably the parent organism from which most of the bacteria which cause infections of the bowel have evolved. Indeed some strains of *B. coli* itself are pathogenic and are responsible for cases of gastroenteritis in infants that may sometimes reach epidemic proportions in hospitals and nurseries. The Gram-negative rods responsible for typhoid and paratyphoid fevers and food poisoning (see page 140) are separate species that have probably evolved from the commensal *B. coli*.

The anaerobic spore-bearing bacilli of the bowel (for example *Clostridium tetani*, see Figure 2.8, and *Clostridium welchii*) are, like most strains of *B. coli*, harmless commensals when they live in the bowel. They are responsible for disease only when they are accidentally introduced into some other tissues of the body, usually by way of wounds. The contamination of wounds by soil is particularly dangerous in this respect, for soil is always likely to contain these anaerobic bacilli from the faeces of animals and man. Contamination of wounds by *Cl. tetani*

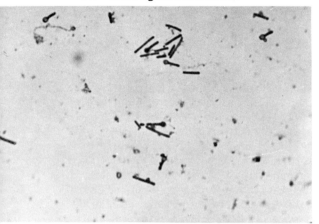

Figure 2.8 Tetanus bacilli with spores. (*By courtesy of WMMS.*)

may produce that dreaded disease called tetanus (see page 69). Contamination by *Cl. welchii* may produce the disease called gas-gangrene, a common complication of war wounds but also seen in civilian practice after severe compound fractures (when bone fragments protrude through the skin) or after criminal abortion, i.e. abortion carried out illegally by the inexperienced and without due antiseptic precautions. If dead tissues in the wound are heavily infected by other bacteria that consume oxygen then the local conditions are ripe for multiplication of these anaerobic bacilli. The proliferating bacilli liberate toxins and these destroy the surrounding living tissue, opening up new areas into which the organisms can advance. This type of infection is rather different from the ones we have previously discussed in this chapter. This infection is produced by the introduction of a harmless bowel commensal into a different and damaged tissue where the anaerobic conditions lead to multiplication, liberation of toxins and disease.

The evolution of pathogens

We have been mainly concerned with the vast and varied commensal population of microorganisms that is harboured by the human body. During the course of human history some of these commensals have given rise to strains of increased virulence. These new strains may no longer inhabit the home of their ancestors, be it the skin, pharynx or bowel. They develop the ability to invade even healthy tissues and cause disease. Even the normal commensal strain may cause disease if it is introduced into tissue which it does not normally inhabit (for example *Cl. welchii*, *Cl. tetani*). The normal commensals

may also be persuaded to invade healthy tissues if there is a reduction of local or general resistance of the body. A good example of the effect of a change in local conditions on the susceptibility to invasion by normal commensals is seen in the case of the human vagina; this situation is discussed in detail in the chapter on fungus infections, page 97.

The evolution of pathogenic strains of bacteria from harmless commensals is followed not only by the ability to invade tissues and cause disease, but also by changes in the biochemistry of the bacterial cell. The pathogens frequently lose the ability to synthesize particular raw materials which are needed for their life processes. They are no longer capable of growth and multiplication outside living tissues which provide these particular requirements. In other words, pathogens tend to become obligatory parasites. They also become less readily grown in the laboratory, where special additions of blood, serum or other delicacies may have to be added to the medium before they can be persuaded to grow and multiply.

Pathogens, of course, vary in their specialization and in their virulence. Some pathogenic strains of staphylococci are harboured by normal skin and may cause harm only if the skin's surface is damaged or if they are transferred to another individual with either a wound or a low resistance to infection (for example the newborn). Yet other pathogens are so specialized and virulent that if they become established in the body they invariably cause disease.

Usually sterile areas of the body

There are many parts of the body that contrast strongly with organs such as the skin, mouth, and bowel in that they are usually sterile, that is they have no population of commensal microorganisms. Contamination of these parts of the body by occasional micro-organisms is usual but the various defence mechanisms of these organs remove such offenders quickly and efficiently. Areas that are usually sterile include the larynx, trachea, bronchi, bronchioles, nasal sinuses, stomach, upper small bowel, liver and gall bladder, the peritoneal cavity, pancreas, kidneys, ureters, bladder, the interior of the eye, brain, blood, and spinal fluid.

The interaction of the commensal micro-flora with invading pathogens

We have seen that parts of the body have their own natural micro-flora. Any invading pathogen may meet a vast and relatively stable population of micro-organisms, interacting with one another to achieve the sort of *status quo* that characterizes any ecological system, be it lake, sea, desert or forest. Pathogenic organisms constantly alight on healthy human skin. However, they do not find ideal conditions for colonization; they meet an already established population in which they must find some niche if they are able to establish themselves. The physical conditions alone may deter colonization—it may be too dry, too unstable (because of continual shedding of the outer layers of the skin), too acid, and so on.

The normal resident flora also gives the skin some defence against colonization by pathogens. The greasy secretion of sebaceous glands contain lipids, which when broken down by some of the Gram-positive members of the normal flora produce unsaturated fatty acids which inhibit the growth of several bacterial and fungal skin pathogens.

A similar state of affairs occurs in the vagina (see also page 97) where the normal flora ferments sugars derived from the shed cells of the vaginal epithelium so as to produce acid conditions which discourage the growth of pathogens. In later sections of the book (page 106) we will see how disturbance of the normal flora of the body, e.g. by antibiotics, can lead to various problems which include the invasion by pathogenic micro-organisms.

How bacteria cause disease

We have seen that certain parts of the body such as the skin and large bowel may be populated by vast numbers of certain bacteria without any disturbance of man's health. There are yet other bacteria whose presence, often in relatively small numbers, causes illness or death. We have now to examine the way in which these bacteria cause illness or death. From the point of view of the survival of a species of pathogenic bacteria it would appear that to kill the host (man) would be a disadvantage. But perhaps a little too much has been made of this argument in the past. Provided that the bacteria can rapidly multiply and spread from their host to other humans it does not matter so much if the host dies. Cholera (page 144) can kill a man within a day, but in that day an individual may pass many litres of diarrhoea each cubic centimetre of which can contain up to a thousand million cholera vibrios. Without strict hygienic precautions, the environment of the rapidly dying case of cholera becomes contaminated by millions of new vibrios within

a matter of hours. This is not to say that a milder and more prolonged attack of cholera may make a man even more likely to spread the infection to others. Many individuals when infected with cholera vibrios do not develop the typical symptoms, and these individuals may be very common during an epidemic of the disease. Their faeces contain much smaller numbers of vibrios than of those who developed typical cholera with copious diarrhoea and vomiting, but in spite of this these 'carriers' may be more important in the spread of the disease, for they are free to move around and can contaminate the environment widely. We will see over and over again similar examples where 'carriers' with mild infections or symptomless 'carriers' of infectious disease can be very important in the spread of disease (e.g. see typhoid fever).

Toxins

The idea that pathogenic bacteria produce harmful effects on the host by way of chemical substances called toxins goes back to the early history of bacteriology. As long ago as 1884, Robert Koch concluded that the symptoms of cholera were due to toxins liberated by the bacteria. The cholera vibrios multiply in the lumen of the bowel and cause illness without invading the wall of the bowel or indeed any other tissue of the body. Koch tested his theory by obtaining cultures of cholera vibrios, filtering the culture to remove the vibrios, and then injecting the filtrate (free of bacteria) into experimental animals. If the symptoms of cholera were due to chemical toxins liberated from the vibrios then this injection should have produced the disease. But the animals which received the injections remained healthy and the idea of cholera toxins was abandoned. We know now that if Koch had given the filtrate by mouth then it would have produced the symptoms of cholera, for the toxins act directly on the wall of the bowel.

In the same year that Koch put forward his ideas about the cause of the symptoms of cholera, another worker called Loeffler made a similar suggestion about the cause of symptoms of diphtheria. Loeffler had found that when experimental animals died after an injection of diphtheria bacilli under the skin the internal tissues of the body were severely affected but diphtheria bacilli could only be found at the place where they had been injected. He concluded that from the point of injection the bacilli liberated toxins that circulated in the blood and damaged other body tissues. He himself was unable to demonstrate this toxin, but a year later Roux and Yersin obtained a substance from cultures of diphtheria bacilli that could kill guinea-pigs in doses less than a milligramme. The discovery of two other bacterial toxins soon followed, tetanus toxin and botulinum toxin.

By the turn of the century the prevailing idea was that the harmful effects of all pathogenic bacteria were due to the effects of toxins liberated from the bacteria. This notion also dominated views on the treatment of bacterial infections. In 1890 Von Behring and Kitasato announced that rabbits and mice that had been inoculated with *small* doses of 'neutralized' tetanus and diphtheria toxins became immune to the toxins (the toxins were neutralized by mixing them with the serum taken from the animals and the mixture was injected back into the animals). By means of these injections of small amounts of 'neutralized' toxins a mouse could survive even after it had been injected with three hundred lethal doses of toxin. These studies were followed by many attempts to prepare 'anti-toxic' serum by injecting small numbers of bacteria or their products into animals. This was the foundation of the new science of immunology, but it turned out that there are few bacterial infections in which the harmful effects of the disease are clearly due to the effects of toxins released from bacteria. The few infections in which toxins are important include diphtheria, tetanus, botulism and plague. Very many other bacterial toxins have since been discovered but their exact rôle in infectious disease is still obscure.

Toxins have been divided into two classes, exotoxins and endotoxins. Exotoxins are those that are released from the bacteria into the surrounding culture medium and these toxins come mainly from Gram-positive bacteria (although at least two exotoxins are produced by Gram-negative organisms—the organisms that are responsible for Shigella dysentery and cholera). Endotoxins were a new class of toxins, first described in 1935, obtained by extraction from Gram-negative organisms, and presumably liberated from the organisms when these died. However, the fundamental difference between exo- and endotoxins is not so much whether the toxin is found inside or outside the bacterial cell but with the chemical structure of the toxin. Exotoxins are protein in nature and they are liberated by the bacteria into the growth medium; an important feature of these toxins is that they can be neutralized by antibody. Endotoxins come from the wall of the bacterial cells. They are complexes of protein, polysaccharide and lipid, and they are released only on the breakdown of bacteria. An important feature of endotoxins is that they are not neutralized by antibody; molecules of antibody attach themselves to protein and polysaccharide but not to lipids.

We do not know why toxins are produced by microbes. The killer toxins produced by the diphtheria bacillus or by the cholera vibrio surely cannot have been selected during evolution to kill the host animal (man). Rapid killing of a host animal by a parasite does not help the parasite to multiply and spread to a new host. It may be that these toxins are mere metabolic by-products of the bacterial cell and serve no function. An explanation that may be more likely is that toxins may be enzymes whose activities we do not yet understand. We will now look at one example of a toxin which is clearly involved in the damage caused by an infecting pathogen; this toxin is that produced by the organism that causes plague. In later sections of the book we will deal with other examples, diphtheria (page 67), tetanus (page 69), botulism and other forms of food poisoning (page 153).

Toxins and plague

In Chapter 16 we shall be discussing the role of arthropods (fleas, lice etc.) in the spread of various infectious diseases. One such disease is plague, the 'black death' that once nearly destroyed European civilization. Major outbreaks of this remarkably virulent infection are now uncommon. The disease 'smoulders' in parts of Asia and is fanned into the flame of epidemics whenever social conditions deteriorate. The holocaust of war in South Vietnam resulted in five thousand cases of plague being reported in 1967 (and how many cases went unreported in the war-torn country can be left to the imagination). Plague is caused by a bacillus, *Pasteurella pestis*, which is spread by fleas living on various rodents, including rats. Interest in the role of toxins in this killing disease stems from observations in Madagascar (now the Malagasy Republic) where the disease is still endemic (i.e. it 'smoulders' with occasional small outbreaks occurring from time to time). Today plague can be successfully treated by means of antibiotics such as streptomycin or chloramphenicol, provided that treatment is begun early in the disease; if treatment is delayed then death may occur. Observations in Madagascar showed that in cases in which death occurred because of delayed treatment, no plague bacilli could be identified in the blood or organs at post-mortem examination.

Presumably these cases died due to the effects of toxins liberated by the bacteria before the latter were destroyed by the antibiotics. Highly purified plague toxin (itself a mixture of at least two proteins) is extremely lethal to rats and mice and about 10^{-7}g (0.1 microgramme) given intravenously will kill fifty out of every hundred mice. The effect of plague toxin on body cells has been studied in detail. The damaging effect of plague toxin on various body tissues—including the heart—is due to an effect of the toxin on those minute structures within body cells that are called mitochondria. Mitochondria are the 'power-houses' of the cell and are concerned with the release of energy from foodstuffs such as glucose. Plague toxin inhibits the mechanism of respiration in the mitochondria and so reduces the energy supplies of the cell.

Other toxins

Some pathogenic bacteria produce a variety of toxins and we do not clearly understand the part played by particular toxins in infections caused by these bacteria. Staphylococci are common commensals of human skin and they are also common pathogens, mainly of the skin (boils, carbuncles and secondary invaders of other skin disorders such as eczema or burns) but sometimes they invade the body to cause a septicaemia (staphylococci in the blood stream) with abscesses occurring in various organs, or they may cause staphylococcal pneumonia or meningitis. Pathogenic staphylococci produce a variety of toxins which are listed below:

1. α toxin—lethal, causes severe damage to the skin and breaks down red blood cells.
2. β toxin—breaks down red blood cells.
3. γ toxin—breaks down red blood cells.
4. δ toxin—breaks down red blood cells.
5. ε toxin—breaks down red blood cells.
6. Hyaluronidase—an enzyme that breaks down the jelly-like material of connective tissue and allows the more rapid spreading of bacteria and their products. This enzyme is called the spreading factor.
7. Staphylococcal coagulase—coagulates plasma.
8. Staphylokinase—breaks down fibrin (the basis of a blood clot).
9. Enterotoxin—causes vomiting.
10. Leukocidin—kills leukocytes (white blood cells).

The significance of these various toxins will depend on the nature of the infection. When food is contaminated by someone whose hands carry staphylococci and the food is then stored, the staphylococci may multiply and liberate various toxins. When this food is eaten it may result in the rapid onset of a type of food poisoning in which early vomiting is a prominent feature (see page 152). In this situation the enterotoxin is important in causing the symptoms, although we are not sure whether the enterotoxin acts directly on the bowel or indirectly by way of an effect upon the nervous system. In another situation where staphylococci infects skin then toxins such as hyaluronidase, coagulase and leukocidin play a part in determining the outcome of the infection. Hyaluronidase, by dissolving the matrix of connective tissues, may assist the spread of bacteria in tissue. The action of coagulase by clotting lymph and blood may reduce the lymph and blood circulation in the area, so thwarting the body's defences—the invasion of the area by white blood cells of various sorts and the supply of the antibodies from the blood. In this thwarting of natural defences, leukocidin, by destroying white blood cells, has a very direct role to play.

We can summarize by saying that there are a few diseases where bacterial toxins are very important in determining the signs and symptoms of the disease, indeed they determine the outcome of the disease. For these diseases, such as diphtheria, tetanus, and botulism, 'antitoxins' either produced by the patient's own defence mechanisms or introduced into him by the doctor are very important in determining successful recovery from the infection. In the case of many other pathogenic bacteria it is by no means clear what role is played by the various toxins they produce. In these diseases 'antitoxins' are not so important in either natural or artificial defence against the pathogens.

What makes bacteria pathogenic?

We have already seen in earlier sections of the chapter that it is often difficult to distinguish between pathogenic and non-pathogenic bacteria. A particular species of bacteria may in one situation be completely harmless, yet if it finds its way to some unusual site it may become a virulent pathogen, particularly if there is some deficiency or disturbance of local or general resistance of the host. The ability of a species of bacteria to produce disease is determined by a complex interaction of factors including features of both bacteria and host. Some important factors are discussed below.

Bacterial factors

1. *Pathogenicity.* This varies not only from one species to another but also between different strains of the same species. Pathogenicity may depend on some special factors such as the production of toxins.

2. *The situation of the bacteria.* Some bacteria that may be harmless on the skin or in the bowel may become serious pathogens if they are introduced into normally sterile areas, for example by injuries or by surgery.

3. *Infectivity.* This is the ability of bacteria to spread from one host to another. Infectivity varies not only between species of bacteria but also between strains of one species. Some infectious diseases, e.g. typhoid or bacillary dysentery (pages 140, 146), need only a small number of organisms to get a foothold in the host. Another bowel infection, paratyphoid fever, needs a much larger dose of organisms to cause disease. Thus typhoid fever can be spread by contaminated water containing only a few bacteria whereas paratyphoid fever is usually spread by means of foodstuffs such as milk, ice cream etc. in which the bacteria can multiply to produce a large infecting dose of organisms.

4. *Invasiveness.* This is the ability of bacteria to spread within the host. Some bacteria that produce extremely potent toxins do not need this invasiveness to produce serious disease, and death from the effects of toxin can occur even with only a local infection by the organisms (e.g. tetanus and diphtheria). These exceptions apart, serious infectious disease is usually linked with the ability of bacteria to spread widely in various tissues in the organism. Invasiveness may be associated with the ability of bacteria to produce enzymes (toxins) that permit them to spread rapidly in tissues, enzymes such as hyaluronidase (which dissolves the jelly matrix of connective tissues) or enzymes called fibrinolysins that dissolve clots of blood or lymph. Once these weapons have breached the wall of blood and lymph vessels then the body's own internal fluid circulations (blood and lymph) may assist bacteria to spread widely and colonize distant organs. Thus virulent staphylococci with their armoury of enzymes may enter blood vessels and be carried widely from a super-ficial boil or carbuncle to many tissues where staphylococcal abscesses may result. This invasiveness of certain species or strains of bacteria is closely linked with the property of bacteria called virulence, the ability to produce severe disease. Highly invasive pathogens are usually highly virulent.

Dosage of bacteria and mixed infections

The number of a particular species of bacteria reaching man may be very important in determining the outcome of the infection and we have already discussed this factor under the heading 'Infectivity'. A mixed infection by two or more bacteria, or by a bacterium and a virus, may produce much more serious effects than invasion by just one kind of micro-organism. We are all familiar with the two stages of the misery of the common cold. First there is the attack by the virus which produces an irritable nose and throat and thin watery secretions; in this stage there may be a slight or moderate fever and a feeling of being generally unwell. After a few days, the epithelium of the upper respiratory tract now damaged by the invasion of virus particles, becomes particularly susceptible to invasion by the common commensals of the nose and throat. The secretions become thicker and yellow because they now contain large numbers of pus cells (dead and dying white blood cells). Many kinds of virus infections are followed by this secondary invasion by various sorts of bacteria, and the secondary infection can often have more serious consequences than the virus infection itself. The damage to the lining of the bronchi and bronchioles by the influenza virus commonly opens the pathway for an infection by bacteria from the upper respiratory tract. This may lead to bronchitis and the appearance of pus in the sputum. Much more serious consequences appear if a virulent staphylococcus invades the damaged mucous membranes; staphylococcal pneumonia is a particularly dangerous secondary infection and can kill within twenty-four hours. The common virus infections of childhood, particularly measles, also lead to secondary infections by various bacteria. Bacterial infections of the middle ear, the throat and bronchial tree often occur during an attack of measles.

Host factors

Many variables in the host and his environment affect the outcome of infection by bacteria and other micro-organisms. Age, sex, drugs, genetic constitution, and the state of nutrition are all important factors that can oppose or encourage infection by bacteria, and we will see many examples of the influence of these variables on the course of various infections in the following chapters. One vitally important host factor is the complex of defence mechanisms that can be brought to bear on invading pathogens. This is such an important and intricate system that it is the subject of a separate chapter.

Before leaving this brief review of the interplay of the various features of bacteria and their hosts in an infectious disease, we must raise the problem of the different susceptibilities of body tissues to invasion by bacteria. Some body tissues contain so little blood or are so shielded from the protective elements of the blood (antibodies and white blood cells) that the introduction of but a few bacteria, even those of low virulence, can have very serious consequences. These tissues are the heart valves, the joint cavities, the brain and spinal cord.

A joint is composed mainly of bloodless tissues—cartilage and fibrous ligaments, and it has a very poor resistance to infection. A soft tissue with a rich blood supply can readily mobilize many forms of resistance to bacterial invasion, including antibodies in the blood plasma and various sorts of aggressive white blood cells. Not so the joint; if bacteria reach a joint cavity either by way of a penetrating injury or from the circulating blood then the organisms may multiply without check and progressively destroy the joint. Joints are so susceptible to infection that surgical operations on these structures are fairly recent developments, following the perfection of aseptic operating conditions (see page 168) and the availability of powerful weapons in the form of various antibiotics.

The heart valves are, paradoxically, in a similar precarious condition. Although the valves themselves are continually bathed with blood, they are fibrous bloodless structures. Normal heart valves have a very smooth surface and there is little tendency for bacteria from the blood to settle down on them. However, if the surfaces are damaged and roughened (e.g. from an attack of rheumatic fever or some congenital abnormality) bacteria are particularly likely to settle down on the valves, where they multiply and progressively destroy the fibrous structure of the valves. This kind of infection is called bacterial endocarditis and the valves may bear soft masses, called vegetations, composed of a mixture of bacteria and fibrin. If this situation is not diagnosed and treated (with appropriate antibiotics) then the valves are progressively destroyed and the strain put on the heart leads to heart failure and death. It is easier to prevent than treat this kind of infection. The presence of bacteria in the blood stream is a commoner event than is often realized. Every bite on a chronically infected tooth may release a small shower of commensal organisms from the dental tissues into the blood stream; a similar thing happens with every dental extraction. These bacteria are usually commensal organisms of low virulence and are rapidly removed from the circulating blood by various defence tissues; however, roughened and damaged heart valves can become colonized by them. Nowadays people with this sort of valvular damage receive special care before and after any kind of dental treatment.

The central nervous system has a special arrangement of blood vessels and tissue so that the blood is separated from nerve tissue by membranes and by a fluid barrier (the cerebrospinal fluid). The membranes that separate blood from nerve tissue are not very permeable to proteins or blood cells, or indeed to many drugs. Only in the presence of severe inflammation do drugs, antibodies, and white blood cells reach nerve tissue in anything like the concentration reached in other tissues of the body. This situation makes the brain particularly liable to infection if bacteria accidentally reach nerve tissue; e.g. from an open wound of the skull or from contaminated needles introduced into the spinal canal for the purposes of diagnosis.

3. Disease-causing micro-organisms II Viruses

The early history of virology

THE STUDIES of Pasteur and Koch formed the foundations of the 'germ theory' of disease. Once that doctors had learned Koch's techniques of growing bacteria outside the body as pure cultures and the methods of staining bacteria before looking at them under the microscope, these faculties were put to use to study very many types of disease. In the late nineteenth century the bacteria responsible for many infectious diseases were isolated from ill patients and grown as pure cultures in the laboratory. When samples of these pure cultures were introduced into the bodies of experimental animals or into men, they produced the same disease as was suffered by the original patient. Koch himself isolated the bacteria responsible for tuberculosis and with great difficulty persuaded these organisms, virulent in man but delicate outside him, to grow in the laboratory on a medium containing serum prepared from cattle blood. After journeys to Egypt and India, and in a race with Pasteur's disciples, Roux and Thuiller, Koch was able to isolate and grow the comma-shaped bacillus responsible for cholera. Dr Fehleisen, one of Koch's students, found minute round bacteria, strung together like beads, from people sick with erysipelas (a skin infection)—St Anthony's fire. These bacteria, now known as streptococci, he injected into patients dying of cancer, on the theory that an attack of St Anthony's fire would cure the cancer. In a few days each of his human volunteers succumbed to St Anthony's fire; this infection did not cure their cancers but the experiment demonstrated the bacterial cause of St Anthony's fire.

From all over the world came reports that bacteria had been isolated from patients suffering from various diseases including cancer, epilepsy, malaria, yellow fever—diseases that we know now have no relation to infection by bacteria—but these 'errors' did not halt the progress of the isolation of disease-causing bacteria. It became clear, however, that there were certain infectious diseases from which no bacteria could be isolated, at least no bacteria which could reproduce the disease when they were injected into animals or men. Pasteur himself met this enigma when he began to study that dreaded disease called rabies (page 191). When Pasteur, Roux and Chamberland looked at brain material from dogs dying of rabies, they could see no bacteria. Yet some infective agent was present for these brain extracts could produce rabies when they were injected into the brain of a healthy dog. For a time Pasteur thought that he had identified the micro-organism responsible for rabies; in the saliva of a child dying of the disease he found a microbe that he called 'microbe-like-an-eight'. But later, with the help of Roux and Chamberland, he found the same microbe in the mouths of many healthy people, and the notion that this microbe was the cause of rabies was abandoned.

Viruses first defined as filter-passing agents

In fact Pasteur never did isolate the micro-organism responsible for rabies; it was far too small to be seen by the most powerful of microscopes available in his time. However, it was a technique developed by Pasteur and Chamberland in Paris that enabled a Dutch worker called Beijerink to visualize the nature of the agents responsible for infectious diseases in which no specific bacteria could be isolated. Pasteur and Chamberland had found that it was possible to remove bacteria from a liquid containing them by filtering the liquid through porcelain. The bacteria were held back in the porcelain and the filtrate was no longer infective. Beijerink was studying an infectious disease of the tobacco plant called mosaic disease that produces a mottled yellowing of the leaves. This disease could be spread to a healthy plant by rubbing it with the leaf from a diseased plant. When he prepared a juice from infected leaves and filtered it through porcelain which would hold back bacteria, the filtered juice was still capable of infecting a healthy plant. Obviously some infecting agent had passed through the filter, i.e. was non-filterable. We now call these non-filterable infecting agents viruses. For many years the detection of these viruses as a cause of disease rested on their effects on the hosts they infected, their distinction from pathogenic bacteria by their ability to pass through filters which would hold back bacteria, and their invisibility under the most powerful microscopes available.

In 1900 two German biologists showed that foot and mouth disease of cattle was also caused by an agent which would pass through a porcelain filter. Many bacteriologists continued to search for infectious diseases for which no specific bacteria could be isolated. It became evident that there were many such diseases. Unfortunately for the progress of these studies, it was found that the invisible agents responsible for two diseases, cow pox and rabies, failed to come through the bacterial filters. We now know that the filterability of viruses is a matter of chance, depending upon the size of the infecting particles and on the size of the pores in a particular filter. The term 'filterable virus' has now been contracted to virus.

The distinctive features of viruses

Viruses certainly are small creatures compared to bacteria but there is in fact a wide range of size in this group of infecting agents (see Table 1 and Figure 3.1). Although most viruses *are* too small to be seen with the aid of the light microscope, some are just visible, particularly if they are heavily stained. But what really distinguishes viruses from other agents that may cause infectious disease (bacteria, protozoa, fungi) is their inability to grow in artificial growth media in the laboratory. We have already seen that pathogenic bacteria have, during the course of their evolution, lost to varying degrees some essential parts of their chemical machinery. They can no longer grow and reproduce using the inanimate matter of salts, water and dead organic matter for their energy and growth needs. These deficiencies in the nature of pathogenic bacteria have to be made good by particular host animals or plants, i.e. they are obligate parasites. However, these pathogens *can* be grown in the laboratory provided that they are supplied with the appropriate chemical and

Table 1 The range of size in some animal viruses

Virus	Approximate diameter of virion (μm)
Vaccinia	200–300
Herpes simplex	120
Newcastle disease	100
Influenza	80
Papilloma	55
Poliomyelitis	30

Figure 3.1 The size, shape, and symmetry of typical viruses. (*Reproduced by courtesy of Prof. R. W. Horne of the John Innes Institute.*)

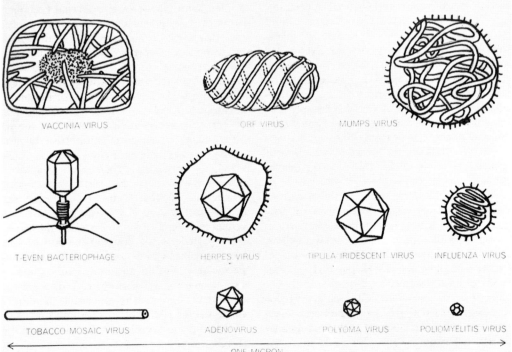

physical conditions, i.e. an artificial non-living system can provide the conditions normally provided by the living host. On the other hand, viruses have carried this specialization of omission to much greater extremes; they can only grow *within* living cells. It is this ultimate in specialization that is the distinguishing feature of viruses. No wonder Pasteur could not culture the rabies virus in his laboratory except by injecting the infecting agents into the brains of susceptible animals.

The development of research into virus infections

The terrible influenza pandemics of 1918 and 1919 certainly gave impact to research on viruses, although it was not until 1933 that evidence clearly pointed to a viral cause for influenza. Laboratory investigation of viral diseases became important during the first two decades of the twentieth century. One important discovery for our understanding of viruses was made in 1915 when it was found that bacteria themselves are liable to be fatally infected with agents that are filterable. These viruses that attack bacteria are called bacteriophages. Their importance for virology is that they are the most suitable viruses for the study of the interaction of a virus with a host cell; but more of bacteriophages later.

At first the study of viruses attacking animals was but a small branch of the science of bacteriology. This was inevitable, for infections caused by viruses were superficially indistinguishable from infections caused by bacteria. Even today we cannot readily separate the two without the aid of laboratory studies. The facilities of bacteriology laboratories proved to be quite inadequate for the study of viral diseases. Viruses could not be purified or cultured, nor could they be seen under the microscope. These limitations resulted in studies of the nature of the effects of viruses on their hosts (man, experimental animals, plants) rather than on the nature of viruses themselves. A study of the nature of viruses had to wait for the development of techniques for culturing viruses in the laboratory and for the revolution in microscopy brought about by the introduction of the electron microscope. In spite of these limitations the early studies firmly characterized several diseases of man and animals as viral infections. The kind of evidence that incriminated a virus as a cause of an infection was the recognition of a distinct human disease of unknown cause that could be transmitted to an experimental animal (or human

volunteer) by the injection of material (e.g. blood, secretions) from a case of the disease. Bacteria, fungi or protozoa could be excluded as a cause of the disease by filtering a suspension of the infective material to produce a microscopically clear filtrate from which no micro-organisms could be grown in the laboratory.

The electron microscope and virus culture in the laboratory

We can now look at two developments in scientific technique which brought rapid advances in our understanding of the structure of viruses and the interaction of viruses with their host cells.

Viruses as distinct particles

We have already seen that most viruses are of sub-microscopic size. A few of the larger viruses, e.g. small pox virus, could be seen as minute dots in the light microscope if the virus had been heavily stained with an appropriate dye. The early workers with viruses did, however, have other techniques which gave them some idea of the size of viruses. One technique depended upon the use of a range of filters of differing pore size. Filters containing the smallest pores allowed only small molecules to pass through them, molecules of water, salts or sugars. Filters with pores of larger size allowed the smaller proteins to pass through them, together with some but not all viruses. In this way it is possible to obtain some idea of the size of viruses by comparing them with the size of identifiable molecules that come through the same filter. Using this technique it was possible to arrange the known viruses in an order of size ranging from 20 nm to about 300 nm. Because of the very small size of viruses we have to use this small unit of measurement, the nanometer or milli-micron (10^{-9} m). To give some idea of the relative size of the smaller viruses, we can compare them to the size of the average molecule of protein, which is about 4 nm across. There was yet another technique available to the early workers with viruses that enabled them to obtain indirect measurements of the size of virus particles. This technique depends upon the fact that the rate at which particles settle down to the bottom of a solution of particles depends upon the size and specific gravity of the particles. A tube containing a suspension of viruses is placed in a high-speed centrifuge, and by measuring the rate at which viruses sediment in the liquid one can come to some indirect estimate of the size of the particles.

Our modern understanding of the nature of

viruses depends upon the belief that all viruses are distinct, minute particles, each virus having its own unique physical, chemical and biological properties. The early studies of the microscopy of the larger viruses, filtration and sedimentation measurements and the culture of viruses in chick embryos (see page 27) all pointed to the real nature of viruses as distinct particles. The development of the electron microscope not only confirmed the particulate nature of viruses and the range of size in this group of micro-organisms, but it also provided some detailed information of the shape and contents of the virus particle.

The first electron microscope pictures of viruses were published in 1938; these confirmed the differing sizes of viruses and their differing outline images. But modern instruments have brought the smallest of animal viruses within the scope of detailed analysis of their structure and their behaviour within cells (see Figure 3.2–3.7).

Figure 3.2 Electron micrograph of tobacco mosaic virus rods. (*Reproduced by courtesy of Prof. R. W. Horne.*)

Figure 3.3 (a) Electron micrograph of influenza virus particle, and (b) model of influenza virus. (*Reproduced by courtesy of Prof. R. W. Horne.*)

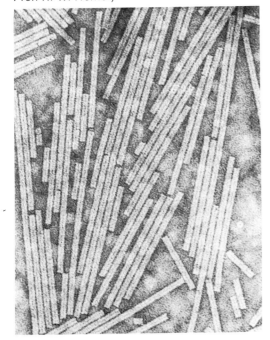

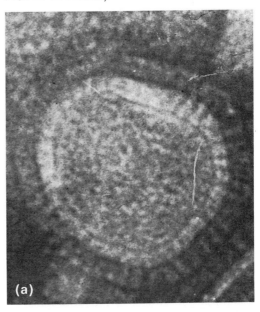

(a)

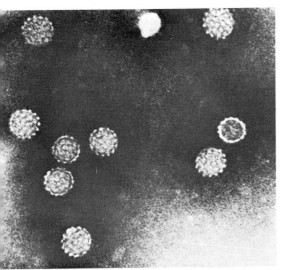

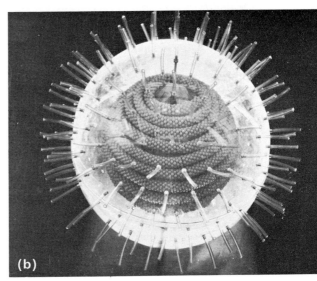

(b)

Figure 3.4 Electron micrograph of wart virus particles. (*By courtesy of the WMMS.*)

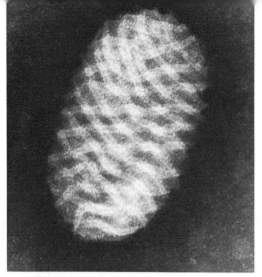

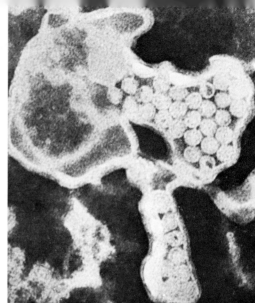

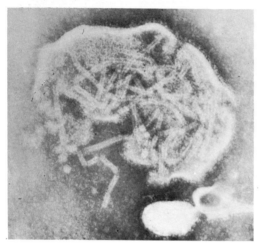

Figure 3.5 (top left)   Electron micrograph of orf virus. (*From Horne, R. W. and Nagington, J., Virology; Academic Press.*)

Figure 3.6 (above)   Electron micrograph of polio virus in cytoplasmic fragment. (*From Horne, R. W. and Nagington, J., J. Molecular Biology, Academic Press.*)

Figure 3.7 (bottom left)   Electron micrograph of mumps virus. (*From Horne, R. W. and Waterson, A. P., J. Molecular Biology, Academic Press.*)

The culture of viruses in the laboratory using whole animals

We know that a characteristic feature of viruses is their inability to multiply except within living cells of a susceptible host. The early workers with viruses were quite unable to grow them in artificial culture media in the laboratory, and they had to use living animals. One animal that has proved to be a boon to virologists is the white mouse. This animal is susceptible to infection by many viruses that cause disease in man. Viruses not only need intact living cells for their multiplication but they often need particular kinds of cells; often the virus must be administered to the mouse so that it reaches the cells that are most susceptible to attack. Thus if one needs to try to isolate a virus as a possible cause of human encephalitis (infection of the brain) then biological material from the human case may be injected directly into the brain of the anaesthetized mouse. As soon as signs of illness appear (usually paralysis) the mouse is killed and the

brain removed and ground up in a suitable fluid. The cell fragments etc. are removed by centrifuging the fluid, and the clear fluid produced can now be injected into the brain of another mouse. This process could go on indefinitely, so maintaining specimens of living virus within the brains of mice. Nowadays stocks of virus can be maintained in a much simpler way by keeping deep-frozen suspensions of brain at very low temperatures ($-50\,^{\circ}$C or lower), but the technique of 'passage' of virus through a series of mice is still performed so that one can culture sufficient virus material for yet other studies which are necessary to try to identify the particular virus.

When one is studying viruses that infect the skin then one may inject suspected material into the hairless skin of the foot-pad of the mouse. Material suspected of containing the influenza virus is dropped into the nose of the anaesthetized mouse so that it reaches the lungs. These kinds of study can tell us if a virus was present in our original material; the presence of a particular kind of virus will produce particular kinds of damage in the mouse—encephalitis, pneumonia, swelling of the foot pad and so on. In addition the mouse may be used as a living culture of viruses so that they can be harvested in amounts needed for detailed studies.

The chick embryo in virology

The embryo chick within its egg shell is another extremely useful culture medium for viruses. Within its egg shell and underlying fibrous membrane the chick is naturally free from infection by bacteria and viruses. Further, the embryonic cells of the chick are much more susceptible to attack by viruses than are the cells of the mature animal. Viruses will behave in embryos in quite a different manner from what they would in the hen or indeed in the cells of the animal which is the natural subject of attack by the virus. These differences are exploited in order to grow large amounts of living virus after 'seeding' the egg with a small amount of virus. In addition one can use the chick embryo to get some measure of the number of virus particles in a sample of material.

The inside of a hen's egg containing a developing embryo is a rather complex place. In addition to the embryo there are a variety of membranes and fluid-filled cavities (Figure 3.8(a)). The embryo itself floats within a fluid-filled cavity, the amnion, which is limited by a membrane. Projecting from the belly of the chick is another membrane-bound cavity, the yolk sac, which contains yolk that is gradually used up during the growth of the chick. Another membrane-bound cavity projects from the belly of the chick—the allantois—and this partly surrounds both the yolk sac and amniotic cavity. The membranes of the chorion and allantois develop a rich blood supply and spread to completely line the shell. These blood-filled membranes act as the 'lung' of the developing chick and exchange gases (oxygen and carbon dioxide) with the air outside the shell.

The first use of the chick embryo was in making estimates of the number of virus particles in a solution, e.g. in a specimen of vaccine to be used to protect persons from smallpox. Various dilutions of the virus suspension are first prepared and samples are dropped onto the chorio-allantoic membrane of chick embryos (see Figure 3.8 for the technique of exposing the membrane). The hole in the egg through which the virus was introduced is now closed, e.g. with wax, and the eggs are returned to the incubator for a few days. Growth of virus in cells causes cell damage and for some reason the substances that leak from the damaged cells cause neighbouring uninfected cells to grow and multiply in an abnormal fashion. This process produces

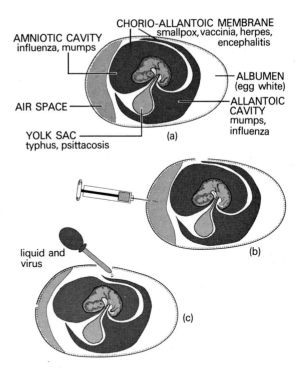

Figure 3.8 (a) Chick embryo in shell showing the various membranes and cavities and the most suitable places for the culture of various viruses.
(b) The preparation of the embryonated egg for the culture of virus on the chorio-allantoic membrane. A hole has been drilled into the shell and the needle of a hypodermic syringe inserted into the air cavity to withdraw air, so allowing the chorio-allantoic membrane to sink into the egg.
(c) A solution containing virus particles can now be dropped onto the surface of the chorio-allantoic membrane, the hole sealed, and the egg further incubated in the warm.

what are called 'pocks', and when the membranes of the chick embryo are examined after several days' incubation, these pocks can be seen and counted (Figure 3.9). Each pock represents the place where a virus particle infected a cell and started the mechanism whereby a visible pock is produced. This is akin to the culture of bacteria on a plate of nutrient medium. Each visible bacterial colony is produced by the multiplication of a single bacterium. Each pock on the membranes of the chick is the result of the activities of a single virus particle. By counting the number of pocks and knowing the volume and dilution of the sample of vaccine applied to the membrane, it is easy to calculate the number of virus particles in the original vaccine. Different parts of the embryo may be more suitable for the growth of other viruses (see Figure 3.8).

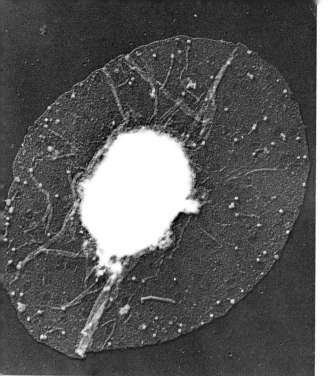

Figure 3.9 Chorio-allantoic membrane removed from a chick embryo after insertion of a solution containing influenza virus particles. The white pocks on the membrane are clearly visible. (*WHO photo.*)

For the influenza virus the amniotic or allantoic cavities are more suitable, and for yet other viruses the yolk sac has certain advantages.

The chick embryo is also used for growing those micro-organisms called rickettsiae which lie between viruses and bacteria in their properties. These are minute bacterium-like organisms but they share the habits of viruses in being intracellular parasites, and they can only be cultured in living cells. All the rickettsiae are primarily parasites of blood sucking arthropods (lice, rat-fleas, mites, ticks—see also page 178) but some half dozen species have become adapted to invade the animal body and cause disease. Human diseases caused by rickettsiae include classical typhus (spread by lice), endemic or murine typhus, Rocky mountain spotted fever (spread by ticks), scrub typhus (spread by mites) and Q fever (spread by ticks—often by inhaling the dried faeces of the cattle tick or by drinking unpasteurized milk from animals bitten by infected ticks, page 128). Although rickettsiae will grow in various parts of the developing chick embryo, the most profuse growth occurs in the yolk sac. The infective material is injected into the centre of the egg through a hypodermic needle inserted into a small hole in the air space at one end of the egg. The embryo usually dies after three to five days, by which time the yolk sac is swarming with rickettsiae.

Bacteriophages

Early in the history of virology (1915) it was shown that bacteria are themselves subject to fatal infections by viruses called bacteriophages (phages). These phages are no academic curiosities; they are of great importance for they provide one of the most suitable materials for the study of the interaction of a virus particle with the host cell. In the last twenty years detailed studies of phages have been made. The success of these studies results from several features of the interaction of phage and bacterium. The bacterial hosts can be cultivated readily in the laboratory under well controlled conditions. Further the bacteria can be readily subjected to physical and chemical analysis during the course of infection by phages. Another important advantage in using phages is that infective phage particles can be counted in a simple and accurate fashion so that the results of experiments can be readily expressed in quantitative terms. Thus a dilution of phage is mixed with a few drops of a concentrated culture of susceptible bacteria and this is poured onto the surface of a culture medium in a petri dish. After incubation the growth of bacteria produces a turbid surface layer on the culture medium except where a bacterium has been infected by a phage. At this point on the sheet of bacteria there is a clear area called a plaque (Figure 3.10). The clear area results from infection of a bacterium by a phage, and multiplication and release of phages which then infect surrounding bacteria. Thus if we count the number of plaques we can readily calculate the number of phage particles in the original sample. This is just one of the advantages of working with the viruses that attack bacteria.

The infection of more complex organisms by viruses does not show the apparent simplicity of the direct invasion of the bacterial cell by a phage, but for all viruses the cycle of infection is similar and consists of the following:

1. entry of virus into the host,
2. multiplication of virus inside the host cell,
3. escape of new infecting particles from the host cell.

However, in order to infect cells the animal virus has to penetrate the outer barriers of the animal body, and then it may have to travel far from the point of entry in order to reach susceptible cells. After the release of new virus particles from the infected cells new cells of the same host may be readily available, but in order to reach a new

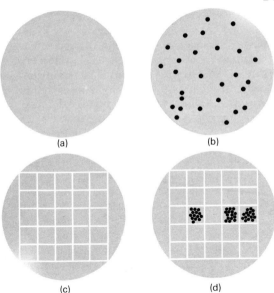

Figure 3.10 (a) and (b) illustrate a method of estimating the number of bacteriophages in a solution. (a) is an agar plate which has been uniformly seeded with bacteria that are susceptible to attack by the bacteriophage to be studied. A known volume of the bacteriophage solution is layered onto the surface of the agar plate which is then incubated.
(b) shows the effect of the bacteriophages. Each dark point is free of growth of staphylococci and is the result of the action of one phage particle.
(c) and (d) illustrate a modern use of bacteriophages in the classification of bacteria. Some bacteria, e.g. the staphylococci, are present as many strains which are indistinguishable by most laboratory tests. One method of classifying and distinguishing them is by 'phage-typing'. There are many different phages that can attack staphylococci but each strain of the bacterium is particularly susceptible to attack only by certain phages. In (a) an agar plate has been uniformly seeded with a staphylococcus of a certain strain, then a drop of each of a variety of phages is placed in a certain position on the surface of the medium before incubation. In this case it is obvious that the strain of staphylococcus is susceptible to attack by only three of the phages, enabling this staphylococcus to be designated phage-type 'XYZ'. Other strains of staphylococci will give a different pattern on the agar plate; they belong to a different 'phage-type'.

host the virus particles have to leave the body of the host and enter the inanimate world.

The use of culture cells in the laboratory

The use of susceptible bacteria in the study of the phage-host relationship provided ideal experimental situations; these were available long

before the development of techniques of the culture of living mammalian cells in the laboratory. However, the study of viruses that parasitize animals requires animal cells. At first these were provided by living chick embryos and intact animals such as the white mouse. Later discoveries made it possible to grow living cells in the laboratory. A suitable solution containing the necessary salts, nutrients and oxygen is seeded with living cells. The suspension of cells will survive and often multiply for several days or weeks. Many viruses can infect these cells and multiply within them so that new virus particles can be harvested from the solution.

The structure and life cycle of viruses

Having looked briefly at the history and techniques of virology, we can examine in some detail the structure and life cycle of viruses. In essence the virus is a microscopic bundle of information; this information is in the form of a chemical code carried by a long molecule of either DNA (deoxyribonucleic acid) or RNA (ribonucleic acid)—but never both (Figure 3.8). When this genetic material, this coded information, enters a living cell it commits this cell to produce more of the same nucleic acid and other components of the virus particle. We call the infective virus particle a virion. This is a packet of viral nucleic acid wrapped in a protein coat, the capsid. Some virions have an outer envelope that may contain lipid, carbohydrate and protein. Table 2 shows the size of various DNA and RNA viruses. Recent work has shown that the larger viruses may be more complex in their structure and may contain one or more enzymes that are necessary for the multiplication of virus within a host cell.

Table 2 Some DNA and RNA viruses

DNA viruses Size (μm)		RNA viruses Size (μm)	
Vaccinia	200 × 300	Rous sarcoma	120
Herpes simplex	120	Newcastle disease	100
Adeno-type 5	70	Influenza	80
Papilloma	55	Poliomyelitis	30

The cycle of virus infection

We will now look at the various stages in the natural history of a viral infection in man; these stages consist of the following:

1. entry of the virus into man by particular routes and the spread of virus within the body to reach susceptible cells,
2. the penetration of cells by virions,
3. the series of events inside the infected cell which culminate in the appearance of new virions,
4. the release of virions from an infected cell, their infection of other cells and their departure from the body when they are potentially capable of infecting new individuals.

Routes of infection

In order that virions can enter and parasitize susceptible cells within the body of man they first have to reach man and then penetrate the 'surface' layers of the body—the skin, respiratory tract, alimentary tract.

Many viruses reach man by way of the mucous membranes of the respiratory tract. The infective virions may be in dust or in tiny fluid droplets exhaled from the respiratory tract of an infected person. Those viruses that are inhaled in dust must be able to survive for periods outside a host and must be able to resist the effects of drying. The smallpox virus is a good example of a virus that is resistant to drying, and the dust from infected personal and bed clothing can spread the disease (page 88). The viruses of measles, influenza and the common cold are less resistant to drying, and probably tiny fluid droplets are important in the spread of these viruses from man to man. Although some viruses that enter by way of the respiratory tract produce infections that are localized to the region of entry (common cold, influenza) other viruses may produce widespread disease after they have entered the body by way of the mucous membrane of the respiratory tract, e.g. smallpox and measles.

Viruses that enter the body via the alimentary tract include the enteroviruses that may cause gastroenteritis (Echo and Coxsackie viruses) and the virus of infectious hepatitis. Yet other viruses enter by way of other mucous membranes such as those of the genital tract or conjunctiva. Although few viruses seem to be able to infect and penetrate unbroken skin, there are many viruses that can enter damaged skin, e.g. rabies virus (from the bite of an infected animal) and Herpes B virus (from the bite of an infected monkey). There is a vast range of pathogenic viruses that enter the body via the bite of an infected arthropod (mosquitoes, ticks, lice etc., see page 178). These are the 'arthropod-borne'

virus infections or 'arboviruses' as they are now called. They are maintained in nature by transmission from one susceptible vertebrate to another by means of blood sucking arthropods, and they multiply in both vertebrate and arthropod hosts. There are some two hundred known arboviruses and slightly over a quarter of these are responsible for human disease, a few of which produce fearsome epidemics. The importance of arboviruses varies greatly in different parts of the world and from one year to another. They produce three roughly defined groups of diseases. The most common and the least harmful produce fevers with or without rashes and arthritis. Another group, the haemorrhagic fevers, are more serious illnesses with a moderate to high fatality rate. The third group produce infections of the brain with or without additional infection and inflammation of the membranes around the brain. We will mention only a few of these arboviruses. Some of them are called after the disease they produce such as the yellow fever virus, dengue virus, type B encephalitis virus of Japan. Later, place names were included, as in St Louis encephalitis virus, Russian spring-summer encephalitis virus, and so on.

Our last example of routes of infection by viruses is by way of the placenta, virus passing from the blood of the mother to infect the foetus in the uterus. Infection of the foetus with the virus of rubella (German measles) has attracted much attention in recent years. This is because an attack of rubella in the mother during the first three months of pregnancy may result in some 10–30 per cent of babies being born with congenital abnormalities (see also page 77).

The spread of virus in the host

The spread of viruses on sheets of cells (e.g. skin and mucous membranes) may be by transmission of virus from cell to cell. In the case of mucous membranes, spread of virus may be much more rapid in the surface film of fluid which in some sites (nose, bronchi) is being constantly moved by ciliary action. Within the body, however, viruses may be rapidly distributed to susceptible cells in the blood or lymph streams. Viraemia (viruses in the blood) is a usual event in most generalized virus infections. Yet other viruses may reach their target organ by migration along nerves; the rabies virus travels from skin to brain in this fashion, as does the virus of varicella (chicken pox) when it travels along nerves to reach and infect the skin to produce herpes zoster (shingles)—see page 81.

The localization of virus in target organs

After they have been distributed within the body, infective virions ultimately settle down in the cells of one or more tissues and undergo their multiplication. We have little understanding of why particular viruses attack particular tissues, but this feature is important in determining the picture of a particular virus infection. Thus the viruses of chicken pox, smallpox and measles have a preference for skin cells so that skin rashes are a prominent feature of these diseases. Yet other viruses (poliomyelitis, some arboviruses) have an affinity for nerve cells, the picture of the disease depending upon the kind of nerve cells that are infected. In the case of the virus of infectious hepatitis, the liver is a very susceptible tissue and liver infection, and damage with jaundice are prominent features of the disease.

The penetration of cells by viruses (Figure 3.11)

Viruses multiply exclusively within living host cells. In order to reach this position they have to penetrate the cell membrane, but we know little of the way in which animal viruses become

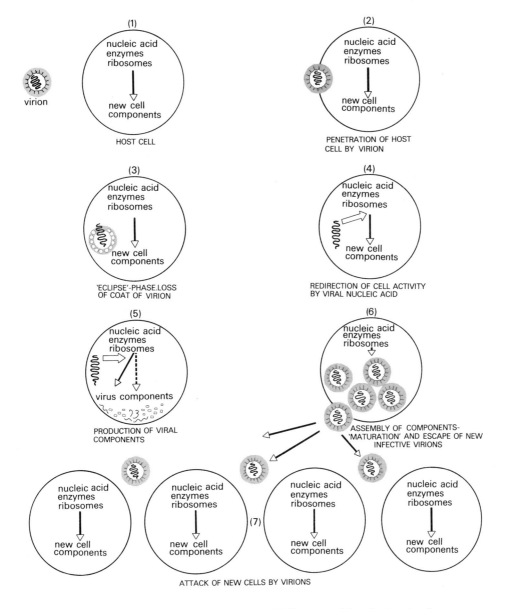

Figure 3.11 The stages of virus multiplication within the host cell.

attached to and breach the cell membrane. It is thought that many viruses are taken into cells by an active process of ingestion of virions, a process called 'viropexis'. The cell membrane in most body cells is not a static structure; the membrane of many cells is in perpetual activity, with infoldings of the membrane producing vesicles that pass into the cell interior, a process called pinocytosis. Certain inorganic salts and proteins can stimulate this activity of the cell membrane and the protein coat of viruses may well have this same property, the virus as it were encouraging the cell to engulf it.

The fate of the virion in the cell interior

Soon after infective virions reach the interior of the cell, they become non-infective to other cells. This is due to the loss of their coat of protein. They have entered what is called the 'eclipse' phase. Now the processes are set in motion which result in the synthesis of new virus components that ultimately leads to the appearance of new virions which will be released from the infected cell. We know that viruses are extremely simple structures, composed as they are of a core of nucleic acid wrapped in protein. In order to reproduce their kind they have to harness the complex machinery of the host cell using not only building blocks (amino acids, sugars etc.) and energy sources of the host cell, but also the array of 'builders' (enzymes, ribosomes etc.) to organize the arranging of the various building blocks into the form of viral nucleic acids and protein. The virus redirects the chemical activities of the host cell so that instead of producing its own components, it produces viral components. These viral components are later assembled to form mature virus particles, a process called virus maturation.

Some details of the formation of virus components

It is beyond the scope of this book to review the enormous advances of recent years in our understanding of the structure and functions of nucleic acids within the cell. This section is included for the benefit of those who have an understanding of nucleic acids.

An important result of the small size of the virion is that it can carry only a limited amount of genetic information in the form of nucleic acid. Thus the smaller viruses of influenza and poliomyelitis can code for only about ten different proteins. Some of these are for the coats of new virus particles, others for enzymes.

After a DNA virus enters a cell and reveals its DNA by shedding of the protein coat, the first stage in virus multiplication begins. The genetic message of DNA is transcribed onto molecules of messenger RNA (m-RNA). This m-RNA then instructs the ribosomes of the cell in the synthesis of new protein. Some of these proteins are enzymes which become devoted to the synthesis of viral nucleic acids and proteins. Thus the enzyme called DNA polymerase, that assembles DNA from its various components, increases very early in the host cell infected by virus. The construction of new virus materials is obviously a highly organized affair and the DNA of the invading virion must code for regulating substances that ensure an order in the sequence of chemical synthesis.

With RNA viruses a rather different process occurs in the infected cell. The invading viral RNA directs the synthesis of viral RNA and protein. This is unusual behaviour for RNA; here RNA is acting both as coded information (genes) and as messenger. It is one of the rare cases where RNA is copied directly from RNA (in animal cells and in DNA viruses the RNA, say of m-RNA, is transcribed from the code of DNA). To accomplish this unique event, RNA viruses carry the code for the construction of an enzyme that can carry out the task. This enzyme is called RNA synthetase.

The union of viral nucleic acid with that of the host cell—'virus integration'

It is known that some bacteriophages can become 'integrated' within the infected bacterial cell. When this happens the infected bacterial cell appears healthy and can continue to multiply. But these dormant bacteriophages *can* become awakened under certain conditions and begin to reproduce in the bacterium.

When a bacterial cell is carrying these dormant bacteriophages it is usually immune to infection with the same bacteriophage. There is a good deal of evidence that this process of 'integration' within the bacterial cell is due to the inclusion of viral nucleic acid into the bacterial chromosome.

Virus integration, cell transformation, and cancer

A similar state of affairs seems to occur when some animal cells are infected by some viruses. These viruses do not reproduce in the cell but they do 'transform' the cell. A feature of normal cells is that when they are in close contact with one another they do not undergo cell multiplication. These cells 'switch off' their synthesis of DNA—for doubling of the DNA content of the cell (doubling of the genetic material) is an important step in cell division whereby each daughter cell can come to carry an identical copy of the genetic information of the mother cell (see page 240). 'Transformed' cells lose this 'contact inhibition', as it is called, and they grow and multiply in a random fashion, doubling their DNA content even under tightly packed conditions. These transformed cells readily form tumours when injected into animals.

There is an increasing interest in viruses that may transform cells and produce cancer. Certainly some viruses can induce cancer in experimental animals—the so-called oncogenic viruses. Very recent studies of the small RNA viruses that have cancer-producing potential have shown that the viruses carry with them an apparatus, in the form of enzymes, that enables a copy of their genetic material to be insinuated into the DNA of the host cell. These enzymes can fabricate a double helix of DNA from the viral RNA and this double helix can in some way be included into the double helix of the host cell's own DNA.

These studies are, of course, very important for an understanding of the cause of at least some human cancers. There is evidence that at least one human cancer, called Burkitt's lymphoma, may be caused by a virus infection. This human cancer has a special geographical distribution, mainly in Africa, but also parts of the Americas and New Guinea. The distribution of this cancer follows closely such features as height, temperature and rainfall, features that also govern the distribution of particular blood sucking arthropods. Perhaps Burkitt's tumour may turn out to be caused by an arbovirus (page 30). Certainly various viruses have been seen in the tissues of Burkitt's lymphoma under the electron microscope. It is only recently that we have acquired some understanding of the complex interaction of animal tumour viruses with their host cells. This understanding has yet to be amplified and applied to the study of human cancer. If and when a human oncogenic virus is discovered, the possibility of control will arise.

The maturation and release of viruses from the cell

We have followed the course of infection of a cell by virions, through the eclipse phase to the redirection of the cell's chemical machinery to the production of new virus components. This production of virus components cannot and does not go on indefinitely. The infected cell may be so damaged that it dies. Even if the cell does not die it may begin to fail to supply all the factors that are needed for virus multiplication. Sooner or later the virus has to leave the cell to reach new cells or indeed new hosts. In the case of the infections of bacteria by some phages, the release of virus from the cell may be an explosive event with sudden disintegration of the bacterium and the release of infective virions. This explosive release of virions does not occur in animal cells.

Different animal viruses mature at different levels in the cell. Some mature within the nucleus and have to pass through the nuclear membrane and cytoplasm before they reach the cell membrane. Yet others mature under the cell membrane. Wherever the various viral components come together to produce infective virions, the first step in the release of virions is their migration to the cell membrane. They often achieve this without the cell showing signs of damage and indeed may be released through the cell membrane without disintegration of the cell. Some cells have bridges connecting one cell with another so that viruses can enter new cells without having to cross cell boundaries.

How viruses produce disease

We can now pose the question, how do viruses produce disease? We have seen how the multiplication of virus within a single cell can damage the cell, but a virus 'disease' involves the whole individual, a whole conglomeration of cells. A particular virus disease, be it influenza, poliomyelitis and so on, is the sum of the effects of damage to many single cells combined with the effect of 'toxic' materials, if any, which may be produced in the process.

There are some virus diseases in which the features of the disease are due to damage to particular types of cells. An important feature of paralytic poliomyelitis is muscle paralysis, and this is due to viral attack on the cell bodies of nerves that supply voluntary muscles, cells that lie within the central nervous system. Other viruses have this affinity for nerve cells, and the effects they produce depend upon the type of nerve cells that are invaded; rabies virus and some of the arboviruses that cause encephalitis attack nerve cells in the brain itself. In yellow fever an important feature of the disease, jaundice, is due to massive liver-cell damage. In these virus infections the picture of the disease is thus to a large extent determined by the multiplication of virus within particular types of cells that are damaged in the process. However, in a disease such as poliomyelitis there is also widespread infection of other cell types, particularly the lymphoid cells in the wall of the bowel and certain fat cells. These cells are attacked in the early stages of the disease; yet there is little evidence of cell damage in these tissues and indeed it is difficult to relate the invasion of these cells with the early symptoms of the disease— sore throat, headache, fever and nausea, symptoms that are so common in any general infection, be it caused by viruses or bacteria. In the case of bacterial infections these general symptoms are often said to be due to bacterial 'toxins' or reactions to foreign protein in the body. In the case of virus infections these early symptoms may be vaguely ascribed to a reaction of the body to the break-down products of infected cells that are released into the circulating blood; but in the absence of any obvious damage to cells in the early course of a viral infection, it is difficult to explain the early symptoms in these vague terms. Later on in the course of the disease, when the virus attacks and damages critically important cells such as the cell bodies of motor nerves in the spinal cord, there is no doubt as to the cause of the symptoms that appear.

We will now go on to look at other viruses that cause illness and death where the effects of the infection cannot be found in the damage to a particular group of susceptible cells that are vital to the function of the body. In particular we will look at smallpox. This virus, like many others that are associated with the appearance of skin rashes (e.g. measles, chicken pox) was once held to show a liking for the tissues of the skin (so called dermotropism). But attack of the skin is only one part of the disease and many body tissues come to contain the virus. Unfortunately no laboratory animal is so susceptible to this virus that it can regularly produce illness and death. We have to infer the way that the smallpox virus can kill man from experiments with related viruses in experimental animals—mouse-pox and rabbit-pox. Injection of these viruses into laboratory animals rapidly results in invasion of nearby lymph nodes where the virus multiplies; new virions are now released in quantity into the circulating blood. These virions may settle down in many body tissues, particularly the liver and spleen. Rapid multiplication of virus occurs, and if this is extensive enough then death occurs.

If the animal does not die at this stage then a second invasion of the blood stream occurs with further tissues being attacked, particularly the skin. In the early phase of virus replication in the lymph nodes there are no symptoms of the disease—this is the incubation period. This is followed by the development of fever and obvious illness—refusal to eat, apathy, weakness, diarrhoea, and so on. Discharge appears from the nose and eyes and large 'pocks' appear on parts of the skin. Death may occur between the seventh and twelfth day of the infection.

We have now to consider why animals die of this generalized viral infection. Certainly death occurs when the heart stops beating, and we have to look for processes that lead to this terminal event. A few infected animals die because the lungs are damaged (assisted by the secondary invasion of bacterial pathogens) and become loaded with fluid that oozes from the inflamed lung tissues. These inflamed water-logged lungs can no longer efficiently exchange gases with the air, and the ever-working heart becomes deprived of oxygen and hence an adequate source of energy. In man pneumonia does sometimes cause death in smallpox but the pneumonia is usually due to secondary invasion by bacterial pathogens. This cause of death may be averted in some cases by the use of antibiotics.

We have obviously to look elsewhere for the cause of death in most pox infections. Our understanding is far from complete but many workers feel that 'shock' of the cardio-vascular system is a common cause of death. The virus particle itself may act as a 'toxin', as indeed may many of the as yet unidentified materials that leak out of cells damaged by virus multiplication. An important site of action of these 'toxins' is the small blood vessels of the body. These become increasingly 'leaky' so that fluid and solutes pass out of the circulating blood and accumulate in the tissue spaces outside the blood vessels. The progressive loss of fluid leads to a fall in the volume of circulating blood. Blood pressure tends to fall, particularly if the heart is unable to adequately increase its output of blood by more vigorous and rapid pumping. This picture is what is understood by the term cardio-vascular shock.

The heart may already be working under the strain of a deficiency of oxygen due to inflammation of the lung, and yet another factor may interfere with the action of the heart—the release of potassium from cells damaged by the virus. This is no place to look in any detail at the function of potassium in the body. We can, however, point out that the main cations (potassium and sodium) of the soft tissues and blood are very unevenly distributed. Potassium is concentrated within the cells, whereas sodium occurs mainly in the blood and in the fluid bathing the cells. This difference in distribution is very closely linked with the function of these ions in the body. When cells are damaged potassium leaks from them into the body fluids. Excitable cells such as muscle and nerve are particularly sensitive to a change in the amount of potassium either inside or around them. In the case of the heart these changes in the distribution of potassium lead to disorders of the action of the heart that can have fatal consequences.

To summarize there is evidence that what we have described as 'shock' is the end result of a number of virus infections—indeed of bacterial infections also. This state of shock is initiated by widespread damage to the small blood vessels of the body, and the progress of this condition is accelerated by factors such as the release of potassium from damaged cells and a deficiency of oxygen supplies because of lung involvement. In certain virus and rickettsial infections the damage to the small blood vessels is a direct one because the infecting particles actually invade and multiply within those cells that line the small blood vessels of the body. Death, when it occurs, may thus be the result of a complex series of interacting events that ultimately lead to heart failure.

The life history of viruses in relation to the treatment of human disease

In other sections of the book we will be considering the methods of prevention and treatment of disease caused by pathogenic bacteria and viruses. However, we should not leave this general study of viruses without pointing out the unique features of virus infections that lead to difficulties in treatment of these infections. Viruses live and multiply within living cells and have to use the chemical machinery of the cell for their own purposes. The virus and host cell become so intimately interwoven that it is obviously a difficult task to attack the virus without at the same time damaging or killing the host cell, indeed all the non-infected cells of the body. Moreover the features of human virus infection often appear only after considerable multiplication of virus particles has already occurred.

For these reasons the treatment of virus infections has always lagged behind the management of infections by bacteria. Pathogenic bacteria live and multiply for the most part outside the cells of the host. They are individual organisms with their own chemical factories for the provision of energy and the raw materials for growth and multiplication. The structure and biochemical activities of bacteria are so different from those of human cells that one can use drugs that preferentially damage or kill bacteria without damaging human cells.

4. Disease-causing micro-organisms   III Fungi

Introduction

THE SIGNIFICANCE of some of the activities of fungi for man are dealt with in various sections of the book—fungi as fairly uncommon causes of human disease (page 94), fungi as a source of antibiotics, alcohol and other chemicals (page 117) and fungi as a cause of food poisoning (page 158). The impact of fungi on man is in fact more profound than these accounts would indicate, in particular with regard to their effects upon plant life. The effects of disease-producing fungi on plants have more than once altered the course of human history. Probably the best documented effect of this kind was attack of the Irish potato crops in the eighteenth century by a fungus called *Phytophthora infestans*. The effects of the destruction of this staple foodstuff led to a famine of almost unbelievable proportions, the exodus of over a million souls to the U.S.A., and a profound effect on British political life.

Growth and multiplication of fungi

The life cycle of fungi consists of two phases. First, a vegetative phase in which the cells of the fungus take up nutrients from their surroundings and use them for the production of new fungal tissues. Second, the reproductive phase which culminates in the production of specialized 'seed-like' structures called spores. These spores, like those of bacteria, may be able to survive unfavourable conditions of drought or cold; they may remain dormant until climatic conditions are suitable, and then germinate and produce new fungi.

Vegetative phase

A few simple fungi, e.g. the yeasts, exist as single cells. These fungi grow to an optimal size and then reproduce by a special form of budding in which a small bulge appears on the cell and eventually becomes separated from it (Figure 4.1). Once separated, the new cell grows and then repeats the process, provided that environmental conditions—moisture, food, mineral

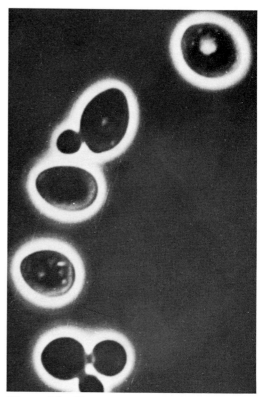

Figure 4.1   Photomicrograph (phase-contrast) of yeast organisms, some of which are budding. Magnification approx. × 1640. (*By courtesy of The Unilever Research Laboratories.*)

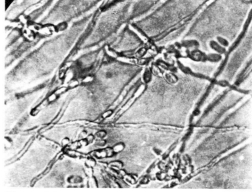

Figure 4.2   Mycelial stage of a yeast species (*Candida tropicalis*) × 600. (*By courtesy of WMMS.*)

salts, oxygen etc.—are suitable. If these fungi are grown on solid media they tend to grow in colonies of separate cells similar to those of bacterial colonies, although sometimes they grow into elongated tubular structures called hyphae which are similar to the structure of more complex fungi (Figure 4.2). Some of these simple fungi are a cause of human disease (see thrush, page 96) and other species play a vital role in alcoholic fermentation.

Hyphae usually branch freely to form a web of fungal tissue that is called a *mycelium*. These slender hyphae, some five to ten microns in diameter, extend themselves over the food material and are able to absorb nutrients over their entire surface. In all but the lower fungi the hyphae are divided by walls called septa. These septa are not in fact cell boundaries, for they carry perforations which permit nuclei and nutrients to pass from one compartment to another. In most fungi there are many nuclei in one compartment, the number ranging from one to a hundred. The hyphae of some species of fungus can fuse together at various points and exchange nuclei, so that a single hyphae can contain nuclei of different genetic constitutions. This phenomenon of exchange of nuclei between hyphae can have important consequences when fungi are used in the production of chemicals such as antibiotics. A mutation occurring in the nucleus of one hypha, which may alter its ability to produce the particular chemical, can rapidly spread to other hyphae in a culture of fungus by means of this nuclear exchange.

The structure of a hypha

The hyphal wall is composed of several layers. The outer layer consists of polysaccharides such as cellulose (a polymer of glucose molecules), mannan (a polymer of the sugar mannose) and chitin (a polymer of molecules of acetyl glucosamine). Under this cell wall of polysaccharides lies the delicate sheath of plasma membrane. Like the plasma membrane of animal, plant or bacterial cells, it regulates the exchange of molecules in and out of the hypha. The plasma membrane envelopes the cytoplasm of the hypha, which contains the usual sort of structures that we associate with other kinds of cells —nuclei, mitochondria, the membranous endoplasmic reticulum, ribosomes, enzymes and so on. Chromosomes have been seen in the nuclei of fungi and the number is typically haploid (see page 241). In fungi that reproduce sexually the zygotes have the diploid number of chromosomes; this state is followed immediately by a

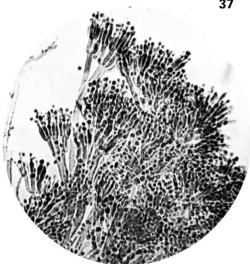

Figure 4.3 Photomicrograph of the mould of penicillium species showing conidiophores and conidia × 375. (*By courtesy of the Beecham Research Laboratories.*)

reduction division so that the sexual spores and the vegetative hyphae that will grow from these spores have the haploid number of chromosomes.

Spores

Spores are the structures by which fungi propagate themselves. They are often produced on a prolific scale so that air, dust and soil may contain large numbers of these structures. Most fungi produce both sexual and asexual spores. Except for the higher fungi such as mushrooms and toadstools (Basidiomycetes) *asexual reproduction* is the more important method of propagating the species. Asexual spores are produced in many ways. Some fungi, particularly when cultured in a sugary medium, produce regularly divided hyphae, components of which round themselves off and separate into a mass of structures called oidia which resemble the buds produced by yeasts. In other fungi some compartments of the hyphae develop rounded, thick-walled resting chlamydospores which outlive the parent mycelium and can germinate later to produce another mycelium. Yet other fungi produce spores in special hyphae that grow upwards from the growth medium into the air, and large numbers of asexual spores bud off from these aerial structures. Figure 4.3 shows one example of this kind of spore production. The spore-producing hypha is here called a conidiophore; it has a branched tip producing a brush-like structure which produces vast numbers of chains of spores called conidia. This is the kind of spore production in the fungi that are used in the production of penicillin. Aspergillus (page 98), an occasional cause of human disease, produces its spores in a similar manner. Other human fungus infections, such as athlete's foot and ringworm of the skin, are transmitted by means of this kind of spore.

Sexual reproduction

As in other organisms, sexual reproduction involves the fusion of two nuclei to form a zygote nucleus. When sex organs are present in fungi, they are given the name of gametangia; these show a whole range of complexity of structure which we will not pursue here. The zygote produced by the fusion of two nuclei then undergoes meiotic division (see page 242) to produce two cells, each bearing the haploid number of chromosomes. These then divide to form other haploid cells which eventually produce the sexual spores. Germination of the spores produces the haploid vegetative hyphae. In the higher fungi such as mushrooms and puffballs there may be millions of sexually produced spores in the fruiting bodies that are visible above the ground.

5. Immunity

Introduction

THE RESISTANCE of the body to invasion by disease-causing organisms is a highly complex system. Indeed, it is composed of a whole hierarchy of systems ranging from primitive reactions that are non-specific and are mobilized on any 'irritation' of tissues (be it physical, chemical or biological), to highly specific reactions which operate against particular chemical substances of micro-organisms. A description of these specific reactions is complicated by the fact that the same reactions are involved in body processes quite unrelated to defence against infection. They are concerned with what has come to be called 'maintaining the integrity of the body', with the 'weeding out' of abnormal cell types that continually arise in the highly complex body of the mammal. We thus find that the same mechanisms that are involved in resistance to infection by micro-organisms also become mobilized when 'cancer' cells arise in tissues or when surgeons transplant into the body of one individual an organ or tissue removed from the body of another individual. These specific defence systems have enormous implications for medicine and surgery, and research is progressing at a fantastic pace to probe their mechanisms and to develop new ways of *promoting* the defences and so increase resistance to infection or to the abnormal cell types of a malignant growth (cancer), and new ways of *blocking* these defences so as to permit organ or tissue transplants. In this field of study there has been a virtual explosion of new information in recent years, so much so that in a book of this sort it is impossible to review the subject comprehensively, For those who are interested in pursuing the subject further, there is a list of some recent publications in the bibliography.

External defence mechanisms

We will first look at the barrier that surrounds the body and then at the reactions that occur when this barrier becomes breached by the action of physical agents (cuts, heat and cold injury etc.), chemicals, or by invading micro-organisms.

The organs of the body are surrounded by various kinds of tissue such as skin or mucous membranes that act not only as a limiting surface but also as a barrier against various agents in the external world, be they animate or inanimate. Let us first look at skin which surrounds the entire body. An important property of skin is its mechanical strength conferred by many layers of epithelial cells and a tough outer layer of dead, keratinized (horny) cells. Intact skin is not only virtually impervious to penetration by micro-organisms but it also has its own mechanisms for decontamination. These mechanisms are both biological (the effect of an established flora of harmless commensal bacteria) and chemical (various chemicals in secretions of the skin); the effects of the mechanisms are discussed on page 16.

The respiratory tract is continuously exposed to large amounts of foreign material—gases (fumes from cigarettes, cars, open fires, industrial fumes etc.), dust, and micro-organisms occurring in dust or in minute fluid droplets. The nose is the first line of defence and it may trap as much as 90 per cent of inhaled particles. Most of the particles are trapped by hairs in the nose and by a moist blanket of mucus which covers all the internal surfaces of the nose and contains a high concentration of the anti-bacterial enzyme called lysozyme, as well as other anti-bacterial substances. This blanket of mucus is in continuous movement, propelled by the action of minute cilia on the cells of the nasal epithelium. The cilia drive the mucus blanket in two directions, downwards to the external openings of the nose and backwards to the pharynx, where the mucus is swallowed. There is a similar mucus blanket in the trachea and bronchi; here the cilia transport the mucus and trapped particles to the larynx where it accumulates until it is coughed into the pharynx and swallowed. Only the smallest of particles reach the end structures of the air passages—the alveoli. Here they meet a further defence mechanism in the form of cells called alveolar macrophages that engulf the particles and kill them if they are bacteria.

The mouth, pharynx, alimentary tract, vagina, and the outer surface of the eye have their own defence mechanisms. Many of these defences are discussed in other chapters but here we can mention the cleansing action of saliva, the effect of stomach acid on swallowed micro-organisms (page 15), antibodies secreted into the intestine (page 51), the cleansing action of tears which also destroy or inhibit bacteria by means of chemical substances such as the enzyme lyso-zyme and antibodies (page 51), and the acid conditions of the adult vagina which inhibits the growth of many pathogens (page 97).

Internal defence mechanisms

Inflammation

The ability of living tissue to react to injury is a very fundamental property. In mammals this is a complex reaction which may begin as a local reaction to damage and then extend to involve many systems of the body. Let us look first at the local reaction of a tissue to injury. This reaction is called inflammation and it continues as long as tissue damage continues. When the local injury stops then the débris of the inflammatory reaction is removed by scavenger cells and, un-less there has been much loss of tissue, the tissue returns to normal.

We are all familiar with the appearance of inflamed tissue, for our skin from time to time becomes cut, scratched, burned, over-exposed to sunlight or is infected by pathogenic bacteria. Whatever the cause of the damage to the skin, the reaction is similar; the skin becomes red-dened, warm and painful, and if the inflamma-tion is more severe then swelling appears. A very basic change in inflamed tissues occurs in the blood vessels. You can readily observe the effect of these changes in blood vessels in your own skin. Expose the delicate skin of the inner side of your fore-arm and then take a fine blunt instrument, such as the head of a pin or needle or even a finger nail, and draw a line a couple of inches in length on the skin. In making this first line use little pressure. You will notice a white reaction along the line of pressure. This white line will increase in intensity for a few seconds and then fade over the next few minutes; it is due to constriction of the capillaries that follows direct stimulation by the instrument. This reac-tion is not very relevant to the process of inflam-mation, so now apply your instrument more firmly to the skin. After this stronger stimulation

you may or may not see a white line, but if it does occur then it is rapidly replaced by a red line. The intensity and duration of this red line de-pends on the amount of pressure that you applied to the skin. The reaction is due to dilatation—opening up—of the capillaries, so that there is more blood in the area. If you now apply an even stronger pressure or repeat the last pressure often enough, then a bright red flush will spread outwards from the red line. This red flare is due to dilatation of arterioles. If the stimulus is even stronger, the red line will become pale and raised above the surface of the surrounding skin. This pale swollen area of skin is called a wheal, and it is caused by the escape of fluid from the capillaries into the tissue spaces around the capillaries. The accumulation of fluid in tissues is known as oedema. After a while the wheal loses its sharpness by becoming wider and less raised, and finally it disappears altogether as the fluid passes back into the capillaries or into the lymph channels of the tissue.

This simple procedure illustrates two impor-tant changes in inflamed tissues—changes in blood vessels and the accumulation of fluid in the tissue spaces. Let us now look at these changes in a little more detail, beginning with the vascular changes. The dilatation of blood vessels that follows the initial constriction persists for the duration of the inflammation, and it affects all of the small blood vessels in the tissue, arter-ioles, capillaries and venules. The dilatation of the arterioles which supply the tissue with blood results in an increased flow of blood to the tissue and a rise in temperature (this rise in temperature is a feature of inflammation near the cooler body surface and is not a feature of internal inflammation). In spite of an increased supply of blood to inflamed tissue, the dilatation of capillaries results in a slowing of the flow of blood. This produces various effects that include an increase in the 'leakiness' of the capillary wall so that the fluid part of blood (plasma) oozes out to accumulate in the spaces in the tissue around the capillaries. There are also changes in the cells that line the capillary—the endothelial cells; these cells become swollen, and white blood cells and platelets stick to the swollen cells. White blood cells now begin to migrate through the capillary wall, squeezing their way between the endothelial cells, to accumulate in the tissues.

The tissue spaces of an inflamed tissue thus come to be filled with a fluid similar to blood plasma and packed with white blood cells of various sorts, particularly neutrophil polymor-phonuclear leukocytes—we will call these poly-morphs for brevity—and monocytes (Figure

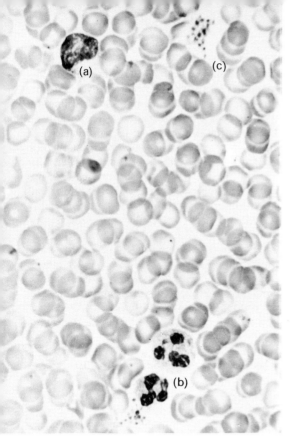

Figure 5.1 Photomicrograph of a film of blood showing red cells, (a) monocyte, (b) polymorphonuclear leukocyte, and (c) platelets. (*From Clegg and Clegg, Biology of the Mammal.*)

5.1). This cell-loaded fluid, the exudate, fulfils a variety of functions. It carries with it any anti-bacterial substances that are present in the blood, either naturally occurring ones such as specific antibodies (see page 48) or any drugs or antibiotics that have been given to the individual. The fluid of the exudate also dilutes any irritant that has been introduced into the tissue, whatever its nature. The exudate also contains the blood protein called fibrinogen, which when converted to fibrin becomes the basis of a clot of blood. This fibrin is often transformed into a clot of fibrin in the tissue spaces. The presence of fibrin clots in the tissue spaces help to unite severed tissues, as in a cut, and they may temporarily act as a barrier against invasion by bacteria. Fibrin clots may also form in the lymph channels of the inflamed tissue; there they obstruct the flow of fluid from the tissues into the lymph stream and so help to prevent the distribution of pathogenic micro-organisms from an infected inflamed tissue.

The accumulation of white blood cells of various sorts in an inflamed area is an important component of the defence system. One important action of the white blood cells is the engulfing of

bacteria, cell débris and the like into the cyto-plasm, a process called phagocytosis; once inside the cytoplasm the material may be digested and destroyed by means of enzymes. The poly-morphs are among the first cells to begin this scavenging activity. Later the monocytes that enter the inflamed area become transformed into cells that can carry out phagocytosis. The scavenger cells that can engulf material into their cytoplasm are called macrophages.

The polymorphs are attracted to any area where there is cell damage, whatever its cause. There are about 25 billion of these cells in the blood of a normal adult, and about a similar number are attached to the lining of blood vessels in the process of moving out into the tissue spaces, where they are eventually des-troyed by other macrophages which are perm-anent residents in connective tissues. For every polymorph in the circulating blood there are about a hundred in the bone marrow so that there are obviously enormous reserves of this defensive cell. The ability of polymorphs to ingest micro-organisms is greatly enhanced by the presence in the plasma of certain antibodies which become bound to the surface of the organisms. The kind of antibodies that have this effect are given the special name of opsonins (see page 49).

If the polymorphs cannot ingest and kill the pathogenic micro-organisms in an inflamed area, then a second line of phagocytic defence is provided by the other macrophages which can carry on a prolonged battle. If a local invasion of pathogens cannot be arrested by these mechan-isms then the general defence mechanisms of the body are activated; but more of these later. If a local invasion has been arrested by the inflam-matory process, the rate at which the tissue returns to normal depends upon the degree of tissue damage. When tissue damage has been slight, the exudate is absorbed back into the blood stream and any fibrin clots are broken down. The blood flow to the area decreases and the tissue resumes its normal appearance. If there has been much tissue damage, this gradual return to normal is not possible. The dead tissues are softened by means of proteolytic (i.e. protein-digesting) enzymes which are released from the dying bodies of polymorphs that have accumu-lated in the region. The fluid that results from this action is called pus and is contained within a cavity called an abscess. As pus accumulates, the pressure inside the abscess rises and the pus then begins to track along a line of least resistance until a free surface (external or internal) is reached. Now the abscess bursts and discharges its fluid-contents—with a dramatic relief of pain—unless this has been anticipated by a surgeon and the abscess drained by cutting into its wall. Sometimes an abscess does not rupture but remains embedded in the tissue; its contents thicken to a porridge-like consistency as fluid is absorbed, and the walls of the abscess become thickened with fibrous tissue.

The cause of inflammation

We have seen that there are dramatic changes in the blood supply and in the character of the blood vessels in an inflamed area. How are these brought about? It is thought that various chemical substances appear in the damaged tissue to trigger off the changes in the blood vessels by means of a direct action on the vessels. Many substances have been isolated from inflamed tissues that have effects on blood vessels, but there is still no general agreement as to which

of these substances are normally responsible for triggering off the vascular changes. Some of the substances such as histamine and 5-hydroxy-tryptamine are pre-formed materials that are stored within cells that occur in most tissues. These chemicals can be released by rupture of the storage cells (see mast cells in Figure 5.2) when the tissue is damaged. Other chemicals are not stored in tissues but circulate in the blood stream in an inactive form. They can be converted into their active form very readily by many factors that can disturb the normal equilibrium of plasma, and it is thought that these active substances appear in inflamed tissues. These chemicals are called the plasma kinins and extraordinarily small amounts of them can produce effects on blood vessels.

Antigens

The defence mechanisms that we have so far

Figure 5.2 Some of the components of loose (areolar) connective tissue as seen at high magnification. The mast-cells are pharmacological 'time-bombs'; when they rupture they release powerful chemicals that can affect various tissues nearby, such as blood vessels or smooth muscle. (_From Clegg and Clegg, Biology of the Mammal._)

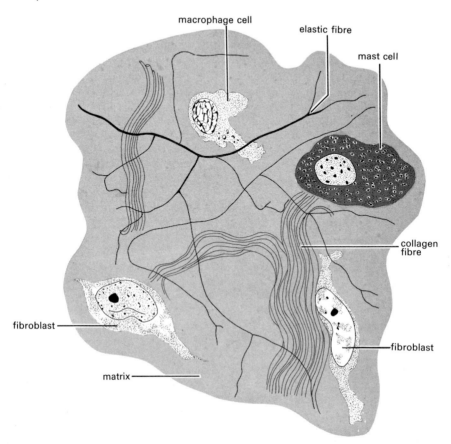

considered—i.e. external 'barriers' and inflammation—are rather non-specific mechanisms in that they can cope with a variety of damaging agents, physical, chemical or biological (i.e. micro-organisms). These are, in terms of evolution, rather primitive mechanisms. We now come to much more sophisticated systems that have become perfected in the evolution of mammals, systems that may have functions much wider than defence against invasion by pathogenic micro-organisms. Animals low down in the evolutionary scale—say insects or crustacea—can tolerate exchanges of tissue between one individual and another. The ability of an organism to *recognize* a transplanted tissue as being different from its own tissues and then to take steps to *reject* this foreign material from its body, appears higher in the evolutionary scale; it comes with the evolution of a cell type called the lymphocyte.

An important feature of these defence mechanisms is that they are specific. This means that the body can develop a mechanism which can protect it from a particular foreign material, be it a particular strain of bacteria, viruses, fungi or the cells of a particular species of animal. Thus the defence mechanism which can protect the body against the smallpox virus are quite ineffective against any other virus, or indeed any other micro-organism. We give the name *antigen* to any substance that can alter the properties of certain body cells so that whenever the antigen is re-introduced into the body these cells can in one way or another 'neutralize' the antigen. We can now look at the nature of antigens, the kind of body cells that respond to them, and at the nature of their response.

The nature of antigens

Antigens are large organic molecules. It was once thought that only proteins were antigenic. Certainly proteins make good antigens, i.e. they provoke marked responses in an animal, but we now know that some carbohydrates are also antigenic. In order that a substance can act as an antigen in an animal, it must be sufficiently different from the body's own chemical substances, i.e. it must be foreign to the animal. If we take a sample of blood from an animal and extract a protein, say plasma albumen, and inject it back into the animal, there will be no disturbance, no response by the immune systems of the body. Similarly if we remove a piece of skin from an animal and sew it back in an abnormal position, the graft will 'take' and the immune systems of the body will not be disturbed. If we repeat these studies using plasma albumen or a skin graft from another animal of a different species then the immune systems are activated and various changes occur in the circulating blood and in the properties of certain cells. The kind of response of the immune system is rather different in the two examples. In the case of the experiment with plasma albumen certain proteins called antibodies appear in the circulating blood, antibodies that unite specifically with the foreign albumen. In the case of the skin graft, lymphocytes with special properties accumulate in and around the graft of 'foreign' skin and ultimately lead to the death of the graft, i.e. its rejection from the body. We thus have two distinct mechanisms in immunity, one in the form of specific antibodies in the circulating blood, the other in the form of various populations of immune lymphocytes, each population of which is generated by the introduction into the body of a particular antigen; both antibodies and immune lymphocytes are capable of reacting with the antigens that caused their production.

The reaction of antigen with cells

There are two main groups of body cells that are involved in the immune responses described above. First we have cells that have the ability to 'recognize' antigens. These cells are called antigen-sensitive or immunocompetent cells. When they come into contact with antigen, one of two reactions occurs. First, the cells can multiply and produce cells that mature into special 'factories' for the production of specific antibodies. These antibodies are liberated into the circulating blood and appear in that fraction of the plasma proteins that are called globulins. A second reaction is that the cells multiply to produce lymphocytes that have special properties; these cells carry the 'memory' of previous contact with the antigen and can react with it whenever they meet it. Thus we have two types of immune responses:

1. cellular—mediated by 'sensitized' lymphocytes.
2. humoral—mediated by circulating antibodies, produced by plasma cells.

There are various other groups of cells that play an important accessory role in immunity. These cells are various kinds of macrophages that can engulf foreign material (antigens); They may travel far in the body, 'processing' antigen and presenting it to the antigen-sensitive cells.

The thymus and immunity

Until a few years ago the function of the thymus, a two lobed structure that lies in the upper part of the chest overlying the heart and great vessels, was a complete mystery. This gland is very prominent at birth but it begins to shrink in size in the early years of life so that only traces remain in the adult (see Figure 5.3). For years the organ had been removed from experimental animals and from human beings during the course of operations of the chest, without causing any ill effects. The reason for our long-continued ignorance of the functions of the thymus is that the gland begins its functions during the embryonic period and these functions are completed fairly soon after birth. Only when in 1961 the thymus was sucked out from the minute bodies of anaesthetized newborn mice did the vital function of this organ become apparent. Although the mice developed normally for a few months, they eventually died. These mice had a deficiency of lymphocytes in the circulating blood and also a deficiency of lymphocytes in the lymphatic tissues of the body, such as the lymph nodes, spleen and bowel wall. There were also defects in the immune responses of the mice, the most dramatic of which was the inability of the mice to reject transplants of the skin taken from other mice, or even from rats! These mice were thus incapable of being able to recognize rat skin as being foreign.

These experiments were the fore-runners of very many studies aimed at elucidating the role of the thymus in immunity. It seems that during embryonic life, and for a period after birth, the thymus becomes populated with what are called stem-cells; these come from the bone marrow. The stem-cells are undifferentiated in form or function but under the influence of the thymus the cells become transformed into immunocytes, a term that we use to describe any cell that is involved in the immune response. Many of the cells mature into lymphocytes, some of which leave the thymus to seed the lymphatic organs of the body—the lymph nodes (Figure 5.4), spleen and intestinal wall. In these situations the lymphocytes continue to divide. In addition to seeding the lymphoid tissues, the thymus produces some chemical substance that enters the circulating blood to stimulate the multiplication of lymphocytes. This hormone also alters the properties of lymphocytes so that they are able to react with antigens.

The thymus is thus a vital structure in the production of antigen-sensitive cells. An important property of these cells is that they do not react with the body's own proteins and other large molecules that would certainly act as antigens if they were injected into another

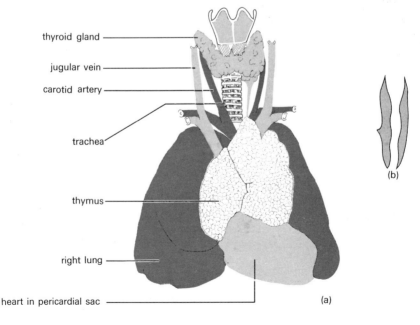

thyroid gland

jugular vein

carotid artery

trachea

thymus

right lung

heart in pericardial sac

(a)

(b)

Figure 5.3 (a) Shows the position and size of the thymus in an infant. (b) Shows the relative size of the gland taken from an adult aged 30 years.

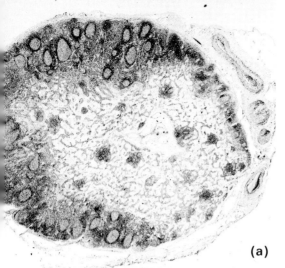 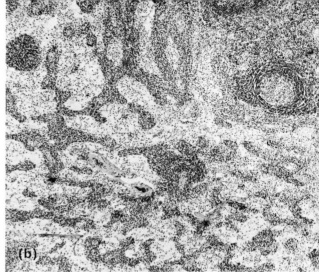

(a)   **(b)**

Figure 5.4   (a) Low power section of a lymph node.
(b) High power view of a part of a lymph node showing a few cortical nodules with germinal centres.
   In (a) note the dense outer rim of the node, the cortex, and the loosely arranged tissues of the core of the gland, the medulla. In the cortex are round structures called nodules. The dark outer rim of each nodule consists of masses of densely arranged small lymphocytes. The paler centre of the nodule is called the germinal centre and it is here that the production of new lymphocytes occurs. Each germinal centre is perhaps a clone of cells developing from a single stimulated immunocyte.
   There is a large traffic of lymphocytes into and out of the lymph node, small lymphocytes entering the gland from the blood stream, and other lymphocytes leaving the node via the lymph vessels. Antigens also reach the lymph nodes and are taken up by phagocytic cells lining the various lymph spaces within the node. Here they stimulate some lymphocytes to multiply and transform into plasma cells which manufacture antibody; the antibody then leaves the node to eventually reach the circulating blood. It is in the loose tissues of the medulla that the plasma cells tend to be found. (*Photographs by Brian Bracegirdle, B.Sc., M.I.Biol., F.R.P.S.*)

person. In the language of modern immunology, this is the ability of the body to distinguish 'self' from 'non-self'. In these processes the thymus plays a vital role. In order to understand the role of the thymus in preventing lymphocytes from responding to the proteins of the body as though they were antigens—a response that would eventually lead to self-destruction—we have to take a brief look at theories of immunity.

A classical view is called the 'instructive theory' which assumes that an immunocyte is incapable of producing antibody until it has been in contact with antigen. According to this view, when an antigen is taken up by an immunocyte the antigen acts as a framework on which the antibody is built. Thus the antigen and antibody unite like a lock and key, and a particular antibody can only get into close contact with one antigen (see Figure 5.5). The instructive theory of immunity described above is no longer acceptable to many immunologists who favour Burnet's theory of 'clonal-selection' or a modification of it. According to the instructive theory the immunocytes of the young mammal are unable to produce particular antibodies until the cells have taken up the antigen and, as it were, 'learned' to manufacture antibody using the

antigen as a template on which antibody is produced. The clonal-selection theory takes an entirely opposite view and regards the body as being capable of producing antibodies against a vast variety of potential antigens, i.e. the ability to produce particular antibodies is genetically determined. Large numbers of small clones, or populations, of cells exist, each of which is capable of producing a particular kind of antibody. When an antigen is introduced into the body it reacts with a particular clone of cells, causing the cells to multiply and transform themselves into the cells that manufacture antibody (plasma cells) or into cells that are the vehicle of cellular immunity. There is considerable support for this view, both experimental and theoretical.

A great advantage of this theory is that it goes a long way to explain the mechanism of self-recognition, as follows. Assume that in the body's population of lymphocytes there exists a vast number of small groups, or clones, of cells, each one capable of reacting with a particular antigen, including the body's own antigens. We know that the reaction of a lymphocyte to antigen depends greatly on the 'dose' of antigen. *Small amounts of antigen*—protein, nucleic acid etc.—

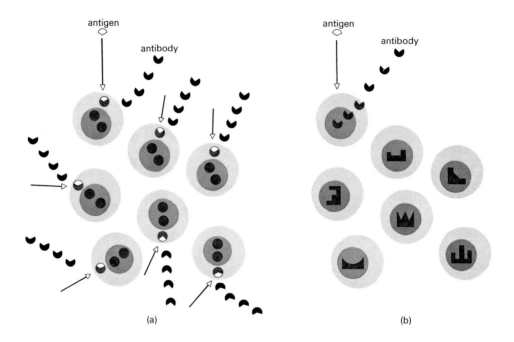

Figure 5.5   The two theories of immunity.
(a) shows the classical instructive theory of immunity. Here all of the immunocytes are capable of response to contact with the antigen. Antigen enters all cells and acts as a template on which an antibody with a complementary structure is manufactured.
(b) shows the 'clonal selection' theory in which only one immunocyte is able to respond to the antigen; this ability is genetically determined. The remaining immunocytes are capable of producing other forms of antibody but they do not do so until they have been in contact with the appropriate antigen.

such as would normally be liberated by bacteria or viruses during the course of infection, stimulate a clone of cells to proliferate to produce large numbers of cells each of which is either capable of reacting with the particular antigen which initiated the process, or capable of producing specific antibody which can combine with the antigen. We also know that a *large* dose of an antigen can have a damaging effect on the immune mechanisms, so much so that the body may tolerate the antigen and come to treat it as a 'self' component. Let us look at one experimental example of this kind of effect using as antigen a pure protein, albumen, prepared from the blood of a cow (bovine serum albumen). No animal can produce antibody until it is a few weeks old, but after an interval the ability to produce antibody rapidly builds up. If we inject a rabbit at a few months old with a small dose of albumen, there is a fairly rapid production of antibody to the albumen. The antibody binds to the albumen and the latter begins to disappear rapidly from the blood of the rabbit. If we repeat this injection after a few months, the production

of antibody is even more rapid and intense and the albumen rapidly disappears from the circulating blood. This is a fairly general reaction to antigens; a first contact with antigen primes the body's defences and a second contact with antigen produces a rapid and vigorous antibody response; this behaviour is made use of in the 'booster' doses of vaccines used to protect individuals against infectious diseases (see Chapter 6).

Now let us look at the effect of *large* doses of albumen on the rabbit. Let us give the first large dose of albumen just after birth when the animal has not yet fully developed the ability to distinguish 'self' from 'non-self'. The albumen produces no antibody response and the albumen is only slowly eliminated from the blood of the rabbit. We can repeat these injections of large amounts of albumen at short intervals of a few weeks; the rabbit continues to fail to respond by the production of specific antibody. However, if a long period, say six months, passes without an injection of albumen and then a dose of the antigen is administered, the animal will respond to the antigen by the production of specific antibody. Thus it seems that continuous and heavy contact with antigen can prevent the body from reacting to it. We have this same state of affairs with the body's own tissue antigens, i.e. they are present in continuous and heavy contact with immunocompetent cells.

What has all this to do with the thymus? It is thought that it is in the thymus that the clones of lymphocytes which are capable of reacting with the body's own proteins and nucleic acid are eliminated. In the environment of the thymus we see the expression of this heavy and continuous contact of body components with lymphocytes. A large number of lymphocytes are destroyed in the young thymus gland where the scavenging macrophages are constantly loaded with the dying and dead remains of lymphocytes. We presume that these lympho-

cytes are the ones that were capable of reacting with 'self'.

We can now summarize the functions of the thymus; this gland receives stem cells from the bone marrow and transforms them into lymphocytes. These lymphocytes form a very mixed population, each small group of which is capable of reacting only with one particular antigen. Within the thymus the lymphocytes are exposed to 'self components' and any of the cells that react with these components are destroyed, thus protecting the body from self-destruction. Only the 'safe' lymphocytes leave the thymus; they go and populate the various lymphoid organs of the body where they multiply and, under the influence of 'thymic hormone' in the blood, become transformed into populations of cells that carry out the immune reactions. The theory that accounts for the role of the

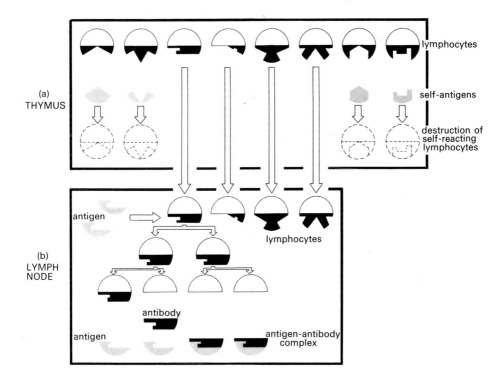

Figure 5.6 (a) A view of the function of the thymus. Large numbers of different populations of cells are present in the thymus (only eight of which are represented in the drawing) each of which is capable of reacting with a particular antigen. In the thymus these cells are exposed to 'self components'. Those cells which are capable of reacting with these 'self components', which are present in high concentration, are destroyed. The remaining cells leave the thymus to populate the lymphoid tissues.
(b) In the lymphoid tissues these cells are ready to meet and react with any non-self component (antigen) that reaches them. Shown here is a particular antigen stimulating a cell to produce antibody which is specific to that antigen. The cell multiplies and the offspring mature into plasma cells that liberate antibody. The antibody unites with the antigen to form a complex, i.e. the antigen is neutralized.

thymus in eliminating 'self-reacting' components is illustrated diagrammatically in Figure 5.6.

Nature of immune reactions

Having looked at the origin of immunocompetent cells, we can now look in a little detail at the nature of the immune reactions of the body. We have already seen that these reactions are basically of two kinds, humoral (i.e. circulating antibodies) and cellular, and we can perhaps best begin by looking at what happens in individuals who lack one component of this two-pronged attack on antigens.

Agammaglobulinaemia

Agammaglobulinaemia is a rare disorder, some cases of which are inherited as a sex-linked recessive condition (the gene is carried on the X chromosomes, see page 248). The basic defect in this disease is an inability of lymphocytes to transform themselves into plasma cells, the cells which manufacture antibodies. Antibodies are mainly found in the fraction of plasma proteins called globulins—hence the name of the disease, agammaglobulinaemia. In these individuals there is no antibody production in response to the introduction of any antigen into the body. This defect shows itself by repeated attacks of infection, particularly in the respiratory tract—bronchitis, pneumonia etc. Before the introduction of antibiotics and other drugs to control infections, sufferers from agammaglobulinaemia used to die early in life, and the disease illustrates the importance of circulating antibodies in resistance to infection. On the other hand the thymus is normal in these individuals and they reject transplants of tissues from other individuals as well as a normal person. Moreover, when they suffer from an attack of measles the illness runs its normal course and they develop an immunity to a further attack of the disease. Obviously there are immune mechanisms other than circulating antibodies. These mechanisms are mediated by cells, principally lymphocytes.

Di-George's syndrome

This disease is the reverse of agammaglobulinaemia. These individuals have normal antibody responses to infections and other antigenic stimulation. The thymus is, however, absent and they show deficiencies in that part of the immune system which is carried out by means of cells.

We can now look at these two mechanisms of immunity, circulating antibody and cell-mediated responses.

Antibody production

When an antigen (bacteria, virus, fungus, foreign proteins in sera, vaccines etc.) appears in a tissue, much of it is destroyed by the various phagocytic cells that appear during the inflammatory reaction (see page 41). Some of the antigen, however, persists in macrophages, remaining there for weeks or months. This antigen is carried away from the scene of the invasion when the macrophages migrate to other tissues, including the spleen, lymph nodes and other lymphoid tissues. Here the antigen seems to persist even though the cells that engulfed it die. It is passed on to yet other macrophages. The persistence of antigen seem to be due to its combination with ribonucleic acid in the cell, a component which protects the antigen from destruction by the enzymes inside the cell. These macrophages are, however, not the cells that manufacture antibody. It seems that the mere contact of the antigen-loaded cells with lymphocytes triggers off multiplication of some of the lymphocytes and their transformation into plasma cells which manufacture antibody. There is no trace of antigen in these plasma cells, which is evidence against the instructive theory of immunity that we have already discussed (page 45). Unlike the lymphocytes with their thin peripheral rim of cytoplasm, the plasma cells carry all the cell machinery which is indicative of an ability for extensive protein synthesis, features such as a rich endoplasmic reticulum bearing ribosomes (Figures 5.7, 5.8).

The following account of a fairly recent experiment will illustrate how the function of plasma cells can be demonstrated in a very direct fashion. The first step is to choose an antigen which is to be injected into an animal to stimulate antibody production. The antigen chosen is the protein extracted from the flagellae of Salmonella bacteria. The choice of this antigen is very deliberate; for the movements of the flagellae enable movement of the bacteria, and union of antibody to the protein of the flagellae will paralyse the flagellae and stop the movement of the bacteria. The immobilization of Salmonella bacteria can thus be used as a very sensitive test for the presence of specific antibody against them. The purified flagellar proteins are now injected into the skin of a rat. After sufficient time has elapsed for the animal to react to antigen (a matter of days), the lymph nodes that receive lymph draining from the skin injected with antigen are removed. The lymph nodes are teased out into individual cells using very fine instruments, the whole process being viewed under a powerful

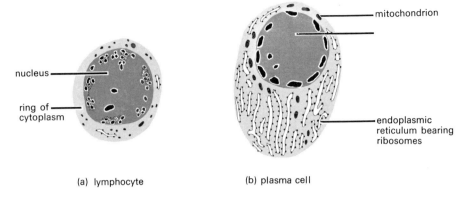

nucleus

ring of cytoplasm

mitochondrion

endoplasmic reticulum bearing ribosomes

(a) lymphocyte

(b) plasma cell

Figure 5.7 (a) A lymphocyte and (b) a plasma cell.

microscope. Using this process it is possible to isolate individual living cells, lymphocytes, macrophages and plasma cells. A single cell can be taken up into a micro-pipette and dropped into a tiny drop of culture fluid hanging onto the underside of a thin strip of glass which is supported on a glass slide. The edges of the slip are now sealed with an oil to prevent the drop of fluid from dying out. The slide bearing its single cell floating in a drop of culture medium can now be incubated at $37\,°C$ and left for a time to allow it to manufacture antibody, if it is capable of this synthesis. The presence of antibody released into the culture medium can now be tested by injecting a few motile Salmonella bacteria into the drop and observing their behaviour. It is found that only slides containing plasma cells are capable of immobilizing the bacteria, and then only the exact strain of Salmonella that was injected into the rat at the beginning of the experiment. Cultures of lymphocytes or macrophages have no ability to immobilize the bacteria (see Figure 5.9).

This sort of experiment demonstrates in a very elegant fashion that antibodies are manufactured by plasma cells. The plasma cells are derived from certain lymphocytes that have reacted to contact with the particular antigen. We have seen one way of detecting antibodies—the immobilization of bacteria. In some cases cells immobilized in such a way stick together; the antibodies that produce such an effect are called agglutinins, i.e. they agglutinate (stick together) particles carrying the corresponding antigen. There are many such names that are given to antibodies according to the kind of visible reaction that they have with antigens, or to their functions in the body. Often these observable results of antigen-antibody union are determined by the physical state of the antigen—i.e. whether

it exists on the surface of cells, particles, as solutions etc.—rather than on the nature of the antibody itself. Some antibodies are called precipitins because a precipitate of antigen-antibody complex may appear when antigen in the form of a colloidal solution is mixed with antibody under suitable conditions. Some antibodies can be seen to produce effects by stimulating macrophages to engulf micro-organisms or particles that carry the antigen; these antibodies

Figure 5.8 Photomicrograph of a film of blood showing red cells, (a) a small lymphocyte and (b) a polymorphonuclear leukocyte. (*From Clegg and Clegg, Biology of the Mammal*)

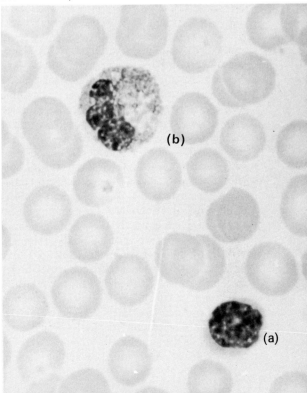

(b)

(a)

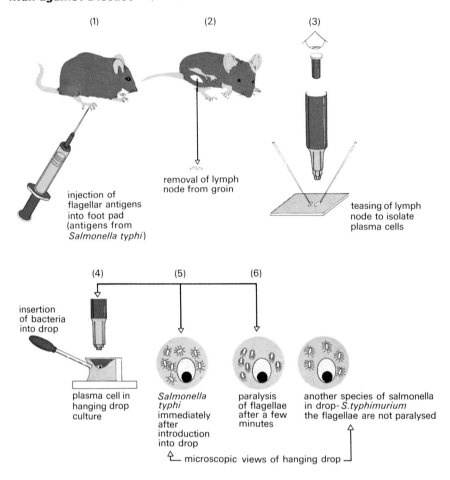

Figure 5.9 An experiment illustrating the function of plasma cells (see text).

are called opsonins. Antibodies that cause micro-organisms to disintegrate are called lysins. *Neutralizing* antibodies are those that either unite with a toxin and inactivate it or combine with a virus to neutralize its ability to penetrate living cells. All these descriptions tell us little of the nature of the antibodies themselves, they merely tell us that antibody has united with antigen to produce some visible or measurable effect. Before we look at the nature of antibodies we might mention that these observable effects of antigen-antibody union do have great practical significance. One use is the identification of strains of a species of bacteria. Thus there are very many different strains of Salmonella bacteria which have an identical appearance under the microscope. Antibodies can be prepared which are specific to each strain by injecting purified proteins from each strain into animals; specific antibodies can later be harvested from the blood of the animals. An unknown strain of Salmonella can be identified by adding some of

the bacteria to a series of tubes each containing a different specific antibody. The bacteria react only with the antibody which is specific to its own strain.

The nature of antibodies

As long ago as the 1930s it was known that antibody was a protein in blood plasma, a protein that belonged to the group called the gamma globulins. For many years antibody was known as gamma globulin. More recent studies of plasma proteins has shown that there are several kinds of globulin that can contain antibodies, and it is now conventional to call these immuno-globulins. The immunoglobulins form a *vast* family of proteins, each member of the family presumably being produced in response to stimulation by one particular antigen. This family of proteins can be subdivided into various groups on the basis of such differences as molecular weight and biological properties.

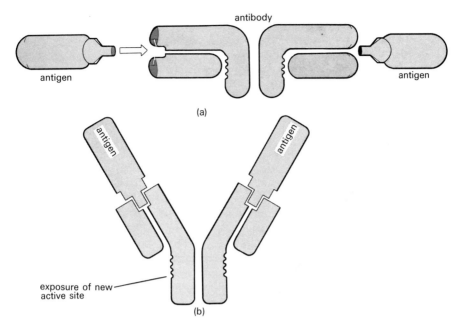

Figure 5.10 The structure of (a) immunoglobulin G and (b) a possible effect of union of antigen with antibody.

Biological properties of antibodies

These major sub-groups are called IgG, IgM and IgA (Ig=immunoglobulin). Because of the enormous number of different antibodies, the chemical studies of antibody structure have been concentrated on certain kinds that can be obtained in relatively large amounts that can be easily purified. Figure 5.10(a) shows the structure of one kind of antibody, IgG. The whole molecule of the antibody can be broken down into four parts, four chains that come in two pairs, a pair of heavy chains and a pair of lighter chains. In any particular IgG antibody the two heavy chains are identical with one another, as are the two light chains. Antibodies have two kinds of function to perform—first they have to recognize a specific antigen: second, they have to do something to the antigen or trigger off some cellular defense response. One suggestion is that the combining site with antigen is shared by the heavy and the light chains (Figure 5.9(a)). IgG antibody is a mixture of very many different antibodies, each specific to a particular antigen, and presumably this specificity is reflected in the structure of the combining site. Figure 5.9(b) illustrates what might conceivably happen when antigen combines with antibody. The molecule becomes transformed, revealing other 'active sites' which may be responsible for triggering off other effects, such as the stimulus which makes lymphocytes multiply and transform into plasma cells that manufacture more of the same antibody.

We have so far been mainly concerned with the role of antibody in the circulating blood, where it does not come into contact with antigen unless the antigen is artificially injected or reaches the tissues in the form of invading pathogenic micro-organisms. Antibodies are, however, much more widely distributed than this. They are, for example, poured out onto the mucous surfaces of the respiratory and alimentary tract, and are present in tears; in these places they act as parts of the first line of defense of the body. Some antibodies cross the placenta to reach the blood of the foetus so that the newly born infant comes to carry a sample of its mother's antibodies. The nature of these antibodies will depend, of course, on the kind of micro-organisms that have infected the mother or the kind of vaccinations she has received. These antibodies are not permanent features of the infant. They are gradually broken down and excreted, as are any proteins of the body. They do, however, give protection against some infections until the infant begins to produce its own antibodies against the micro-organisms that it meets. This kind of temporary protection is called passive immunity. In this case it is conferred by antibodies that have passed across the placenta from the blood stream of the mother. In some mammals passive immunization of the offspring is transferred by way of the first secretion of the mammary glands that we call colostrum. These kinds of passive immunity are given the name 'natural' to distinguish them from the artificial passive immunity that results when we try to protect an individual from developing an infection by injecting immunoglobulins that have been extracted from the blood of another individual, often from an individual who is convalescing from an attack of the infection (see also page 77). These kinds of passive immunity must be clearly distinguished from the immunity that results from an infection or from the administration of a vaccine (see Chapter 6). In the latter case the individual produces his own antibodies from his own plasma cells. This is *active* immunity and differs from passive immunity in another important respect, for the body's ability to produce antibody persists for long periods, often for a lifetime. After an initial contact with the antigen there is a mobilization of the immunological defense mechanisms in which a particular set of lymphocytes is stimulated to divide and transform into plasma cells that manufacture specific antibody. The antibody produced in this first reaction to the antigen performs its function, i.e. the control of the infection, and then the level of antibody in the blood gradually falls over months or years. However, the memory of this first contact persists, perhaps in the form of a small group of lymphocytes that are, as it were, committed to producing this particular antibody. If there is a second contact with the same antigen then these lymphocytes multiply rapidly and transform into plasma cells; the production of antibody is more rapid and more intense than in the first contact with the antigen.

Cell mediated immunity

We now come to the second type of immune response that is carried out by cells, a response that can occur in the absence of any circulating antibody. The study of this kind of immunity is still in its infancy but without any doubt this will become a very important branch of immunology, for it is the kind of immune response that is involved in the destruction of an organ or tissue grafted from one individual to another, and is probably also involved in the body's defenses against internal hazards in the form of cancer cells.

The kind of cell that determines this form of immunity is the lymphocyte. If we inject some foreign cells into an animal we can later remove lymphocytes from the animal which, when added to the same foreign cells growing in artificial culture in the laboratory, will 'recognize' these cells, move closely to them and cause their destruction.

Although the discovery of the wide significance of cellular immunity is a recent event, the first hint that cells had a direct role to play in immunity came from studies made as long ago as 1880. There are some infectious diseases, such as tuberculosis, in which an infection may produce a long-lasting immunity without any protective antibodies appearing in the blood stream. Clues as to the nature of this immunity came when Koch discovered an unusual reaction in guinea-pigs suffering from tuberculosis.

He found that if he injected living tubercle bacilli into the skin of animals suffering from tuberculosis, then a severe localized inflammation occurred at the point of injection and this damage progressed to produce an ulcer. This reaction was very different from that in uninfected animals in which the inoculation site healed rapidly, perhaps to develop some ten to fourteen days later a small nodule. In tuberculous guinea-pigs the same severe local inflammation occurred even after injection of killed tubercle bacilli or a cell-free extract of the bacteria. This reaction was later used as a test for the presence of tuberculosis in man and animals (see page 45) and is called the Mantoux test, after the man who first used it for this purpose.

Because of the delay of hours or days in the development of the response described above, the reaction has come to be known as 'delayed hypersensitivity'. Delayed hypersensitivity has been found to occur with antigens other than those of the tubercle bacillus—antigens from other bacteria and from fungi and viruses. It is possible to transfer the ability of tissues to react in this way to an antigen by transferring lymphocytes (but not plasma) from one animal to another. Thus a guinea-pig without tuberculosis can be made to respond to an injection of tubercle bacilli with a vigorous but delayed local inflammation by previously injecting into the skin a suspension of lymphocytes taken from another guinea-pig suffering from tuberculosis (Figure 5.11).

The real significance of this particular reaction is unknown. Animals and man can become immune to tuberculosis and yet the blood contains no antibodies against the tubercle bacillus. In animals with experimental infections of tubercle bacilli, the unrestricted multiplication of the bacilli stops when delayed hypersensitivity appears in the tissues of the animal. Thus in tuberculosis delayed hypersensitivity develops

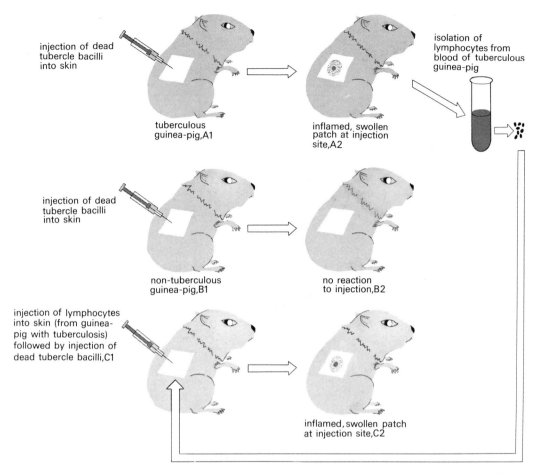

Figure 5.11 The delayed hypersensitivity reaction. In A1 a guinea-pig with tuberculosis receives an injection of dead tubercle bacilli into the skin. After a few days an area of inflammation appears at the site of injection, A2. A guinea-pig not suffering from tuberculosis does not react in this way (B1 and B2) but it can be made to do so by injecting into the skin lymphocytes that have been isolated from the blood of an animal suffering from tuberculosis (C1 and C2).

in parallel with immunity, and it is tempting to think that the one is the cause of the other. At the site of a delayed hypersensitivity response there is a striking accumulation of macrophages. This accumulation is no doubt due to the presence of 'sensitized' lymphocytes which, in contact with tubercle bacilli, release a substance that immobilizes macrophages. In the laboratory a single sensitized lymphocyte will, when in contact with the products of tubercle bacilli, release enough material to immobilize one hundred macrophages.

We have already hinted at the importance of lymphocytes in the destruction of transplanted foreign tissue and of cancer cells. It is impossible here to consider even the basic evidence for the role of lymphocytes in these reactions, but references from the explosively expanding liter-

ature in this new field are given in the bibliography.

Auto-immune diseases

There is increasing evidence that a variety of human diseases are the result of a failure of the immune mechanisms to eliminate lymphocytes that have the ability to react with the antigens found in the tissues of the body. In these diseases, appropriately called auto-immune diseases, one or more of the body tissues such as thyroid gland, adrenal cortex, joints etc., become progressively damaged by the appearance of specific antibodies or sensitized lymphocytes that react with the tissue. Part of the treatment of these diseases is the use of drugs that suppress immune mechanisms.

6. Vaccination (immunization)

Introduction

IN THE last chapter we looked at the body's defence mechanisms against pathogenic micro-organisms. We saw that after the successful control of an infection caused by a particular micro-organisms, the defences may be so primed that a second infection does not occur in the individual's life-time, at least rarely so. We say that the individual is immune to the particular disease. This long-lasting immunity is particularly striking after diseases such as smallpox, diphtheria, measles, mumps, chicken pox, and poliomyelitis, although for reasons which we will discuss in later sections, a permanent immunity does not usually follow influenza or infections by staphylococci or streptococci. The term vaccination describes the technique of artificially introducing the antigens of pathogenic micro-organisms so that the body's defences are stimulated and immunity achieved without the penalty of having to suffer the effects of infection by the living virulent pathogens. This technique of artificially and safely producing immunity against certain infections is called vaccination for historical reasons. A more modern and perhaps more rational name is immunization, which describes both the aim and the result of the procedure. These two names, vaccination and immunization, are interchangeable. In this chapter we will be looking at the history of this technique, which is possibly the greatest achievement of modern medicine.

Variolation

The first way in which immunity was artificially produced was by the technique called variolation. A person was inoculated with material (containing living virus) from the skin rash of a patient suffering from a mild form of smallpox. The inoculated person developed smallpox, usually, but not invariably, in a mild form; following this mild infection the person was immune to even the most virulent and dangerous form of smallpox. This technique goes back to ancient times and it was practised in India and

in China. It was introduced into Europe in the early part of the eighteenth century by a Lady Mary Wortley Montagu who was wife of the British Ambassador in Turkey. She wrote from Turkey to her friends in England telling them how, in Turkey, groups of people collected together to be visited by an old woman who brought with her a nutshell full of the matter taken from the skin of the best form of smallpox. She used a needle to make a scratch in the skin and then introduced a small amount of the pox matter into the scratch. The aim of this procedure was to produce a mild form of smallpox and so develop an immunity which would protect the individual against the severe forms of the disease. The procedure was, in fact, far from safe; some people became seriously ill and perhaps three in a hundred died. However, in these times naturally occurring smallpox was a common illness having a mortality of some 20–30 per cent; obviously variolation was an improvement on this, and was probably worthwhile until something better was introduced. Variolation became so popular in England that even George I was persuaded to have some of the royal family treated. Inoculation centres were set up in various parts of the country for the purpose of variolation. Of course, opposition developed when some variolated person died or when smallpox in a variolated person spread to other people in whom it sometimes produced a more severe form of the disease.

Vaccination

Variolation was gradually replaced by the much safer technique of vaccination, introduced mainly due to the efforts of Edward Jenner of Berkeley, Gloucestershire. In vaccination the skin was inoculated not with material from a human case of smallpox, but with material from the udder of a cow suffering from a related disease called cow pox. Inoculation with this material produced only a small localized pustule on human skin, but afterwards the individual had a high degree of immunity to human smallpox. Jenner cannot be credited with the

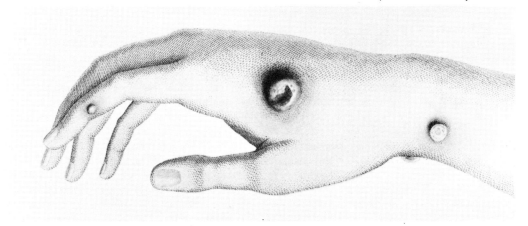

Figure 6.1 The hand of Sarah Nelmes. (From Jenner, *Inquiry*, 1798, plate 1. *By courtesy of the Wellcome Trustees.*)

discovery that infection with cow pox produces immunity to smallpox, but his scientific approach to the problem did a great deal to popularize the procedure and establish it as a safe way of preventing smallpox. In country districts the 'superstition' was often held that those who contracted cow pox by milking cows infected with the disease were subsequently immune to the ravages of human smallpox. When a local milkmaid—Sarah Nelmes—developed a typical sore of cow pox on her hand (Figure 6.1) Jenner took some of the material from the sore and scratched it into the skin on the arm of a healthy boy, James Phipps. On the boy's arm a sore developed where the material had been introduced into the skin (Figure 6.2), but otherwise the boy remained well. Then six weeks later Jenner put the superstition to the critical test. He inoculated into Phipps' arm material from the skin of a case of smallpox. Nothing happened to Phipps! Again, months later, Jenner repeated the test, but the boy remained immune to smallpox. Jenner then repeated these tests on a number of other subjects. The results were the same. Infection by cow pox produced immunity to smallpox. Jenner published his findings privately (his paper on the subject was rejected by the Royal Society because of the 'lack of adequate proof') and in spite of various objections from doctors who were not entirely successful in repeating his work, the popularity of vaccination grew and grew. Special sessions were held for the purpose of vaccination in different parts of the country. In recognition of his services parliament granted him £10 000 in 1802. However, it was not until 1840 that the dangerous practice of variolation was made illegal in England. The use of vaccination in the control of smallpox is discussed in Chapter 8.

Pasteur's contribution

Jenner's success, although founded on a scientific test of the validity of country 'folk lore', was not based on any understanding of microorganisms, and he did not know why vaccination prevented smallpox. The scientific basis of artificial immunization against infectious disease was established by Louis Pasteur who developed the 'germ theory' of disease (Chapter 1).

Figure 6.2 Jenner inoculating James Phipps. (From a drawing by William Thompson, *c.*1880. *By courtesy of the Wellcome Trustees.*)

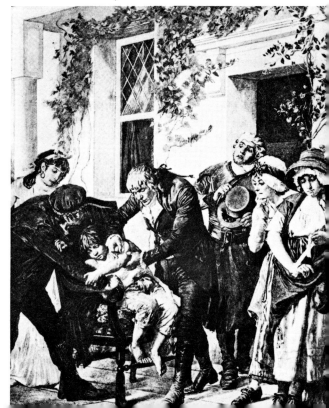

Pasteur's first studies of the ways in which animals and men could be protected from attack by microbes was in the field of infections in poultry. At that time fowl cholera was a serious threat to poultry in France. Pasteur's discovery of a method of making poultry immune to cholera was in part due to an accident. He had previously been able to culture the cholera bacteria in his laboratory, and whenever he wished to produce cholera in chickens all that he had to do was inject a small number of the bacteria from his laboratory cultures. The bacteria, however, had to come from a fresh culture; old cultures failed to produce the typical disease in many of the chickens and most of them recovered. On one occasion when Pasteur wished to inject fresh cultures of virulent cholera bacteria into chickens, his technicians gave him birds that had survived after an injection from an old culture of cholera bacteria. He found that these birds were resistant to the virulent bacteria and after a mild illness they recovered. These birds had obviously been rendered immune to cholera by the previous injection of old bacteria. Soon, these suspensions of bacteria from old cultures were being used in France to protect poultry from cholera.

Later, Pasteur was able to produce a vaccine to protect animals from the killer disease anthrax. Because anthrax bacilli produce resistant spores (Chapter 1), old cultures of the bacilli were useless as vaccines for they were as dangerous as fresh cultures. He found, however, that if cultures of anthrax bacilli were kept at 42–43 °C for about a week (instead of at 37 °C, the temperature of the human body) the virulence of the bacteria was reduced and they lost their ability to produce resistant spores. The virulence of these modified (attenuated bacteria) was related to the period at which they had been held at 42 °C, and the longer they had been kept at this temperature the less virulent they became. He was thus able to produce samples of anthrax bacilli of varying virulence. He immunized farm animals by first injecting them with a suspension of bacteria of low virulence, and following this twelve days later by an injection of bacteria of greater virulence. About a month after these injections, the animals—sheep, goats, cattle— could be given injections of anthrax bacilli of full virulence without them succumbing to anthrax. These living attenuated anthrax vaccines radically reduced the mortality of farm animals in France. In these early studies several accidents occurred; many animals died because anthrax bacilli were used which had not been sufficiently attenuated.

Several years later, in 1885, Pasteur produced what is perhaps his greatest achievement, a living attenuated vaccine for rabies (a virus infection, see page 191). Pasteur was quite unable to see the minute rabies virus but he was able to establish that it lived and multiplied in the brain and spinal cord of infected animals. The vaccine he used to protect men and dogs from this terrible disease contained living virus that had been weakened (attenuated) by passage through the brains of a whole series of living rabbits. He injected rabies virus (from an infected dog) into the brain of a rabbit, then later he killed the animal and took a small amount of its brain substance for injection into the brain of another living rabbit, and so on until he produced a virus of reduced virulence for dogs and man. The virulence of the virus was further reduced by drying the spinal cord of the infected rabbits in sterile air over a desiccating (drying) agent at room temperature. The longer the spinal cord was dried, the less virulent was the virus it contained. After fourteen days of drying, the rabbit's spinal cord was not infective and was used as the first dose of a course of injections.

On the following days cord was used that had been dried for shorter periods, thirteen days, twelve days, eleven days and so on until the final dose, the fourteenth, was of fully virulent fresh spinal cord. Using this method Pasteur was able to save the lives of dogs that had been bitten by another animal infected with rabies. Rabies is a disease with a long incubation period, and provided that the course of injections were started soon after the bite then few animals died.

In 1885 Pasteur tested this method of vaccination on a nine-year-old boy, Joseph Meister, who had been brought to him from Alsace for treatment. The boy had many wounds inflicted by a dog suffering from rabies and he would almost certainly have died. Pasteur gave this child a course of his vaccines and he survived. Further human cases received the same treatment, although not all were saved, either because the vaccination was started only after some days delay or because the rabies virus had been introduced close to the brain from bites on the face. The death rate of those who received Pasteur's vaccine after the bite of a rabid animal was less than one per cent compared with the death rate of 15–20 per cent of those who received no treatment after the bite. Of course not everyone who is bitten by a rabid animal develops rabies, but all of those who do develop rabies die of the disease.

The use of dead micro-organisms and the contribution of Almroth Wright

The vaccines we have seen so far are composed of living micro-organisms. In the case of fowl cholera, anthrax or rabies the micro-organism has been attenuated by changes in the culture of the organism in the laboratory—ageing the organism, growing it at high temperatures, or repeatedly passing it through the brains of rabbits. Vaccines against tuberculosis, brucellosis, yellow fever, poliomyelitis, german measles (rubella) and measles also contain living micro-organisms, the virulence of which has been modified by various procedures (see Table 3). Injections of dead micro-organisms may also produce some immunity against a particular infectious disease, although the immunity may not be as complete or as long-lasting as that which follows the use of living, attenuated micro-organisms.

The first disease to be attacked by means of injections of dead organisms was typhoid fever, and the success of this venture was due to the work of a British bacteriologist, Sir Almroth Wright. Wright started his researches on vaccines in 1892 at a time when it was believed that any vaccine likely to be effective must contain living organisms. He began his studies of the effects of dead vaccines in the prevention of a prolonged, weakening infectious disease that attacked the garrison troops in Malta, a disease appropriately called Malta fever (=brucellosis, see page 128). This illness with its prolonged fever was often confused with other diseases such as typhoid fever or tuberculosis. After some preliminary research on monkeys, Wright demonstrated his faith in vaccines in a most realistic way by injecting himself with the dead bacteria that were the cause of Malta fever, followed at a later date by an injection of living bacteria. Unfortunately the injection of dead bacteria did not produce enough immunity and Wright succumbed to Malta fever, with a prolonged illness. This experience did not, however, deter him and he next made plans to prepare a dead vaccine for immunization against typhoid fever.

His first experiments with a vaccine prepared from dead typhoid organisms were made on himself and other volunteers at the Royal Victoria Hospital at Netley. Although the vaccine made some of the volunteers rather ill, soon there was evidence that the blood of Wright and his other volunteers had developed the ability to destroy typhoid bacteria. Because of the rather severe reactions to the vaccine, further experiments were needed to find out how small a dose of the vaccine could protect individuals from typhoid fever. The chance to make these experiments soon occurred when an outbreak of typhoid fever appeared in an asylum in Kent. Wright prepared a vaccine from cultures of typhoid bacteria in a broth. The bacteria were killed by heating to 53 °C and by the addition of 0.4 per cent lysol. Although there were still local reactions at the site of injection of the vaccine (swelling and discomfort) and general reactions (fever etc.) the blood of those who received the vaccine developed a marked ability to destroy the typhoid bacteria.

At this time the Boer War (1899–1902) was in progress, a war in which there were 58 000 cases of typhoid (15 per cent of all troops) with about 9000 deaths, more deaths than were due to wounds (8000). Wright was unable to persuade the War Office to inoculate all troops embarking for the Boer War. However, compulsory vaccination was later introduced for troops leaving for India and other foreign countries. By 1909 nearly all the British soldiers in India had been inoculated with typhoid vaccine, and this

Table 3 Types of vaccine

1. Living attenuated micro-organisms

Rabies	Tuberculosis
Brucellosis	German measles (rubella)
Yellow fever	Measles
Poliomyelitis	

2. Dead micro-organisms

Typhoid and paratyphoid fevers	Influenza
Cholera	Whooping cough
Plague	Leptospirosis

3. Toxoids

Diphtheria	Tetanus

produced a reduction in hospital admissions due to typhoid fever from 8.9 per thousand (with a death rate of 1.58 per cent) to 2.3 per thousand (with a death rate of 0.25 per cent) in 1913. After the introduction of Wright's vaccine no other British Army campaign suffered the misery and death due to typhoid fever that had harassed the soldiers in the Boer War. In the First World War (1914–18), when typhoid vaccination was compulsory, only 2.35 per thousand soldiers suffered from typhoid fever, compared to 10.5 per thousand in the Boer War. This reduction in typhoid fever was achieved in spite of the insanitary trench warfare of the First World War (see transmission of typhoid, page 140). After 1916 paratyphoid organisms were included in the typhoid vaccine, which came to be known as T.A.B. vaccine. After the First World War there were considerable improvements in this vaccine, particularly in the strains of bacteria that were used in its preparation.

Modern vaccines against typhoid fever reduce the risk of developing the disease by about 75 per cent. Since protection is not absolute, unnecessary risks from drinking water and food that are likely to be contaminated by typhoid organisms should still be avoided. Immunity is not permanent and booster doses need to be given from time to time. Because paratyphoid fever is usually less severe than typhoid fever, the paratyphoid organisms are now omitted from *some* modern vaccines. These vaccines also cause less severe local and general reactions than T.A.B.

Filtrates (toxins and toxoids) as vaccines

We have seen that early in the history of immunization, living attenuated organisms or dead organisms were used in the production of vaccines. A new milestone in preventive medicine appeared when it was discovered that whole bacteria, either living or dead, were not necessary for immunization against certain infectious diseases, such as diphtheria and tetanus. In these diseases, the bacteria produce their damaging effect by the liberation of toxins (see also page 17). These toxins were discovered early in the history of bacteriology. As long ago as 1888 two of Pasteur's followers, Roux and Yersin, produced a bacteria-free filtrate of a broth culture of the diphtheria bacillus which contained a chemical toxin that could produce effects in animals identical to those produced by living virulent bacteria. Similar powerful toxins

were isolated from cultures of tetanus bacilli. It was found that when animals were injected with small doses of toxins, they developed powerful substances in the circulating blood which could neutralize the effects of toxins. These substances in the blood stream were called anti-toxins. They could be extracted from the blood of animals (mainly horses) to treat cases of diphtheria or tetanus (see Figure 6.3). Each anti-toxin is specific to the kind of bacterial toxin that stimulates its manufacture in the body. Injections of diphtheria toxin result in the appearance of anti-toxin which neutralizes only diphtheria toxin, and the same holds for tetanus toxin.

In addition to this use of anti-toxins in the treatment of established cases of disease, anti-toxins had another use. It was found that if toxin and anti-toxin were mixed together, the combination lost the damaging effect of the toxin but still retained its ability to stimulate the body to produce anti-toxin. Anti-toxins could then be produced by injecting horses with safe mixtures of toxin and anti-toxin; later blood was removed for isolation of serum (i.e. blood minus cells and fibrinogen) containing anti-toxin. For many years these 'sera' have been used in the treatment of various bacterial infections, mainly diphtheria and tetanus but also staphylococcal infections, gas-gangrene and botulism. For various reasons these sera have almost disappeared as methods of treatment (see also page 69). Diseases such as tetanus and diphtheria are more easily prevented than treated (see below for immunization) and the use of horse serum carries risks for some individuals who are allergic to horse serum and who may have alarming reactions after injection of the material. For other diseases, such as staphylococcal infections and gas-gangrene, much more effective methods of treatment are now available.

Immunization against diphtheria and tetanus in man

The discovery that mixtures of toxin and anti-toxin could safely be injected into animals and still stimulate the manufacture of anti-toxins had far reaching effects on the prospects of the eradication of diphtheria and tetanus from human populations. In 1901 Von Behring was awarded a Nobel prize in Physiology and Medicine for his work on immunization of animals by injection of toxin + anti-toxin mixtures. A few years later this work was applied to man and in 1913 he used a toxin + anti-toxin mixture which produced rapid, lasting and fairly

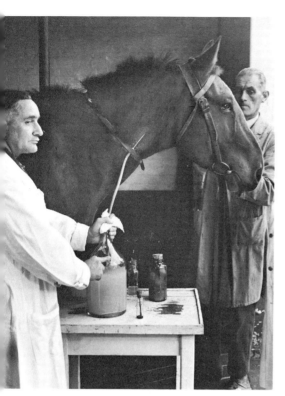

Figure 6.3 A horse being bled for the production of anti-toxins. (*Photograph generously supplied by Prof. L. H. Collier of the Lister Institute of Preventitive Medicine.*)

safe immunity to diphtheria in man. A even safer method of inactivating toxin was discovered by Alexander Glenny. Glenny was puzzled when he found that a certain batch of diphtheria toxin had very little damaging effect in animals although it produced as strong an immunity against diphtheria as did highly toxic batches. His safe toxins had been stored in containers that had been sterilized with formalin. The formalin had in some way 'detoxicated' the toxin and yet left its ability to make the animals immune to diphtheria. These inactivated toxins are called toxoids and are used nowadays in vaccines for immunization against diphtheria and tetanus in man.

The use of a vaccine against diphtheria is a classic example of the dramatic possibilities for the prevention of infectious disease. We have already seen the early work on the preparation of a vaccine by modifying diphtheria toxin so that it could safely be injected into the body to produce a prolonged immunity to diphtheria. There were early trials, in the 1920s and 30s, of the use of diphtheria vaccines in various institutions and training centres in Britain. All of these various projects were successful in the preven-

tion and control of diphtheria, but a mass immunization campaign was a late development in Britain. There were various mishaps in immunization campaigns in certain parts of the world which were very discouraging. In some of these accidents, laboratories carelessly issued toxin alone as a vaccine, omitting the anti-toxin which would have produced a safe mixture. Such an accident occurred at Baden, Austria where seven infants died, and this was followed by the forbidding of immunization in Austria. Other accidents were due to bacterial contamination of the vaccines which produced serious and sometimes fatal infections in the vaccinated. This sort of error led to the famous Bundaberg accident in Queensland, Australia, when the omission of a preservative from diphtheria vaccine led to a large multi-dose container of vaccine being contaminated by a virulent strain of *Staphylococcus pyogenes*. This error led to the death of twelve children. When we look at the development of vaccines against many infections, we will see that the early stages of the formulation of the vaccines has often led to various sorts of accidents that have hindered, at least for a while, the general acceptance of the vaccine. Partly as the result of the various accidents with the early diphtheria vaccines, the British Therapeutic Substances Act was passed in 1925; the purpose of this was to control the quality of all the vaccines and antisera prepared for use in this country. This Act of 1925 has been reviewed and modified continuously since it first became effective in 1931.

The British Ministry of Health at last supported large-scale vaccination against diphtheria in 1941, and for the first time the materials were issued free by the Government. Now the control of diphtheria changed from the treatment of established disease by antisera (which were sometimes dangerous in themselves and often ineffective against some strains of diphtheria bacilli) to active immunization of a large proportion of the young population of the country with toxoid. Anti-toxin itself did indeed save many lives, reducing the mortality from around 30 per cent to 8 per cent, but it did not reduce the incidence of the disease; in the years before 1940 there was an average of 58 000 cases of diphtheria a year with 2800 deaths per year. By the end of the 1939–45 war, over 60 per cent of the child population had been actively immunized with toxoid, producing a dramatic fall in the number of cases of diphtheria (see Table 4).

Immunization against diphtheria with toxoid is so successful that there can be little doubt that if sufficient numbers of children received the

Table 4 Deaths and cases of diphtheria

Year	Number of cases per year	Deaths per year
1946	11 986	472
1960	49	5
1964	20	–

protection of toxoid, then the disease would disappear from our country. That the disease has not disappeared is in no small measure due to apathy or ignorance on the part of parents who fail to take their children for immunization or fail to ensure that they complete the course of injections. Unfortunately individuals who are immune to the disease can still 'carry' virulent strains of diphtheria organisms in the nose or throat and can thus infect other individuals who have not had the benefit of immunization. For these reasons diphtheria has not been completely conquered in this country. In 1970 there were twenty-two cases of diphtheria with three deaths. This was an increase over the previous two years in which there were seventeen cases in each year with no deaths.

At the time of writing there was a recent out-break of diphtheria within Manchester in February 1971. There were four cases in children, three of whom were admitted to hospital with a 'membranous tonsillitis'. Fortunately in none of the cases was the illness severe. Three of the children had never been immunized and one child had received only a primary course. Throat and nose swabs were taken from over 2000 children and family contacts of these cases. This resulted in the detection of twenty-six carriers of a virulent strain of diphtheria; these individuals were admitted to hospital for observation and treatment to eradicate the organisms. As a result of this outbreak over 7000 children attending the local schools or who lived in the neighbourhood of the cases received immunization against diphtheria.

This great achievement, the virtual eradication of diphtheria from Great Britain, does not end our story of the conquest of infectious diseases by vaccines. Later years saw the beginning of the conquest of tuberculosis, measles, and German measles, but we will leave our account of particular vaccines here and discuss them in the context of the management of particular infectious diseases (see Chapters 7, 8, 10).

Schedules of immunization

The kinds of vaccine that a child may receive have changed considerably since the introduction of the first vaccine—that against smallpox. New vaccines against particular diseases have been introduced from time to time, together with improvements in the nature of particular vaccines. The vaccines in routine use today in Great Britain are:

1. Smallpox vaccine.
2. Vaccines against diphtheria, tetanus and whooping cough, usually combined in a single injection but sometimes used separately.
3. Live poliomyelitis vaccine, given orally.
4. Live measles vaccine.
5. Live tuberculosis vaccine—B.C.G.
6. Live German measles vaccine.

Additionally, vaccines such as those against yellow fever, typhoid fever, and cholera have to be given if an individual travels to an area where these diseases are common.

The effectiveness of a particular immunization programme in a child depends upon many factors. The age at which vaccination begins is important because antibodies transferred from the mother to the child by way of the placenta can neutralize the effect of vaccines. A period has to elapse before vaccination begins to allow for the disappearance of these maternal antibodies from the body of the child. Once immunization has begun many factors now operate to determine the effectiveness of the vaccination, factors such as the size of the dose, the interval between doses and the use of combined vaccines (e.g. diphtheria-tetanus-whooping cough) in which the balance of the different components is critically important. Not all children are automatically given a course of vaccination that includes all of the six vaccines listed. Before each child begins its vaccination programme, careful consideration has to be given to whether a particular vaccine will carry more risk for the child than the disease which he *may* develop if he is not protected by vaccine. There are special contra-indications for certain vaccines and some of these will be discussed in the appropriate sections of the book. Here we can mention the dangers of whooping cough vaccine in children who have a history of convulsion or the dangers of smallpox vaccination in individuals who suffer from eczema.

The following is a recommended schedule of immunization to be given where there are no special reasons for avoiding a particular vaccine.

Age	*Immunization*
3 months	Diphtheria-tetanus-pertussis (whooping cough) mixture plus oral polio. 1st dose.
4½–5 months	Diphtheria-tetanus-pertussis mixture plus oral polio. 2nd dose.
9–11 months	Diphtheria-tetanus-pertussis mixture plus oral polio. 3rd dose.
15 months	Live measles.*
5 years or at school entry	Diphtheria-tetanus-pertussis booster.*
10–13 years	B.C.G. (against tuberculosis).
15–19 years	Diphtheria-tetanus plus oral polio booster doses.*

N.B. This schedule does not include the recently introduced vaccine against German measles (rubella). The main aim of this vaccine is to produce immunity in *women*, thus preventing the possible damaging effect of rubella on the foetus (see page 78). Immunization against rubella can be carried out at any age (preferably after the first year of life since below this age the presence of maternal antibodies in the blood can reduce the immune response) but pregnant women must not be vaccinated because there is a risk that the foetus could be infected and damaged by the attenuated virus. Women of child-bearing age must not become pregnant for at least two months after this vaccination. Vaccination against rubella is now routinely given to girls at 11–13 years.

In view of the proven value of the various vaccines in preventing serious infectious diseases, it is indeed surprising that all children do not benefit from this protection. A few children do not receive their vaccination schedules, or do not complete them once begun, because of special contra-indications. The vast bulk of omissions, however, is due to apathy or ignorance on the part of parents. The number of children immunized varies from one part of the country to another, ranging from as high as 95 per cent of all children to as low as 20 per cent, and for vaccination against smallpox the figures are much lower than these. The persistence of diphtheria in these islands, a disease that *can* be eradicated by 100 per cent vaccination, provides a cautionary tale to all parents and all those involved in health education.

Recent attitudes to smallpox vaccination in Great Britain

Since 1967 when the World Health Organization's smallpox eradication scheme was introduced (page 88) the incidence of the disease has progressively fallen and many countries are now free of the disease. In view of this success, attitudes to vaccination have changed remarkably, attitudes reflected in the internal policies of nations and in the requirement for international travel. At the time of writing the Department of Health has accepted a recommendation by the Joint Committee on Vaccination and Immunization that *routine* vaccination against smallpox should now be abandoned. The U.S.A. no longer requires an International Certificate of vaccination against smallpox, except for individuals who have recently been in an endemic area (this does not, however, mean that independent airlines will transport individuals to the U.S.A. without a valid vaccination certificate!).

This decision has been made in Great Britain because the risk of dying of the complications of vaccination are now greater than those of dying from smallpox. In England and Wales smallpox ceased to be endemic in 1935. All cases since that date have been imported ones; between 1951 and 1970 the disease was imported thirteen times, giving rise to 103 cases of smallpox with thirty-seven deaths. During this same period there were about 100 deaths in England and Wales due to the complications of vaccination. The moral is obvious; routine vaccination of infants has been abandoned and vaccination is reserved for certain travellers or for certain groups, such as doctors and nurses, who are at special risk.

---

*See page 93 for note on the achievement of eradication of smallpox from the world.

7. Some common and important bacterial infections

Tuberculosis

IN THE 8th Report of the World Health Organization Expert Committee on Tuberculosis (1964) is included the following comment—'tuberculosis is generally conceded to be the most important specific communicable disease in the world as a whole, and its control should receive priority and emphasis both by W.H.O. and by governments'. Tuberculosis is indeed a major public health problem in the world, although some developed countries have achieved marked success in the control of the disease. Conservative estimates put the number of cases of active tuberculosis in the world today at 10-20 million cases with more than three quarters of these cases being in developing countries. Each year between one and two million persons die of the disease and their place is taken by two or three million new cases of the disease.

Cause and nature of the disease

The disease is caused by the mycobacterium tuberculosis discovered by Robert Koch in 1882 (Figure 7.1). Two types of mycobacteria may cause the disease, the human and the bovine form (see also page 126). Infection with the bovine variety is now uncommon in countries such as the U.S.A. and Great Britain, but it is still common in countries where the slaughter of tuberculous cattle and pasteurization of milk (page 126) are not required by law.

The entry of tubercle bacilli into the body is not always followed by serious disease. The outcome of an infection is influenced by the size of the dose of bacilli, their virulence and factors in the host such as age and the state of nutrition. Inhalation and swallowing (e.g. infected milk) are the commonest ways in which the tubercle bacilli obtain entry into the body. Tuberculosis can involve almost any tissue or organ in the body—lymph glands, peritoneum, liver, central nervous system, bones and joints, kidney and genital organs, eye—but disease of the lung is by far the most common form and is the easiest to trace in historical records of the disease. Some-

times in one individual many organs become involved in the infection by spread of the bacilli in the blood stream from an infection of the lung or other organ; this widespread infection is much more likely to occur when tuberculosis occurs in the first few years of life.

As we have already mentioned, the outcome of an infection by tubercle bacilli depends upon a variety of factors, including the age of the patient, social class and state of nutrition, the presence or absence of immunity conferred either by a previous infection or by vaccination with attenuated tubercle bacilli (B.C.G.) and the use of specific drugs to attack the bacilli or surgical measures such as removal of diseased tissues, drainage of abscesses and the like. Without the benefit of modern drugs or surgery the victory of the body's defences against tubercle bacilli may only be a temporary affair. Living tubercle bacilli may persist in the body tissues for many years in an inactive form. These dormant bacilli may become active later on in life when

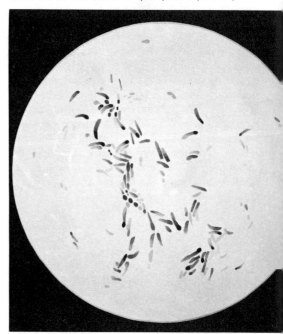

Figure 7.1 A drawing of tubercle bacilli as seen under the microscope. (*WHO photo.*)

the general health and resistance is undermined by the degenerative processes of ageing. Indeed, nowadays tuberculosis in Great Britain is becoming a disease of the elderly, particularly the elderly male.

The early signs of pulmonary tuberculosis

A study of the various ways in which tuberculosis develops in all the various tissues of the body could take up almost this entire volume. We will confine ourselves by looking at how pulmonary tuberculosis, the commonest form, shows itself. Despite the presence of progressive destruction of lung tissues by tubercle bacilli, the patient may not be aware that anything is amiss. This state of affairs may be particularly true of elderly patients where a cough with sputum tends to be attributed to bronchitis, and loss of appetite to the decline in physical activity that follows retirement, the loss in weight then being regarded as the result of loss of appetite. Sometimes the symptoms of tuberculosis are dramatic ones such as coughing up blood or chest pains, and these usually take the patient rapidly to the doctor. More commonly, however, the disease shows itself by the presence of vaguer symptoms that are the result of chronic infection, symptoms such as loss of appetite and weight and excessive sweating. Quite commonly there are no symptoms from early tuberculosis and the disease may be diagnosed accidentally by a routine chest X-ray.

Trends in tuberculosis in Great Britain

Figure 7.2 shows the number of reported cases of pulmonary tuberculosis and the deaths from this cause since 1932. The deaths from pulmonary tuberculosis have progressively fallen from 27 000 in 1932 to 1526 in 1970. Note the temporary rise in the number of deaths during the period of the Second World War. In contrast to this progressive fall in the death rate from pulmonary tuberculosis, there was little change in the notifications of the disease until the 1950s in a period when B.C.G. vaccination was being introduced (see page 65). This failure of the decline in the number of notifications of the disease may have been partly due to improved methods of diagnosis, in particular the mass screening of individuals—mass radiography (Figure 7.3). The decline in mortality from pulmonary tuberculosis shown in Figure 7.2 is

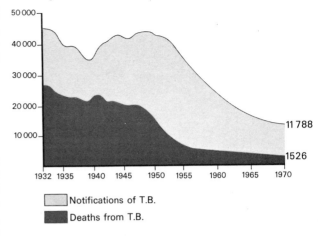

Figure 7.2 Notifications and deaths from pulmonary tuberculosis, 1932–70.

that of the whole population. When we look at different age groups and social conditions, including occupation, the decline shows inequalities. In young adults the decline has been most rapid; modern methods of treatment, particularly with drugs, are highly successful in young adults but less successful in the middle-aged and elderly. Nowadays death from tuberculosis is most common in the elderly and in the Chief Medical Officer's report on The Health of the Nation for the year 1967 (Ministry of Health, 1968) there is the comment that 'respiratory tuberculosis in males is now a disease in which the incidence increases in direct proportion to age'. Tuberculosis has always been commoner in the lower social classes and in certain occupations, e.g. miners exposed to silica dust.

The control of tuberculosis in developed countries of the world is the result of a variety of factors, not the least of which has been a progressive improvement in standards of living, including nutrition. Specific measures which have been introduced in the last twenty-five years include the following:

1. The eradication of tuberculosis in cattle and the pasteurization of milk (see page 126). These measures have virtually eliminated tuberculosis of bovine origin in certain countries.

2. The development of effective drugs (e.g. streptomycin, isoniazid, para-amino-salicylic acid) which control the disease in the individual patient and in so doing reduce the 'reservoir of infection' in the population. In tuberculosis the reservoir of infection is what is called the 'open case', the patient who has pulmonary tuberculosis and who is coughing

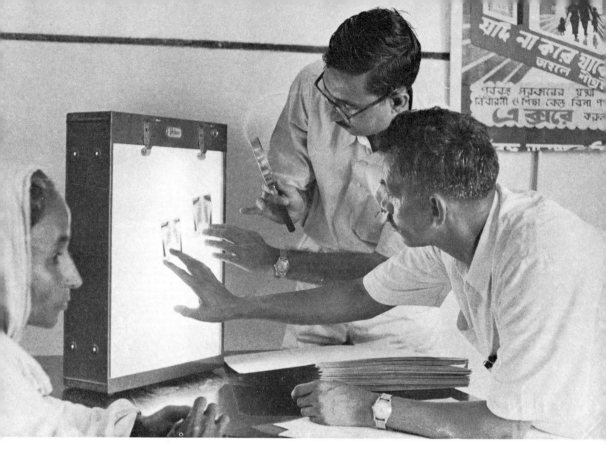

Figure 7.3   Mass radiography in the detection of tuberculosis in Pakistan. Note the miniature X-ray films being examined in front of an illuminated screen. (*WHO photo by Eric Schwab.*)

up living tubercle bacilli. Improvements in surgery and anaesthesia have also increased the prospects of cure for the individual.

3. The detection of new infectious cases on a large scale by mass radiography and chest-clinic services. Like the use of drugs, this process protects both the individual—by recognizing the disease which can then be treated—and the community, by reducing the reservoir of infection. The reservoir of infection of tuberculosis consists of two distinct parts, the *known* cases of open tuberculosis who are undergoing treatment (at the moment about 12 000 cases in England and Wales) and the *unknown* cases of open tuberculosis at large among the public. This unknown reservoir is difficult to estimate but it may be as high as one in every five hundred or so of the population. With the known reservoir of infection much can be done to reduce the chance of the individual from infecting others. He can be, and often is, treated at home with modern drugs that render him non-infectious, and much can be done by instruction in personal hygiene, particularly the disposal of sputum. Members

of the unknown reservoir are much more dangerous, for obviously nothing can be done to reduce the chances of their infecting others.

Nowadays mass radiography of the general population in Great Britain reveals very few numbers of active pulmonary tuberculosis, and this service is to finish in many areas. However, screening on a smaller scale of special groups such as immigrants or patients with chest symptoms has more rewarding results.

4. The last control measure to be introduced was an effective vaccine to prevent tuberculosis and this continues to play its role in the prevention of the disease.

Vaccination against tuberculosis

The development of an effective vaccine against tuberculosis is due to the work of two French scientists—Albert Calmette and Camille Guerin. Following in the footsteps of Pasteur who developed effective vaccines consisting of living attenuated micro-organisms (see page 55) they tried to attenuate (i.e. make less virulent) a bovine (=from the cow) strain of tuberculosis by repeated sub-culture in a medium consisting of a glycerine-potato culture medium to which ox bile was added. Ox bile was used because it was known to produce changes in the appearance and virulence of some laboratory strains of tubercle bacilli. Beginning in 1906 they sub-cultured (i.e. removed a sample from a culture and added it to a fresh culture medium) their tubercle bacilli every three weeks over a period of thirteen years! They continued their work throughout the German Occupation of their city of Lille, and after the 1914–18 War the strain of the tubercle bacilli was considered to be in a permanently attenuated state. A vaccine consisting of these attenuated organisms was tested in various animals. Guinea-pigs, a species which is very susceptible to tuberculosis, were unharmed by the injection and moreover these guinea-pigs later resisted the effects of an injection of living virulent bovine bacilli. The vaccine was now named—B.C.G. (Bacille Calmette Guerin).

This vaccine was first used in man in 1921 when it was given by mouth to a newborn baby whose mother had died of tuberculosis. The baby was not harmed by the vaccine and did not develop tuberculosis. This was the first of many cases treated with the vaccine. By 1925 over a thousand newborn babies (many of whom had been in contact with tuberculosis) were given the vaccine. In this group there were only ten deaths from tuberculosis at the end of six months. Mass vaccination of the infants with B.C.G. by mouth soon became popular in France. Abroad, however, there was much suspicion about the safety of the vaccine, for an American bacteriologist, S. A. Petroff, claimed that the bacteria in the vaccine were not permanently attenuated and that he had isolated a virulent strain from a culture of B.C.G. Petroff's warning seemed to be justified by the Lubeck disaster of 1930. After some 250 infants in this German town were given B.C.G. by mouth, 83 per cent developed tuberculosis and 27 per cent died of the disease. However, an investigation showed that it was not a virulent strain of B.C.G. that had been the cause of the disaster. In the laboratory that had provided the vaccine there was a culture of virulent human tubercle bacilli, and it was this culture that had been issued instead of B.C.G. The vaccine of Calmette and Guerin was thus completely vindicated.

The administration of B.C.G. by injection into the skin was pioneered by Scandinavian workers and this has become the routine way of administering the vaccine. Many studies confirmed the

Table 5 B.C.G. Vaccination, Medical Research Council 1950–63

	Incidence of tuberculosis per 1000
Unvaccinated	1.91
Vaccinated	0.4

safety and value of the vaccine. In Great Britain the vaccine was not investigated until 1950 and the final report did not appear in print until 1963. The results of this detailed study are shown in Table 5. Over 50 000 healthy children were used in these studies. The trials also showed that the benefits of vaccination last for a long time and that there was still substantial immunity after ten years.

Before treating an individual with B.C.G. vaccine it is important to test whether or not they are already suffering from tuberculosis or have recovered from tuberculosis, and thus have a natural and substantial immunity to reinfection. The basis of this test is the reaction of the skin to an injection of the products of dead tubercle bacilli (tuberculin). Individuals who have tuberculosis or who have recovered from the infection react violently to tuberculin and

Figure 7.4 Tuberculosis—the Mantoux test. The standard Mantoux test consists of the injection into the skin of a small amount of tuberculin, derived from a culture of tubercle bacilli. In the past the tuberculin was injected into the skin using a hypodermic syringe and needle. Nowadays an instrument called a Heaf gun is being increasingly used. With this technique the tuberculin is first smeared onto the skin and then the Heaf gun is applied to the area. This gun carries a number of needles which penetrate a short distance into the skin, carrying in some of the tuberculin. The Heaf gun can also be used to administer BCG vaccine. (*Photograph reproduced from a film strip by Diana Wyllie Ltd, Vaccination and Immunization.*)

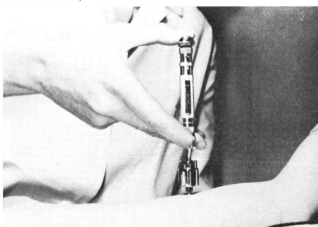

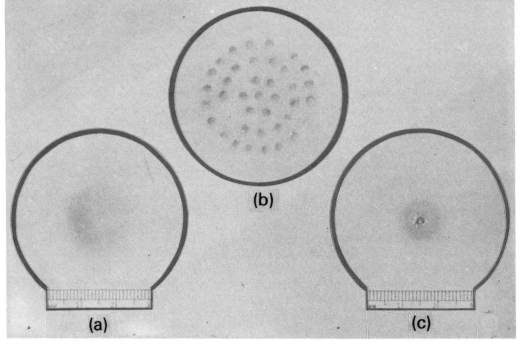

Figure 7.5 The reactions to tuberculin testing and BCG vaccination.
(a) in the left circle is a positive reaction following an injection of tuberculin,
(b) the result of BCG vaccination with the Heaf gun (5 weeks after vaccination), and
(c) the result of BCG vaccination by injection with a syringe. (*Photographs reproduced from a film strip by Diana Wyllie Ltd, Vaccination and Immunization.*)

the skin swells and reddens at the site of the injection of a small amount of tuberculin (see also page 52 and Figures 7.4 and 7.5). In the absence of tuberculosis, present or past, the skin shows no visible reaction to the injection.

The use of B.C.G. vaccination in Great Britain today

Vaccination against tuberculosis is undertaken by local health authorities or by family doctors in children aged twelve to thirteen years; as many as 75 per cent do in fact receive the vaccine. First of all a tuberculin test is carried out and only negative reactors are vaccinated. Nowadays about ten per cent of children are naturally tuberculin positive at this age. In some parts of the country the tuberculin-positive children are X-rayed to exclude the presence of active pulmonary tuberculosis, but in fact very few of these children have active tuberculosis.

In addition to this routine vaccination of young teenagers, certain special high-risk groups, such as medical students, laboratory technicians and nurses, are vaccinated at the beginning of their training, provided they are tuberculin negative. Also contacts of cases of tuberculosis, e.g. children born to families in which there is tuberculosis, are also vaccinated.

Ill-effects of vaccination are very rare and usually take the form of a persistent sore at the injection site or a local abscess; this can readily be controlled by local application of drugs that are active against tubercle bacillus. The only cases in which serious or widespread tuberculosis has resulted from vaccination with the attenuated strain is in individuals who have defective immune mechanisms, e.g. agammaglobulinaemia, see page 48. However, these rare ill-effects apart, B.C.G. vaccine is probably the safest of any vaccines that are in use today.

Summary

We have seen that the control of tuberculosis in developed countries is the result of the interaction of social and medical progress. The cost of this progress is of course enormous, and the control of the disease in developing areas of the world where tuberculosis is still rife requires the most efficient spending of any resources that are available. The efficient control of tuberculosis in these areas is discussed in detail in the W.H.O. Expert Committee on Tuberculosis, Technical Report Series, No. 290.

Diphtheria

Diphtheria is an infectious disease caused by a bacterium called *Corynebacterium diphtheriae* (Klebs-Loeffler bacillus) in which a *local* infection (usually of the nose, throat or larynx) releases a powerful toxin that can kill by damaging important tissues such as the heart,

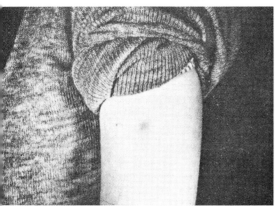

Figure 7.6 Photograph of a patient showing the skin lesion produced by injection of BCG vaccine. (*From Clegg and Clegg, Biology of the Mammal.*)

nerves or adrenal glands.

In developed countries of the world this disease has been virtually eradicated by means of vaccination, so much so that nearly all the doctors trained in these countries in the last twenty or so years have never seen a case of diphtheria. However, the disease remains a continuing problem in the tropics and it has been estimated that there are about 1 270 000 cases in the world each year, with about 127 000 deaths. This figure may well be underestimated since the diagnosis of the disease can be missed even when good laboratories are available.

Features of the *Corynebacterium diphtheriae* and the disease it produces

There are three types of the diphtheria bacillus, gravis, intermedius and mitis, which can be distinguished from one another by their different staining properties and their culture and behaviour in the laboratory. These strains also differ in the severity of the disease they cause and in their response to treatment by anti-toxin. Gravis and intermedius types are highly toxic, and infections by them do not respond readily to anti-toxin treatment. It is important to note that diphtheria is purely a human disease and the human carrier of the bacilli (in nose or throat) is the only reservoir of infection in the community. Individuals who have developed anti-toxins in their blood stream (i.e. those who have been immunized or who have suffered the natural disease) can carry the bacilli in their nose or throat with as little damage as is caused by any of the other commensals of the nose or throat (see also page 14). If, however, these bacilli reach individuals who have not developed anti-toxic immunity, then a serious disease results

which commonly results in death. Moreover, vaccination does not always produce *full* immunity, and individuals with partial immunity can develop mild atypical forms of diphtheria that are difficult to diagnose but which are nonetheless infectious to susceptible individuals.

Infection of tissues by diphtheria bacilli produces only a local infection. This local infection usually is in the respiratory tract (nose, tonsils, larynx or trachea) but it may also be of wounds, skin infections, the eye or genital tract. The incubation period of the disease is usually one to three days, after which local signs appear (depending on where the organisms are growing) and toxic reactions—on the heart, nervous system (paralyses of various kinds) and on the kidneys and adrenal glands. At the site of the local infection a 'false membrane' is formed which consists of dead epithelial cells embedded in a mesh of fibrin. In this web the bacteria multiply and release their toxin. They do not penetrate deeply into the tissues, nor does this local infection usually cause much of a fever.

Diagnosis and treatment

The disease is diagnosed by the appearance of the local infection and toxic reactions and by the isolation of diphtheria bacilli from the patient. In any suspicious case treatment should not await the results of culture of the bacteria in the laboratory. Treatment consists in the administration of anti-toxin. Modern anti-toxins (prepared from horse blood after stimulation of the production of anti-toxins by injections of toxoid) are relatively safe (Figure 7.7). However, some people are allergic to the horse proteins in the product and small test doses have to be given first. The bacteria are themselves sensitive to various antibiotics (penicillin and erythromycin) so that it is usual to give anti-toxin and antibiotic. Even mild cases of diphtheria are admitted to hospitals so that the first signs of nerve or heart damage can be detected. It is necessary to make sure that the nose and throat (or other infected areas) become free of diphtheria bacilli before patients are discharged from hospital.

The Schick test

This is a simple skin test to discover whether or not a person is susceptible to diphtheria, and it may be used to check the success of vaccination. If an individual has no anti-toxins against diphtheria in his blood, the injection of a small dose of diphtheria toxin into the skin produces a reddening of the skin. In immune individuals

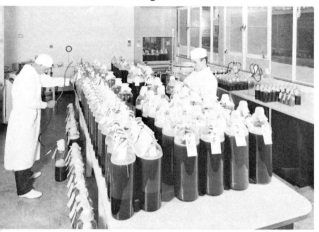

Figure 7.7 Preparation of refined anti-toxins . Oxalated blood taken from horses immunized with diphtheria toxin is allowed to settle overnight. Then the clear plasma is decanted from the red cells and is used in the preparation of refined anti-toxin by the peptic process. (*By courtesy of the Wellcome Research Laboratories.*)

the injected toxin is neutralized by the circulating anti-toxin and there is no damaging effect of toxin on the skin, i.e. no red patch develops. The Schick test can also be used in a quantitative manner to measure the level of circulating anti-toxin; this is done by injecting different doses of toxin into different areas of the skin and noting the result.

Spread of diphtheria

Diphtheria is usually spread by 'droplet infection', i.e. from the air. Usually it is the symptomless carrier of the disease who contaminates the air and infects others, for obvious cases of diphtheria are generally isolated before they have much chance to infect others. The organisms can survive in dust or on articles such as pencils, toys etc. Occasionally milk-borne epidemics have been described, the milk usually being infected by a human carrier of the disease.

The history of diphtheria in Britain

Diphtheria seems to have been almost unknown to doctors in Britain until 1855 after which the numbers of people affected reached epidemic proportions. At this time diphtheria was overshadowed by scarlet fever as a cause of death in children, but it took the lead in about 1890 and it remained a leading cause of death in children up to 1941. In the early outbreaks in the 1860s, the death rate from diphtheria was about 800 per million living and it stayed at about this level

until about 1900, a time when anti-toxins were introduced as a method of treatment; then the death rate fell to about 300 per million, a rate which persisted until 1940. The use of anti-toxins was probably responsible for this fall in the death rate due to diphtheria. Anti-toxin is a form of what we call 'passive' immunization and consists in the artificial introduction into one individual (man) of anti-toxin (antibodies) made by another individual (in this case a horse, Figures 6.3 and 7.7). This anti-toxin does not persist long in the human body and immunity disappears with the loss of anti-toxin. Anti-toxin reduced the death rate from diphtheria but it did not reduce the number of cases of diphtheria. This step in the control of the disease had to await the introduction of active immunization by means of injections of diphtheria toxoid (see page 59) which produces a long-lasting immunity. Mass immunization was begun in 1940 and the dramatic effects in the number of cases can be seen at a glance at Figure 7.8. Other countries in Europe did not, at this time, share this method of prevention. Virulent diphtheria moved with the German armies and in the occupied countries there was a sharp increase in the death rate from diphtheria during the years of the Second World War.

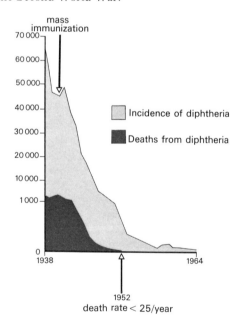

Figure 7.8 Diphtheria in England and Wales (incidence and deaths), 1938–64.

Immunization of children against diphtheria has never been compulsory, but in 1940 it was not difficult to persuade parents to have their children immunized when they could see the devastating effect of this disease on children in their neighbourhood or in their own families. Nowadays we have an influx of doctors and parents who have never seen this disease, and recent outbreaks of diphtheria make it all too clear that ignorance or apathy on the part of parents could all too readily lead to a resurgence of this disease even in developed countries (see page 60).

Tetanus

Tetanus is a disease caused by an anaerobic spore-forming bacterium that occurs widely in soil, road dust and the bowel content of many animals. The spores are extremely resistant to sterilization by heat or by chemicals. The disease occurs when wounds become contaminated by these bacteria or spores. Because the organism is anaerobic, the wounds that are most likely to result in tetanus are those that are devitalized by infection with other bacteria and where there is much dead tissue (i.e. tissue without a blood supply bringing oxygen to the area). If tetanus bacilli colonize such a wound, they do not invade the body but they produce their damage of various tissues by means of a toxin.

After a variable incubation period, the disease begins to show itself by restlessness and irritability followed by spasms of the muscles of the mouth which make it difficult for the patient to open the jaw or chew (hence the alternative name of lock-jaw). Soon spasms spread to other muscles and the entire body may be involved in attacks of muscular spasms. Generalized convulsions appear. In fatal cases these generalized convulsions follow one another in such rapid succession that the patient dies of exhaustion or asphyxia (lack of oxygen).

Although tetanus can and does occur in civilian populations it is typically a disease of war, because of the large numbers of contaminated wounds. In some parts of the world it is a common disease of infancy because of infection of the stump of the umbilical cord. In some cultures it is common practice to apply cow dung to the newly cut end of the cord! In rural India tetanus is thought to be one of the four main causes of death, where it replaces tuberculosis as a leading cause of death. Many of these cases are due to infection of the umbilical cord of infants. A similar state of affairs occurs in Latin America, where two-thirds or more of deaths due to tetanus occur in newborn infants. Over 50 000 persons die of tetanus each year, although thanks to vaccination only about thirty of these cases occur in England and Wales.

Treatment of tetanus

Obviously tetanus is a dangerous disease and needs highly skilled care. Anti-toxin (from horses or human volunteers injected with toxoid) is an important line of treatment, and the sooner it is given the better. Once anti-toxin has been injected into a vein to neutralize any circulating tetanus toxin, then other lines of treatment can commence. Spasms can be controlled by a variety of muscle-relaxing drugs. If necessary the patient has to be completely paralysed using tubocurarine (similar to the arrow-poison of South American Indians) and breathing has to be performed mechanically through a tube inserted through an opening cut into the trachea. The tetanus bacillus is sensitive to a number of antibiotics including penicillin. The infected wounds harbouring the tetanus bacilli also need special attention. These wounds are treated by surgery and all dead tissue and foreign bodies are removed. Survival depends on constant medical care and expert nursing.

Prevention of tetanus

Like diphtheria, tetanus is a disease that is far easier to prevent than treat. The first experiments in the immunization of man against tetanus were carried out in the Pasteur Institute in Paris during 1927. The volunteers for these studies were soldiers. The promising results of these experiments were confirmed by British studies in 1938, and active immunization became an official policy for the British Army—one year before the start of the Second World War! After a course of two injections of tetanus toxoid there were yearly 'booster' doses of toxoid to maintain immunity. This immunization produced a dramatic fall in the number of cases of tetanus compared to the First World War. In the soldiers who were evacuated from Dunkirk there were no cases of tetanus in more than 16 000 men, all of whom had been immunized with toxoid. In the 1800 men who had not been actively immunized against tetanus there were eight cases of the disease.

The British Army were reluctant to rely entirely on tetanus toxoid in the prevention of the disease, particularly when anti-toxin had proved its worth in the 1914–18 War. Accordingly a dose of anti-toxin was given routinely after wounding. In the opinion of some, the results would have been better if the anti-toxin had been withheld, for many individuals react even to the highly refined (pepsin-treated) horse serum.

Following the success of tetanus toxoid in the Second World War, the vaccine was introduced to civilian use and nowadays all children receive, or should receive, tetanus toxoid and booster doses in their first years of life (see immunization schedule, page 60). Reactions to toxoid are rare and usually trivial. If someone who is already immunized by tetanus toxoid becomes injured then a dose of toxoid rapidly boosts the immunity. In addition, wounds should be carefully cleaned and antibiotics given if appropriate. The problem arises in the treatment of wounds in individuals who have never been immunized against tetanus. In the past it was customary to confer passive and temporary immunity on the patient by injecting a dose of anti-toxin. However, the number of cases reacting to horse serum has deterred many doctors from carrying out this treatment, and many now rely on the careful cleaning of wounds and the use of penicillin (provided the patient is not sensitive to penicillin). In addition an injection of tetanus toxoid is given for active immunization, but it must be emphasized that this injection is just the initial course of a series of injections and full immunity will not develop for some months, i.e. the injection of toxoid will not effect the outcome of the present wound infection.

Whooping cough

Whooping cough, like measles, has been a common infectious disease of children for at least 200 years, and probably for much longer. Throughout the nineteenth and early twentieth centuries whooping cough was one of the most lethal of the common infections of childhood, particularly of the very young. Despite a sharp fall in the number of cases in recent years with a fall in mortality—mainly due to the immunization programme since 1946 in Britain—it still remains a potentially serious infection. There are many possible complications of this disease, particularly lung collapse and bronchopneumonia—which may lead to permanent disability or death.

Early medical writings give little reference to the disease, perhaps because it was not recognized as a disease in its own right but rather as a complication of other diseases. In the early part of the nineteenth century it came to be recognized as an important cause of death in childhood, and whooping cough and measles together began to replace smallpox as the main killing disease of young children. The number of cases of whooping cough between 1943 and 1964 is shown in Figure 7.7. In 1940 there was one death in every seventy cases of whooping cough and in 1955 this figure fell to only one death for every 900 cases. The dramatic fall in the death rate is due to two factors, first the use of effective treatment of complications of the disease with antibiotics, and second the introduction of a vaccine. It is easier to develop a vaccine for a 'toxic' disease such as diphtheria or tetanus, and it is probable that the number of cases of whooping cough will not be reduced as dramatically as was the case with diphtheria, certainly not with the killed vaccines that are in use today.

The cause and features of whooping cough (pertussis)

The organism that causes whooping cough is the minute Bordet-Gengou bacillus named after the Belgian workers, George Bordet and Octave Gengou, who first saw it in 1900, and succeeded in culturing it in a special medium in the laboratory in 1906.

The disease is present in the community throughout the year, but there are periodic flare-ups with the appearance of epidemics which are perhaps due to the appearance of virulent strains of the bacteria. After infection there is a delay of ten to fourteen days, the incubation period, before symptoms appear. A simple cough appears which gradually worsens with the appearance of attacks of a whole series of coughs in the form of expiratory grunts, followed by a typical 'whoop' which results from the drawing in of breath through a narrowed airway in the larynx. There may be as many as forty of these attacks in a day and the patient becomes exhausted. Vomiting often occurs at the end of an attack. Very gradually the attacks become reduced in number and severity but a cough with a 'whoop' may continue for many months.

A variety of complications can and do occur during an attack of whooping cough and these include pneumonia, collapse of lung tissue, convulsions and various mechanical effects due to the raised pressure in the chest during a sustained attack of coughing. Obviously this disease needs very careful nursing, and the outcome has been greatly improved by the advent of various antibiotics which can attack the Bordet-Gengou bacillus itself, or other bacteria that invade the damaged tissues of the respiratory tract.

Vaccination

Attempts to prepare vaccine against whooping

cough were made soon after it became possible to grow the bacteria in the laboratory (1906). For various reasons, which included differences in the nature and culture of the bacteria and the number of bacteria used in a single dose of vaccine, it was difficult to assess the effects of the various vaccines, and statistically controlled trials were not carried out until 1946. Between 1946 and 1959 the Medical Research Council carried out large and statistically controlled trials of various different vaccines. Effective vaccines arose from these trials and are now in general use. Vaccination is given routinely in the third or fourth month of life and usually the dose of pertussis vaccine (containing 20 000 million killed organisms) is given, combined with diphtheria and tetanus toxoid. A total of three injections at monthly intervals is usually given (see immunization schedule page 60). Unfortunately the infants that are most at risk are those in the first six months of life when protection from immunization has either not commenced or is still incomplete. The safest way to protect these infants is to ensure that all other children in the family are fully immunized before a new baby is born.

It was, of course, hoped that routine mass use of this vaccine would virtually eradicate the disease. The disease fell to its lowest level in 1962 (see Figure 7.9) but the number of notified cases increased in following years. This change is perhaps the result of the appearance of new strains of the bacteria against which the strains that are used in the vaccines could not be expected to produce full protection. There is an obvious need for continuous review of the effectiveness of vaccines that are in present-day use. Although the number of cases of whooping cough have been reduced, there were nevertheless 19 482 notified cases in 1966 in this country. Studying the cases of whooping cough it is common to find that at least 30 per cent have a history of completed immunization. We are dealing here with a killed bacterial vaccine of limited potency, although when whooping cough does occur in the immunized it often takes the form of a mild illness, especially in younger children when the disease is most dangerous.

We should here consider the possibility of the risks that are associated with the use of vaccines. Occasionally whooping cough vaccine causes convulsions and very rarely may produce permanent brain damage. The number of cases of brain damage after this vaccine is very small compared to the large numbers of children who have been vaccinated (about 1 in 50 000 vaccinations). As long as there is a high risk of children developing whooping cough the risks of the disease are far greater than that of immunization. However, should one injection of vaccine cause symptoms in the nervous system then no further injections should be given. Children with a history of convulsions should not receive the vaccine and indeed any children with another illness should not be immunized until they have recovered from it.

Infections with streptococci

The streptococci are a large and varied group of bacteria with a tendency for the organisms to stick together to form chains (Figure 2.1). The individual cocci of the chain are spherical or oval bodies about 1 micron in diameter. We are here concerned with one group of pathogenic streptococci. These streptococci are called beta-haemolytic streptococci, which means that when they are cultured on an agar medium containing blood, the organisms produce chemicals (haemolysins) which break up the red cells suspended in the agar; each colony of haemolytic streptococci becomes surrounded by a clear area of blood agar. Even within this group of streptococci there are, in fact, many sub-groups which can be distinguished from one another by studying the nature of the proteins and carbohydrates in the bacteria.

Infections caused by haemolytic streptococci (in future we will call them just streptococci) do not always produce the same pattern of disease.

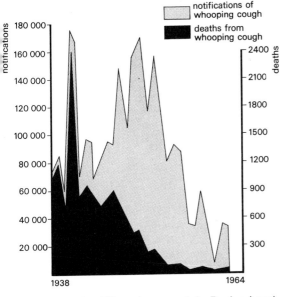

Figure 7.9 Whooping cough in England and Wales (notifications and deaths), 1938–64.

The effect of infection by streptococci depends upon the type of streptococcus and the way it enters the body. Tonsillitis, scarlet fever, puerperal fever (infection of the womb after childbirth or abortion), erysipelas and impetigo (both of the latter are skin infections) are different diseases caused by streptococci. Streptococci continue to be among the commonest causes of bacterial infection in man. Furthermore, streptococcal infections can be followed by rheumatic fever or nephritis, which are not infections of body tissues but are conditions in which the body tissues are damaged by reactions of circulating products derived from streptococci (antigens) with antibodies that are bound to the surfaces of certain body cells.

Unfortunately the body does not develop any relatively permanent immunity to many types of streptococci so that repeated infections, e.g. tonsillitis, with the same organism, may occur. Fortunately there are several potent, safe antibiotics that can be used against streptococci; penicillin, still the safest and most useful of all antibiotics, maintains its activity against the streptococcus, even after many years of use. This situation contrasts strongly with that of staphylococcal infections (see page 74) where continuous ingenuity is needed to provide a supply of antibiotics which are active against these micro-organisms.

Streptococcal tonsillitis and scarlet fever

We consider these two diseases together because in fact the diseases are identical, except that in scarlet fever the streptococcal infection causes a lobster-red rash over much of the body. This rash is caused by a particular toxin, appropriately called the erythrogenic toxin, produced by the streptococci. Individuals can become immune to the effect of this toxin so that repeated streptococcal infections no longer produce the rash, explaining why a patient with a streptococcal tonsillitis without a rash can infect another in whom the full picture of scarlet fever develops.

The severity of scarlet fever has changed dramatically in the last century. After a mild phase of the disease lasting until about 1830 the disease began to increase in severity, and for a generation scarlet fever became the leading cause of death amongst the infectious diseases of childhood. In 1863 the death rate from scarlet fever reached its peak when in children under fifteen the disease killed 4000 per million living per year. In the four-year period 1866–70 there was a marked fall in the death rate from scarlet fever, and this decline has followed steadily ever since; by 1951–55 the death rate had fallen to 0.6 per million living under the age of fifteen years. It is thought that the decline in the severity of the illness is due to a reduced virulence of the streptococcus, and certainly the decline occurred long before the introduction of sulphonamides and penicillin. Should the virulence of this pathogen ever increase again we have now very efficient weapons in the form of antibiotics, particularly penicillin, to deal with it.

Individuals usually become infected from 'carriers' of the bacteria who harbour the streptococci in the nose or throat. Spread of the bacteria occurs in fine droplets in the air or by contaminated objects or by food such as milk. Usually the streptococci enters the body via the throat but scarlet fever can occur from infections of wounds or the uterus (puerperal fever) with the organisms. As in all infections by cocci, the incubation period is short, usually only two to four days. The disease usually begins abruptly with a sharp rise in temperature, sore throat and perhaps vomiting. The tonsils become enlarged and vividly inflamed. The tongue becomes coated with white 'fur' through which project inflamed papillae of the tongue—producing the typical 'white strawberry' stage. Later this changes to the 'red strawberry' by peeling of the white fur from the tip and edges of the tongue (colour plate 1). If the individual is not immune to the effect of the erythrogenic toxin then a skin rash appears a day or two after the change in the mouth and throat. This rash usually begins on the neck and then spreads downwards in the next few days over the trunk and limbs. When examined closely the rash consists of very many closely arranged fine red points, but at a distance the skin looks uniformly lobster-red. The skin may scale as the rash clears up.

Complications of the disease

In the past severe attacks of scarlet fever were accompanied by invasion of streptococci into the blood stream and lungs, and death was caused by pneumonia or septicaemia. These severe complications are rarely seen nowadays, and they certainly can be prevented by early treatment with penicillin. Complications that are more likely to occur today are due to the local spread of streptococci into the bony sinuses of the skull (air-celled cavities in various skull bones), into the middle ear cavity (producing an infection called otitis media) or into the lymph glands of the neck. All these complications can be prevented or treated by the prompt use of penicillin. If untreated, the infection of

PLATE 1

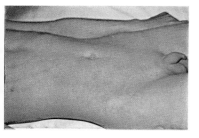

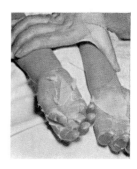

a.   The rash of scarlet fever.

b.   Close-up of rash of scarlet fever.

c.   Peeling of skin commonly follows scarlet fever.

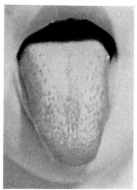

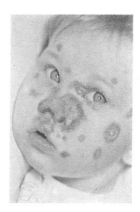

d. & e.   The tongue in scarlet fever. During the early stage of 'white-strawberry' tongue the enlarged papillae project through the thick fur but peeling produces rapid transition to the 'red-strawberry' stage.

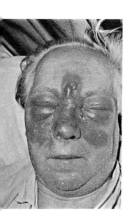

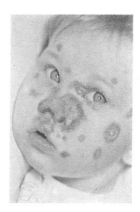

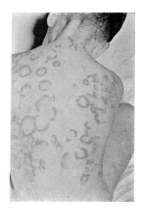

Facial erysipelas with 'butterfly' distribution. Note oedema of eyelids and formation of bullac.

g.   Impetigo.

h.   Erythema marginatum may accompany acute rheumatism. In common with other sensitisation rashes it may fade and recur.

PLATE 2

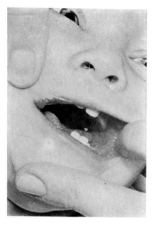

a. Koplik's spots appear as minute white granules on a red-velvety background of inflamed mucous membrane.

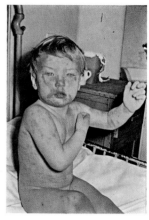

b. Puffiness of eyelids with a blotchy eruption on the face is typical of early measles.

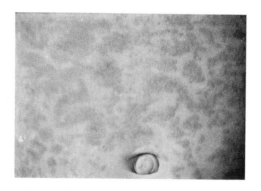

c. The rash of measles consists of dusky-red macules and maculo-papules which coalesce.

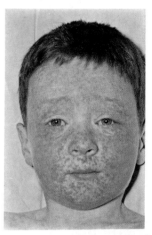

d. The brilliant phenomenon of 'staining' occurs characteristically in measles.

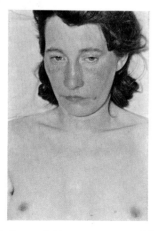

e. In rubella the peach-bloom appearance of the face and mild conjunctival inflammation contrast with the more florid appearance in measles.

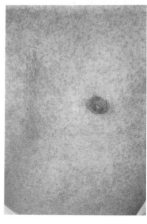

f. During the second day of rubella the skin spots join together to produce a red rash which may be mistaken for scarlet fever.

PLATE 3

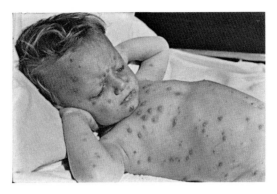

a. Chickenpox showing distribution of rash and cropping.

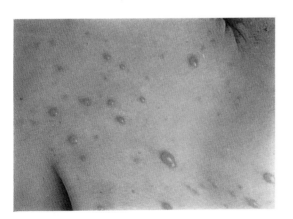

b. The rash of chickenpox in close-up.

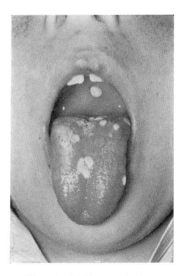

c. The rash of chickenpox. Lesions are frequently present on the palate and sometimes on the tongue.

the middle ear may spread to the air-filled cavities of the mastoid bone (that bony prominence felt behind the lobe of the ear) and from here into the skull cavity and brain.

Other complications that arise later (rheumatic fever and nephritis)—the 'post-streptococcal state'—are due not to infection of internal organs but to abnormal reactions of the tissues to the presence of circulating streptococcal antigens (see below).

Erysipelas (colour plate 1)

This disease results from infection of the skin and underlying tissues with the haemolytic streptococcus. It occurs most commonly in older age groups in which the pathogens can more readily penetrate the elderly skin. In former times outbreaks of the disease occurred in overcrowded institutions or in hospital wards.

After a short incubation period the disease begins abruptly with fever, headache and perhaps vomiting. Changes in the infected skin now appear; the skin, at first uncomfortable and warm, rapidly becomes inflamed, and the red inflamed area gradually grows, its growing edge being raised and firm. When the disease occurs on the face, the cheeks and nose are often affected—the 'butterfly area'—and the eyelids may become so swollen as to be closed. Blisters may appear on the surface of the inflamed skin.

Treatment with penicillin usually rapidly clears up the infection, but in the untreated case invasion of the blood stream by streptococci may lead to infection of internal organs, producing meningitis or bronchial pneumonia.

Impetigo contagiosa (colour plate 1)

Unlike erysipelas in which the streptococci spread through skin and underlying connective tissues, impetigo is a superficial infection. It can be caused by either streptococci or staphylococci, and although these bacteria can infect healthy skin, the diseased skin—e.g. by scabies, lice, eczema etc.—is particularly likely to be infected. At the site of the infection on the skin there is an oozing out of a protein-rich fluid; this dries to form a thick crust which is typically yellowish or golden in colour in the case of streptococcal infections. Where staphylococci are the cause of the infection then the appearance is more likely to be one of blisters full of pus which burst and then dry to form crusts. Usually the skin infection begins around the nasal openings or around the mouth, but it can spread rapidly to other parts of the face or to other parts of the body.

This skin infection is highly contagious and can spread rapidly around schools and nurseries. It is a much more serious condition in infants where the blood stream can become invaded by the organisms; this can have fatal results, particularly if staphylococci are the cause (see staphylococcal resistance to common antibiotics, page 75). In newborn babies the treatment of staphylococcal impetigo is urgent, and appropriate antibiotics are given by mouth or injection. Infected babies have to be isolated and every attempt made to find the carriers in nursing and medical staff.

In children there is far less danger and treatment consists in local application to remove crusts. An antibiotic cream or lotion is often used; the choice of the antibiotic is critical, because many antibiotics (such as penicillin, streptomycin and neomycin) commonly cause allergic reactions if the drug is applied to the skin. Once an individual becomes 'sensitive' to a particular antibiotic in this way, then it may be impossible to use the antibiotic again, even for life-endangering infections.

The 'post-streptococcal' state, e.g. rheumatic fever, nephritis, chorea (St Vitus dance)

These diseases may appear one or two weeks after a streptococcal infection. We do not fully understand the cause of these diseases but they seem to be due to some uncommon reaction of the body to the presence of streptococcal antigens in the blood stream. Estimates of the number of cases of acute streptococcal infections which are followed by rheumatic fever vary from as high as 3 per cent in some military communities to as low as 0.1–0.3 per cent in the general population. In the case of kidney damage (acute nephritis) only some strains of haemolytic streptococci seem to be involved, and after infections caused by these strains the occurrence of nephritis has been estimated as affecting between 1 and 10 per cent of individuals.

The most effective way of preventing these diseases is the efficient treatment of all streptococcal infections. This means that an antibiotic, usually penicillin (provided the patient is not allergic to this drug), must be given in sufficient dosage for at least ten days. Unfortunately a course of this length is sometimes not prescribed, and even when it has been prescribed the parent may discontinue treatment of a child after the acute symptoms of, say, tonsillitis have subsided, particularly if some minor reaction, such as diarrhoea, is caused by the antibiotic.

Rheumatic fever is such a serious disease, because of the permanent damage to the heart valves which often accompanies the inflamed joints, that efficient treatment of streptococcal infections should be given priority. After one attack of rheumatic fever, the risks of a second attack following a further streptococcal infection are so high that treatment with penicillin or another antibiotic may have to be continued for years to prevent repeat infections.

Summary

Streptococcal infections are of world-wide importance and are common infections in childhood and adults; they may reach epidemic proportions in groups such as schools, prisons and military camps. Symptomless carriers of the streptococci are important in causing outbreaks, and an explosive outbreak in which many people are involved suggests a food-borne or milk-borne epidemic. During these epidemics, mass treatment with an antibiotic may be the best solution to the problem, together with the detection of carriers. These common infections must be regarded seriously because of the risk of the 'post-streptococcal state' and they need adequate treatment.

Staphylococcal infections

Pathogenic strains of staphylococci (see Figure 2.1(a) produce two quite distinct diseases in man. One disease is an acute gastro-enteritis caused by eating foods in which certain strains of staphylococci have multiplied and produced their toxin. This disease will not be discussed further here, for it is dealt with in the chapter on food hygiene (page 152). The second disease produced by pathogenic staphylococci consists of various septic lesions ranging from infected pimples, boils, carbuncles of the skin and underlying tissues, abscesses of internal tissues, pneumonia, meningitis etc.

There is some doubt about the role of immune mechanisms in resistance to staphylococcal infections. Like the situation with streptococcal infections one attack of staphylococcal disease does not appear to give immunity to further attacks, even with the same strain of the organism —as anyone who has suffered from repeated attacks of boils will readily confirm.

Our understanding of the reasons why many healthy people carry pathogenic staphylococci on various parts of their body surface (see pages 14–17) is very incomplete. In some groups of people epidemics of staphylococcal infection is common, and these infections often occur after surgical operations. Certainly individuals differ in their susceptibility to staphylococcal infection, and the micro-organism itself exists as a variety of strains which differ in their virulence. These sub-populations of this common pathogen are indeed legion. Most pathogenic staphylococci produce golden-yellow colonies on agar (hence the name *Staphylococcus aureus*) but a more reliable guide to their pathogenicity is their ability to clot blood plasma by means of an enzyme called coagulase. Once a staphylococcus is identified as pathogenic, it can be subdivided according to its antigenic structure or according to its sensitivity to various antibiotics. However, the most sensitive method of classification is that called 'phage typing'. We have already seen that bacteria may be parasitized by viruses, called bacteriophages (see page 28). Each strain of *Staphylococcus aureus* can be destroyed by several distinct bacteriophages, and if one uses a combination of a variety of bacteriophages it is possible to identify several hundred strains of *Staphylococcus aureus*, although there will always be some particular staphylococcus that cannot be typed by this method. Figure 3.10(c) and (d) illustrates this modern method of typing of pathogenic staphylococci. This type of classification is important in practice, for it becomes possible, for example, to find the source of a particular outbreak of staphylococcal infection by matching the phage types of carriers with infected cases.

The kinds of staphylococcal infection

1. In the general population

The commonest kind of staphylococcal infection in the general population takes the form of boils, a skin infection that begins around the root of a hair follicle. Some people may have several of these skin infections or suffer from repeated attacks over months or years. Usually the source of infection is in the patient's nose or the nose of a member of the family or other close contact. Estimates in Great Britain show that up to 9 per cent of the population may suffer from one or more minor skin infections with the staphylococcus in the course of a year, and most of these are boils or infected wounds. Another skin infection caused by staphylococci is impetigo (see page 73).

In the general population serious staphylococcal infections are rare; they may take the form of a septicaemia (i.e. staphylococci in the blood stream) following a superficial infection, and staphylococci may then settle down in the internal organs, e.g. bone, to produce a local abscess. In young adults dying of influenza the commonest cause is staphylococcal pneumonia, an uncommon but extremely serious illness.

2. Hospital populations

Various types of staphylococcal infections are common in hospitals. Minor septic lesions of the skin are fairly common in newborn infants and at times these reach epidemic proportions. In newborn babies there is a risk that staphylococci will enter the body to infect the lung, bones or other tissues. The number of babies who are reported to have minor infections varies from one report to another, but figures of 4–28 per cent have been quoted. In epidemics the number of cases in a nursery may rise to as many as 40 per cent. Surgical wounds and burns are also liable to infection by staphylococci; the number of cases involved varies from hospital to hospital, and even in a particular hospital there may be wide variations from time to time. The consequences of these infections may be trivial or they may be disastrous.

Not only are hospital patients more exposed to the risk of staphylococcal infection (because of the various procedures to which these patients are exposed, or because of the use of drugs in which a depression of the resistance to bacterial infection is an unwanted side-effect) but they are also exposed to strains of staphylococci that are different from those in the general population in one important respect. This difference is in their sensitivity to the commonly used antibiotics. 'Hospital staphylococci' are commonly resistant to several antibiotics so that there may be problems in the management of the infection, (see Resistance to antibiotics, page 104). The medical profession has tried to safeguard patients suffering from staphylococcal infections by keeping certain antibiotics 'in reserve' for these kind of infections; by restricting their general use it was hoped that this would retard the emergence of strains of staphylococci resistant to the antibiotics. Unfortunately an inability to control the prescribing habits of doctors and the overcrowded nature of many hospital wards has made a mockery of many good intentions. Thus when cloxacillin was first introduced (a penicillin derivative effective against penicillin-resistant staphylococci, now commonly found in hospitals) many doctors advised that this antibiotic should not be used in wards where there was a possibility that cloxacillin treatment of a patient with staphylococcal disease might lead to the emergence of cloxacillin-resistant strains which could infect many other patients in the same ward or even in the same hospital, so rendering the new potent drug valueless. However, few hospitals have facilities for the isolation of patients receiving these new antibiotics, and quite soon after their introduction the drugs were in use in general wards.

Unfortunately an outstanding feature of these 'hospital staphylococci' is their ability to survive in hospitals for long periods. Carriers of the organisms, particularly in the hospital staff, serve to maintain the continuity of infection to successive intakes of patients. In addition to their resistance to commonly used antibiotics, hospital staphylococci may have great virulence and may spread rapidly. A striking example of this is a staphylococcus called phage-type 80–81 which was first found in Australia in 1954; this organism became world-wide distribution within two years.

Hospital workers are now taking special measures to reduce the dangers of hospital-acquired infections of all kinds. These measures are many and varied and include ventilation of operating theatres with air that does not contain staphylococci, the avoidance of overcrowding in wards, the 'barrier' nursing and the isolation of infected patients, the isolation of patients at special risk, and the treatment of those carriers of staphylococci in the nursing staff who have been shown to be the cause of infections in patients, particularly of those staff who work in special 'ultra-clean' units or in nurseries for the newborn. There is little that can be done at the moment to increase the resistance of a normal person to staphylococcal infection, but research is in progress to estimate the value of staphylococcal toxoids in increasing immunity.

8. Some common and important virus infections

Measles (colour plate 2)

MEASLES is a virus infection present in the community throughout the year but with a tendency for epidemics to occur every second year. The disease is commoner in the crowded conditions of urban areas when most children develop the disease before they enter school. The virus probably enters the body by way of the respiratory tract. The incubation period of the disease is about ten to fourteen days, during which the virus is multiplying in the cells of both the respiratory and gastro-intestinal tracts. The illness begins with fever and catarrh and harsh coughs. At this stage the eyelids may be puffy and there may be a blotchy reddening of the face. Inside the mouth an internal rash appears called Koplik's spots; these spots appear as tiny white granules which show up very clearly against the background of the inflamed mucous membrane of the mouth, particularly opposite the back molar teeth. The patient at this stage may be irritable and react strongly to light and sounds. There may be an abrupt rise in temperature before the typical skin rash appears. During this stage a convulsion may occur, but this is not a special feature of measles and convulsions are likely to occur in any childhood infection in which there is a high fever. The rash of measles now appears, beginning along the hair line and behind the ears, quickly spreading over the face then downwards over the body. The individual components of the rash are dusky red, large, flat areas (sometimes the edges of these areas may be slightly raised); often there are so many of these areas that they fuse to form an irregular blotchy area. In the absence of complications, cases generally completely recover within about a week of the appearance of the rash, when the patient can be regarded as non-infectious.

Complications of measles

Measles, like whooping cough, is more dangerous in the younger age group. In measles the damage to the mucous membrane of the respiratory tract extends from the mouth to the bronchi, and the cells damaged by the invasion of virus are liable to be secondarily infected by pathogenic bacteria, producing for example a bronchial pneumonia. In the young infant, inflammation and swelling of the vocal cords can cause alarming signs of obstruction of respiration —crowing breathing noises (croup) appear. This condition needs urgent attention in a children's hospital where equipment is available if it proves necessary to clear the airway. The middle ear is also likely to be infected, often by staphylococci, and in every case of measles there is almost invariably a reddening of the white of the eyeball that can proceed to bacterial infection of the surface of the eye. The inflamed mucous membrane of the mouth may also become secondarily infected, particularly if hygiene of the mouth is neglected. Vomiting, diarrhoea and abdominal pain may occur during the course of the disease. A very uncommon, though much feared, complication of measles is inflammation in the central nervous system, so-called post-infectious encephalomyelitis in which drowsiness, convulsions or coma may occur. Complete recovery is the usual rule but there may be permanent damage shown as mental or personality changes.

In view of these various complications, it will come as no surprise that measles is an extremely important cause of death in the undernourished and underprivileged infants and young children in the developing areas of the world.

Measles vaccination

One attack of measles usually produces life-long immunity. Thus in the Faroe Islands, after sixty-five years freedom from the disease, there was a great epidemic in 1846 when 78 per cent (6000) of the 7782 inhabitants developed this disease. None of the ninety-eight persons who had had measles previously developed a second attack.

The first attempt to protect individuals was the use of blood serum from a person convalescing from the disease. This kind of protection is short-lived, lasting until the antibodies in the serum are removed from the circulating blood; it may be long enough to protect a child in a poor state of health after contact with a case of measles or during an epidemic of the disease. This kind of temporary protection was introduced into Britain in 1925. In the 1930s this treatment resulted in a disaster in which thirty-seven patients who had received serum developed jaundice and seven of them died. This accident arose because the serum was a mixture from various convalescent donors and one or more of these donors carried a particularly virulent virus in the blood stream, a virus that produces what we call serum hepatitis. This kind of risk from human blood is now all too evident in hospital units that handle large amounts of blood for haemodialysis of patients with kidney failure. Only a small amount of blood from a carrier is needed to transmit the infection, less than 0.01 cm^3.

Later developments avoided this complication. Whole serum was no longer used to protect individuals from measles. The active principle of blood—gamma globulin—was isolated from the serum. Gamma globulin is still used to protect ill individuals who have been exposed to various infections. However, it is a scarce product and very expensive to produce. The successful use of gamma globulin in Southern Greenland is a classic in medical history. In 1951 measles was introduced to this area where epidemics of measles do not usually occur. 99.9 per cent of the whole unprotected population *at all ages* developed measles. The Danish authorities rapidly organized protection with gamma globulin and the treatment of complications of the disease with penicillin. The death rate was only 1.8 per cent in those receiving gamma globulin and penicillin for complications. In those who did not receive gamma globulin the complication rate was 45 per cent. We can estimate the effect of protection by gamma globulin by comparing the death rate in Greenland of 1.8 per cent with the death rate in the Fiji Islands when measles was introduced in 1875; in Fiji the death rate was about 20 per cent.

Little progress was made with the development of a vaccine to produce prolonged active immunity until it became possible to culture the measles virus in the laboratory. The measles virus was first isolated by Enders in America during 1954. He was able to grow the virus in cultures of human kidney, and after over fifty passages through kidney cultures the virus was able to grow in the chick embryo. The Edmonston 'B' strain of attenuated measles vaccine, from which most other strains are developed, came from the name of the patient from whom the virus was isolated—John Edmonston. This

achievement was followed by trials in the U.S.A. with this strain of attenuated virus. In almost every child who was injected with the virus there was a fever and a rash, although the illness did not spread, like natural measles, to susceptible contacts. These experiences were followed by further manipulations of the virus in the laboratory to make it safe and acceptable for routine use. At the same time attempts were made to immunize with inactivated or killed virus vaccines, but these did not give satisfactory protection against the disease.

Measles vaccine is now available and in general use in Great Britain. Although measles causes only about eighty deaths a year in Great Britain it produces many complications, loss of schooling time and a great demand on medical services, particularly during epidemics. For these reasons many authorities recommend measles vaccination in Great Britain. Although some may have reservations to the use of the vaccine in this country there is no doubt of the importance of its role in undeveloped parts of the world where measles is responsible for one-half of the deaths due to infection in infancy and childhood.

The vaccines in present use produce a mild fever in some 30 per cent of cases, and a smaller number have a modified measles rash. About one in a thousand have a minor convulsion during the fever but this compares with seven per thousand in natural measles. Two vaccines are available in this country, a live attenuated vaccine and a killed vaccine.* The live vaccine may be given alone as a single injection, or it may be preceded four to six weeks earlier by a dose of killed vaccine with the intention of reducing the number and severity of the reactions to the live vaccine. There are various contraindications to the use of this vaccine, such as a history of convulsions, the presence of another infection and pregnancy. If a weak child cannot be given vaccine and yet has been in contact with measles, temporary protection with gamma globulin is available.

The duration of immunity following immunization against measles is uncertain and no policy has been formulated regarding booster doses. However, bearing in mind that the vaccine is a living attenuated virus, it is likely that immunity will be prolonged.

Rubella (German measles) (colour plate 2)

Rubella is a virus infection which for most of its victims produces a mild and uncomplicated illness. The disease is not notifiable so that

*1971. The killed vaccine is no longer available.

figures of the number of cases are not available. It tends to occur in epidemics every seven to ten years. In general the virus attacks older children and young adults, and in an epidemic there are probably many mild and undiagnosed cases. Furthermore, many other disorders in which rashes are present may be wrongly diagnosed as rubella.

After the virus enters the body by way of the respiratory tract, there is a long incubation period of seventeen to eighteen days, sometimes exceeding twenty-one days. The infection of the throat and larynx with the virus usually produces some throat discomfort and a mild catarrh. There is always some enlargement of the lymph nodes in the neck, and the glands in the nape of the neck are also enlarged. The eyes are often reddened and feel gritty. A rash appears on the first or second day of the illness, starting on the face and spreading down. The components of the rash are small pink areas which are not raised above the surface of the surrounding skin. On the second day these pink areas merge together, and at this stage the rash may be wrongly diagnosed as the scarlet fever rash. The rash quickly fades after the third day, leaving no peeling or staining of the skin. Usually patients recover rapidly and are regarded as free of the infection by the sixth day. Complications are usually rare except in certain epidemics of severe disease. The commonest complication is pain or swelling of some joints and the rarest complication is encephalitis. There is no specific drug for this disease and one is left with alleviating the various symptoms by drugs such as aspirin.

Rubella in pregnancy

The only reason for immunization against this normally mild disease is because of the potentially disastrous effects of rubella when it occurs during a woman's pregnancy. About 20 per cent of women infected during the first four months of pregnancy will bear babies which are affected by one or more of the features of what are called 'the congenital rubella syndrome'. These defects in babies are due to infection by the rubella virus when they are in the uterus. The greatest risk of rubella is in the first few weeks of pregnancy when 50–60 per cent of infants will be affected. This figures falls to 4–5 per cent in rubella affecting the mother in the fourth month of pregnancy. About 15 per cent of all women of child-bearing age in Britain lack antibody in their blood against the rubella virus and are therefore at risk.

Congenital rubella shows itself in many ways (see Figure 8.1) the commonest features being cataracts, deafness and defects in the heart. In some cases defects in any one child may be multiple. Furthermore, infants born with rubella defects may excrete the virus for long periods after birth, and so are a potential source of infection in a maternity hospital in which there may be women at many different stages of

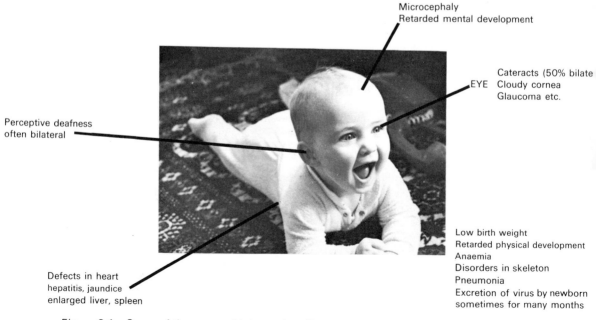

Microcephaly
Retarded mental development

Cateracts (50% bilate
EYE Cloudy cornea
Glaucoma etc.

Perceptive deafness
often bilateral

Low birth weight
Retarded physical development
Anaemia
Disorders in skeleton
Pneumonia
Excretion of virus by newborn
sometimes for many months

Defects in heart
hepatitis, jaundice
enlarged liver, spleen

Figure 8.1 Some of the areas which can be affected by the congenital rubella syndrome shown on a normal baby. (*By courtesy of Jonathan.*)

pregnancy. It has been estimated that 200 damaged babies are born in the United Kingdom each year because of rubella infections, and this figure may rise steeply during epidemic years.

Active immunization

Various live attenuated vaccines have been developed and tested in many countries. Live attenuated virus stimulates the formation of anti-bodies in at least 90 per cent and sometimes nearly 100 per cent of subjects who are not immune to rubella, and satisfactory antibody levels are maintained for several years. Experiments have shown that this antibody does give protection against rubella, even when the wild virus is instilled into the nose.

The side-effects of the vaccine are mild and resemble a mild form of the natural disease; these reactions usually appear between one and two weeks after vaccination, taking the form of fever, enlarged glands and sometimes a slight rash. Reactions are more common and more severe in adults, when painful joints or a

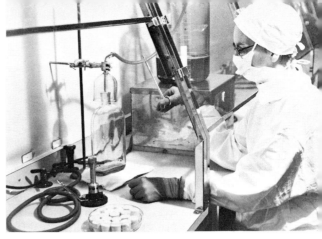

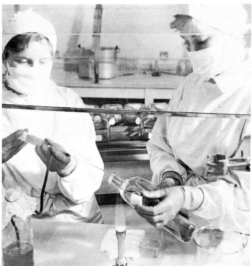

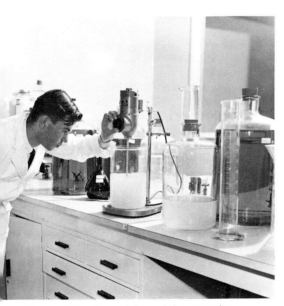

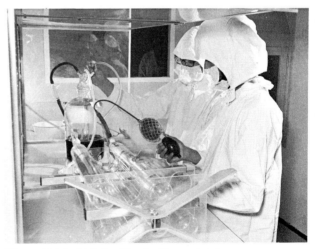

Figure 8.2   The mixing of the complex nutrient solution (containing scores of ingredients) in which living cells, in which virus will multiply, are suspended. (*By courtesy of The Pfizer Group.*)

Figure 8.3 (top right)   A suspension of living cells in the nutrient solution is now dispensed from the large container on the right into a bottle. The cells will grow to form a thin continuous sheet of cells on the glass surface. The bottles are kept in an incubator room while this growth takes place. (*By courtesy of The Pfizer Group.*)

Figure 8.4 (middle)   The bottle containing living cells is now inoculated with a suspension of living virus particles and undergoes further incubation. Note the antiseptic conditions under which this manoeuvre is carried out. (*By courtesy of The Pfizer Group.*)

Figure 8.5 (bottom)   This photograph illustrates the harvesting of rubella virus vaccine. (*By courtesy of the Wellcome Research Laboratories.*)

temporary arthritis may appear. However, they lead to no permanent effects and they are no worse than the normal mild disease that women used to be eager to suffer for the sake of their future children, when they had 'rubella tea-parties' around the sick bed of someone suffering from the natural disease.

There are certain clear contra-indications to receiving this vaccine. First the woman must not be pregnant or become pregnant for two months after vaccination, as it is still uncertain whether attenuated strains of the virus can infect the foetus and cause abnormalities of development. In addition there is the usual precaution in using any live virus vaccine, that the vaccine should not be given to anyone who has impaired immune responses. The vaccines contain traces of antibiotics that are used to suppress the growth of bacteria during the culture of the virus in cells or embryo. Some individuals are 'hypersensitive' to one or more antibiotics and may suffer severe reactions following their use. One rubella vaccine contains a small amount of the antibiotic neomycin and another contains, in addition to neomycin, a small amount of the antibiotic polymyxin.

The vaccine was made available in Great Britain in 1970 and at first was used for immunization of all girls in their fourteenth year. Now it is used as part of the normal immunization programme for all girls between eleven and fourteen years. Because of the often doubtful histories of attacks of rubella, all individuals should receive the vaccine. In any case the vaccine is harmless to anyone who possesses antibody against rubella and it can act as a useful booster of immunity. The vaccine is not yet recommended as a routine injection for women of child-bearing age. Some special groups may be suitable for vaccination, such as women without rubella antibody (detected by a blood test) who are in contact with children at work or in their own families.

Two types of vaccine are in use in Great Britain at the moment. One called 'cendevax' is produced from a particular strain of virus that has been passaged in rabbit kidney. Another strain of the virus is cultured in human cells ('almavax')—see Figures 8.2–8.5, illustrating vaccine production.

The treatment of rubella when it occurs during pregnancy

If a pregnant woman develops rubella or comes into contact with a case of rubella the only treatment available is to try to protect the foetus by treating the women with 'immunoglobulin' (see page 50), so conferring temporary passive immunity to rubella. Theoretically at least, this should be given only to women who do not already have antibodies in the blood stream from a previous attack of the disease. However, it is unwise to wait for the few days needed for receiving the result of antibody measurements before starting immunoglobulin treatment. This kind of treatment by no means offers complete protection against developing the infection or foetal damage; because of the long incubation period much viral multiplication has already occurred when the first symptoms of rubella appear. A diagnosed rubella infection during the first few months of pregnancy is therefore a recognized indication for legal abortion.

Mumps

Mumps is a virus disease present in most urban communities throughout the world, with epidemics occurring at irregular intervals. Sixty per cent of adults have a history of having mumps and study of the blood shows that many more individuals possess antibody to the virus, so that there must be many mild or undiagnosed cases of the disease.

Mumps is only moderately infective, and the virus is spread by droplet infection or by mouth contact with articles contaminated by infected saliva. The virus enters the body through the upper respiratory passages and later is spread via the blood stream. Many different tissues may become infected with the virus, which is excreted in urine and saliva. Mumps is thus a generalized virus infection, and although the salivary glands are the organs usually involved in the disease many other organs may show evidence of infection; these organs include the testes, pancreas, central nervous system, ovaries, heart, joints, eye and ear.

The incubation period of the disease varies from twelve to thirty-five days with most cases having an incubation period of about twenty days; at the end of this period most people develop a fever and feel unwell; soon, usually within a day, there is stiffness of the jaw and discomfort on chewing. Within a few days the parotid salivary glands become swollen and often painful. The parotid gland is at the side of the face, in front of the ear and overlying the angle of the jaw. The swelling of the gland may reach from the temple to the neck. Sometimes other salivary glands are also affected.

Because other organs may be involved in a similar process, the symptoms of mumps can be very varied. By far the commonest of these other complications is inflammation of the testes (orchitis); it rarely affects boys before puberty but it affects 25 per cent of male cases after puberty. This may be a most distressing complication affecting one or both testes.

In spite of the widespread and varied complications that are possible in this virus infection, nearly all cases recover within one to two weeks. When the parotid glands only are involved death is extremely rare. Some atrophy of the affected testis may occur after orchitis but sterility, due to bilateral orchitis is rare.

There is no drug active against the mumps virus; the treatment is aimed at relieving symptoms as they occur.

Vaccination

A living attenuated vaccine is under trial in the U.S.A. and the U.S.S.R. The results of these trials have been very promising and it is likely that a similar vaccine will be introduced into Great Britain. An attack of mumps can have various complications (see the previous section) but the number of these cases is small, especially in children, and an acceptable mumps vaccine will have to be very safe and give prolonged protection.

Chicken pox and shingles (Herpes zoster) (colour plate 3)

Chicken pox and shingles are considered here together because it is most probable that both of these diseases are caused by the same virus. Chicken pox is an acute infectious disease of children and young adults in which the virus settles mainly in the skin. Shingles is a disease typically affecting the elderly in which the virus attacks one or more sensory nerves and the skin supplied by the nerves. Children and adults who are in contact with cases of shingles may develop chicken pox, although the reverse is rather rare.

Chicken pox

Chicken pox virus is present in the community throughout the year and the virus is spread from person to person by droplets in the air. It is a highly infectious disease and even patients who are incubating the disease can readily spread the virus to other susceptible persons. The incubation period of the disease is usually just over two weeks (fifteen to sixteen days). Before the typical rash appears, adults may feel ill for one or two days with fever, headaches and a sore throat.

The rash of chicken pox first appears on the chest and abdomen and on the inner side of the thighs, and then during the next day or so the face, scalp and the upper parts of the arms and legs are affected. Each element of the rash passes through stages of development—a flat red patch which then thickens and accumulates fluid (a small blister or vesicle) whose contents then become clouded. This progression may be very rapid so that the first elements that may be noticed are vesicles. In many cases these same elements are found in the mouth and larynx. Gradually the small blisters dry out and form a scab. The blisters may be very itchy; if they are scratched they are likely to become secondarily infected by bacteria. Crops of new blisters may appear at intervals for about a week; as soon as this cropping stops the patient begins to feel well again.

In children the general effects of the disease are usually mild, and complications are rare. Adults sometimes suffer from a more severe effect of the disease which may be complicated by invasion of the lung by the virus (virus pneumonia). There are no drugs available which attack the chicken pox virus. Antibiotics are used only to treat infections that arise from contamination of the skin rash with pathogenic bacteria.

Shingles

Many sufferers from shingles have had chicken pox previously. It has been suggested that during an attack of chicken pox the virus in the skin may enter some nerve endings and migrate up the sensory nerve fibres, ultimately coming to rest in the cell bodies of the sensory nerves which lie just outside the central nervous system. Here it is presumed the virus lays dormant, and is protected from the effect of antibody circulating in the blood stream. At some later time, perhaps when the immunity to the virus is waning, the virus becomes active again, multiplies and spreads down the nerve fibres to invade the skin which is supplied by the particular nerve. In the skin the rash is similar to that of chicken pox.

In a few cases the patient may be generally unwell before the appearance of the rash, perhaps with fever and headache. More often the first symptom is the appearance of pain over the area of skin supplied by the infected nerves. After a few days the rash appears. The infection may damage the nerves so that there is a loss of sensation in the area or it may cause prolonged attacks of pain in the affected area—the so-called post-herpetic neuralgia. Usually it is a patch of skin on the chest which is affected (in over 50 per cent of cases). Unfortunately, in some cases the virus affects a sensory nerve supplying the head, in which case the eye may be involved.

In the early phase of the disease when pain is the only symptom, diagnosis may be a problem, but the appearance and distribution of the rash (i.e. in an area of skin supplied by a particular sensory nerve) clinches the diagnosis. Local treatments—of which there are many—have no proven value, and the only measures to take are those which keep the affected skin dry and the pain under control. However, special treatment may be necessary if the eye becomes involved.

No vaccine is available to protect individuals from chicken pox or shingles.

Influenza—The sweating sickness

The influenza virus was first isolated in 1933 and our understanding of the disease dates from this time. By 1947 three basic types of influenza virus had been isolated, called influenza A, B and C. The disease caused by these different types of influenza virus is similar; the difference lies in the pattern of the infection in a community— i.e. in the epidemiology of the disease. Virus A is the one that is usually found in major epidemics, and may spread across continents producing what we call pandemics. Virus B tends to occur in localized outbreaks of the disease such as schools and military camps. Influenza C causes relatively minor respiratory illnesses that resemble the common cold.

Although the virus responsible for the diseases was isolated only in 1933, the history of this disease probably goes back to 1510. In 1841 during the early years of the General Register Office, there were 1659 deaths registered from influenza. In the years 1847–8 there were epidemics of the disease and 15 000 deaths from influenza were recorded. After 1860 the disease declined in importance until the pandemics of 1889–92; these pandemics seem to be the beginning of a new epoch in the history of the disease throughout the world. Following the pandemics there were recurring waves of the disease, and in 1918–19 there was one of the greatest outbreaks of infectious disease which the human race has experienced, comparable in effect to the Black Death. In England and Wales about 150 000 people died of the disease, and in the world it has been estimated that the total deaths from influenza reached 15 million. A very special feature of this pandemic was that it tended to kill the young and vigorous rather than the elderly. After the pandemic the disease persisted at a fairly high level but it soon lost its effect on the young, and the elderly were once again the most seriously affected by this infection.

In more recent history pandemics occurred in 1957 and in 1968–69. These pandemics are known to be due to the emergence of new variations of the influenza A virus, which can spread rapidly in populations because they have no immunity to the new variant. The original A virus persisted until about 1946, when it gradually became replaced by a variant called A1. In 1957 yet another variant called A2 appeared in the Kwei-Chow province of China, and within months the virus had spread throughout the world to become the dominant strain of influenza. This became known as Mao flu. Yet another variant, 'Hong Kong flu', appeared in 1968. This again spread rapidly across continents. Britain was severely affected in 1968–9, with a prolonged epidemic lasting from December to April. During this period there was an excess of over one million claims for sickness benefits, an excess of about 1000 deaths due to influenza, and an excess of deaths due to bronchitis and pneumonia of over 12 000. In this first year of Hong Kong flu, about a quarter of the whole population appears to have been infected. This did not prevent a further explosive epidemic of the same variety of influenza in 1969–70, with an excess of 10 000 influenza deaths.

We do not know why the influenza virus can produce so many variations. Certainly it is an advantage for the virus itself, for each new variation in antigenic structure (for definition of antigen see page 42) enables the virus to spread rapidly in human populations. The virus can attack individuals who have already suffered one one or more previous attacks of influenza, for the influenza antibodies in the blood of these individuals is effective only against the 'old' strain of the virus. In terms of human misery and economic losses this facility of the virus to present itself in new forms is a grave disadvantage. Moreover the situation creates immense problems in the preparation of effective vaccines, but more of this later.

The nature of the disease

Influenza is transmitted by way of 'droplet' infection, the virus entering the body through the respiratory passages. Overcrowding is thus a very important factor in determining the spread of the disease. The virus attack is a fairly localized one on the epithelial lining of the upper and lower respiratory passages. This epithelial damage paves the way for secondary invasion by bacterial pathogens, and accounts for many of the complications of the disease.

The incubation period is usually about two days. The illness begins suddenly, often with dramatic speed, with headache, sore throat, shivering, backache and nasal congestion. In the first day the temperature rises rapidly and may reach 104 °F (40 °C). Pain in the back and limbs is a very common early symptom in adults. The duration of this acute illness is variable, but usually it does not last long and the temperature falls on the third or fourth day. Cough becomes a more important symptom as the disease progresses because of the damage to the epithelial lining of the trachea and bronchi, and there may be an ache behind the breastbone due to inflammation of the trachea. In children the illness is usually mild and they recover rapidly. Recovery in older adults may be prolonged, and symptoms of fatigue and depression may be present for some time.

The outcome of the disease and complications

The mortality of influenza varies in different epidemics. In recent years the mortality rate has been low—less than one death per 10 000, although in the pandemic of 1918 rates as high as two per 100 were recorded in Europe and North America and many of these were in young adults.

The common complications of influenza are bronchitis, bronchiolitis and pneumonia. The appearance of these complications depends not only on the strain of the virus but also on the age and previous health of the patient, e.g. the chronic bronchitic or the patient with chronic heart disease may be severely affected. Influenzal pneumonia occurs most frequently in young children and in adults over fifty, particularly those with chronic lung or heart disease. Invasion of the damaged lung by the *Staphylococcus aureus* (page 74) is the most feared type of pneumonia and can rapidly be fatal. Infection of the sinuses or of the middle ear are also common complications. The Asian influenza epidemic in 1957 had an unusually high number of cases of complications in the nervous system such as meningitis.

Treatment

Recent research with a drug called Amantadine offers some hope of prevention and treatment of influenza during epidemics. However, at the moment treatment is aimed at making the patient comfortable—nursing in a warm room, aspirin to relieve headache and muscle pain, a sedative cough linctus to suppress a dry cough etc.—and the use of antibiotics to treat any secondary bacterial infection such as bronchitis, sinusitis or pneumonia.

Influenza vaccines

Influenza is a very common illness. During epidemics there is considerable disruption in the national economy and a nearly intolerable strain on the health services. In the elderly or those already damaged by previous lung or heart disease there is also a risk to life. It is obvious that any measure to reduce the frequency of this disease would benefit both individuals and the community at large. Killed influenza vaccines (see Figures 8.6–8.10) have been in limited use for several years; this has failed to have any noticeable effect on the spread of the disease in the population. The vaccines have not been used on a mass scale for various reasons. There has been a general lack of confidence in the ability of the vaccines to produce lasting immunity. One of the reasons for the failure of the natural disease or killed vaccines to produce lasting immunity lies in the periodic major changes in the nature of the virus, particularly influenza A. When a new strain of influenza virus appears, this strain has to be isolated and cultured and added to the mixture of variants present in existing vaccines. However, this takes considerable time and effort so that vaccines containing new variants may not be prepared in sufficient amounts before an epidemic appears in any one country. The World Influenza Centre in London and the International Influenza Centre for the Americas at Atlanta, U.S.A., collect and examine the strains of viruses that are causing infections at any one time. This information and a specimen of the new virus is made available to research and vaccine-producing laboratories all over the world, with the collaboration of the World Health Organization (W.H.O.). Another factor limiting the widespread use of the vaccine is that in children it is likely to produce a fever.

Because of these various problems, influenza vaccination has tended to be restricted to individuals at special risk (e.g. those with chronic lung and heart disease) or to important groups such as nurses, doctors, transport workers.

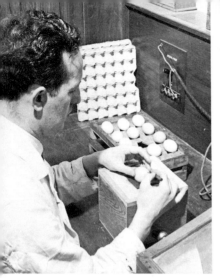
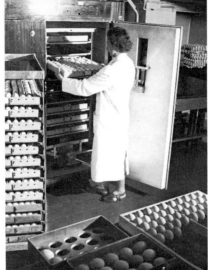
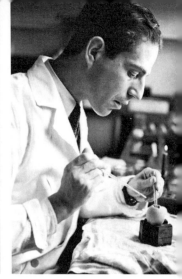

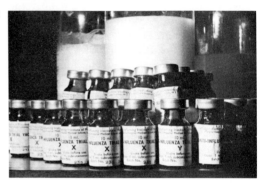

Figure 8.6 (top left)   Stage 1 in the production of influenza vaccine
Samples of throat washings are flown to the World Influenza Centre, London, as soon as an outbreak of influenza occurs in any part of the world. In order to determine the strain and type of the virus it is injected into fertile eggs which are then placed in an incubator to allow the virus to multiply. Here they stay for 2–3 days after which the eggs are opened and the fluid extracted. This photograph shows 'candling' of the eggs—shining a light through them—to determine the position of the embryo before inoculation. (*WHO photo.*)

Figure 8.7 (top middle)   Stage 2 in the production of influenza vaccine
After injection of material containing virus into the amniotic cavity of the embryo the hole in the egg is sealed and the batch of eggs is placed in an incubator for several days. (*WHO photo.*)

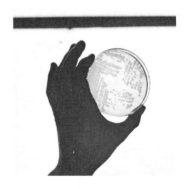

Figure 8.8 (top right)   Stage 3 in the production of influenza vaccine
After incubation the fluid contents of the amniotic cavity are removed for the preparation of vaccine. Here Dr A. Isaacs, assistant to the Director of the World Influenza Centre, extracts the fluid. (*WHO photo.*)

Figure 8.9 (opposite, middle)   Stage 4 in the production of the influenza virus
Samples of the vaccine for trial. (*WHO photo.*)

Figure 8.10 (opposite, bottom)   Photograph of an agar plate with a culture of bacteria coming from the throat swab of a case of influenzal pneumonia. Most deaths attributed to influenza are in fact due to invasion of the damaged respiratory system by pathogenic bacteria, particularly staphylococci.

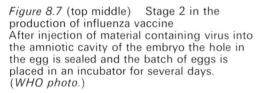

Various types of influenza vaccines are available. In the first vaccines a suspension of killed virus particles in saline was used and these vaccines are still produced by various pharmaceutical firms. Large amounts of virus have to be given before there is a significant rise in the amount of circulating antibodies. These vaccines must also be given yearly to maintain antibody levels. The protective value of the vaccines is far from complete and estimates give figures ranging from 40 to 60 per cent protection. Various attempts have been made to improve the effectiveness of influenza vaccines. Mineral oil was one addition to saline vaccines which enabled the use of smaller amounts of virus, at the same time increasing the antibody response of the body and reducing the frequency of both local reactions (e.g. inflammation and discomfort at the site of the injection) and general reactions (e.g. fever) to the vaccine. However, a few individuals develop lumps and sterile abscesses at the injection sites, and the production of these vaccines has been halted. Other modifications such as the administration of the vaccine in emulsified peanut-oil or the splitting of the virus particles produce advantages similar to those mineral-oil killed vaccines without the disadvantages of the latter.

Living attenuated influenza virus administered by a nasal spray has been in use for some years in the U.S.S.R. and is on limited trial in Britain. Russian studies have shown that the use of living viruses can reduce the number of cases of influenza by up to one-third or one-quarter of that in vaccinated controls.

Note that influenza vaccines are cultured in hens' eggs so that the vaccines contain traces of chick protein. They are thus not to be used in patients who are allergic to eggs.

The common cold

The common cold is so familiar to everyone living in an industrialized community that it really does not merit description. Each year every one of us suffers from at least one and often several attacks of this fairly brief misery. Most cases of this viral attack of the upper respiratory passages clear up within a week, although severe attacks may produce symptoms which last considerably longer, particularly if the middle ear cavity or one of the air-filled cavities in the facial bones becomes secondarily infected by bacteria.

A large variety of different viruses may produce head colds, but the commonest culprit is a group of viruses called the rhinoviruses. The first evidence that common colds are caused by viruses was in 1953 when Andrewes and his colleagues succeeded in producing colds in human volunteers with fluid from cultures of human embryo lung tissue which had been inoculated with material from a case of the common cold. Rhinoviruses have since been grown in various tissue cultures in the laboratory and have been photographed under the electron microscope—although they are very small particles, less than 30 nm in diameter.

Infection by a rhinovirus that produces the symptoms of the common cold also results in the appearance of specific antibody in the blood stream. In addition living or inactivated rhinovirus vaccines, when given by intramuscular injection, will also result in the production of antibody that is specific to the virus; this antibody will also protect the individual if the living virus is instilled into the nose. Why then do we not become immune to the common cold, and why cannot we use vaccines to protect individuals? The answer to this question lies in the large number (approximately 100) of types of rhinoviruses that can cause the common cold. Antibodies against one strain of rhinovirus do not protect the individual against attack by another strain. It would be quite impractical to prepare a vaccine against all the known rhinoviruses that can cause the common cold or include the many other viruses that sometimes cause upper respiratory infection.

Poliomyelitis (infantile paralysis)

Although poliomyelitis has almost certainly existed throughout the ages (the mummy of Rameses II shows evidence of the disease), it was not recognized as a clear-cut entity until 1840. The disease typically occurs in epidemics, large and small, and because children were the usual victims, infantile paralysis became the common name for the infection. However, this name has now fallen into disuse because older age groups are now often attacked, particularly in developed countries of the world. In 1916 a major epidemic occurred in the U.S.A. where 27 000 people were paralysed and 6000 died; many of these cases were adults.

There are three strains of the virus of poliomyelitis; all of them are parasites of man and the main source of the virus is the human intestine. No animal is known to harbour the virus, although flies are important in the passive transfer of the virus from human faeces to food (see also Chapter 16). Usually the virus either gains entry to the body in contaminated food and water or it is inhaled into the respiratory tract. In countries where sanitation is primitive, contact with the virus occurs very early in life and antibodies against all three strains of polio virus appear in the blood stream, usually before the age of two years.

After entering the body multiplication of virus occurs, mainly in the pharynx and intestine from which virus particles enter the blood stream. The blood distributes the virus around the body and virus particles may settle down in various parts of the nervous system to attack and damage vital nerve cells. The incubation period of the disease varies widely, but usually it is about two weeks. The majority of persons infected suffer only a minor illness which may be very similar to influenza, with fever, headache and general aches and pains. Usually the fever settles down after a few days. In some cases there may be tonsillitis or an episode of gastro-enteritis, i.e. diarrhoea and vomiting. These vague symptoms seldom lead to a diagnosis of poliomyelitis unless they occur during an epidemic of the disease when samples of faeces may be taken for culture of viruses.

In only a few cases does the disease progress to involve the nervous system. The first symptoms may be those of meningitis—inflammation of the membranes that cover the brain and spinal cord. The symptoms of meningitis, and these are common to any infection of the meninges whether it is caused by bacteria or viruses, include pain in the neck and back, headache, irritability and vomiting. These symptoms are not diagnostic of poliomyelitis and other causes have to be eliminated. Sometimes the illness may end here with a full recovery. In some cases the patient may begin to improve for a few days before developing weakness of various muscles. The kind of muscles involved depends upon where the virus has attacked the nervous system. The most feared effects are paralysis of the muscles that are involved in breathing or swallowing; if these muscles are involved then highly skilled nursing and medical care is needed to support the patient until the recovery of muscle function. There is no specific drug which is available to combat the infection. If the patient survives the following three weeks then there is no further danger of spread of paralysis to involve other muscles; the patient now ceases to be infectious from the respiratory tract although virus still continues to be excreted in the faeces for some time and the faeces need to be sterilized.

Poliomyelitis is a common disease in the world, commoner than the number of reported cases of paralytic polio would suggest. The paralytic form of the disease is becoming increasingly important in many tropical and subtropical areas of the world, particularly since 1950. The number of cases dying of paralytic polio—the tip of the iceberg of this disease—has been estimated to be about 30 000–40 000 per year; this figure may be a very conservative estimate. In developed parts of the world the disease has fortunately been controlled by the use of safe and effective vaccines. In Great Britain, major epidemics occurred during the period 1947–50 when the peak numbers of notification of the disease rose to over 10 500 cases per year and the deaths approached 700 a year. Since the introduction of a vaccine in 1956 the number of cases and deaths has progressively fallen; by 1961 there were less than 1000 cases a year and in 1970 poliomyelitis had become a rare disease.

Vaccines against poliomyelitis

There is a long history of the development of vaccines against polio, a history that is punctuated by failures and tragedies. The first vaccines to be used were composed of suspensions of the spinal cord of monkeys that had been infected with polio. It was thought that this virus had been attenuated and thus made harmless to man by repeated passage through monkeys and by chemical treatment of the suspensions of monkey tissues containing the virus. When this and another 'killed' vaccine prepared from the spinal cord of monkeys were used in over 100 000 children, there were twelve cases of paralytic poliomyelitis and six deaths. Both vaccines were withdrawn from use.

A great step forward in the development of polio vaccine was the technical ability to grow the virus in tissues that did not belong to the nervous system. This was achieved in 1949 by Enders, Robbins, and Weller in the U.S.A. The virus was grown in various monkey tissues, especially the kidney. This culture of the virus in the laboratory was an essential stage in the large-scale production of vaccine.

Inactivated killed vaccines. Salk vaccine

In 1954 there was a nation-wide trial in the U.S.A. of a 'killed' vaccine. This vaccine, which included all three strains of the virus, had been developed by Jonas Salk. 650 000 children received the vaccine in 1954 and the results showed a reduction in the number of cases of paralytic polio to about a quarter of the number in an unvaccinated control group of children. Unfortunately the vaccine varied in its potency and some batches conferred no protection at all. Soon tragedy occurred; a batch of vaccine prepared by a Californian laboratory was found to contain living polio virus. The use of this batch resulted in the development of polio by 204 vaccinated persons and their family contacts. This accident led to much research on the processing and testing of Salk vaccine, and the regulations governing the manufacture of the virus were revised. The Salk vaccine continued to be used and caused no further problems. A similar vaccine was used in Great Britain in 1956, although a less virulent strain of type 1 virus was introduced instead of the American strain. The results of a campaign using this vaccine were good. By 1957 out of a total of 184 684 children who received Salk vaccine paralytic polio occurred in 2.68 per 1000 compared to 11.57 per 1000 in a control group who did not receive the vaccine.

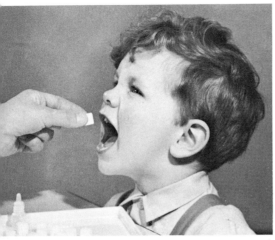

Figure 8.11 Administration of live attenuated polio vaccine. Drops of a solution containing virus are placed on a sugar lump. (*By courtesy of the Wellcome Research Laboratory.*)

Live vaccines (oral)

Although the potency of the Salk vaccine has been considerably improved in recent years, it has been almost entirely replaced by living attenuated vaccines which were introduced in 1962. This live vaccine has a variety of advantages over the killed vaccines. First, it can be given orally, thus making it easier to persuade an individual to complete a course of immunization. Second, the two vaccines differ in their mode of action. Both vaccines stimulate the production of antibodies which protect the vaccinated from paralysis. However, the attenuated living vaccine has an added effect; the virus in this vaccine colonizes the intestine and prevents any virulent 'wild' vaccine from establishing itself in the bowel. Oral vaccines thus give two lines of defence, one in the bowel and the other in the blood stream. The simplicity of administration of the attenuated living virus is shown in Figure 8.11. The possibility that living attenuated vaccine might cause paralysis in vaccinated persons, or in their close contacts, has been constantly reviewed. The risk is so small as to be considered insignificant (less than one case per million doses of vaccine). In all countries using the oral vaccine on a large scale, the number of cases of polio have been reduced to very low levels and they have remained low. In 1961, the last year before live vaccine was used on a large scale, there were 707 new cases of paralytic poliomyelitis and fifty-nine deaths in England and Wales; all were due to wild virus. In 1969 there were only nine cases, and there have been no deaths due to polio since 1966.

Warts

This harmless virus infection is included not only because it is a very common infection, but also because most students of health education seem to feel that a text without an account of plantar warts is most incomplete. The common wart, which can occur on any part of the skin surface, is certainly due to a virus infection (Figure 3.4) but in spite of many attempts it is doubtful if the virus has ever been grown in the laboratory.

Plantar warts (verrucae)

When warts occur on the under-surface of the foot where the skin is thick and exposed to pressure, the warts differ in their appearance from those that occur on other parts of the skin surface. The plantar wart does not project above the skin surface and it seems to be buried deep in the thick epidermis of the sole of the foot. In contrast to warts in other situations, plantar warts are painful, particularly if they are squeezed from side to side. Sometimes there may be several plantar warts, either separated by areas of normal skin or fused together to form a large area of wart. Plantar warts have a clearly marked outline and are covered by hard cornified skin which does not carry the normal ridges of the skin. They have to be distinguished from corns and callosities (large areas of thickened skin). The lack of growth of the wart above the surface of the skin is due to the effect of pressure on the wart; when a patient with a plantar wart rests in bed, the wart now grows to project above the skin surface and comes to resemble warts on other parts of the skin.

After infection of the skin by the virus it may take anything up to eight months for the wart to develop, but the interval is usually two to three months. Epidemics of these warts may occur in communities such as schools and barracks and seems to be related to the use of communal showers, swimming baths and other bare-footed activities. People do, however, vary in their susceptibility to infection; those with warm, moist feet seem to be those most likely to develop a wart.

Treatment

Before embarking upon treatment an accurate diagnosis is essential, and a number of rarer skin diseases must be excluded before one can regard a hard lump in the skin of the foot as being a verruca. There are many treatments for warts (and plantar warts), including 'wart charming', hypnosis, soaking of the area in 3 per cent formalin every night, covering the wart with plaster, destruction by chemicals (trichloroacetic acid, salicylic acid, silver nitrate etc.) or by physical means (e.g. freezing the wart with carbon dioxide snow or liquid nitrogen and scooping the wart out using a spoon-like instrument with sharp edges). Usually simple local treatments are tried first; these will clear up to 50 per cent of cases. More resistant warts may need chemical or physical destruction.

Genital warts

Warts around the genital organs are caused by a virus that is often transmitted during sexual intercourse. These warts tend to spread over the skin and they may be very numerous. They have to be distinguished from other skin conditions such as those of secondary syphilis (page 321). Treatment involves scrupulous cleanliness of the area and local applications which, if unsuccessful, have to be replaced by physical destruction of the warts, e.g. by heat (electric cautery) under the effect of a local anaesthetic.

Smallpox

Smallpox is a highly contagious and serious infectious disease caused by a virus. In unvaccinated individuals the disease has a high mortality—up to 50 per cent of those infected ultimately die. There are, in fact, two viruses which can cause the disease. One virus gives rise to the classical severe form of the disease which is called variola major. The other virus is a modified or attenuated strain and gives rise to a milder form of the disease called variola minor or alstrim.

Distribution of the disease

Smallpox was once endemic throughout the world but its distribution is gradually becoming restricted, mainly because of intensive public health measures in various countries and also because of the activities of the World Health Organization which has begun programmes of smallpox eradication in many parts of the world —but more of smallpox eradication in a later section.

The disease is no longer endemic in Great Britain, mainly because of vaccination (sometimes compulsory), but also because of the energetic management of the disease when it has occasionally been re-introduced into the country. In 1920 variola minor was introduced into Great Britain where it became endemic. It did not disappear until 1934. The disease was imported again in 1951 in Rochdale, Lancs, and persisted until April 1952 with a total of 135 cases, but fortunately no deaths. The disease is still endemic in many parts of the world, Asia accounting for more than two-thirds of reported cases of smallpox, most of which are in India, Pakistan and Indonesia. In North America the disease is no longer endemic but it still occurs in Central and South America. In Africa smallpox is endemic in most countries south of the Sahara.

Some features of the disease

It is thought that the virus enters the body through the respiratory tract and for a time the virus multiplies in the lymphoid tissues around the respiratory organs. At this time there are no symptoms due to invasion of the body by the virus. This is the silent period of the disease, the incubation period. The incubation period of the disease is very constant from one case to another and this knowledge is an important factor in the management of an epidemic of smallpox. The period is eleven to thirteen days. In the next phase of the illness virus particles begin to enter the blood stream from the lymphoid tissues where they have been multiplying. The patient now develops a fever, headache, backache and perhaps vomiting. Of course, these symptoms are by no means peculiar to smallpox and they may be present in the early stages of many different infectious diseases. However, these non-specific symptoms, as they are called, lead one to suspect smallpox when they occur in someone who has recently been in contact with a known case of smallpox. After three or four days of these symptoms the true nature of the disease reveals itself by the appearance of a typical rash (Figure 8.12), appearing first on the face, forearms and hands, and the mucous membrane of the mouth and pharynx, later spreading to the trunk and lower limbs. This rash is due to the settling down of virus particles in the skin. The character of the skin eruption evolves from flat elevations of the skin to a more raised kind of spot which begins to accumulate fluid—the vesicles. The fluid in these vesicles, although initially clear, gradually becomes yellow as pus cells appear in response to invasion of the vesicles by bacteria from the skin surface— usually streptococci and staphylococci. In the recovering case these pustules, as they are now

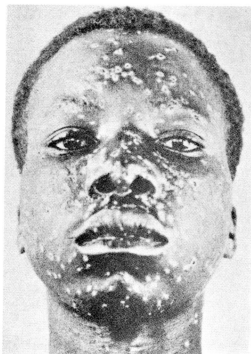

Figure 8.12 A patient with smallpox showing the typical rash. (*From Clegg and Clegg, Biology of the Mammal.*)

called, begin to dry—so-called crusting of the rash occurs—and by the third week of the illness the crusts have mainly separated. This is a description of a typical development of the rash of smallpox, but many variations may occur which we cannot pursue here. Previous vaccination can considerably modify the course of the disease. Indeed, in well-vaccinated individuals the disease may be so mild that no rash appears. These cases may be very important from a public health point of view, for they may not be diagnosed as smallpox and may be allowed to move about freely and cause spreading or prolonging of an epidemic of smallpox.

The treatment of patients with smallpox demands a very high standard of nursing and medical care. Care of the skin, mouth and eyes are particularly important for the rash may involve all these areas. Antibiotics may be necessary to control secondary infection of the rash on the skin and mucous membranes by invading staphylococci and streptococci, to prevent or treat boils, abscesses, bronchitis and bronchopneumonia. Death may occur for many different reasons. The invasion of the rash by pathogenic bacteria can lead to blood stream infection and many different organs may be infected by way of the circulating blood. There is no really effective drug which one can use to attack the virus itself.

One is left with treating the various complications which arise, such as secondary infections or heart failure. We have already seen, however, that the disease can be prevented, or its effect considerably lessened, by the technique of vaccination (page 54). The following table shows the effect of vaccination on the mortality of smallpox in Madras (India) from 1961–67.

Table 6 Mortality of smallpox in vaccinated and unvaccinated in Madras

	Vaccinated patients	Unvaccinated patients
Total number of cases	3375	3518
Mortality (%)	6	35.5

The transmission of smallpox

Family groups

The only natural source of the smallpox virus is man himself. Other animals do not harbour the virus. As in the case of most infectious diseases, the household is the fundamental unit in considering the spread of the disease, and spread is most frequent in the close association of the family group. By no means do all members of a household develop the disease when there is one infected member of the group. Thus in a study in India only 37 of 103 unvaccinated family contacts developed the disease. The probability of spread of the disease depends on the infectiousness of the case (e.g. determined by the extent of the rash), the susceptibility of the contact (determined, e.g. by vaccination status, nutrition, presence of other diseases) and the various features of the home environment such as closeness of contact, overcrowding, bed sharing).

All cases of smallpox are infectious from the first appearance of the rash until the last scab separates from the skin. It seems that transmission of the disease occurs mainly from shedding of virus from the respiratory tract, and the virus can be recovered from the skin, clothes and bedding of patients. The room or house occupied by a patient with smallpox can be made safe by proper disinfection. If this is not done then the possibility of infection persists for some time.

Spread of the disease in a population

The factors involved in the spread of smallpox within a community are, in general, the same as those involved in spread of the disease within a family. Spread from one country to another or from one community to another is usually caused by an infected individual who has travelled while incubating the disease. Air travel is particularly important here; because of the speed of air travel a person can acquire the disease in one country and travel to another country before the earliest symptoms of the disease appear.

In places where smallpox is endemic, cities, and particularly their slum areas, offer many chances for personal contact and tend to maintain a smouldering reservoir of smallpox. In many parts of the world unskilled labour in towns and cities is provided by villagers. When such workers become ill they often return home to their village, taking the disease with them. In cities and towns congestion of population is an important factor in determining contact between families. Children are important in the spread between families because of their mobility and because children tend to form the un-vaccinated part of the population. Local customs in caring for the sick are also important in determining the spread of the disease. In some parts of the world relatives from neighbouring villages come to help to care for the sick or to bury the dead, and this behaviour encourages the spread of smallpox between communities.

Hospitals have also been places where spread of smallpox has occurred. Spread of the disease to other patients or nursing staff has usually happened before the disease has been diagnosed and the patient isolated.

A well-known way in which smallpox can spread in a population is by way of the clothing and bedding of an infected person. This means that laundry workers can be under a high risk of exposure to the disease.

The control of an epidemic of smallpox—the 'expanding ring technique'

The very first step in the control of an epidemic of smallpox—as in any infectious disease—is early and accurate diagnosis of the disease. All general practitioners should immediately report a suspected case of smallpox to their local Medical Officer of Health. Apart from the actual medical care of sick individuals, the management of an outbreak of suspected smallpox is entirely his responsibility. He can, if he wishes, call on the services of one of a panel of consultants who have special experience in the diagnosis of smallpox, consultants who are employed by the Ministry of Health.

The first duty of the M.O.H. is to vaccinate what are called the 'inner ring' or class 1 contacts of a suspected or confirmed case. These people are members of the same household, people working closely to the patient in the early stages of the illness, and neighbours or visitors who have been in actual contact with the patient, his room, clothes or bedclothes. The discovery of all of these important contacts may involve considerable detective work on the part of the M.O.H. and his staff—public health inspectors, district nurses etc. It is important to contact and vaccinate *all* inner ring contacts early—preferably within six hours. In addition it is important that these contacts should be closely followed up, not only to ensure that vaccination has been successful but also to check the appearance of any suspicious symptoms or signs (fever, rash, etc.) which may indicate that the contact is developing smallpox. If this were the case then they would have to be removed to a 'special' hospital.

The M.O.H. or members of his staff should also vaccinate 'outer ring' or class 2 contacts. These are relatives and visitors who have not been in contact with the sick person or his bed-room but may have entered the house, and it also includes persons at the same workplace who have not been close to the patient. Where housing and environmental conditions are poor then these cases should be included in the inner ring and managed with the same urgency. Class 3 contacts include hundreds of *possible* contacts, e.g. crowds at sports gatherings, dances, public meetings, shopping centres etc. These provide difficult problems in tracing but they are less important than class 1 and 2 contacts.

The M.O.H. must notify all other M.O.H.s in the country that there is a case of suspected smallpox. It is also his duty to organize a special hospital to receive cases suspected of smallpox. In all regions of the country there should be special hospitals which, although normally un-occupied, are regularly maintained as regards heating, plumbing, telephone etc. This building should have a resident caretaker, always available. When this or other hospital buildings are in use for cases of smallpox, every person entering the hospital grounds must be vaccinated at the gate and sign the visitors book so that they can be followed up. All persons passing through the porter's lodge must put on a gown, a head covering and wellington boots. On leaving the hospital they disrobe, have a bath and wash their hair.

Transport of cases to hospital

Probably enough has already been said about the details of care which are needed in the management of a suspected case of smallpox. These details extend to transport of suspected cases to hospital (special ambulances appropriately disinfected after transport of the case and manned by crews with a high state of immunity to smallpox by regular vaccination) and to the disinfection of the premises and contaminated articles from a suspected case. Disposal of the dead also presents special problems; cremation is preferable and this is facilitated by order of the M.O.H.

Controls at ports and airports (See also notes on International Health regulations, page 112)

Since August 1963 all persons entering Great Britain need a valid certificate of vaccination against smallpox (Figures 8.13 and 8.14) if they arrive from smallpox infected local areas or from regions where the disease is endemic. If these travellers do not have a valid certificate of vaccination they must be regarded as suspected cases and offered vaccination. If they refuse to be vaccinated they may be compulsorily isolated for fourteen days—the incubation period of the disease.

However, a valid certificate of vaccination is no guarantee that the traveller was effectively vaccinated or that he is not already infected with smallpox. If a ship or aircraft arrives in this

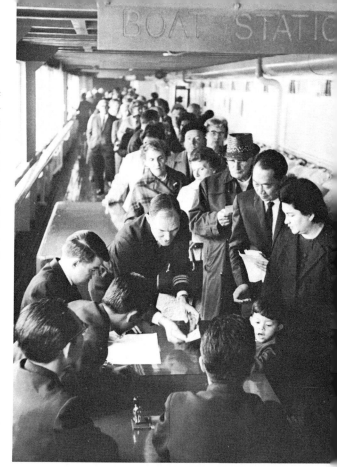

Figure 8.14 Sea port quarantine in Yokohama harbour; checking on vaccination certificates. (*WHO photo by Takahara.*)

Figure 8.13 International Certificate of vaccination against smallpox. (*WHO photo.*)

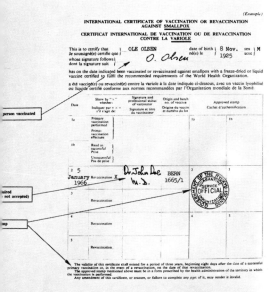

country carrying a known or suspected case of smallpox on board then disembarking passengers are offered vaccination or are held under observation for fourteen days. The port or airport medical officer then informs the Ministry of Health, giving details of the case and the names and addresses of the travellers who may have come into contact with the case. For those passengers who are proceeding immediately to other countries particulars are sent to the World Health Organization, so ensuring that these persons are kept under supervision. Greater problems arise when a case of smallpox is discovered *after* the passengers have already dispersed to their various destinations. The help of television, radio and the press may then be needed to trace contacts of the case.

The eradication of smallpox from the world

No infectious disease has been treated with so much concern as smallpox, and many countries have carried out some kind of vaccination programme for decades. Even in those countries

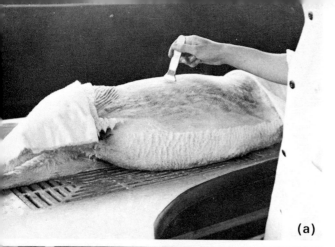

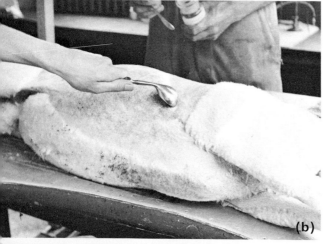

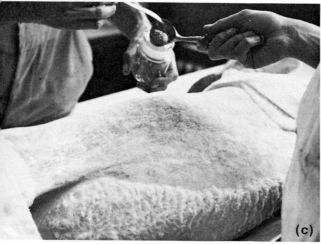

Figure 8.15 Modern production of smallpox vaccine using the sheep.
(a) Under general anaesthesia the shaved skin of the sheep is scarified (scraped) and then seeded with living variola virus.
(b) Collection of skin 'pulp' by curettage (using a sharp edged spoon) on the fourth day after inoculation. The sheep is dead.
(c) The 'pulp' is now placed in a bottle for the preparation of vaccine—a suspension of living variola virus. (*By courtesy of Prof. L. H. Collier, Lister Institute of Preventitive Medicine.*)

where smallpox has been eradicated (Great Britain, most of Europe, and N. America) constant vigilance is necessary to prevent the re-introduction of the disease from areas of the world where it is still endemic. Because of this constant threat of re-introduction of the disease into non-endemic areas, and because of the success of vaccination programmes even in countries with limited health services, the Eleventh World Health Assembly in 1958 proposed that smallpox should be eradicated on a global basis.

The objective of smallpox eradication is brought about by reducing the number of cases of the disease to such a low level that spread of the disease from individual cases can be checked (see management of a suspected case of smallpox, page 90). It is only when cases of smallpox are infrequent that the public health measures we have already discussed can be effective.

The number of cases of smallpox in a country can be reduced to such a point by systematic mass vaccination of the population with a potent vaccine (Figures 8.15, 8.16). For this purpose the 'calf lymph' used in this country is of little use. Liquid vaccine undergoes rapid deterioration at ordinary air temperatures, even faster in tropical and subtropical countries. For this purpose freeze-dried vaccine is used (Figure 8.17). This vaccine when stored at 10 °C or lower, keeps its potency for years. Before use it is reconstituted with sterile water. Then it is no more stable than liquid vaccine and it can lose its potency within hours if it is exposed to sunlight.

In addition to mass vaccination a system must be set up for detecting and reporting each case of the disease. Public health measures must also be set up to contain the disease once it is diagnosed. When the incidence of smallpox in a country is high then the detection of every case becomes virtually impossible. It is only when mass vaccination has reduced the numbers of cases of the disease that the need to trace the source of each infection becomes of the greatest importance. When this state has been reached then the isolation of patients and the disinfection of houses, clothes etc. become vital. Vaccination must be maintained in non-endemic areas to keep up the level of immunity. Unfortunately, for reasons already discussed, it is difficult to achieve vaccination of the majority of infants in a country such as Great Britain, where the chances of meeting a case of the disease are remote.

No country in which smallpox is now non-endemic can relax its vigilance until the disease

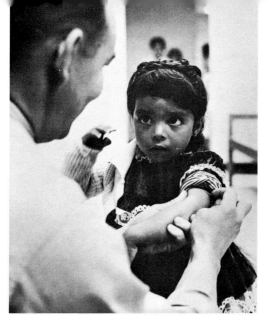

Figure 8.16 Smallpox vaccination in Mexico. The living variola virus is introduced into skin which has been damaged by the *pressure* of a needle over a small area. (*WHO photo by Paul Almasy.*)

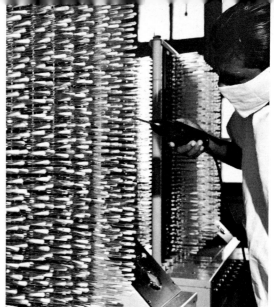

Figure 8.17 Modern freeze-dried vaccine production in India. (*WHO photo by Sharma.*)

has been eradicated from the entire world*. Some countries have in fact become free of the disease only to become re-invaded when circumstances changed. Thus smallpox was eradicated (by means of mass vaccination), from Indonesia, where the disease ceased to be endemic in 1937. However, during the second world war there was a complete break-down in the programme of vaccination and revaccination. In the post-war period smallpox was present in neighbouring countries and the disease was re-introduced into Indonesia in 1947; in 1951 over 100 000 cases were reported. Endemic smallpox persists there at the present time.

Not all smallpox eradication schemes have succeeded. The reasons for this tend to be complex. In some countries there has been inadequate supervision of the programme. Thus supervisors have not checked at the level of the family that a wide vaccination cover of the population was achieved. Further, because of lack of inclination or inadequate travel expenses, supervisors were reluctant to travel to remote areas, concentrating their attention instead on much more easily reached groups of the population such as school children. In some countries

cases of smallpox have been deliberately concealed or at least not reported promptly, resulting in epidemics which public health authorities could probably have contained. Further, although laws which insist on the transfer of all suspected cases of smallpox to hospitals are designed to limit the spread of infection, they can actually lead to concealment of illness and spread of the disease if the hospitals are so primitive that patients are afraid of being admitted to them.

Since the first edition of *Man Against Disease* was published the WHO had declared the eradication of smallpox from the world. This major achievement is the result of the work of the WHO in collecting and integrating data from all countries of the world, combined with the use of mass vaccination against the disease. The WHO still carries millions of doses of vaccine in reserve, against the possible survival of the virus in some remote area or the evolution of related pox viruses that affect other primates into a form infective to man.

Vaccination against smallpox is now no longer required; indeed for some time the risks of vaccination have been greater than the risk of contracting smallpox. For virtually all countries of the world the International Certificate of Vaccination Against Smallpox is no longer required.

*See account of recent changes in attitudes to vaccination in Great Britain and other countries where smallpox has been eradicated, page 61.

9. Diseases caused by fungi

Introduction

COMPARED with the legions of bacteria and viruses that can parasitize man and cause illness and death, very few of the fungi disturb human health. These fungi fall into three main groups.

1. *The dermatophytes.* These fungi infect skin, hair and nails. They cause most of the common mycoses (fungal infections) that are seen in Great Britain and many other countries. Although some of these infections may be highly contagious and irritating, they do not cause serious illness.

2. *Infections by yeasts (candidiasis) and aspergillus (aspergillosis).* These fungi are normal saprophytes of the human skin, mouth, respiratory tract or vagina. Under certain circumstances, when the resistance of the tissues is lowered, these fungi can invade tissues and cause disease. The disease is usually only a local one; in candidiasis, for example, infection is usually of the vagina, mouth or skin. Only very rarely do these fungi spread widely in the body to produce what is called a systemic mycosis.

3. *The systemic mycoses.* Although in candidiasis a systemic (generalized) infection is a very rare event, there are other fungi in which infection of the internal organs may be fairly common. These infections include actinomycosis, cryptococcosis, sporotrichosis, histoplasmosis and coccidiomycosis. They are fortunately rare in Great Britain and are usually contracted abroad. For example, only seven cases of widespread histoplasmosis have been reported in Great Britain. Infections with these fungi are commoner in the U.S.A. Coccidiomycosis (San Joaqum fever) for example is widespread in California's San Joaqum valley and in other parts of California, Arizona and Texas. Most of the population in these areas have been infected at one time or another. The initial infection is usually self-limiting but some cases are unable to resist the fungal attack which now produces a generalized infection with a high mortality rate in the untreated. We will not consider these systemic mycoses further except to mention that an antibiotic called amphotericin B is now available to treat the infection; this is a very toxic drug and is reserved for life-endangering infections.

Dermatophytosis—ringworm infections of the skin, hair and nails

Three groups (genera) of fungi can cause these infections (Microsporum, Trichophyton and Epidermophyton) and each group may contain several different species of medical importance. As we will see later it is often important to know the particular species which is causing an infection.

Ringworm of the scalp

This is a disease of children, especially those between five and fifteen. Often the disease is a sporadic one, but because of its highly contagious nature (via direct contact, combs, brushes, caps etc.) epidemics may occur, particularly in schools and other institutions. The disease may be caused by several different fungi. One fungus (*Microsporum audouini*) is a purely human parasite. Another (*Microsporum canis*) is contracted from cats and dogs. Yet another fungus that may attack the hairs of the scalp comes directly or indirectly (e.g. from rubbing posts) from infected cattle. The appearance, progression and treatment of the disease depends upon the species of the fungus, so that in any suspected case hairs should be examined under the microscope and an attempt made to culture the fungus in the laboratory so that the species may be identified. This information will help to eradicate the source of the infection if it is coming from cats, dogs or cattle.

In ringworm caused by the human parasite, the earliest stage appears as a small scaly spot about a centimetre or so in diameter with a few broken hairs on its surface. This small spot can easily be overlooked because of a covering of hair. Older patches are covered with greyish scales which may be thicker at the edge of the patch to form a distinct margin. In later cases there may be several infected areas of various sizes, but broken hairs are present on all the patches. The fungus grows in the shaft of hair which becomes weakened and fractures near the base of the shaft. In the case of cattle ringworm the patches may be considerably inflamed.

Treatment of scalp ringworm

In the past a variety of forms of local treatment have been used. One treatment was to remove infected hairs by plucking them out using forceps. More drastic methods of removing infected hairs was the temporary removal of all scalp hairs by a dose of X-rays sufficient to damage the hair roots so that all hairs fell out. In addition there were a variety of ointments and creams to apply to the infected areas. The treatment of ringworm of the scalp—indeed of ringworm on all parts of the body surface—has been considerably simplified by the introduction, in 1959, of an antibiotic called griseofulvin. This has special activity against the dermatophytes and there has been little evidence of the appearance of strains of these fungi which have developed resistance to the drug. A most important feature is that this is an extremely safe drug. We do not know how the drug acts, but its effect appears to be due to the incorporation of the drug into keratin (the horny substance of skin, hair, nails) as it is being formed. Unfortunately the drug is not active when applied locally, so it has to be taken by mouth.

Not all cases of ringworm need treatment with giseofulvin. Some species are fairly readily eradicated by the local application of fungicides. In the case of ringworm contracted from cattle the lesions are often so inflamed that the fungus is eradicated by the host's own defence mechanisms, but if the drug is given in cattle ringworm then it will prevent the appearance of new lesions. Most school authorities exclude children with scalp ringworm until the infection is cleared, and other members of the class may be examined to exclude infection in them.

Ringworm in the beard area

This is generally contracted by farmers and labourers in contact with infected animals. The appearance is generally similar to that of ringworm of the scalp, but if the cattle ringworm is the cause then there may be severe inflammation and swelling.

Ringworm of the skin

This can be caused by any of the fungi that infect the scalp; indeed both scalp and skin lesions may co-exist in the same individual. The lesions of *Microsporum audouini*, the common cause of scalp ringworm in children, are often seen as pale scaly discs on the body skin. Sometimes these have a thicker, coloured edge. In skin ringworm caused by fungi from animals there is more inflammation, particularly at the edges of the lesion, which may be swollen, red and blistered. A special site for ringworm of the skin is the groin; here the warmth and moisture of the skin combined with the effects of scratching may cause inflammation, blistering and oozing of the affected skin. In the tropics these infections of the skin of the groin are called 'Dhobie itch' because it was thought that infection was caused by the dhobie—native washerwoman—using her feet in washing clothes. This form of ringworm may also come from infected showerbath floors, bath mats and possibly towels and borrowed clothing. The infecting agents are spores produced by the fungi. Treatment of ringworm of the body skin is similar to that of the scalp—griseofulvin and/or the local application of fungicides. The offending fungus should be identified and if it is of animal origin, the animal should be treated by a veterinary surgeon. In the case of small animals, griseofulvin is used. This treatment proves rather expensive for large animals such as cattle, when one may have to rely on anti-fungal dips and local applications of fungicides.

It is important to note that there are many skin diseases showing individual round lesions with perhaps a raised edge. The task of distinguishing ringworm from these other skin diseases (which are usually not of an infective nature) is usually that of the specialist dermatologist.

Ringworm of the feet—Athlete's foot (*Tinea pedis*)

The term athlete's foot is a euphemism for fungus infections of the feet. It is by no means restricted to athletes but it is more common in individuals who, like athletes, use communal changing and bathing facilities—school children, miners etc. It is a fairly common disease, even in temperate climates. There are, however, many other disorders of feet which may cause a somewhat similar picture to athlete's foot—disorders such as excessive sweating, and dermatitis due to dyes from shoes and socks or chemicals in shoe leather. Athlete's foot can only be firmly diagnosed by the isolation of fungus from the diseased skin. In its commonest form, the infection shows itself by the presence of sodden, peeling and cracking skin between some of the toes (usually between the fourth and fifth) persisting throughout the year. The infection is usually more irritating in the summer, when sweating of the feet adds to the problem. The broken skin barrier can be invaded by pathogenic bacteria and this secondary infection, as it is called, may cause an additional burden or difficulty in diagnosis.

The treatment of athlete's foot depends upon its severity. When symptoms are few, griseofulvin is usually withheld; for some unknown reason the cure rate in fungus infections of the feet is rather low, although the drug will control an acute attack of fungus infection. Many mild local fungicides are available, but if secondary infection by bacteria occurs then a more vigorous treatment may be needed. There is little that can be done to prevent those who use communal baths from contracting the infection, although any person known to be infected should be excluded from gymnasia and communal baths.

Ringworm of the nails

Ringworm may infect the nails of both hands and feet, although it is infection of the former that usually brings the patient for treatment because of the unsightliness of infected finger nails. Nail infection may well be associated with infections elsewhere, the nails becoming infected from scratching skin infections. Usually the infection of nails progresses slowly; small infected areas gradually enlarge and become dark, soft and crumbly; the infected nail has been described as being like 'worm eaten wood'. Infection may persist for years. Fungus infection of the nails must be distinguished from many other causes of disturbance of nail growth.

It seems that infection of the nails is easier to prevent than treat. Prevention lies in the early treatment of ringworm infection elsewhere for, as mentioned above, nail infection is often secondary to infection in some other region. Infected, disfigured finger nails need at least six months treatment with griseofulvin. It is fortunate indeed that griseofulvin is a very safe drug! For toe nails, over a year's course of griseofulvin is necessary. It is, however, doubtful if such a long and expensive course of treatment is justified for toe nails. Return of the disease may occur after griseofulvin treatment—or

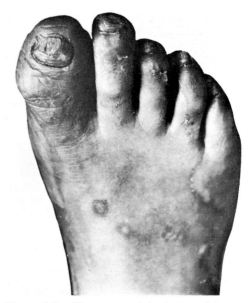

Figure 9.1 Ringworm of the foot and toe nails. (*WMMS photo by Professors Laccaz and Pupo, Sao Paulo.*)

indeed after surgical removal of the nails.

Candidiasis

This infection is caused by a yeast-like organism, *Candida albicans*. The organism is a yeast-like cell, 2–4 micrometers in diameter, that reproduces by budding. An apparent mycelium (in reality elongated cells joined end to end) may be present with buds along its length. The organism is a common, harmless commensal of man and can be found in the mouth and faeces of most normal individuals. Infections by these yeasts is usually due to some local or general reduction in the resistance of tissues to infection. Two causes of a general reduction in resistance to infection may be mentioned. First, the prolonged use of wide-spectrum antibiotics. These antibiotics damage or destroy a wide range of bacteria and can considerably disturb the normal pattern of the bacterial flora of the skin, intestine, mouth and respiratory tract. Following this disruption of the normal flora there may be an overgrowth of micro-organisms which are unaffected by the antibiotic, and these may include yeasts. Patients on long-term treatment with these antibiotics may thus develop yeast infections in one or more parts of the body—mouth, intestine, vagina etc. These infections may clear up when the normal flora re-establishes itself, i.e. when there is a return to the normal competition between the components of the normal flora, but the infections may need treatment with drugs which specifically attack the yeasts (see below). One other general disturbance is the use of those drugs called corticosteroids, drugs such as cortisone, hydrocortisone, prednisone. These drugs are used for *many* conditions in medicine, mainly because of their ability to suppress inflammation in tissues, whatever the cause. The drugs disturb resistance in many ways. When applied directly to the skin, e.g. for eczema, they so reduce the normal inflammatory responses of skin that local invasion by bacteria and fungi *may* be a problem. When given by mouth, corticosteroids also depress general defence mechanisms by destroying lymphocytes and by causing a shrinkage of lymphatic tissues, those tissues which are so important in immunity (Chapter 5).

Candidiasis is usually a local infection of some part of the body. Treatment of the disease involves not only an attack on the fungus with a specific drug but also some attention to the underlying predisposing cause. Systemic (widespread) candidiasis is very rare and is almost invariably secondary to some underlying disease process or to a profound general disturbance of resistance. Whenever there is a local invasion by yeast organisms, there appear similar lesions which have a 'thrush breast' appearance. Like the white patches on the breast of the thrush, clusters of yeast organisms form fluffy white patches; under each white patch is a red inflamed base. A severe irritation may result and the scratching which it leads to may modify the appearance of the infection. Below are listed some local sites of infection and the factors which predispose to infection.

1. Vagina and external genitals in the female. Yeasts are a common cause of infection of the vagina. The normal healthy vagina in the adult female is fairly resistant to any infection by pathogens. It possesses its own normal commensal flora of Gram-positive bacilli and it has a fairly low pH of 4.5. This acid quality of normal vaginal secretions is due to the action of the Gram-positive Döderlein's bacillus on simple sugars which are break-down products of glycogen in the epithelial cells shed from the wall of the vagina. The cells of the vaginal epithelium accumulate glycogen under the influence of the sex hormone oestrogen which is secreted by the ovaries (and in large amounts by the placenta during pregnancy). Thus the adult female vagina has an acid secretion which does not encourage the growth of bacterial pathogens. The vagina of the child or the woman after the menopause is much less resistant to infection. This is due to an inadequate amount of oestrogen which deprives the vaginal epithelial cells of glycogen—from which the normal flora produce the acid conditions.

Yeasts however, seem to thrive in acid conditions, especially when there is an abundance of carbohydrate present. These two conditions are *par excellence*, found in pregnancy; large amounts of oestrogen are in the blood stream which ensure a high glycogen content of the vaginal epithelial cells. This glycogen is available for the Döderlein's bacilli to ferment into acid and also for the needs of the yeasts. These optimum conditions for yeast growth also occur in diabetes mellitus, a disease in which large amounts of sugar may be present in the urine. Thus vaginal candidiasis is common in pregnancy and in diabetes mellitus. Wide-spectrum antibiotics and the taking of contraceptive pills containing oestrogen can also cause this vaginal infection.

2. Yeasts may also infect another mucous membrane—that of the mouth. This is a fairly common infection of infants who are presumably infected from the vagina of the mother during their progress through the birth canal. In adults thrush of the mouth is usually secondary to some other disorder, e.g. after the use of wide-spectrum antibiotics.

3. Infection of the healthy skin by yeasts is an extremely rare condition. Almost invariably there is some predisposing factor which reduces the local resistance of the skin. These predisposing factors include maceration and destruction of keratin of the skin by water, alkalis, detergents or some local disease such as eczema or a poor local blood circulation in the elderly. Common sites of infection are the nail folds, finger or toe clefts and the skin under heavy breasts or overhanging folds of abdominal fat.

Treatment of thrush

In treating thrush, search must be made for some underlying predisposing factor which if attended to may clear up the infection. Before the era of antibiotics a range of local applications was used, and some of these may still have a place today. Solutions of gentian violet or magenta paint were effective although they are rather too colourful for the patient of today! We now have a safe and effective antibiotic called nystatin, so called because it was discovered in the laboratories of the New York State Department of Health. The drug is remarkably non-toxic, but absorption of the drug from the intestine is too limited to be of any practical importance. The drug is used locally in the form of lotions, creams, pessaries (for vaginal use) although it is sometimes given by mouth for heavy infections of the bowel. It can also reach infected bronchi in the form of aerosols.

Aspergillosis

The fungus aspergillus is a very widespread saprophytic fungus. This fungus has a mycelium and propagates itself by means of spores. It occasionally infects the outer ear canal, perhaps as a secondary invader after the local resistance has been reduced by bacterial infection. Many kinds of dust, from hay, bird seed, animal houses etc., may contain the spores of aspergillus —indeed the spores of many other fungi. These spores may be found in the sputum of healthy individuals exposed to this kind of dust. If the bronchi or lungs are already diseased then aspergillus may establish itself to produce the disease called aspergillosis. In the treatment of this infection, antibiotics such as nystatin or amphotericin B may be inhaled in the form of aerosols or injected into the pleural cavity around the lung.

Farmer's lung

The presence of fungal spores in dust can cause disease in a different way, i.e. not by infection of the tissues by the fungus. The lung may be damaged because the tissues are 'hypersensitive' to the fungus and the lungs become severely inflamed when the person is exposed to dust containing fungal spores.

The growth of fungi in hay occurs best under moist conditions so that farmer's lung is commoner after wet summers. The patient usually becomes ill in the winter, when the present year's mouldy hay is fed to cattle in poorly ventilated buildings. The affected individual may become severely ill with fever, rapid heart rate, rapid shallow breathing and a cough with sputum. Repeated attacks produce progressive lung damage and heart failure. Thus farmer's lung is an occupational disease. The sufferer must avoid further exposure to the dust of mouldy hay and it may be necessary for him to give up farming, certainly to give up the handling of hay.

Conclusions

We have seen that in Great Britain there are only two fungal infections of any importance—ringworm and thrush. Ringworm fungi are not normal saprophytic inhabitants of the human body. They are strict pathogens and are highly infective, attacking normal hair or skin. In Great Britain the number of infections, certainly of epidemic proportions, has declined in recent years. The disease is, however, of world-wide occurrence and there is little information available on the prevalence of the disease.

The yeast organisms (*Candida albicans*) and aspergillus are common saprophytic fungi and may be harmless commensals or contaminants of the human body. They produce infections when the defense mechanisms of man are disturbed. They provide a good example of the fine balance that exists between man and the micro-organisms he harbours and how this balance can be tipped in favour of infection. In addition we have various human diseases, e.g. farmer's lung, which are not fungus infections in the strict sense of the word but are severe allergic reactions to the presence of fungi in the air we breathe.

10. The treatment of bacterial, fungal, and viral infections

The importance of the prevention of infectious diseases

THE beginning of man's direct control of infectious disease was with the development of vaccines and anti-toxins. Today, vaccines play an important role in protecting both the individual and the community from infectious disease; if a high proportion of the individuals in a community are protected against a particular disease by vaccination, then there is less chance of an epidemic appearing and this itself protects even the unvaccinated. It is certainly easier to prevent many infectious diseases than to treat them; notable examples are diphtheria and tetanus. Even in the case of infections for which no fully effective vaccine or anti-toxin is available, appropriate public or personal health programmes can do much to prevent the diseases —measures which are too numerous to mention here and which range from pasteurization of milk, chlorination of water supplies, hygienic disposal of faeces and urine, food hygiene etc. to the proper management of established cases of infection, e.g. by isolation, quarantine, disinfection.

The treatment of established infections

Chemotherapy

We are now going to look at the treatment of established cases of infectious disease by various synthetic or naturally occurring chemicals. We now have a vast and powerful armoury of these drugs, but this armoury has developed only during the last forty years.

Sulphonamides

The chemotherapy of infections was virtually non-existent until about 1935 when it was announced in Germany that a red dye called prontosil could cure infections by haemolytic streptococci (page 71). Within less than a year it was shown by workers in France that this substance was broken down in the body into two compounds, a dye which was inert and a substance called para-aminobenzene-sulphonamide (sulphanilamide) which was the component active against bacteria. Many different derivatives of this compound were synthesized in the succeeding years, and we use the term sulphonamide for the whole family of chemicals. These compounds revolutionized the treatment of many bacterial infections such as streptococcal and some staphylococcal infections, cerebro-spinal fever (caused by an organism called the meningococcus), urinary infections and some bowel infections. The early sulphonamides reduced the mortality of pneumonia to near its present level, long before the introduction of antibiotics. Likewise they provided the first ever available means of rapidly terminating an attack of gonorrhoea.

Three things about the action of sulphonamides gradually became clear. First, the drugs were not equally active against all pathogenic micro-organisms. Viruses were usually unaffected by the drug; indeed we still have very few drugs capable of dealing with virus infections, and most of these are of limited use. Bacteria are the most susceptible of all pathogenic micro-organisms to attack by sulphonamides. Second, all bacteria are by no means equally susceptible to the effect of sulphonamides and some are completely resistant to the effect of the drug. The term 'spectrum of activity' describes the range of micro-organisms that are susceptible to a particular drug. Nowadays we have a host of drugs with differing spectra of activity—and this feature of drugs is an important consideration in determining the choice of a drug to deal with a particular infection. A third feature of sulphonamides became all too soon apparent. This was the appearance of strains of micro-organisms which were resistant to the effects of the drug. During the decade 1935-45, when sulphonamides were the only anti-bacterial drugs generally available, resistant strains of all the more important susceptible groups of pathogenic bacteria began to emerge. It has been suggested that but for the introduction of antibiotics, the sulphonamides would now be virtually useless. Sulphonamide-resistant

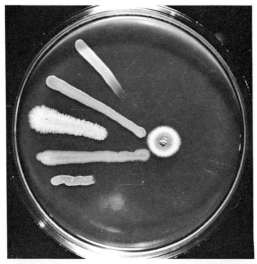

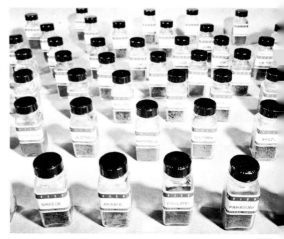

Figure 10.2 A collection of soil samples for Pfizer Laboratories. Suspensions of these soil samples were cultured to discover whether they contained antibiotic-producing moulds. (*By courtesy of Pfizer Laboratories.*)

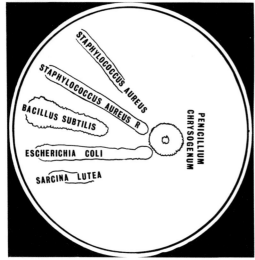

Figure 10.1 Penicillin mould versus bacteria. On an agar plate containing a growing patch of penicillin mould, are cultured five different kinds of bacteria. The bacteria were streaked along a line radiating from the edge of the plate to the mould. The growth of certain bacteria is inhibited by substances released by the mould into the agar, while other bacteria are unaffected. (*By courtesy of the Beecham Research Laboratories.*)

strains first appeared and progressed most rapidly in the gonococcus—the organism responsible for gonorrhoea. Nowadays there are only a few infections for which sulphonamides are the drugs of choice. Although these drugs are fairly cheap and can usually be taken in the convenient form of tablets, antibiotics of one sort or other will produce their effects more quickly and more certainly.

This decline in the importance of sulphonamides is due not only to the presence of sulphonamide-resistant strains of common

pathogenic bacteria, but also reflects the mode of action of drugs that are used in chemotherapy. Sulphonamides do not kill bacteria, they merely arrest their growth and multiplication; the pathogenic bacteria have to be removed by the body's own defence mechanisms. Drugs that produce their effects in this way are called 'bacteriostatic'. Some of the antibiotics that have been introduced since the sulphonamides owe part of their rapid and powerful action to the fact that they actively destroy bacteria, i.e. they are bactericidal. This kind of action is particularly important in treating infections of certain body tissues such as joint cavities or the central nervous system, where the natural local defence mechanisms are poorly developed (see also page 21).

Recent years, however, have seen a resurgence of sulphonamides, used not alone but in combination with another synthetic drug called trimethoprim. Used alone each of these drugs is bacteriostatic, but used together the action becomes bactericidal and the spectrum of action of the mixture is greater than the sum of its two components. These combinations are used for the treatment of infections of the chest and urinary tract and also for the treatment of malaria (see page 215).

Antibiotics

Antibiotics are chemical substances produced by various species of micro-organisms (fungi and bacteria) that suppress the growth of other micro-organisms and may destroy them. This 'golden age', the antibiotic era, began with the chance observations of Sir Alexander Fleming in 1928 (see page 100) of the effect of a contaminating growth of fungus on an agar plate containing a growth of *Staphylococcus aureus* (Figure 10.1). This observation was not exploited until 1941 when the drug began to be produced commercially. This was followed by a systematic search for other micro-organisms that could produce antibiotics, and it led to the appearance of a whole family of these compounds which are now in regular use. Each type of antibiotic has its own special use, depending upon its spectrum of activity, its safety, whether it can be given by mouth or has to be injected, and whether its action is bactericidal or bacteriostatic. There is little to be gained in a book of this kind by looking in detail at these characteristics of various antibiotics, and we will restrict ourselves to some general considerations of the modern use and abuse of these drugs.

Production of antibiotics

Let us first look at the techniques of antibiotic manufacture. First we have to have a sample of a fungus or bacterium that is known to produce an antibiotic. The discovery of such an organism may involve the culture of thousands of different soil samples. Figure 10.2 shows a collection of soil samples for Pfizer Laboratories obtained from all over the world for culture to detect whether or not they contain antibiotic producing moulds. Figures 10.3, 10.4 show pure cultures of two moulds, one producing penicillin and one producing tetracycline. The commercial exploitation of these moulds needs large-scale equipment for growing the moulds in broth culture and the isolation of the pure antibiotic from the broth (Figure 10.5).

The finished product, the pure antibiotic, may be issued and used as such. However, increasingly the natural antibiotic is subjected to chemical modifications to improve the properties of the drug, in making it absorbable when taken by mouth, in altering its antibacterial spectrum or in making it active against resistant strains of bacteria. Thus the original penicillin G which had to be given by injection and which had a restrictive spectrum of action, mainly against Gram-positive and Gram-negative pathogenic cocci, has now been replaced by a whole family of penicillins. Major achievements in the modification of penicillin arose when the 'nucleus' of the penicillin molecule was isolated —6-aminopenicillanic acid (Figure 10.6). Now it became possible to produce semi-synthetic penicillins by adding different chemical groups to the penicillin nucleus. Penicillins are now available that can be taken by mouth, that preferentially attack Gram-negative bacilli or that are resistant to the destructive effect of those staphylococci that can destroy penicillin by means of an enzyme called penicillinase (Figure 10.7). Below is a list of some of the penicillins available.

1. Benzylpenicillin—the original penicillin. Active mainly against many Gram-positive and Gram-negative cocci. Many Gram-negative bacilli are resistant.
2. Phenoxymethyl penicillin—similar activity to benzylpenicillin. Resistant to acid and can be taken by mouth.
3. Phenethicillin—similar to phenoxymethyl penicillin.
4. Propicillin—similar to above.

Figure 10.3 (below, left) Growth of the mould *Penicillium notatum* on a culture plate. This mould produces penicillin. (*By courtesy of the Beecham Research Laboratories.*)

Figure 10.4 (a) (below, middle) Growing in this test tube is a culture of the mould *Streptomyces riseus* used to produce the broad spectrum antibiotic terramycin. (b) (below, right) Another view of the mould *Streptomyces riseus* on a plate of culture medium. (*By courtesy of The Pfizer Group.*)

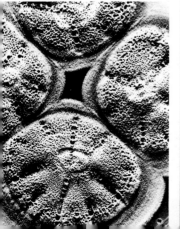
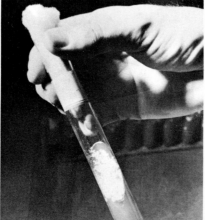
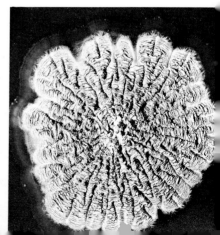

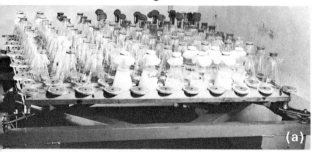

(a)

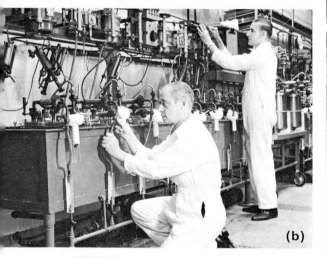

(b)

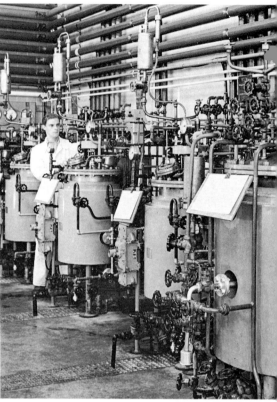

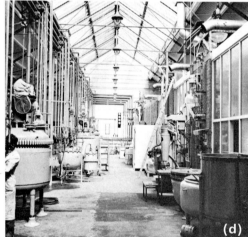

(d)

Figure 10.5 Production of penicillin.
(a) (top left) small scale production of penicillin in flasks.
(b) (left, middle) 10-litre fermenters at the Micro Pilot-Plant, Brockam Park. The fermenters in which the mould grows are housed in a long tank.
(c) (above) 100-litre and one 300-litre fermenters.
(d) (opposite) Pilot Plant, Brockam Park.
(e) (bottom left) A 30 000-litre fermenter about to be installed into the Worthing factory

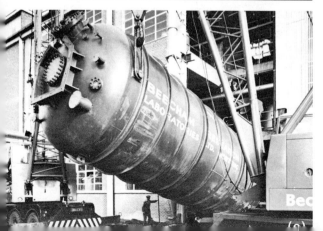

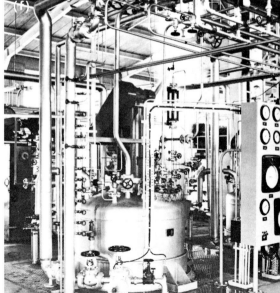

(f)

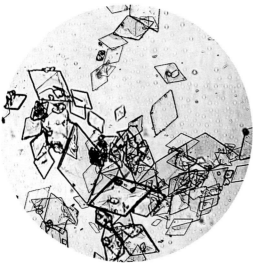

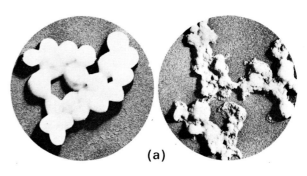

(a)

for the production of penicillin. This fermenter extends through 3 floors.
(f) (bottom right, page 102) Part of the Worthing plant showing the top of one fermenter and the control panels. (*By courtesy of the Beecham Research Laboratories.*)

Figure 10.6 (above)   Photomicrograph of crystals of 6-aminopenicillanic acid.

Figure 10.7 (*opposite*)   (a) Electron micrograph of staphylococci, normal cells $\times 10\,350$ on the left and after contact with cloxacillin sodium (10 μg/cm^3) on the right. (*By courtesy of the Beecham Research Laboratories.*)
(b) Electron micrograph of *Escherichia coli*, $\times 10\,350$ on the left and after coming into contact with ampicillin (10 μg/cm^3 for 40 min) on the right). (*By courtesy of the Beecham Research Laboratories.*)
(c) (bottom right) The disc on the left shows a culture of a staphylococcus isolated early in the days of penicillin therapy, showing its sensitivity to penicillin and other antibiotics. Zones of inhibition of bacterial growth surround each paper disc which has been impregnated with a particular antibiotic.
CB = Methicillin   TE = Tetracycline
P   = Penicillin G   S = Streptomycin
E   = Erythromycin   C = Chloramphenicol
The disc on the right shows a staphylococcus typical of those found in hospital today. It is sensitive to methicillin (and cloxacillin) but is resistant to penicillin G and the other antibiotics tested.

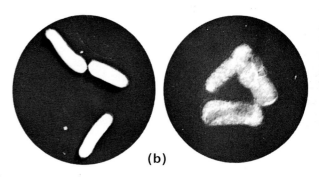

(b)

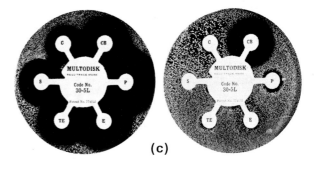

(c)

5. Methicillin—a penicillin resistant to penicillinase producing staphylococci. Given by injection.
6. Cloxacillin—an oral penicillin resistant to staphylococcal penicillinase.
7. Flucloxacillin—similar to above.
8. Ampicillin—has increased activity against Gram-negative bacilli but is inferior in action against Gram-positive cocci.
9. Purified penicillin G.
10. Carbenicillin—active particularly against certain Gram-negative bacilli. Inferior in action against Gram-positive cocci.

The mechanism of action of antibiotics which damage bacteria

Antibiotics damage bacteria by interfering with some stage of bacterial metabolism. Some antibiotics, such as penicillins or the cephalosporins, interfere with the synthesis of components of the bacterial cell wall—a vital structure for the integrity of these organisms (Figures 10.6, 10.7). Other antibiotics attack the bacterial cell at a deeper level, attacking the cell membrane (e.g. polymyxins, novobiocin), the ribosomes which form the machinery for protein synthesis (e.g. chloramphenicol, tetracyclines, streptomycin) or the metabolism of nucleic acid. Antibiotics that can be safely used in man carry out these forms of attack on bacteria without seriously influencing the metabolism of human cells. Pathogenic bacteria for the most part lie outside the body cells, in the tissue fluids, where they can be readily reached by antibiotics in the circulating blood. Moreover the metabolism of bacterial cells is sufficiently different from human cells to enable damage of the one to occur with only minimal effects to the other. Of all the antibiotics, only the penicillins can differentiate virtually completely between parasitic bacteria and host (i.e. man). Sensitive bacteria can be killed by concentrations of penicillin as low as 10^{-9} g/cm^3 whereas many tens of grammes may be injected into a mammal over a fairly short period without evidence of damage to the animal cells.

Resistance of bacteria to antibiotics

The origins of antibiotic resistance (see page 10), the dangers for man of treating food animals with antibiotics (page 11) and the significance of antibiotic resistance for the treatment of human disease (see staphylococcal infections, page 75) have already been discussed. This phenomenon of antibiotic resistance is shown dramatically in Figure 10.7. The two agar plates have been uniformly seeded with pathogenic staphylococci, A with a staphylococci isolated in the early days of penicillin treatment and B with a staphylococcus typical of those found in hospitals today. A disc has been placed in the centre of each plate and each arm of the disc has been impregnated with a different antibiotic. If the staphylococcus is destroyed by a particular antibiotic then there is a clear area of agar around the arm in which there are no bacterial colonies, see also Figure 10.8. The restricted antibiotic sensitivity of the modern hospital staphylococcus is all too evident.

The nature of antibiotic resistance is not completely understood. Certainly it varies from one organism and one antibiotic to another. Some form of penicillin resistance in staphylococci are due to the secretion of an enzyme by the organism which destroys the penicillin—a penicillinase. In the case of other resistances it seems that the micro-organisms 'find' other ways of completing the metabolic pathway which was previously interrupted by the antibiotic.

The significance of this phenomenon of drug resistance for the treatment of disease is profound. New antibiotics or new variations of old antibiotics have to be produced in an attempt to keep up the race with bacteria evolution (see also page 10). Some diseases now respond so poorly to present-day drugs, e.g. bowel infections (except typhoid), that many doctors feel it is of no value to use the drugs, and indeed that they may be a positive hazard (page 10). Certainly this problem is not helped by the indiscriminate use of antibiotics for conditions such as sore throats and colds which are caused by viruses and are not susceptible to any antibiotics. The more an antibiotic is used, the greater is the chance of the appearance of resistant strains of pathogenic bacteria, and we know that antibiotic resistance can be transferred to pathogens from the normal commensal body flora (see page 10).

It is indeed fortunate that some pathogens have shown no evidence of the appearance of strains resistant to commonly used and safe antibiotics; haemolytic streptococci and *Leptospira pallidum* (the organism responsible for syphilis) still remain sensitive to the original penicillin even after nearly thirty years of the use of this drug.

The choice of an antibiotic

The choice of an antibiotic for treating a patient

ANTIBACTERIAL SPECTRUM OF OLD AND NEW PENICILLINS

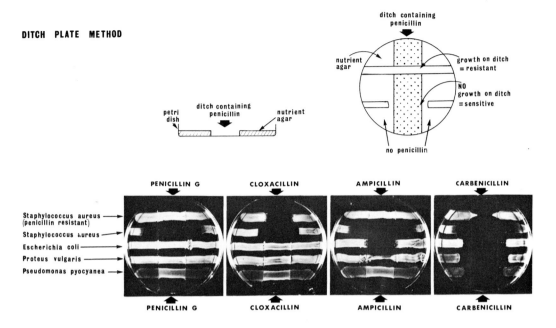

Figure 10.8 Antibacterial spectrum of old and new penicillins shown by the ditch plate method. (*By courtesy of the Beecham Research Laboratories.*)

may be quite a simple and empirical affair, particularly in general medical practice. If a patient suffers from a certain type of tonsillitis, erysipelas or scarlet fever then it is quite rational to immediately treat the patient with penicillin G, since the haemolytic streptococcus is almost invariably involved in these diseases and it is known that virtually all strains of this organism are sensitive to penicillin G. Similarly in the case of syphilis. In the case of middle-ear infections, bronchitis or urinary infections it is known that Gram-negative organisms are very likely to be involved; instead of penicillin G then ampicillin, a tetracycline or a trimethoprim-sulphonamide mixture would be a drug of first choice. In these and other infections the antibiotic is given without first culturing the pathogenic bacteria and determining their sensitivity to various antibiotics (as in Figure 10.8). For other infections it is vital to isolate the bacteria responsible, for one may have to use potentially highly toxic antibiotics, the use of which would not be justified without prior knowledge that the bacteria are sensitive to the antibiotic. Of course the patient may be so ill that it is impossible to wait the day or two needed for the results of laboratory tests on the bacteria. In this case several antibiotics may be given first to 'cover' the possible bacterial sensitivities. When the results of laboratory tests become available then appropriate changes in treatment can be made, if these are necessary.

Toxic effects of antibiotics

No drug and certainly no antibiotic is completely without unwanted side-effects in some individuals. For any one antibiotic there is a long list of possible side-effects, ranging from skin rashes, diarrhoea, deafness, to fatal reactions such as immediate death due to anaphylactic shock or a more delayed death due to suppression of the function of the bone marrow. Antibiotics differ widely in the seriousness and frequency of these side-effects, and some of them are so toxic that they are used only under close medical supervision and often only for life-endangering infections. Obviously, anyone prescribing an antibiotic has to be aware of the possible side-effects and take all possible steps to minimize the risk of their occurrence, and be capable of treating them should they occur.

Antibiotics that act on fungi

Antibiotics that are used in the treatment of bacterial infections have, in general, no action on fungi. Indeed fungal infections, usually by yeasts, are a recognized complication of treatment with 'broad-spectrum' antibiotics. It is believed that fungal infections arise in these cases because 'broad-spectrum' antibiotics suppress the growth of the normal commensal bacterial flora and thus allow other micro-organisms to find a 'niche'. There are, nevertheless, other antibiotics of quite a different chemical character which have a powerful action on pathogenic fungi, with little or no action on bacteria. Some of these, however, are so toxic that they must only be used in life-endangering infections. For ringworm of the skin, hair and nails (see page 95) there is a safe antibiotic called griseofulvin. For infections with yeast organisms an antibiotic called nystatin is used, although this drug is not absorbed from the intestine and can only be used locally on skin or on mucous membranes. When we come to widespread fungal infections of internal organs—systemic mycoses—the antibiotic which is available, amphotericin B, is a highly toxic drug that is given only under close medical supervision and then only for serious infections.

The treatment of virus infections

Introduction

The treatment of virus infections has always lagged behind that of bacterial infections. The reason for this state of affairs lies in the unique features of virus infections in which viruses live and multiply within living cells and have to use the chemical machinery of the cell for their own purposes. The virus and host cell become so intimately interwoven that it is obviously a difficult task to attack the virus without at the same time damaging or killing the host cell, indeed all uninfected cells of the body (see Chapter 3). Furthermore, the features of particular virus infection often appear only after considerable multiplication and spread of virus particles in the body has already occurred. For these reasons there are only a few drugs that are available for the prevention or treatment of specific virus infections. However, if present trends continue there is likely to be an increasing number of available anti-viral agents. At the moment the most effective method of control of virus infections is by means of vaccines.

Figure 10.9 shows the phases of viral multi-plication in the body and indicates the points at which anti-viral agents are thought to act.

Gamma globulin

The success of some viral vaccines in the prevention of certain virus infections means that they probably stimulate the production of a fairly potent antibody and/or cellular immunity and it would seem logical to use gamma globulins extracted from human blood in the prevention or treatment of virus infections. Antibody acts by combining with the virus and so preventing penetration of the virus into the cell. This means that once virus particles have penetrated the cell, antibodies no longer have an opportunity to attack them until new virions are released from the infected cells; this latter action can prevent the infection of new cells.

Human immunoglobulin can be used in various ways in the control of virus infections. Two forms of human immunoglobulin are available. One, normal gamma globulin, is a preparation containing almost all of the gamma globulins of normal human plasma, together with smaller amounts of other proteins of the blood. The antibodies are concentrated between ten and twenty times more than those that are present in the plasma of normal human adults. A second variety of human gamma globulin is known as hyper-immune immunoglobulin and is produced from the blood of patients who are convalescing from a particular infection. Human gamma globulin has been used without a great deal of success for some years to try to protect pregnant women who have been in contact with a case of German measles (see page 77). A more successful use has been the protection of individuals against infectious hepatitis, e.g. in contacts of the disease in nurseries and mental institutions, or for people travelling to places outside Europe or North America where the chances of exposure to the disease is high. Human immunoglobulin is, however, a scarce and expensive commodity and has limited uses. Its use is mainly in the prevention rather than the treatment of established infections.

Interferon

This substance, discovered in 1957, is a low molecular weight protein produced in living cells when they are infected by viruses. The action of this natural anti-viral compound is to limit the ability of the virus to multiply and spread to infect new cells. Its action appears to be at the level of the ribosomes in the cell where the

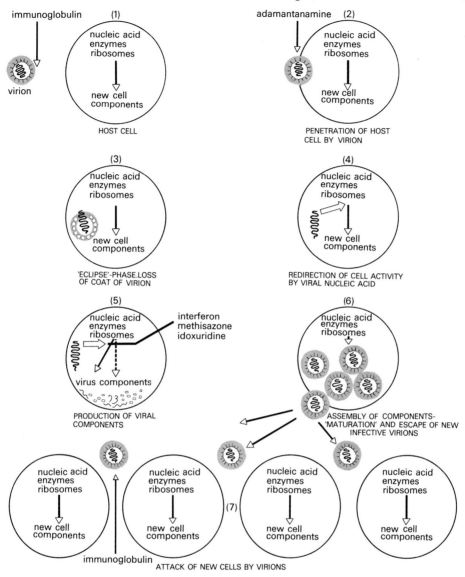

Figure 10.9 The stages of virus multiplication in body cells and the points at which anti-viral agents are thought to act.

production of new viral nucleic acid is inhibited. The discovery of interferon raised great hopes for the treatment of virus infections, for the material is active against essentially all viruses. Unfortunately it is only active in the species in which it is produced, i.e. in man only human interferon is effective. This material, which is prepared from cells in culture in the laboratory, is extremely costly to produce and its action after injection is very brief. Because of these problems, increasing attention is being paid to the action of certain substances which can be injected into the body to stimulate the production of more interferon by a patient suffering from a virus infection. These substances which stimulate interferon production are not necessarily viruses and include some bacteria and fungal extracts.

Synthetic chemicals

In spite of extensive research there are at present only three substances or classes of substances which have any clinical use. These are thiosemicarbazone for the prevention of smallpox, adamantanamane for the prevention of influenza, and metabolic inhibitors such as idoxuridine for the treatment of superficial infections caused by the herpes simplex virus. Thiosemicarbazone and adamantanamane are of use only in the *prevention* of smallpox and influenza and they have little place in the treatment of established infections. Apart from the established viral vaccines, these then are the limited weapons available for the prevention or treatment of virus infections (see Table 7).

Isolation and quarantine in infectious disease

There are various measures that must be considered in any infectious disease with the aim of protecting susceptible individuals in the same family or indeed in the general community. These measures include isolation of the infected patient (and sometimes the contacts of the patient) and other procedures such as notification of the disease to the Medical Officer of Health and disinfection of the room or home of the infected person. The urgency and stringency with which these measures will be applied depend on the seriousness of the disease and upon the risk of spread to the community. It is impossible to deal with every infection in detail, and indeed there are often no hard and fast rules. Each case should be considered in the light of the risks of spread of the infection; thus the quarantine of nurses or of infants returning to a nursery or of someone returning to the food industry may be more strictly applied than in the case of an adult returning to work with other adults in the general population.

Let us now consider these terms quarantine and isolation. Quarantine describes the limitations imposed on the free movement of contacts of a case of infectious disease; to be fully effective the period of quarantine must be the longest incubation period of the particular disease to which they have been exposed. The aim of quarantine is to reduce the risks of a person infecting other individuals during the period when he is incubating a disease, i.e. before the typical features of the disease have appeared. Isolation describes the separation of the infected patient or the carrier of a disease. A more limited practice is now replacing isolation and quarantine for many diseases; this is called surveillance and describes the practice of keeping contacts of a disease under observation during the incubation period of the disease, without imposing restrictions upon their movement.

Table 8 gives general guidance for the isolation and quarantine of individuals in the case of various infectious diseases and the place of immunization of contacts. Table 9 is reproduced by kind permission of Dr A. B. Stewart, Medical Advisor to the Inner London Education Authority, and provides the instructions for this authority for the exclusion of children from day schools on account of infectious disease. The control of any disease depends upon our understanding of the natural history of the disease, which includes methods of transmission, the degree of infectiveness of cases of the disease, the duration of the incubation period, the persistence of the infecting agent in the environment, and so on. In recent years our increased understanding of the natural history of infective diseases has changed our attitudes about the value of isolation and quarantine for particular diseases. Anyone following Tables 8 and 9 should refer to more detailed accounts of

Table 7 Vaccines and drugs in the control of virus infections

Vaccines	*Drugs*
Smallpox	Immunoglobulin
Rabies	Interferon – still experimental
Yellow fever	Amantadine – prevention of influenza—still experimental
Western equine encephalitis	
Eastern equine encephalitis	Methisazone, prevention of smallpox
Venezuelan equine encephalitis	Idoxuridine – treatment of *Herpes simplex*
Influenza A and B	
Poliomyelitis	
Measles	
Mumps	
German measles	

Table 8 Isolation, quarantine, immunization, and disinfection in various infectious diseases

Disease	Isolation of infected case	Quarantine of contacts	Immunization of contacts	Disinfection of home if death should occur	Additional notes
Brucellosis	0	0	0	0	
Chicken pox	Until scabs have shed (about 21 days)	Advice varies from 0–21 days see notes	0	0	Patients are highly infective early in the disease even when without symptoms. Quarantine thus has little value in preventing spread in schools
Diphtheria	Until virulent bacteria have disappeared from the patient. Isolation in hospital	7 days	Passive and/or active	Bed and furniture	
Dysentery bacillary	Until faeces free of the pathogenic bacteria. Usually a few days	7 days See notes	0	0	Quanrantine period varies depending upon whether the disease occurs in the home, hospitals or schools
Erysipelas	0	0	0	0	
Gonorrhoea	1–2 weeks	0	0	Bed and furniture	
Impetigo	Until skin healed	0	0	Bed and furniture	
Influenza	Until end of symptoms	0	0	Bed and furniture	
Infective hepatitis	Until end of symptoms	0	P in hospitals	0	
Measles	Until end of symptoms	0	P for infants at special risk	Bed and furniture	
Mumps	Until end of symptoms	0–28 days	0	0	Mumps is only moderately infectious and fairly close contact is needed. Hence wide range of advice for quarantine of contacts See notes for school children
Ringworm	0	0	0	0	
Poliomyelitis	21 days	0–21 days	0	0	
Rubella	7 days	0–21 days	P. see notes	0	Note the need for passive immunization for women contacts who are pregnant
Scarlet fever and other streptococcal infections of the upper respiratory tract	Until the streptococci have disappeared from the nose and throat	0	0	0	In epidemics penicillin may be given to *contacts* to prevent infection
Smallpox	Transfer to special hospital	16 days	Active	Disinfection of room	
Tetanus	0	0	0	0	
Tuberculosis	Varies	Surveillance	0 or Active (B.C.G.)	0	
Typhoid fever	21 days	Until no *Salmonella typhi* in faeces	0	Bed and furniture	
Whooping cough	Varies depending on whether the infection occurs in hospital or in a home with a young infant	0	0	0	

Table 9 Inner London Education Authority School Health Service
Instructions with regard to the exclusion of children from day schools on account of infectious diseases

Disease (1)	Period of exclusion of child suffering from the disease (2)	Action necessary when child has been in contact with the disease at home or otherwise outside the school (3)	Action necessary for other children in the school (4)
Chicken pox	Exclude for 14 days from the date of appearance of the rash	No exclusion	No action
Diphtheria	Exclude for one week after discharge from hospital and until principal school medical officer permits return	Exclude until principal school medical officer agrees that child may return to school	*N.B.* If smallpox is prevalent in the district special arrangements will be advised by principal school medical officers Nose and throat swabs of other members of the class and immunization as advised by principal school medical officer
Dysentery	Exclude for period to be decided by principal school medical officer	May attend school unless instructions to the contrary are received from principal school medical officer	No action
Enteritis and gastro-enteritis	Exclude until recovery or discharge from hospital	May attend school unless instructions to the contrary are received from principal school medical officer	No action
Erysipelas	Exclude until recovery or discharge from hospital	No exclusion	No action
Impetigo or purulent eczema	Exclude at discretion of the principal school medical officer	No exclusion	No action
Influenza	Exclude sufferers until recovery	No exclusion	No action
Infectious sore throat	As for scarlet fever	No exclusion	No action
Infective hepatitis	Exclude until recovery	No exclusion	No action
Measles	Exclude for 10 days after the appearance of rash and then admit if child appears well	No exclusion	No action
Meningitis	Exclude until recovery or discharge from hospital	May attend school unless instructions to the contrary are received from principal school medical officer	No action
Mumps	Exclude until 7 days from the subsidence of all swelling	No exclusion	No action
Ophthalmia or purulent conjunctivitis	Exclude until cured	No exclusion	No action
Poliomyelitis Polioencephalitis (Infantile paralysis)	Exclude until recovery or discharge from hospital	Exclude for 21 days	No action
Ringworm of body	No exclusion, but lesion should be treated and covered	Do not exclude. Examine at once	Examination of other members of the class and other close contacts
Ringworm of the feet	No exclusion. Child not to attend baths or gymnasium classes	No exclusion	No action
Ringworm of scalp	Exclude until cured	Do not exclude. Examine at once	Examination of other members of the class and other close contacts
Rubella (German measles)	Exclude for 7 days from appearance of the rash	No exclusion	No action
Scabies	Exclude until child is treated	Exclude until pronounced free from infestation	No action

Disease	Exclusion of patient	Exclusion of contacts	Action
Scarlet fever and other streptococcal infections of upper respiratory tract	Exclude until pronounced by a medical practitioner to be free from infection	No exclusion	Routine examination as advised by principal school medical officer
Smallpox	Exclude for 17 days	Exclude for 17 days	Review vaccination state of each child and where unsatisfactory principal school medical officer to decide as to action
Tuberculosis	Exclude at discretion of principal school medical officer	No exclusion	Investigations to be carried out as arranged by the principal school medical officer when a case occurs in children or staff
Typhoid, Paratyphoid (or Enteric fever)	Exclude until recovery or discharge from hospital	May attend school unless instructions to the contrary are received from principal school medical officer	No action
Whooping cough	Exclude for 10 days after which the child may be re-admitted providing attacks of coughing have ceased	Exclude children under 7 years who have not had the disease for 21 days from the date of contact with the disease	No action

Where the regulations require exclusion, the instructions in column 3 should be applied as follows in respect of flats and tenement houses :—

(a) In the case of blocks of flats, only children from the same flat (or self-contained tenement) as that in which the case of infection occurs need be excluded.

(b) In the case of an ordinary dwelling-house sub-let, children from the whole house should be excluded, except in cases where the tenements are absolutely self-contained and each family has its own domestic and sanitary conveniences, in which case rule (a) will apply.

Note. The London borough councils are empowered, with the sanction of the Minister of Health, to make any infectious disease compulsorily notifiable as regards their respective areas. Head teachers are required to report, on S.H.S. 366 to the Principal School Medical Officer, who is also the Borough Medical Officer of Health, all cases of infectious diseases whether notifiable or non-notifiable, all cases of suspected infectious illness, and all children absent from school on account of infection in the home.

Table 10 Notifiable diseases in Great Britain

Anthrax	Food poisoning	Ophthalmia neonatorum	Trachoma
Cerebro-spinal fever	Gastro-enteritis, up to 2 years only	Pemphigus neonatorum	Tuberculosis
Cholera	Glandular fever	Plague	Typhus
Continued fever	Hepatitis	Poliomyelitis	Undulant fever
Diphtheria	Leptospiral jaundice	Psittacosis	Vincent's angina
Dysentery	Leprosy	Relapsing fever	Whooping cough
Encephalitis	Malaria	Scarlatina and scarlet fever	Yellow fever
Enteric fever (typhoid fever)	Measles	Smallpox	

Note. There are slight differences in the notification requirements from region to region of Great Britain.

particular infectious diseases in various sections of the book.

Public Health Regulations

In addition to the various measures of isolation, quarantine, surveillance or immunization of contacts which may be recommended by family or hospital doctors, there are various Public Health Laws that are aimed at preventing the spread of infectious disease in a community. One of these measures is the compulsory notification of certain infections, notification being made by the person in charge of the patient or any medical practitioner called upon to visit the patient. The list of notifiable diseases in England, Wales, Scotland and Northern Ireland is given in Table 10. From time to time other diseases may be made notifiable in a certain area.

There are other Public Health Laws which prevent the sale or loan of articles liable to carry infection, the control and disinfection of houses, the removal of certain infected persons to hospital and the control of infected food handlers etc.

International Health Regulations

New international health regulations were adopted by the World Health Assembly in May 1970 and these are now in force. The need for revision of the regulations resulted from an increased understanding of the epidemiology of infectious diseases and the rapid changes in the patterns of world travel and trade. The increased use of containers and other kinds of unit loads has altered the handling of these cargoes such that infected cargoes or vectors of disease (rats, arthropods etc.) may be overlooked. The speed and volume of international air travel has increased enormously (from 7 million in 1951 to 50 million in 1966) and this is paralleled by an increased risk of the spread of infectious diseases.

The new regulations have reduced the reliance on international declarations of health and medical inspections of ships and aircrafts and their passengers, and have increased the emphasis on the international surveillance of disease. All members of the World Health Organization (131 members with additional associate member states) must immediately report the presence of any serious infectious disease within their borders so that the information can be made available to countries all over the world. Provided with this information, countries can now act with intelligent foresight and take measures to prevent the importation of the disease. It is unfortunate that some countries take such stringent measures that they discourage other countries from reporting cases of infectious disease, as happened in 1970 when cholera spread from its ancient nest in the East to involve Russia, the middle-East and Africa.

The International Certificate of Vaccination has been slightly modified; the certificate now requires that the doctor who performed the vaccination must sign the form and his official stamp is not accepted as a substitute. There were six quarantinable diseases under the old regulations—plague, cholera, smallpox, yellow fever, louse-borne typhus and relapsing fever; these have now been reduced to four since typhus and relapsing fever are no longer regarded as a serious threat to international health. In view of the increasing volume and speed of air travel other diseases such as typhoid fever, influenza, poliomyelitis and malaria now form part of the international surveillance of the World Health Organization.

11. Useful micro-organisms

Introduction

AFTER perusing much of this book one could be forgiven for gaining the impression that mankind must wage a ceaseless war against *all* microbes on this planet. Fortunately nothing could be further from the truth. It would be rather an unequal struggle, for the total mass of microbes on earth is enormous; it has been estimated at over twenty times the total mass of *all* animal life, both on land and in water. Only the minutest fraction of this mass of microbes can invade human tissues and cause disease. The bulk of microbes are of enormous economic importance for all living things on earth, and without them the higher organisms, including man, would rapidly die out.

Microbes, then, can be—and indeed usually are—useful organisms and play an irreplaceable role in the balance of life on this planet. Before we look at the ways in which man has learned to exploit the activities of microbes to his own advantage, we will take a brief look at some of the vital activities of microbes which have contributed to the economy of life from time immemorial, long before man himself existed.

The nitrogen cycle

The most important activity of microbes is the part they play in the general 'turnover' of some vital elements which are incorporated into the stuff of all living matter, be it animal or plant. Consider the element nitrogen. All living things contain nitrogen as a component of protein. Of course, proteins are large complex molecules containing many other elements, but about 10 per cent of every molecule of protein is composed of nitrogen. How do living things obtain this element for the manufacture of protein? Of course, air contains large amounts of nitrogen—the element forms four-fifths of the atmosphere. Most living things cannot use this inert gas as a source of nitrogen for the manufacture of protein. Nitrogen, in fact, tends to be passed on from one kind of living thing to another in the form of chemical compounds containing nitrogen. When animals and plants die, they decompose and the nitrogen they contain becomes available for other living things. The decomposition of dead plants and animals is mainly the result of the actions of microbes. This paramount useful activity of microbes can be highlighted by considering what might be the state of the earth if the carcasses from billions of years of life still littered its surface; instead, the putrefying microbes *do* destroy the remains of dead animals and plants, and they gradually return the components of dead tissues to the soil. The nitrogen of proteins in the dead tissues is released in the soil in the form of the compound ammonia (NH_3). Although plants can use ammonia as a source of the nitrogen which they need for the synthesis of their proteins, in fact they prefer the nitrogen in the form of nitrates, and there is a group of soil bacteria which can convert ammonia into nitrate by way of nitrite.

Thus plants use nitrogen in the form of ammonia and nitrate—which have been derived from the putrefied frames of dead organisms—for the synthesis of their own proteins. The nitrogen of plant proteins is then passed on to other organisms, namely herbivorous animals which eat the plants. When these herbivorous animals are eaten by carnivores the nitrogen that we have traced from dead carcasses through ammonia, nitrates, plant protein and herbivore protein ultimately appears in the flesh of the carnivore. All living organisms ultimately die and so the nitrogen is again returned to the soil.

This cycle of soil → plants → animals → soil is complicated by other living processes which affect the distribution of nitrogen. A group of soil bacteria use nitrate instead of oxygen to oxidize organic foodstuffs and so obtain their energy needs. The oxygen present in the nitrate is removed by the activities of the bacteria, leaving nitrogen which eventually returns to the atmosphere as a gas. The amount of 'fixed' nitrogen which is present in a soil, i.e. as ammonia or nitrate, is a critical factor in determining the productivity of the soil, i.e. the amount of plant life that the soil can support. This, of course, also limits the number of animals that can live off the plants. Anything which encourages the supply of fixed nitrogen to a soil increases its productivity. We have seen that the putrefying organisms break down dead organisms and liberate their contained nitrogen as ammonia, and that other soil organisms convert this ammonia into nitrate which can be used by plants for the synthesis of their proteins. However, the activity of these 'useful' bacteria, which encourage the turnover of nitrogen on earth, is opposed by the activity of the de-nitrifying bacteria which use nitrate as we use oxygen. If their activity were unopposed the nitrate content of soils, and hence their productivity, would progressively decline. Fortunately their activity is opposed by yet another group of soil organisms called the nitrogen-fixing micro-organisms. These convert free atmospheric nitrogen into nitrate, some of which they use to manufacture their own protein and some of which is available to other organisms. Some of the nitrogen-fixing organisms are free living in the soil, e.g. some blue-green algae. These blue-green algae are very important in determining the productivity of the soil in the Antarctic, and in the water-logged rice fields of the East they provide the main source of nitrogen for the rice crop. But the most important nitrogen fixers for the economy of the soil are not free living. Instead they live inside the roots of plants. The plant responds to the presence of the bacteria inside its roots by the formation of nodules (Figure 11.1), and inside these structures the

Figure 11.1   Root nodules of clover.
(*Photograph by Brian Bracegirdle, B.Sc., M.I.Biol., F.R.P.S.*)

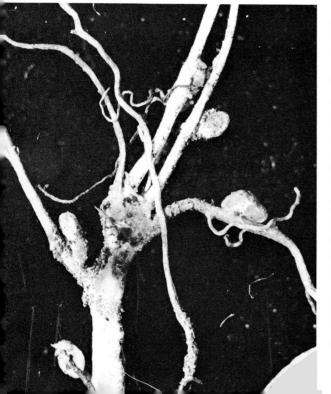

combination of activities of plant and bacteria fixes atmospheric nitrogen. The plant supplies the bacteria with sources of energy—carbo-hydrates—and the microbe uses this energy to fix free nitrogen which can then be used for the synthesis of both bacterial and plant protein. The best known examples of these plant-bacteria combinations are the leguminous plants (plants with seeds in pods) such as clover and lucerne, but there are in fact nearly two hundred different plants which can fix free nitrogen with the aid of microbes. Many of these microbes are in fact bacteria, but yet others are fungal in nature or are algae. We can now summarize the transformations of nitrogen diagrammatically (Figure 11.2).

Microbes in the gut of mammals

We will now turn to microbes which play a useful role on a smaller scale, that is inside the bodies of living animals. We have already seen that our skin, hair, mouth, teeth and alimentary tract are populated by enormous numbers of microbes. On the whole these neither damage the host nor do they contribute anything to it—animal and microbes live together in a state of mutual tolerance. But some of these microbes do make an invaluable contribution to the life of their host. The natural diet of herbivorous animals consists of grasses or other vegetation which contain large amounts of the plant carbohydrate which we call cellulose. We know of no mammal which can produce an enzyme (a cellulase) which is capable of breaking down the large molecules of cellulose into a form which can be absorbed by the animal. Instead, the animal has to rely upon microbes in the bowel to perform this task of the break-down of cellulose. Under the warm, moist conditions inside the bowel with a plentiful supply of fermentable material, the microbes grow and multiply rapidly. The animal obtains its energy sources from the products of bacterial fermentation and by the digestion of bacterial protoplasm. The position of these useful microbes in the bowel varies from one kind of animal to another. In the rabbit, for example, the microbes are located in the large caecum (Figure 11.3), but in ruminants such as the cow they occur inside the specialized stomach of these animals.

In non-ruminant animals such as the horse and the rabbit, the microbes in the caecum ferment the cellulose in the diet. Most of the products of this fermentation are presumably absorbed through the wall of the caecum. In the

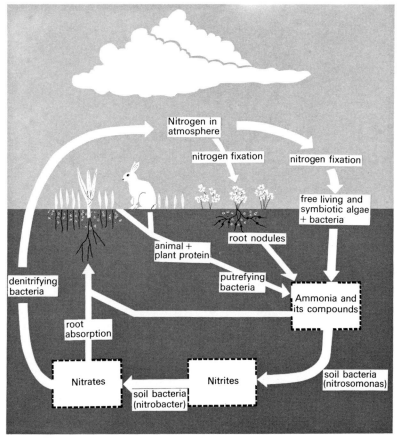

Figure 11.2 The nitrogen cycle.

rabbit, however, there is a specialized habit, called refection, which permits the material in the caecum to be exposed to the action of the small bowel so that the bacterial products can be more fully utilized. During the night the rabbit produces faeces which are large and creamy white. The animal sleeps with the mouth close to the anus and these night faeces are swallowed. The faecal pellets which are produced in the day are dark brown in colour and are of a firmer consistency; the material in these faeces has been twice through the alimentary canal.

In ruminants such as the cow the bacteria are housed in a specialized stomach. After the initial chewing of the food it is passed into the first part of the stomach, called the rumen, which is a large bag where juices are added and where bacterial fermentation of the food begins. Here the cellulose, and also starch, are fermented to yield short chain fatty acids—acetic, propionic and butyric—methane gas and carbon dioxide. The fluid in the rumen contains vast numbers of organisms—up to 10^{10} microbes/cm³. Gas

production is vast—hundreds of litres a day! In the presence of this methane and carbon dioxide the fermentation process is completely anaerobic. In addition to the products of fermentation, the cow obtains extra sources of energy from the bacteria themselves; any bacteria which pass from the rumen into the true stomach are killed by the acid secretions and their protoplasm is digested. This provides a good source of protein for the cow, particularly since the bacteria can manufacture protein using nitrogen from various sources.

The bowel of man also contains vast numbers of microbes—a rod called *Escherichia coli*, gas-producing bacteria of the clostridium group, methane-forming organisms, yeasts, non-pathogenic protozoa etc. Unlike the ruminant, man does not rely on these organisms to digest his foodstuffs; he relies on sources of energy other than cellulose. The organisms in the bowel do ferment any vegetable matter, producing gas in the process. During the course of their fermentation these microbes produce several substances which are very important for nutrition.

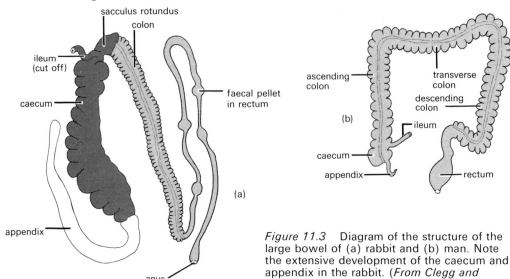

Figure 11.3 Diagram of the structure of the large bowel of (a) rabbit and (b) man. Note the extensive development of the caecum and appendix in the rabbit. (*From Clegg and Clegg, Biology of the Mammal.*)

In particular they produce vitamins such as the B vitamins (including vitamin B_{12}) and vitamin K. These vitamins supplement the vitamins which are taken in the diet. The importance of the microbial source of vitamins is sometimes seen when patients are treated for long periods with wide-spectrum antibiotics. These antibiotics destroy many of the normal bacteria in the bowel and the production of vitamins is reduced. Symptoms of deficiency of vitamin B and K may now appear, particularly if intake of vitamins in the diet is reduced by loss of appetite or vomiting. Moreover the normal micro-flora of the bowel may become disturbed by the overgrowth of organisms which are resistant to the effect of the antibiotic. There may be an overgrowth of yeasts in many parts of the bowel from mouth to anus, resulting in local inflammation and irritation.

Microbes in the production of beer (Table 11)

We can now turn to ways in which man has learned to utilize the activities of micro-organisms to his own advantage. The oldest example is the production of alcoholic beverages; some kind of beer was made about 6000 years ago by the ancient Egyptians. The main ingredients of beer are barley and water. The raw material for the production of alcohol is present in the form of grains of starch in the barley. In this form it cannot be used by the microbes—yeasts—which produce alcohol as a by-product of their energy-releasing processes; the starch has first to be converted into a sugar.

The first stage in the production of beer is the treatment of the barley grains so that their energy stores are changed into a form that can be used by yeasts. First the barley grains are steeped in water for a day or two. Then the barley is allowed to sprout (germinate) by leaving it in a warm moist place for a few days. During the process of sprouting, intense activity is occurring inside the grains of barley. The sprouting grains

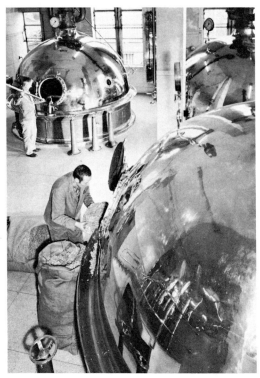

Figure 11.4 Copper wort boilers.

Table 11 The commercial exploitation of micro-organisms

Product	Micro-organism	Use of product
Beer	Yeasts	
Wine	Yeasts	
Cider	Yeasts	
Vinegar	Bacteria—*Acetobacter*	
Cheese	Fungi e.g. *Penicillium camemberti* and *Penicillium roqueforti*	Drinks, foods and flavouring
Soya sauce	Fungus—Aspergillus species	
Tempeh	Fungus—Rhizopus species	
Miso	Fungus—Aspergillus species	
Yeast	Saccharomyces species	
Penicillin	Fungus—Penicillium species	
Cephalosporins	Fungus—Cephalosporium species	
Griseofulvin	Fungus—*Penicillium griseofulvam*	Antibiotics used in the treatment of various infections
Streptomycin	Fungus—*Streptomyces griseus*	
Polymyxin	Bacterium—*Bacillus polymyxa*	
Bacitracin	Bacterium — *Bacillus subtilis*	
Colistin	Bacterium — *Bacillus colistinus*	
Tyrothricin	Bacterium—*Bacillus brevis*	
Citric acid	Fungus—*Aspergillus niger*	Soft drinks
Dextrans	Bacterium — *Leuconostoc mesenteroides*	Replacements for blood or plasma
Riboflavin	Yeast — *Ashbya gossypii*	Medicine
Vitamin B$_{12}$	Bacterium—*Bacillus megaterium*	Medicine
Giberellin	Fungus — *Giberella fujikuroi*	Stimulation of plant growth
Vitamin C	Bacterium—*Acetobacter suboxydans*	Medicine
Cellulase	Various fungi	
Pectinase	Fungus—*Aspergillus niger*	
Protease	Fungus—*Aspergillus niger* Bacterium—*Bacillus subtilis*	Enzymes used in various industries e.g. laundries, hide-production, food industries.
Invertase	Yeasts	See text
Amylase	Fungus—*Aspergillus niger* Bacterium—*Bacillus subtilis*	

produce enzymes—those catalysts of chemical reactions in living organisms—which convert the starch in the grains into soluble sugars which can be extracted from the barley. The sprouted barley is now killed by drying it in warm air. During this process not all of the enzymes of the sprouted barley are destroyed, and their action continues into the next phase of beer production when the barley is soaked in water to extract soluble materials—sugars, amino acids and minerals—which are needed for the activity of the yeasts. The dried sprouted barley is now ground and added to large vessels called mash tuns where hot water is added. The resulting extract, called 'malt wort' is eventually boiled (Figure 11.4). This boiling halts further enzymic activity, and most important it sterilizes the wort, i.e. it kills unwanted microbes which

might multiply and 'spoil' the beer. During the boiling, hops are added to impart the bitter flavour of the finished product. Hops also contain substances which help to prevent bacteria from multiplying during the stage of fermentation.

The next stage is that of fermentation (Figure 11.5). The boiled wort is first cooled and then bubbled with air to encourage the multiplication of yeasts. Yeasts are now introduced into the wort, where they multiply using the nutrients derived from the barley. Although the initial growth and multiplication of the yeasts is aerobic, conditions gradually become anaerobic as the yeasts utilize the oxygen which was introduced into the wort by bubbling it with air. Under these anaerobic conditions the yeasts are unable to break down the sugar of the wort

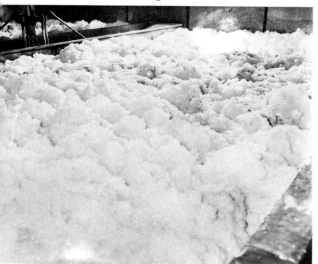

Figure 11.5 Beer wort fermentation. The frothy head is composed mainly of yeasts. *(By courtesy of Dr J. G. Carr.)*

completely, and alcohol and carbon dioxide accumulate as by-products of incomplete oxidation of sugar. The fermented liquor is now beer, which is stored for a time to allow the yeasts to settle. Various refinements are now used depending upon the kind of beer that is to be produced. Hop oil may be added for flavour, colour may be added and carbon dioxide may be added to give 'fiz'. Beer which is to be stored in bottles or cans has to be sterilized to remove microorganisms which would 'spoil' the product. The modern way to sterilize beer is by the method of 'flash' pasteurization; the beer is heated to a temperature of 68 °C for a few seconds and then it is cooled. It can now be stored for long periods.

The production of wine

Wine is the fermented juice of grapes. All the ingredients which are necessary for wine production are in the grape. On the skin of the grape are 'wild' yeasts which will carry out the fermentation; thus yeasts do not have to be added as they do in the production of beer. Inside the grape are the raw materials—sugars, organic acids, amino acids, vitamins, minerals and water— which will nourish the yeasts and allow them to produce alcohol. These materials are extracted by crushing the grapes; traditionally this was done by bare feet, but it is nowadays carried out out by mechanical means, and the juice is allowed to ferment in large vats. The growth of undesirable bacteria in the fermenting juice can be prevented by 'sulphuring' the grape juice, that is by the addition of sulphur dioxide, which

is more toxic to bacteria than it is to yeasts. The colour of the wine, white, red or rose, depends on whether or not coloured skins of the grape are added to the fermenting juice. White wine is made from grape juice which has been separated from skin and pips at an early stage in the process. Red wines are fermented in the presence of skins and pips which provide pigments which colour the wine. Rose wines are more like white wines, and are made either from pink grapes or by removing the skin and pips from red grapes from the fermenting juice after only a small amount of pigment has been extracted.

After fermentation, the wine is stored in vats where the wine 'matures' and sediment settles out. After one or two years in vats, from which sediment is periodically run off, the wine is filtered and bottled. Various substances may be added before the wine is bottled. Wines may be now blended together to improve their flavour. Some wines, called fortified wines, have sugar and alcohol added to them. Fortified wines include port, sherry and madeira.

Cider making

Cider is fermented apple juice. The production of cider is very similar to that of wine. Apples are first ground to a pulp and then the juice is extracted in large presses, leaving behind the skin, cell walls, pips etc. Like grape juice, apple juice contains sugars, organic acids, amino acids, vitamins and minerals, which form the nutrient medium for yeast growth and fermentation (Figure 11.6).

The apple juice is fermented in large vessels. The yeasts which carry out the fermentation come in part from the fruit itself, that is wild yeasts on the skin. Other yeasts come from the presses which are used to extract the apple juice. Improvements in hygiene in cider factories has so reduced the numbers of yeasts which contaminate the apple juice from pulpers and presses that it is often necessary to add a suitable yeast to the apple juice. In England the cider is fermented until all the sugars of the apple juice have been used up by the yeasts. This is done to prevent spoilage of the cider by a particular group of bacteria which tend to grow in sweet cider and produce a disease called 'cider sickness'. Sugar is added to the dry cider, if necessary, before it is bottled. If the cider is to be canned or bottled for prolonged storage, it is first filtered or treated by 'flash' pasteurization to destroy spoiling organisms. The cider is also usually 'carbonated' by chilling it and injecting carbon dioxide. As an extra precaution to prevent

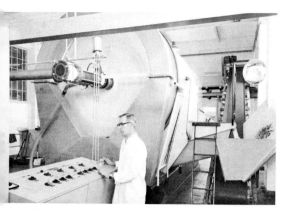

Figure 11.6 Expressing apple juice from the pulp by hydraulic pressure. (*By courtesy of Dr J. G. Carr.*)

the growth of spoiling organisms some sulphur dioxide is also added to the cider.

Vinegar making

Wines and beer are sometimes invaded by a group of organisms—the acetobacters—which oxidize ethyl alcohol to produce acetic acid. This contamination of wine produces unwanted acidity and souring of the wine. This kind of contamination is not acceptable to wine or beer drinkers, but we can deliberately encourage this change if we want to produce vinegar. French wine vinegar is produced by a simple process— the Orleans process (Figure 11.7). In this process a cask is partly filled with wine. In the presence of air in the cask, acetobacters oxidize the alcohol of the wine to acetic acid. When the

wine has been converted into vinegar it is run off from the bottom of the cask and new wine is added. In Britain vinegar is usually made from beer. The process—the so-called quick process —is shown in Figure 11.8. The alcohol of beer is converted into acetic acid in a large wooden vat packed with beechwood shavings or the like, on the surface of which the acetobacters grow. The beer is introduced into the vat through a revolving hose which distributes the beer over the surface of the shavings. As the beer trickles down over the surface of the shavings, the bacteria convert its alcohol into acetic acid. The liquid that accumulates at the base is pumped back to the top of the vat; the beer is thus in continuous circulation until all of the alcohol has been converted into acetic acid. The conversion of alcohol to acetic acid results in the liberation of heat (i.e. the reaction is an exothermic one) and the vat is cooled by ventilation with air from below.

Production of chemicals and drugs

Micro-organisms—bacteria, yeasts and fungi— are now utilized in many industrial processes to manufacture chemicals which either cannot be produced synthetically or can be produced in this way only at great expense (see Table 11).

Antibiotics (see also page 101)

The first antibiotic to be discovered was penicillin. This was discovered as long ago as 1928 by Sir Alexander Fleming. Whilst he was

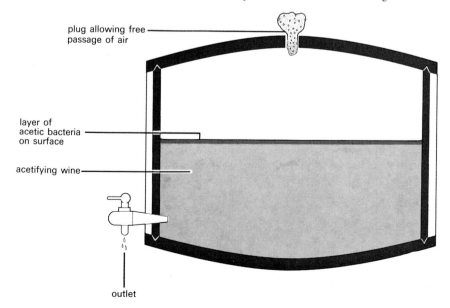

plug allowing free passage of air

layer of acetic bacteria on surface

acetifying wine

outlet

Figure 11.7 Orleans vinegar process. (*By courtesy of Dr J. G. Carr.*)

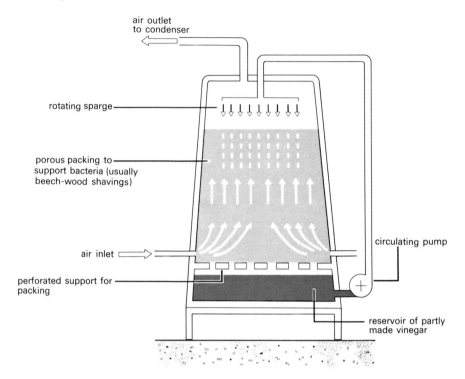

air outlet
to condenser

rotating sparge

porous packing to
support bacteria (usually
beech-wood shavings)

circulating pump

air inlet

perforated support for
packing

reservoir of partly
made vinegar

Figure 11.8 A quick vinegar generator. (*By courtesy of Dr J. G. Carr.*)

working at St Mary's Hospital, London, on the problem of staphylococci, he noticed that on an agar plate on which staphylococci were growing, the chance growth of a blue fungus had produced dramatic changes in the colonies of staphylococci which surrounded it; around the patch of fungus on the agar plate the colonies of staphylococci were destroyed (Figure 10.1). He found that if he grew this fungus in a broth then a substance appeared which could destroy many pathogenic organisms. This discovery of an anti-bacterial substance produced by a fungus remained dormant for many years, and it was not until 1941 that penicillin was produced commercially on a large scale for use in the treatment of human disease caused by infections with various micro-organisms.

Penicillin is so-called because the blue-green fungus which produced it belongs to a group of fungi called the Penicillia. Several different strains of this group produce penicillin. One of the best strains for the production of penicillin was found by growing the fungus from the stem of a mouldy melon found in the fruit market in Peoria, Illinois, U.S.A. This strain was made even more effective in penicillin production by bombarding the fungus with X-rays; a very efficient mutant strain was produced which is now used in the manufacture of penicillin all over the world.

Penicillin was the first antibiotic to be discovered; it is still the safest and most generally useful of the antibiotics. There are now many different kinds of penicillin which are produced by making chemical modifications of the original penicillin molecule. These penicillins are thus semi-synthetic and they have different properties from the original penicillin G. For example, penicillin G—the original penicillin—has to be given by injection since if it is taken by mouth it is destroyed by the acid in the stomach, but chemical modifications of the penicillin molecule have given several penicillins which are resistant to acid and which can therefore be given by mouth—much more convenient and much less painful! Other modifications of the penicillin molecule have produced penicillins which are active against different kinds of micro-organisms and thus which can be used for disease which are unaffected by the original penicillin G.

The exploitation of the fungus which produced penicillin was followed by a systematic study of thousands of other micro-organisms to try to discover other antibiotics. A group of fungi called the Actinomycetes have been found to produce a wide variety of antibiotics. *Streptomyces griseus* which is present in manure, compost and soil produces an important antibiotic called streptomycin; when this antibiotic was introduced into medicine it radically changed the outlook for those suffering from tuberculosis. Hundreds of tons of this antibiotic are now produced annually. Streptomyces also produce other antibiotics such as chloramphenicol, tetracyclines and neomycin. Chloramphenicol is now manufactured synthetically but it is the only antibiotic to be manufactured in this way; all other antibiotics are produced by living micro-organisms which are grown in special nutrient broths from which the antibiotic is eventually extracted. So far we have only mentioned antibiotics which are produced by fungi, but some bacteria also produce antibiotics such as gramicidin, polymyxin, and bacitracin.

We do not really know why micro-organisms produce these chemical substances which can damage and destroy other micro-organisms. It has been suggested that the Streptomyces, for example, which are slow-growing soil fungi, produce antibiotics to destroy soil bacteria which live in competition with them. However, in their natural environment—the soil—they do not appear to produce enough antibiotic to affect neighbouring bacteria. Whatever may be the significance of these substances for the micro-organisms which produce them, there can be no doubt that the technological exploitation of this activity in the production of large amounts of pure antibiotics has revolutionized the management of many infectious diseases, in particular those which are caused by bacteria and fungi.

Other chemicals

A large variety of other chemicals are manufactured with the aid of micro-organisms. Various vitamins are manufactured in this way, including vitamin C (only one stage of the production is assisted by bacteria) with the aid of a bacterium (*Acetobacter suboxydans*), vitamin B_2 by the aid of yeasts, vitamin B_{12} by the aid of bacteria and yeasts, and carotene by the aid of a fungus. Citric acid is a very important substance for the soft drink industry, and enormous amounts of the acid are prepared by the action of a mould, *Aspergillus niger*, on sugar. Dextrans—starch-like materials obtained from sugars—can be used in emergencies as a substitute for blood or blood plasma in transfusions. Dextrans are prepared by the action of the bacterium *Leuconostoc mesenteroides* on sugar.

Of increasing importance is the extraction of enzymes—those catalysts of biochemical activity—from cultures of bacteria and fungi. Enzymes have very wide uses. The markets are being flooded with 'biological' washing powders containing bacterial enzymes which help to separate

dirt and stains from fabrics. The enzymes in the class called amylases (i.e. those which break down starches) are used in the paper industry to dissolve starch from fabrics before these are used to manufacture paper. Amylases are also used in laundries to break down starch on clothes. Pectinases are enzymes which break down the pectin of fruits—the component which causes jams to set. These pectinases are used in industry to stabilize fruit juices. Proteinases—the enzymes which break down proteins—are used to remove traces of meat and hair from hides before the hides are tanned. This class of enzymes is also used for clarifying beer and for removing stains from clothes in laundries.

Some microbial enzymes are also used in medical practice. One enzyme called hyaluronidase breaks down the jelly-like substance of connective tissue. If this enzyme is present in a solution which has to be injected under the skin, it allows a very rapid spread of the fluid through the tissues. Other proteinases (e.g. streptokinase) have also been injected into patients to try to 'dissolve' blood clots. These enzymes to be used in man have to be in a very pure state to avoid untoward reactions in the patient. The efforts needed to produce highly pure preparations make them relatively expensive drugs.

Micro-organisms and the disposal of sewage

We have already considered briefly the role of microbes in the processes of decay which returns the materials of dead organisms to the soil so that they can undergo the various transformations into other living systems. We can make use of this activity of micro-organisms in the composting of garden refuse. On a much larger scale we can use them to assist in the disposal of sewage. We will discuss the health aspects of sewage disposal in a later section (Chapter 13). The ways in which man deals with his excreta varies greatly, depending upon local circumstances and economics. In primitive or isolated communities excreta may be passed into and stored in pail closets or earth closets. A pail closet is merely a receptacle, such as a bucket with a lid; this is emptied periodically and the contents dug into the soil or burned. A refinement of this system is the addition of soil to the bottom of the pail—the earth closet; the earth helps to keep down the odours and assists in the break-down of the faeces. Both these systems of disposal carry the risk of contamination of water supplies if the excreta is dug into the soil near a shallow well or near a defective water pipe. A modification of the system is in fairly common use in temporary dwellings—caravans and camps. The excreta is passed into a chemical closet. This is a container fitted with a seat and lid and containing a pail of some sort which has a layer of disinfectant and deodorant solution. The liquid is either an alkaline emulsion of coal tar or a strong solution of caustic soda. The contents are periodically emptied and buried in the soil. Unfortunately, disinfection of the solid material is not always complete. Instead of emptying the contents of pail closets into the soil, the contents can be drained into a large underground water-tight tank called a cesspool. These have to be emptied periodically. Cesspools are usually made of bricks and they have a ventilated cover. Unfortunately these brick built stores of sewage often leak into the surrounding soil and thus carry a real risk of contaminating water supplies. They should certainly not be sited near a well or water pipes.

Much of the civilized world has a water-borne sewage system in which excreta (urine and faeces) is carried in water—from lavatories, sinks, bathrooms etc.—through a system of drains (the term drain describes pipes leading from one set of premises) and sewers (the large pipes with which individual drains are connected). These sewers must be soundly made to prevent leakage of their contents and the risk of pollution of water.

This water-borne sewage is dealt with in various ways. In coastal areas sewage is almost invariably discharged directly into the sea. The sewage is not usually treated before its discharge, but some local authorities homogenize the solid matter so that if winds and currents do bring the sewage onto the beach then one is not presented with the distasteful sight of intact faeces. Normally this does not occur because the sewage is passed into the sea through a long pipe (an outfall) which is long enough to ensure that the sewage is not washed ashore. Residents of coastal regions are becoming increasingly dissatisfied with this type of sewage disposal and from time to time claims are made that it is a danger to health. It seems, however, that sea water is a good sterilizer of sewage; certainly people who live on the coast do not suffer more from those sewage-borne diseases such as typhoid or infectious hepatitis than those who live inland.

In inland regions water-borne sewage cannot be discharged in untreated form into rivers because of the very real risk of contamination of water supplies, apart from the unimaginable pollution of the water which would occur if

bacteria and algae grew in this rich brew of nutrients. One of the first ways of dealing with water-borne sewage in Britain was by 'sewage farms'. The sewage was discharged onto land used for agriculture—hence the name 'sewage farm'. This process fertilized the soil and the water of the sewage became purified as it percolated through the soil. However, there was a serious risk of polluted water reaching wells and water pipes, and only a few sewage farms still exist in Great Britain.

We will look now at the techniques of disposal in a modern sewage works (Figures 11.9 and 11.10) which uses the great technological advances that have been made in recent years—including that of automation. We have seen that sewers contain excreta and a large amount of water from various sources—amounting to volumes as large as thirty to fifty gallons per person per day. The sewage also contains other materials—paper, food debris, hair, detergents and other chemicals. Industries may also discharge various wastes into the sewers and this can complicate the process of sewage treatment. This mixture of materials is first received into large settling tanks in which the solid materials gradually settle to the bottom to form a sludge—'settled sludge', as it is called. The liquid from the settling tanks is then run into large ponds where the water is stirred and aerated. This treatment encourages the growth of aerobic bacteria which oxidize much of the organic matter in the water; the latter disappears as carbon dioxide to the atmosphere. Many bacteria have grown in this bath of liquid nutrients and these are allowed to settle down to produce a second kind of sludge. Some of this sludge is removed and added to other aerating ponds to hasten the process of oxidation of the organic matter. Yet more of the sludge—called activated sludge—is dried and sold as fertilizer.

The liquid part of the sewage has now been considerably purified although it is not yet pure enough to be discharged into waterways. It is now spread by rotating sprays over beds of porous material such as coke. In these beds the porous material becomes covered by a film of bacteria and fungi, and the activities of these organisms further purifies the water as it trickles down through several feet of this 'living' filter. The water can now be run into a river or into the sea.

We have yet to describe what happens to the solid part of the sewage—the settled sludge. This semi-liquid sediment is pumped into large vats called digesters which may hold hundreds of gallons of sludge. The vats are not aerated

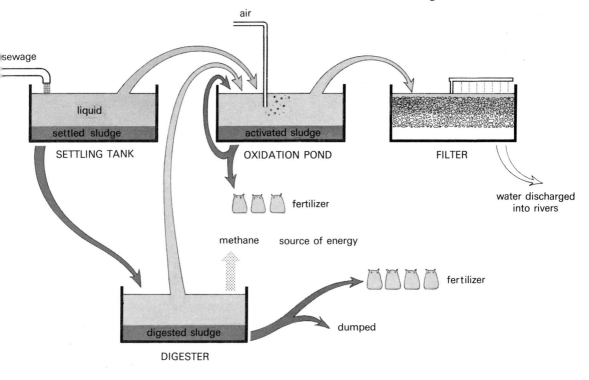

Figure 11.9 Scheme of activated sludge method of sewage processing.

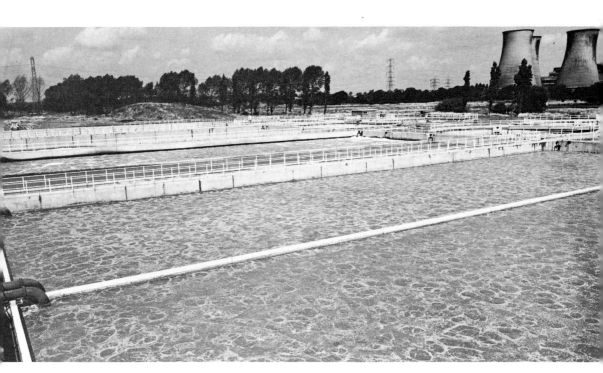

Figure 11.10 Activated sludge processing. (*By courtesy of Activated Sludge Ltd.*)

and anaerobic conditions prevail. Numerous micro-organisms of various kinds appear in these vats. Thus the methane bacteria break down organic matter and in the process liberate the gases methane and carbon dioxide, and the cellulase bacteria destroy the paper in the sludge. Every day more settled sludge is added to the 'digester'. The methane produced during the process of 'digestion' can be a valuable source of power which can be used to drive stirrers and pumps in the sewage works. It can also be compressed in cylinders and used as a fuel for lorries. The digested sludge is now run off into tanks and allowed to settle; a deposit accumulates at the bottom of the tank which consists of a mixture of bacteria and solids which have resisted the bacterial attack. This digested sludge can be dried and used as fertilizer for the land but often it is dumped into the sea—at a specified distance from the shore.

Problems caused by the discharge of industrial effluents into sewers

We have already mentioned that effluents from a variety of industries may be discharged into sewers. Depending upon the kind of material in the effluents, they may cause problems at sewage processing plants. Some industrial effluents contain chemicals which are toxic to micro-organisms and these can drastically interfere with the workings of an activated sludge process. Chromium-plating industries, for example, produce effluents which are highly toxic to micro-organisms. These effluents must be carefully regulated if they are not to disturb the working of a sewage plant. An industry may be obliged to set up its own treatment plant for

dealing with special toxic wastes. Fortunately microbes exist which can deal with all sorts of chemical substances. By choosing the appropriate group of microbes, the effluents can be purified sufficiently to be discharged into sewers or into rivers. Thus one kind of chemical factory produces effluents containing phenols, which are used as antiseptics; some microbes can oxidize phenol, and these are established in activated sludge plants to remove the phenol from the effluent.

Another kind of nuisance is created by industries which produce effluents very rich in organic water, e.g. dairies and abbatoirs. The average sewage works cannot deal with these effluents unless they are diluted by large volumes of water. Household effluents may also cause problems if they contain chemicals which cannot be broken down in the sewage plant. In particular, many detergents are resistant to bacterial attack and pass over with the sewage water when this is ultimately discharged into rivers. They may thus appear in our drinking water if this is taken from such rivers. The problem created by detergents is discussed in more detail on page 138.

Summary

We have seen that micro-organisms form a large fraction of the total organic life on earth; without them the higher organisms could not exist. Man is making increasing use of the activities of diverse groups of micro-organisms in a variety of industries, not the least of which is that concerned with the disposal of his waste materials.

12. Milk as a source of human disease

Micro-organisms in milk and their effects

Spoilage

CLEAN fresh milk which is taken from a healthy cow is a valuable food for all human beings. Modern conditions of life in which most of the population lives in industrial communities means that freshly drawn milk is not normally available. Milk is collected from distant farms and is transported, usually with supplies from neighbouring farms, to distributing centres where the milk is processed. After processing, the milk is bottled and then distributed to the individual consumer. At all these various stages, milk may be contaminated by organisms which 'spoil' its quality. Milk is a solution of proteins containing a suspension of fat globules, mineral salts, vitamins, and milk sugar. It provides an ideal medium for bacterial growth and multiplication. Some of the products of bacterial metabolism, notably lactic acid produced by the acid-forming bacteria such as *Streptococcus faecalis* and *S. lactobacilli*, can so alter the chemistry of the milk that 'spoiling' rapidly occurs. The solubility of the proteins in milk is critically dependent upon the pH (i.e. the acidity or alkalinity) of the milk. Lactic acid produced by the above organisms reduces the pH of the milk to the point where the proteins precipitate out of solution. Thus the bacteriology of milk is very important from an economic point of view. These organisms may cause the 'spoiling' and thus wastage of large amounts of milk unless the milk is initially relatively clean and is further treated to reduce the number of 'spoiling' organisms.

Human disease

The micro-organisms in milk are important not only from an economic point of view; they may also be responsible for transmitting a variety of diseases to man. Some of these organisms come from the cow itself and include *Mycobacterium bovis* (which produces bovine tuberculosis in man), Brucella (producing undulant fever in man) and streptococci and staphylococci, which in the cow may come from infections of the udder (mastitis) and cause a variety of disturbances in man, including septic sore throats and scarlet fever. These organisms are present in milk at its source but many other kinds of organisms may be introduced into the milk, either on the farm or in the processing plant. The latter may come from human carriers or cases of the disease, contaminated water, dust etc. and include *Mycobacterium tuberculosis* (human tuberculosis), Shigella (bacillary dysentery), infectious hepatitis virus, *Salmonella typhi* and *S. paratyphi* (which cause typhoid and paratyphoid fevers), other Salmonella organisms which cause food poisoning, and the diphtheria bacillus.

Hygienic milk production and processing

In the production of safe, clean milk we need to consider two fairly distinct aspects of handling of milk; first, standards on the farm (condition of the cows, methods of milking etc.) and second, the methods of handling and processing of the milk after it has arrived at the distributing centre. Both aspects are important, for no amount of processing in the distributing centre can make dirty milk clean, although it may make it relatively safe.

Cows, farms, and farmers

Even under the cleanest conditions milk which is freshly drawn from a healthy cow is never sterile. A mixed population of bacteria is always present in the milk ducts and teat canals of the udder of a healthy cow, and freshly drawn milk contains about 20 000 bacteria per cubic centimetre of milk. These bacteria are obligatory tissue saprophytes and do not cause human disease, nor are they very important in the 'spoiling' of milk. Large numbers of other bacteria can, however, enter the milk during the process of milking or during the transfer of milk to storage containers. These bacteria may come from the hide of the cow (earth, dung), from dust and dung in the cow shed, from the vessels used for collection and storage of milk, from the hands and clothes of the milker, and from contaminated water used for washing utensils or cooling the milk. Cow dung contains over a million bacteria per gramme, and the litter in a dirty cowshed may contain more than ten times this population per gramme; it is obviously important to prevent the contamination of milk from these sources. These bacteria, although they may contain no human pathogens, are important for the economics of milk production, for they can greatly reduce the market-life of the milk. They ferment milk sugar into lactic acid, which results in the souring and eventually the clotting of milk. Clean milk will keep for several days in cool conditions, but dirty milk will be spoiled and unsaleable in less than a day.

T.T. milk

We have already listed the bacteria which may enter the milk from the cow, either from infections of the udder and teats (streptococci and staphylococci) or from generalized infections of the cow which are associated with the presence of bacteria in the blood stream, and hence in the milk of the animal. The most dangerous human pathogen which enters the milk in this last way is *Mycobacterium bovis* which causes tuberculosis in cattle and man. *M. bovis* does not actually multiply in the milk or in milk products, but it is a very resistant germ and can remain alive for long periods in milk, cream, butter and cheese. During the process of the separation of cream from milk, the bacilli tend to become concentrated in the cream. This means that cream and butter may be more dangerous than milk itself. Bovine tuberculosis is a disease of serious economic importance to breeders of cattle, and the disease has been responsible for a large amount of human illness, particularly in children.

All milk today is produced from cows which have been 'tuberculin tested'. A cow which is infected, or has been infected, with *M. bovis* becomes what we term 'hypersensitive' to the products of living tubercle bacilli. One can make use of this fact in detecting cows which are suffering from tuberculosis. In the laboratory the bacteriologist cultures the bacilli responsible for bovine tuberculosis in a special fluid medium in which the products of the activities of the bacilli are concentrated. After a certain time the culture fluid is concentrated by evaporation and the bacilli themselves are removed from the fluid by filtration. The concentrated fluid is called tuberculin and it can be further purified to provide material which can be used in the tuberculin test in animals or men. A small amount of purified tuberculin is injected through a fine needle into the skin. If an animal or man has tuberculosis (or has previously had tuberculosis), then the individual is sensitive to tuberculin and reacts, after an interval, to the presence of tuberculin in the skin by a local swelling and redness at the site of the injection. If a cow reacts in this way it is called tuberculin positive, and is no longer used for milk production. Cattle need to be tested in this way at regular intervals to make sure that they are free of tuberculosis (see also tuberculin test in man, page 65).

Since all milk is now produced from cows which are tuberculin tested, and since some 90 per cent of the milk sold by retailers is further processed to destroy at least 99 per cent of all bacteria, including all pathogens, milk is no longer a significant source of bovine tuberculosis for man. Nowadays brucellosis is a greater hazard from milk; in 1961 it was estimated that 15 per cent of herds in England and Wales were infected with brucellosis and 5 per cent of milk samples contained living Brucella organisms. Of course this applies only to non-processed milk (i.e. milk that has not been pasteurized or sterilized). We will look further at brucellosis and other milk transmitted diseases at the end of this chapter.

Processing of milk

We have looked at the factors which determine the cleanliness and safety of milk which arrives at central processing and bottling plants from surrounding farms. The milk has usually been pooled from a number of farms and may have been transported some distance to the processing plant. Some milk is still bottled on farms without further processing. This milk, of course, comes from cows which have passed the tuberculin test. It still contains varying numbers of bacteria which cause spoiling and it *may* contain bacteria which are pathogenic for man, coming either from the cow or from contamination of the milk after it has been drawn.

At central processing and bottling plants, milk is subjected to some form of heat treatment which destroys the bulk of 'spoiling' organisms and pathogens. Three heat processes are in use:

1. Pasteurization,
2. Sterilization,
3. Ultra-high temperature.

Pasteurization

Milk is pasteurized by heating it for a certain time, at a certain temperature, and then immediately cooling it. This destroys about 99 per cent of the bacteria, including the pathogens. Pasteurization does not alter the flavour of milk and the loss of nutritive value is very slight (e.g. loss of a little of some vitamins). There are several different kinds of pasteurization. In one process milk is maintained at a temperature of 63–66 °C for at least thirty minutes, and in another the milk is held at 72 °C for at least 15 seconds. In both processes the milk is cooled immediately after pasteurization to a temperature not more than 10 °C.

No matter what pasteurization process is used, care must be taken to prevent contamination of milk occurring after the heat processing, e.g. during cooling (coolant water should be bacteriologically pure) and bottling (the equipment and containers used must be clean). After bottling, pasteurized milk should be stored at a sufficiently low temperature to prevent multiplication of any organisms that may have survived pasteurization or that may have contaminated the milk after the pasteurization process.

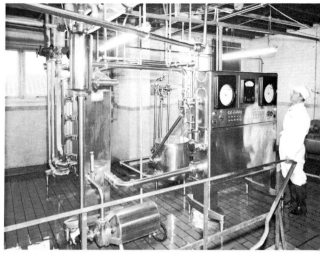

Figure 12.1 A modern pasteurization plant. (*By courtesy of the APV Co. Ltd., Manor Royal, Sussex.*)

Tests for the efficiency of the process

Pasteurized milk must satisfy two tests—the phosphatase and methylene blue tests. The phosphatase test depends on the fact that milk is a biological fluid containing various enzymes. One such enzyme is called phosphatase. All enzymes are destroyed by sufficient heat. Phosphatase is made completely inactive by the minimum temperature and time of exposure required by legal pasteurization. The amount of this enzyme can readily be measured in the laboratory. If pasteurized milk is found to contain a significant amount of this enzyme, it means either that the milk has not been adequately pasteurized or that it has been mixed with unpasteurized milk. The methylene blue test gives a measure of the degree of bacterial contamination of milk. The activities of bacteria reduce the colour of this indicator dye so that it eventually becomes colourless. For the test a small volume of milk is added to a tube containing a quantity of methylene blue. The tube is then plugged and incubated in a water bath at 37 °C. Bacterial action decolourizes the methylene blue. The more bacteria present in the milk, the faster the decolourization occurs. A control is carried out using a sample of milk which has been boiled to destroy all bacteria; no decolourization should occur in this control tube.

Pasteurization reduces but does not prevent 'spoilage' of milk. Further, pasteurization can fail if milk is heavily contaminated with material such as cow dung, straw dust and pus (from infected udders). These materials in milk can protect bacteria from destruction by being deposited as a protective coating around them. It has been said that pasteurization encourages farmers to neglect some of the basic aspects of hygiene in milk production. There may be a tendency to reduce efforts to produce clean raw milk if the farmer knows that the milk is going to be subjected to the 'magic and certain' process of pasteurization. In spite of advances in the processing of milk, there should be no weakening of efforts to produce initially clean raw milk. No one wants to drink a pasteurized solution of cow dung, however few living bacteria it contains.

Sterilized milk

Sterilization of milk is carried out by heating bottled milk to a prescribed temperature and then cooling it so that at the end of the process the bottles of milk are not only hermetically sealed but are sterile. The milk has a typical cooked flavour which is not acceptable to some people. It also has a darker colour than raw milk.

Ultra-high temperature process

This process produces milk which is, for all practical purposes, sterile. The milk is rapidly heated to not less than 133 °C for not less than one second. It is then cooled and transferred to sterile containers under aseptic conditions. This process kills all bacteria, including spores, without very appreciable changes in flavour or colour.

Untreated milk

Milk which has not been processed in one of the above ways can be made safe by boiling it and then rapidly cooling it. This procedure is of particular importance when the milk is to be consumed by babies and young children.

Milk products

Milk products include

1. unsweetened condensed milk,
2. sweetened condensed milk,
3. dried milk,
4. fermented milk,
5. butter,
6. cheese.

Unsweetened condensed milk

After the milk has been concentrated by evaporation of water, it is placed in tins that are hermetically sealed and then sterilized in an autoclave (page 170). The bacteriological properties of this milk are thus very similar to those of sterilized milk.

Sweetened condensed milk

This milk is not sterilized and its keeping properties are due to:

1. The initial pasteurization of the raw milk.
2. The high sugar content of this product.

Some moulds and yeasts can, however, tolerate such conditions. Because the milk is not sterilized, pathogenic staphylococci may sometimes be a problem, and sweetened condensed milk can contain appreciable amounts of staphylococcal toxin responsible for food poisoning (page 152).

Dried Milk

This is produced by first concentrating milk by evaporation of water and then dehydrating it by pouring it over hot rollers or more usually by 'spray drying'. During the initial concentration of milk, staphylococci may produce the toxins which persist in the dried product. Further, in the process of spray drying the temperature in the centre of the droplets of milk stays at 60–80 °C for only a short time and bacteria which are susceptible to heat can survive. These do not usually undergo multiplication in the dried product because of the lack of water, but they will multiply if milk reconstituted from the powder is left standing at room temperature.

Fermented milk

In fermented milk products, e.g. yoghourt, the micro-organisms which are responsible for the fermentation greatly lower the pH of the milk (i.e. make conditions acid). This produces conditions in which multiplication of pathogenic organisms is impossible. However, the pathogens which were originally present in the milk are not destroyed so that preliminary pasteurization of the raw milk used to make the yoghourt is advisable.

Butter

Farm butter, made from unpasteurized milk, is potentially dangerous since it contains any pathogenic bacteria that may have been present in the milk from which it was made. Indeed, some organisms may become concentrated in cream during its separation from milk so that butter may contain a higher concentration of organisms than the original milk. However, butter prepared from pasteurized milk presents no risk to health provided, of course, that hygienic precautions are maintained during its manufacture, packing and storage.

Cheese

Cheese is prepared by curdling milk with lactic ferments or rennet, or both. Whenever possible cheese should be made from pasteurized milk. In order to limit the multiplication of any pathogens in the milk, the fermentation process should be as rapid as possible.

Some types of cheese are liable to dangerous contamination. Cream cheese sometimes contains Salmonella organisms, staphylococci toxin or tick-borne encephalitis virus. Soft or semi-hard cheese made from cow's, goat's or ewe's milk may be contaminated with Brucella organisms. Some cheese may contain *Cl. botulinum* spores or botulinum toxin (page 153).

Some important diseases transmitted by milk

Brucellosis

This is the name given to a disease which occurs in many species of animals and man. Usually man contracts the disease from animals. The Brucella micro-organism is a Gram-negative bacillus. There are various species of Brucella and not all of them occur in Great Britain. Here the species is called *Brucella abortus*. It produces contagious abortion in cattle and undulent fever in man. Cattle form the main reservoir of infection. When the disease is introduced into a new herd of cattle it spreads rapidly, producing an epidemic. Pregnant animals are very likely to abort (i.e. suffer miscarriage).

Man acquires the disease in two main ways, by drinking infected milk or cream and by direct contact with infected animals. The disease is an occupational risk of farmers, veterinary surgeons, slaughterers and meat packers. Before cattle were vaccinated against the disease, over a fifth of the total number of cows in Great Britain were infected and contagious abortion was the most important single factor in causing loss of cattle.

After man has been infected with *Br. abortus*, several months may elapse before symptoms appear but the incubation period is more usually two to four weeks. There are few diseases which can show such a wide variety of signs and symptoms, and this makes diagnosis difficult. In some cases symptoms appear suddenly with high fever, severe chest or abdominal pain, sweating and bronchitis. But the undulant type of brucellosis is most commonly seen in Great Britain. The temperature runs an irregular—undulant—course, with some days of normal body temperature in between periods of high fever. This fever follows a period of weeks or months of vague ill health. The fever is associated with generalized aches and pains, headache and drenching sweats. Some cases who remain undiagnosed may suffer from the effects of the disease for years. They may have such vague symptoms of ill health that they may be labelled 'neurasthenics'—suffering from imaginary illness. Such a fate overtook one of the bacteriologists working on the problem of brucellosis who showed that contagious abortion of cattle and undulant fever in man are caused by the same organism. This doctor suffered from the disease for over five years before the disease was diagnosed.

If brucellosis is suspected in man it can be diagnosed in several ways:

1. Blood, pus or secretions are taken for culture in the laboratory in a suitable medium.
2. The blood of a patient suffering from brucellosis develops antibodies against the organism. In the laboratory, suspensions of Brucella bacilli are agglutinated (clumped) by these antibodies. A positive agglutination test in the laboratory thus indicates the presence of antibodies against Brucella

organs in the blood of the patient. This means that the patient has, or has had, an infection with Brucella.

3. Just as patients who have, or have had, tuberculosis develop a hypersensitivity to products of tubercle bacilli which can be detected by a skin test (page 65), so does the patient with undulant fever develop a hypersensitivity to the products of Brucella bacilli. Hypersensitivity is shown by a positive reaction—a raised tender area on the skin—following injection of Brucella proteins into the skin.

Treatment of undulant fever is made difficult because the organisms live *inside* cells, which means that they are not exposed to drugs in the cirulating blood. Drugs which have some effect in undulant fever include tetracyclines, streptomycin and sulphonamides.

Prevention of brucellosis

Undulant fever in the general population can be prevented by pasteurization or sterilization of milk. This does not, however, prevent transmission of the disease to those in contact with

Figure 12.2 One method of mass screening of herds for the presence of brucellosis—the milk ring test. If a cow has brucellosis then its blood and milk come to contain antibodies against the bacteria. The presence of this antibody can be detected in milk by incubating a sample of milk with a coloured Brucella antigen. Antigen and antibody unite producing a dark ring in the test tube, i.e. a dark ring in the tube indicates brucellosis. (*By courtesy of the Milk Marketing Board Veterinary Research Laboratory, Worcester.*)

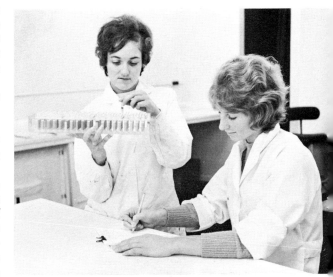

cattle. In order to prevent this direct transmission, contagious abortion of cattle has to be
eradicated. In small herds, improved standards
of hygiene together with regular skin testing of
cattle with Brucella proteins, and the slaughter
of all those that become positive reactors, may
eradicate infection from a herd. With larger
herds these methods are not so effective. A real
problem is the infected animal who does not
have a positive skin response to Brucella proteins
and thus is allowed to roam freely in the herd
and spread the infection.

There has been some success using living
Br. abortus vaccines. These vaccines do not
prevent the infection in the animals, although
they reduce its severity and thus the number of
organisms which are distributed by the infected
animal, i.e. they reduce its infectivity. These
measures are, however, temporary ones. The
policy of the Ministry of Agriculture is towards
total eradication of infectious abortion and the
setting up of registered herds of cattle which are
free of the disease (Figure 12.2).

Typhoid fever

Typhoid fever is essentially a water-borne
disease, and we will be looking at it in some detail
in Chapter 13. The bacterium responsible—
Salmonella typhi—may also be transmitted by
milk and milk products. The bacteria are able to
multiply in milk without producing any detectable change in the nature or taste of the milk.
The bacteria may reach the milk in various ways

including:

1. *Direct* contamination from a human 'carrier' of the disease.
2. *Indirect* contamination from:
   (a) flies that have fed on human faeces,
   (b) sewage-polluted water used for cleans-
       ing and rinsing utensils in the dairy,
   (c) dried earth and shed hairs from the
       hide of a cow that has been in contact
       with sewage-polluted water.

Causes (b) and (c) are the most likely ones to
produce widespread milk-borne epidemics of
typhoid fever, since they alone permit the
necessary degree and duration of contamination
of the milk with *S. typhi*. No surface water in
England is certainly safe from contamination by
water polluted by sewage containing *S. typhi*
(from faeces from human 'carriers' of the
disease). These organisms are relatively resistant
ones and remain alive in milk, cream, ice cream,
butter and cheese. In frozen ice cream the
organisms remain viable for over a year, and they
can remain alive for months in butter kept under
normal market conditions.

Milk-borne typhoid fever can be prevented
by various hygiene measures and by pasteurization of milk. Cattle should not be allowed
access to streams and ponds unless the quality
of the water is checked by regular bacteriological
analyses. Only tap water should be used in the
milking parlour. No 'carrier' of *S. typhi* should
be employed anywhere in the milk industry—
nor, for that matter, in any food industry.

13. The need for pure water

Introduction

AN ADEQUATE supply of water fit for drinking, cleansing and industrial processes of all kinds is the most important single requirement for any community. In Great Britain an average supply of water is about thirty to forty gallons (140–180 dm³) per person per day. Only a small fraction of this water is used for drinking, the rest being used for flushing of toilets and sewers, laundry, personal washing etc.; however, we will not attempt to list here all the purposes for which water may be used. The supply of water may rise to as much as eighty to one hundred gallons per person (360–460 dm³) per day, depending upon the kind and number of local industries. Some industries, e.g. atomic power establishments, use enormous amounts of water for cooling purposes. In spite of the fact that only a minute fraction of the water supplies is used for drinking, *all* water supplies must be safe and must always meet certain standards of quality. The provision of such volumes of pure water presents considerable technical and financial problems, particularly in arid parts of the world. These needs must be met. Because of the problems associated with provision of large amounts of pure water, in some parts of the world water of two qualities has been supplied to homes, one for drinking and one for household purposes. Wherever this has been done it has proved to be a serious risk to health, because of the danger of confusing the two supplies, and the practice has now been abandoned in most areas. The only exception is in some dry coastal regions of the world where pure fresh water may be supplied for drinking, cooking and washing, and sea water supplied for other purposes. These two types of water are so different in taste that they cannot easily be confused. The possible grave effects of pollution of water on the health and well being of the public means that the control of water pollution must be given a very high priority.

What is safe, pure water?

Pure water does not occur in nature except perhaps as rain water as it leaves clouds. All other waters, both salt and fresh, contain some inorganic and organic substances which can support some form of microscopic life. As rain falls through the air it picks up substances from the atmosphere, and the more polluted the atmosphere is, the more polluted will be the water as it falls onto the land. As rain water seeps through the ground it dissolves other substances, both inorganic and organic, and it picks up living micro-organisms. This water ultimately reaches either surface waters—streams, rivers, lakes etc.—or passes down to deep waters. It is mainly the activities of man which are responsible for the extensive and often dangerous contamination of these waters with such materials as sewage and industrial wastes.

Water authorities are required to provide a supply of 'pure and wholesome' water and sanitary authorities are required to make sure that every dwelling house has a supply of 'wholesome water'. These terms 'pure' and 'wholesome' are not as yet defined by law, but they are generally recognized as meaning water which cannot transmit such diseases as typhoid fever and cholera. The water must be free of chemical poisons, be bright and clear, free from suspended matter, reasonably soft and without excessive amounts of salts in solution.

There are enormous numbers of possible contaminants of water, but the number of substances in water which are regulated is kept to a minimum, because if standards were created for all possible contaminants then this would mean that periodic analyses would be necessary to make sure that the standards were being complied with. It would obviously be an impossible task to perform regular water analyses for hundreds of possible pollutants of water. However, several general tests are regularly carried out which make it unnecessary to test for a large number of different micro-organisms and individual chemical substances.

Bacteriological examination of water

Particular pathogenic bacteria, e.g. *Salmonella typhi*, the causative organism of typhoid fever, are rarely found in water samples even when a particular water source has caused an outbreak of disease. The pathogenic bacteria are present in very small numbers and, because of the interval between the initial contamination of water and the outbreak of disease, they may already have disappeared from the water supply when this is tested, i.e. contamination may be intermittent.

So instead of looking for particular pathogenic bacteria, *routine* tests look for evidence of water pollution by sewage. If water is contaminated by sewage it is potentially dangerous. The tests look for bacteria which originate in faeces, e.g. coliform bacilli, faecal streptococci and *Clostridium welchii* (see page 15). Coliform organisms are a diverse group of bacteria which come from different sources so that *Bacillus coli* of intestinal origin has clearly to be distinguished from coliform organisms which occur in vegetable matter and soil. One way of distinguishing these kinds of coliform organisms is to culture water samples on agar at 22 °C and 37 °C. Most of the bacteria which grow at 22 °C come from soil and vegetable matter and do not indicate faecal contamination of the water. Those bacteria which multiply at 37 °C are mainly intestinal in origin. The ratio of the count of bacterial colonies growing on agar at 22 °C to that at 37 °C is useful for explaining sudden changes in the number of bacteria in a water supply.

The higher the ratio the more likely it is that the bacteria have come from soil, e.g. after a period of heavy rain, and thus are of little significance.

The results of a bacteriological analysis of water have to be interpreted in the light of the source of the water and the treatment it has received, e.g. source from surface or deep water, recent rainfall or floods and whether the water has been chlorinated or not. Water intended for supply to the public is expected to reach certain bacteriological standards. Coliform bacilli (indicating sewage contamination) should be absent from 100 cm³ of the water, but this ideal is rarely attained consistently. The following is a rough classification of the nature of water according to the number of coliform organisms it contains.

		Coliform count/100 cm³ water
1.	Very satisfactory	Less than 1
2.	Satisfactory	1–2
3.	Suspicious	3–10
4.	Unsatisfactory	More than 10

In the course of a year 50 per cent of water samples should fall into class 1; 80 per cent

should not fall below class 3 and none should be in class 4. If the samples are taken from water which has already been chlorinated then *all* should come into class 1.

Group analysis of water

Instead of analysing water for individual substances it can be examined for groups of substances. If the results of group analysis are suspicious then one can go on to measure individual substances. One group analysis consists in the evaporation of a sample of water to dryness to measure the total amount of dissolved solids. This gives a measure of total inorganic pollution. Pollution by organic chemicals can be measured by passing water through carbon filters and then extracting the filters with an organic solvent such as chloroform. Potable (drinkable) water is generally considered to be a colourless clear solution without unpleasant odour and containing no more than 1500 mg/dm³ of total solids and no more than specified amounts of certain pollutants. International standards have been set up for many pollutants of water. There are, however, many pollutants for which limits have not yet been specified. Thus water which does conform to international standards may in fact be unsafe and produce long-term ill-effects on health. We will be looking in more detail at the pollution of water in a later part of this chapter.

Water supplies

Our supplies of water on the land come ultimately from the seas. In ways we cannot pursue here, water evaporates from the surface of the seas and eventually falls onto land in the form of rain, snow and hail. This water is free of salts and pollutants, but as it passes through the air it dissolves various gases and as it percolates through the soil it picks up additional substances. All of this water ultimately reaches the seas again, but some is temporarily trapped in surface and subterranean lakes and some is artificially trapped in reservoirs and canals.

We can classify water supplies into two main groups, surface waters and deep waters. The superficial waters include lakes, reservoirs, rivers and springs. The deep waters are formed by the downward percolation of rain waters through the earth or by water flowing down natural clefts in the earth. The nature of the earth through which the water descends to deep levels has an important bearing upon the quality of the water. Some kinds of earth are impervious to water while others are permeable to varying degrees. Some, indeed, are so porous or fissured that they present no barrier to the downward movement of the water. Semi-permeable strata act as very efficient mechanical filters so that the water loses most of its suspended particles, including bacteria. Deep water of this kind is a very safe source of water. Fissured and porous strata, e.g. chalk, are so permeable that surface water can flow downwards without undergoing any filtration. Thus deep water in chalk and limestone regions may not be safe from bacterial contamination, particularly when a period of heavy rainfall follows a drought which has dried the subsoil and caused cracking.

Our supplies of water are drawn from the following:

1. lakes—natural or artificial,
2. rivers and streams,
3. wells, deep and shallow,
4. springs,
5. reservoirs.

Lakes

Many large towns and cities obtain their supplies of water from lakes, many of which are artificial ones created by damming a mountain valley. Liverpool obtains its water from artificial lake Vyrnwy in Central Wales, Birmingham from artificial lake Ruador in the same region, Manchester from natural lakes in the Lake District and Glasgow from natural Loch Katrine. These lakes are in uninhabited regions of the British Isles. The land surrounding the lakes is uncultivated and is protected from trespass by human beings and cattle, thus reducing the risk of pollution of water as it drains into the lake. This water has to be piped from the lakes to the cities, often over distances of hundreds of miles. Great care has to be taken to ensure that water in these pipes is not polluted on its way to the city. The greatest risk occurs if sewage systems run close to the water mains, for if both were to fracture in the same region the water could be dangerously contaminated. Both water mains and sewers are liable to fracture because of the effect of surrounding stresses in the soil, e.g. vibration from traffic and faults in the pipe. Several epidemics of typhoid fever have been caused by such accidents.

A growing problem of waters in lakes and reservoirs is that called eutrophication. This is the growth of enormous numbers of microscopic plants (algae) in the water. These plants obtain their nourishment from mineral salts dissolved in the water. Overgrowth of algae occurs when a body of water receives wastes which contain plant nutrients, particularly phosphates. Sewage contains large amounts of phosphates, but the most likely source of excess phosphate for water which is conserved for human use is drainage water from agricultural land, particularly when phosphate fertilizers have been applied to the land.

Eutrophication may cause great damage to lakes. Not only does it make them unsightly—the water is green and cloudy—but it can seriously interfere with the use of the water for domestic and industrial processes. Some algae are poisonous, and there have been reports of death of fish and aquatic birds from this cause; some algae give water an unpleasant taste which is very difficult to remove from the water. These heavy growths of algae eventually die and decay, and the putrefaction of large masses of these microscopic plants creates anaerobic conditions. The water may become foul smelling and contains high concentrations of iron and manganese which have been leached from the bottom of the lake under the anaerobic conditions.

Rivers

The water supplies of many cities and towns come from rivers. London takes the bulk of its public supply from the Thames; the remainder comes from deep wells. Shrewsbury takes water from the Severn and Rugby from the Avon. All these rivers receive sewage effluents and are heavily polluted with dangerous bacteria and undesirable organic matter. Thus water taken from these sources *must* be purified. Purification of water occurs in three stages—sedimentation, filtration and chlorination. First the river water is stored in reservoirs where solid mineral and organic matter settles to the bottom. In these reservoirs many of the bacteria contained in the water gradually die. Water from the sedimentation reservoirs is then filtered either through beds of sand or through mechanical filters. As the water seeps slowly through the thick beds of fine sand, suspended matter is filtered out and organic matter is oxidized by the action of bacteria coating the sand. Finally the water is chlorinated. The minimum amount of chlorine is added which will make the water safe and then any excess chlorine is neutralized by the addition of ammonia, which results in the formation of harmless ammonium chloride. Only minute amounts of chlorine (about 0.5 parts per million of water) are present in the water which is

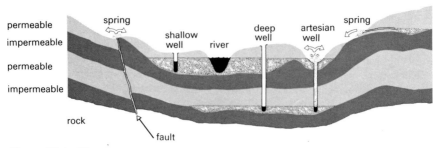

permeable

impermeable

permeable

impermeable

rock

fault

Figure 13.1 The nature of deep and shallow wells, an artesian well, and springs.

delivered to the public. This amount cannot be detected by taste or smell and it is not injurious to health. Certainly chlorination is the only certain way of making dangerous water safe to drink. Even this process, however, can fail under certain circumstances, but these circumstances are not likely to occur in Great Britain, because of the great care exercised in controlling water purity by regular and frequent bacteriological and chemical analyses.

Wells

Deep wells

Deep wells, i.e. those more than 13 metres in depth, usually provide a supply of safe water. There are, however, exceptions, particularly in chalk and limestone districts, where deep wells can become polluted by water which has run directly from the surface through fissures in the subsoil; this is particularly likely to occur after a period of heavy rainfall. The source of the pollution may be at some distance from the well itself for the water in deep wells has travelled many miles underground. Also, pumping of water from the well draws water by capillary force from the surrounding water-bearing stratum, and during the construction of a deep well there may be fissuring of surrounding rock strata, or the drilling may actually follow the line of existing natural fissures. This means that pollution near the deep well can affect the deep water. Thus the safety of a deep well depends upon its location and on the nature of the subsoil.

Artesian wells are a special kind of deep well. If the impervious strata where the water collects are at a higher level than the well itself then the water will rise to the surface without pumping. London supplements its water supply from an artesian well lying beneath the city. The outcrops of this well are in the downs surrounding the London basin.

Shallow wells

Shallow wells are still used in many country districts in Britain, supplying villages, farms and isolated houses. Wherever they occur they must be regarded with suspicion, for they are liable to dangerous contamination. They may be contaminated from the surface—from wind-blown soil and vegetation, from surface water washing into them during heavy rains and from contaminated water (faeces and urine) draining through a depth of subsoil which is inadequate for purification of the water. They may also be contaminated at deeper levels from seepage from defective drains or from a cesspool. Figure 13.2 shows the structure of a kind of well which is found in many country districts. The well has no water-tight cover so that surface water, rain, dust (often contaminated by manure and human faeces), vegetation, insects and even rats all have access to the well. The walls of the well have gaps in the stonework so that contaminated surface water can seep into the well. Any human or animal excreta which is deposited on the topsoil within fifty to a hundred metres radius of the well is liable to contaminate the well water, particularly after heavy rain.

All wells of this kind should be examined by a water engineer and samples of the water investigated by a bacteriologist before the water can be regarded as safe for drinking. Figure 13.3 shows a modern shallow well in which various of the above defects have been corrected. The top of the well has a surrounding wall with a concrete base together with an efficient cover. There is a water-tight lining for the upper 6 metres of the well so that all water which enters the well has to percolate through a considerable depth of subsoil. The well is also sited at a distance from cesspools, farm manure dumps—in fact at a distance from any source of pollution by excreta from man or animals, and these include rivers, streams, estuaries, human dwellings and animal houses.

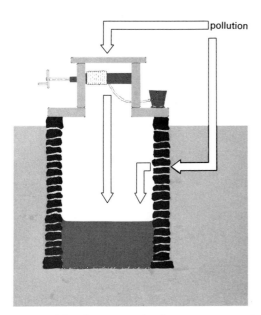

Figure 13.2   Structure of a dangerous type of shallow well.

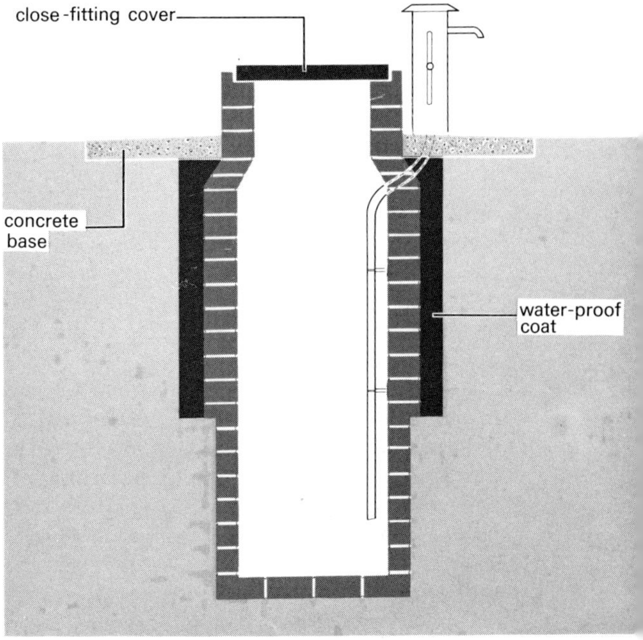

Figure 13.3   Structure of a modern shallow well.

Springs

Many small towns and villages obtain their water from springs. Some of these springs provide adequate amounts of safe water but others are likely to intermittent contamination. The purity of spring water depends upon the situation of the spring, the nature of the subsoil and the depth from which the water rises. Figure 13.1 shows two kinds of spring, a shallow spring occurring where there is an outcrop of impermeable strata and a deep spring where a geological fault brings permeable and semi-permeable strata into apposition.

Purification of water

We have already discussed the bulk purification of water for distribution to the general public (page 133). This consists of sedimentation, filtration and chlorination. On a small scale the purification of water involves similar principles. Purification of domestic or personal supplies may be necessary on camping holidays, when water has to be used from suspected sources, and in times of emergency when sanitation and water supplies are damaged by natural disasters or by the effects of war. Bacteria, but not viruses, can be removed from water by passing the water through filters with sufficiently small pores. One

kind of filter is made of unglazed porcelain. The porcelain filters can be obtained in various grades and the finest will hold back most viruses. The apparatus has to be dismantled every few days and the filter washed and sterilized, e.g. in an autoclave. Unfortunately it is difficult to provide large volumes of purified water using this kind of purification because the filtration process is slow and has to be assisted by pressure. Easier ways of small-scale purification involve either chlorination or boiling. A variety of substances can be added to water to kill micro-organisms, e.g. ozone and chloramine, but chlorine remains the cheapest and probably the most effective way of purifying water. The usual source of chlorine is bleaching powder. Chlorine is neutralized by organic matter in the water, so that enough bleaching powder should be added to leave some free chlorine in the water. With a free chlorine concentration of one part in a millions parts of water, the water will be sterilized in about thirty minutes. This amount of free chlorine can be obtained by first making up a stock solution of bleaching powder containing 9 cm^3 of bleaching powder in a litre (1 dm^3) of water and then adding a tea-spoon (5 cm^3) of the stock solution to every forty-five litres of water which is to be sterilized. Alternatively water can be boiled. All vegetative bacteria and many spores are killed by five minutes' boiling. Boiling will also remove temporary hardness from the water.

Water pollution

The most serious pollution of our environment
—air, water, soil—is the direct result of the
activities of man. The term environmental
pollution describes the unfavourable alteration
of our surroundings by agents such as faeces,
urine, chemicals, micro-organisms, radio-active
materials, smoke etc. These changes in the
environment affect man in many ways. They
can affect his water, food, agriculture, his
opportunities for leisure and his appreciation of
the beauty of nature.

As soon as man lived in large settlements and
towns, there was the problem of disposal of
domestic wastes—particularly human excreta.
Earth closets and the burying of excreta in soil
have been sanitary measures since ancient times,
indeed many ancient cities had an elaborate
system of sewers. The earliest reference to
industrial pollution is in the sixteenth century
and describes the effects of tin mine wastes in
Cornwall. Tin is usually associated with metals
such as lead and zinc, and the presence of such
substances in the wastes from the tin mines no
doubt had devastating effects on river life. In
the eighteenth century there was the development of large industrial cities and towns where
garbage and human excreta accumulated in the
streets. More and more of this filth found its way
into the rivers, particularly after the introduction of sewers which discharged completely
untreated excrement into the rivers. Even now
in the twentieth century, untreated or only
partially treated sewage is discharged into the
sea close to land. From time to time human
faeces, tea bags and other objects which pass
down our water closets are washed up onto our
beaches—mingling with the oil discharged from
ships!

In the early eighteenth century the condition
of our rivers was deteriorating rapidly. Salmon
disappeared from several rivers, notably the
Thames, and outbreaks of cholera occurred in
London. A series of Acts of Parliament appeared
in an attempt to regulate the pollution of rivers
and certain Acts related to the handling of
sewage. The civilized, so called 'developed',
countries of the Western World have to a large
measure solved the problems of contamination
of water by sewage. Death from water-borne
diseases such as cholera and typhoid fever have
been replaced by deaths from cancer, strokes
and coronary artery disease. As we shall see, the
pollution of water by sewage has been replaced
by pollution by industry and agriculture. The
state of environmental hygiene which is des-

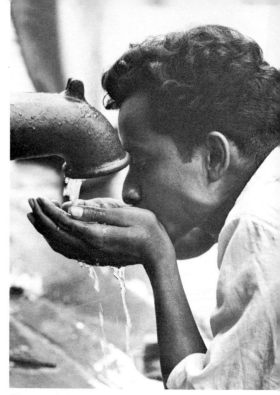

Figure 13.4 Water needs are tremendous
and the persistence of many diseases is
greatly affected by the nature of water
supplies. Photograph shows a water tap in
Calcutta. (*WHO photo by Paul Almasy.*)

cribed by modern Western textbooks describes
a world which is inhabited by less than one-third
of the people of the globe. For the other 2000
million people of the world the standards of
water supplies and sewage disposal present a
dismal picture. In South-East Asia 61 per cent of
the population is not served by piped public
water supplies. Although 86 per cent of the
urban population of South America is served
from piped supplies, these supplies are often
only intermittent and the quality of the water
often leaves much to be desired. Populations
and industry are expanding so rapidly that
supplies of water to urban populations in much
of the world are a potential danger to health and
economic development. With regard to the
removal of human excreta from continuous
contact with man, the world situation is even
more appalling. Waste disposal has always
lagged behind community water service in every
country in the world. In large regions of the
world which have recently been surveyed
(including South America, Africa, South Asia
and the Far East) only 24 per cent of the urban
population is connected to sewers, 25 per cent
have privies, and 51 per cent are not served at all.

Even in developed countries where water
supplies and sewage disposal have reached
acceptable standards, neither homes nor

industry can operate without producing polluting effluents which have to be discharged somewhere. The standards of freedom from water pollution that have been achieved represent a compromise between ideals and practicalities. Apathy and ignorance still play an important role in water pollution. Most English rivers still contain some fish in spite of 200 years of industrialization. It is estimated that the population of Great Britain—45 million—produce 7000 million litres ($7 \times 10^6 \text{m}^3$) of sewage each day, and more than three-quarters of this (together with effluents from industries) are discharged into our fresh waters. This amount of pollution is likely to increase rather than decrease because of the expanding population and increasing industrialization. Some of our rivers, e.g. the Don, are so heavily polluted with industrial wastes, household detergents and sewage effluents that no life can survive in the smelling, foaming, putrid waters. More and more of our rivers are likely to suffer a similar fate.

Water pollution is, of course, not restricted to Great Britain (Figure 13.5). It is becoming an increasing problem in almost every country of the world. A marked growth in the size of populations, rapid growth of towns and industries and an increase in irrigation, all call for increased supplies of water and all cause an increasing pollution of water. The importance of controlling pollution of water has generally only been realized after damage has already been done. Serious pollution accidents occur with increasing frequency. In Delhi in 1955–56 there was an explosive outbreak of infectious hepatitis involving tens of thousands of cases due to faecal pollution of the water supply. The most recent European pollution accident occurred in June 1969 when Rhine water was contaminated by some potent insecticide. The total number of dead fish floating down the Rhine was estimated at the staggering figure of forty million—practically the entire fish population of the river. Whole cities which obtained their water supplies from the already polluted Rhine had to turn to emergency supplies of water. A case of similar magnitude occurred in 1961 in the U.S.A. when a rainstorm washed a large quantity of DDT into the Colorado river, killing the fish population for 200 miles below Austin, Texas. Smaller comparable incidents have occurred in Great Britain, one when there was a discharge of cyanide into the river Chealmer in Essex and another the 'Smarden incident', when a drum of highly poisonous insecticide leaked into the soil killing livestock and plant life.

Figure 13.5   Water pollution in Europe—the waters of the Rhine.
(a) (below, left) From the St. Gotthard Glacier to the dykes of Rotterdam, the Rhine—flowing through sixty cities and out into the busiest sea in the world—drains a catchment area of 224 000 square kilometres inhabited by 44 million people. On its banks a flourishing chemical industry has developed. Its waters are now blackened with coal, polluted with ammonia, and charged with salt and phenol. The photograph shows barges and shipyards near Duisberg. (*WHO photo by Jean Mohr.*)
(b) (below, top right) Shows the muddy liquid that is swallowed by the purification plants along the Rhine. (*WHO photo by Jean Mohr.*)
(c) (below, bottom right) Shows Rhine water before and after purification.
(*WHO photo by Jean Mohr.*)

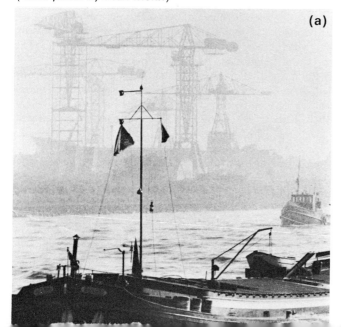

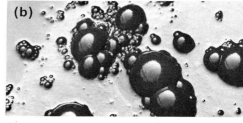

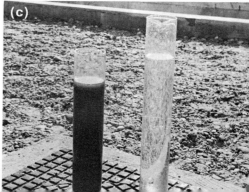

Sources of pollutants in water

The contaminants that enter the surface and underground waters of the earth do so in three main ways:

1. wastes and waste waters from sewered and unsewered communities,
2. wastes and waste waters from industry not connected to public sewerage systems,
3. surface run-off and underground seepage from rainfall collected by the drainage systems of urban and rural areas.

Nature and amounts of pollutants

The danger of pollution of water is determined by the nature and the degree of pollution with sewage and chemicals and the size of the population which is at risk. Another factor is the ease with which chemical pollutants can either be extracted from the water or so modified to make them non-toxic.

Synthetic detergents

The history of the pollution of waters by detergents serves as an example of the possible consequences of the introduction of a new contaminant into water and the ways in which one can solve the problems associated with the introduction of the new contaminant. About fifteen years ago the household detergent mixtures which were marketed contained as their active component a substance called an alkylbenzene sulphonate. This kind of detergent is very persistent in water, mainly because it resists decomposition by bacterial action. In this property these early detergents differed markedly from soap, which undergoes rapid decomposition in water and does not give rise to any particular difficulties in waters into which soap is discharged.

Because of their resistance to attack by bacteria, these early detergents—so called 'hard' detergents—were only partly decomposed during the treatment of sewage, and about half of the original amount of detergent was later discharged in the sewage effluents. During the processing of sewage, air is bubbled into tanks of sewage to encourage the purification of water by bacterial action. Bubbling of air into sewage containing 'hard' detergents merely froths up the detergent until the foam overflows from the processing tanks. Moreover the foam interferes with transfer of oxygen from air bubbles to solution in the liquid sewage, thus hindering the purification of the sewage. This foam has been known to reach heights of ten to twelve feet on aeration tanks in sewage disposal plants. Moreover the sewage residues discharged into surface waters caused a serious deterioration in the quality of the water. Rivers became unsightly with foam, particularly below turbulent stretches of a river. Of equal importance, the presence of the foams reduced the oxygenation of river water and slowed the process of self-purification of water (by aerobic bacterial action). Moreover, low concentrations of detergents are toxic both to animal and plant life in the river. When river water is used for domestic purposes the presence of detergents is obviously undesirable.

Increasingly these 'hard' detergents are being replaced by 'soft detergents' which are more susceptible to bacterial attack and which are thus less persistent. Some governments have in fact banned the use of 'hard' detergents.

Pollution by other synthetic organic substances

The presence of persistent synthetic organic substances in water are a potential health hazard to man when they are present in water which is taken for municipal supplies. Where water has been taken from rivers contaminated by sewage effluents, the evidence indicates that treated water has no adverse effects on human health—provided of course than it has been adequately sterilized before distribution to the public. Thus London takes part of its supply of water from the Thames, which has received sewage effluent, and part from deep wells. There does not seem to be any significant difference in the health of the communities served by these two sources.

There has, however, been a rapid increase in the amounts of persistent organic materials which are discharged into water systems from all kinds of industrial processes. One example of this group of compounds are certain pesticides which are widely used in agriculture, horticulture, home gardens, food storage and veterinary practice. These pesticides are a hazard not only to man but also to all our wild life. Although many of the pesticides that are used in agriculture are relatively toxic to vertebrates, including man, they decompose quickly and leave no harmful residues in the plants or on the soil. Paradoxically it is a group of less toxic pesticides which are potentially the most dangerous. These compounds, e.g. the chlorinated hydrocarbons—DDT, aldrin and dieldrin—are toxic because they are very persistent compounds and can accumulate in the tissues of animals, so creating long-term problems. DDT is the most persistent of the chlorinated hydrocarbon pesticides, and as much as 35 per cent of DDT applied to soil may still be present after five years. Unless they actually live in the soil, larger animals are usually affected only by pesticide residues in the food they eat, e.g. in insects. Fish are very sensitive to DDT and can be killed by the compound when water drains into streams and ponds from treated soil. Birds can be killed by feeding on seed treated by insecticide, or on insects contaminated by the compound. These birds, when eaten by carnivorous animals such as eagles and hawks, pass on the contaminating insecticide; the food chain (herb-herbivore-carnivore) is a concentration mechanism for DDT. It is becoming increasingly obvious that the widespread use of pesticides is having serious adverse effects upon our wild life. The question at issue here is what effects may these insecticides have on man, who is at the end of the food chain. It would be foolish to deny the enormous economic advantages that have followed the introduction of pesticides into agriculture and veterinary practice. It has been estimated that if DDT and BHC pesticides were to be withdrawn from use in agriculture in England and Wales, there would be a potential annual loss of about 100 000 hectares of crop production. However, much of this loss could be made good by using less persistent pesticides which are already available.

When animals are fatally poisoned by these organochlorine pesticides, the function of the nervous system is profoundly disturbed. They die of convulsions—'fits'—or in the case of DDT with widespread muscle tremors and uncoordinated muscular activity. Many men engaged in public health programmes to eradicate malaria by destruction of mosquitoes (page 211) have been poisoned by pesticides to the extent of having serious convulsions. What we are more concerned with is not the effects of sudden accidental overdosage with pesticides in a few exposed individuals, but the effects of insidious long-term contamination of water and foodstuffs by minute amounts of these chemicals. It is quite clear that no one as yet knows what might be the effects of this low-dose, long-term, contamination of our environment with persistent pesticides. Over fifteen years ago it was reported that DDT was present in the body fat of the general population of America. More recent studies in Germany and the United Kingdom have confirmed these findings. Other insecticides such as dieldrin are also laid down in body fat. We do not know what may be the long-terms effects of this contamination but we do know that some animals show various defects in their metabolism; rats, for example, when fed on diets containing minute amounts of DDT (ten parts per million) show a disorder of the storage of vitamin A in the liver.

Obviously, far more information is needed on the potential long-term effects of these small amounts of persistent insecticides. Increasing attention is also being paid to the development of less persistent insecticides. In many parts of the world there is an increasing pressure on government agencies to ban the use of some of these pesticides. Because of the accumulation of DDT and other compounds in inland lakes, the Swedish government has put a two year ban on the use of organochlorine pesticides. The Arizona pesticide control board has also banned the use of DDT in commercial agriculture for one year.

Other pollutants

We have given most of our attention to contamination of our water by sewage, detergents and pesticides; there are, however, hundreds of other possible pollutants of water from industrial processes, not the least of which is radio-active material. There are at least fifty metals which may contaminate water by industrial effluents. Lead and mercury continue to be the most important ones but other metals such as arsenic, beryllium and cadmium are becoming important. Exposure to water containing traces of these metals usually does not cause clear-cut toxic effects in man, but it does cause an accumulation of these metals in the body. Occasionally outbreaks of human disease are caused by heavier contamination of water. Thus in Japan coastal waters have been contaminated by mercury from industrial wastes. This pollution caused disease and deaths from eating fish taken from these waters. The fish had absorbed enough mercury to become toxic foodstuffs. It is not known whether the water itself would have been toxic to man, because being sea water it was not used for drinking.

Health aspects of water pollution

The extent to which the contamination of water with human excreta is a hazard to health depends upon the prevalence of certain diseases in a given area. In many developing countries the prevalence of typhoid fever, bacillary dysentery, infectious hepatitis etc. may be ten to one hundred times that found in more advanced countries. Further, situated as they mainly are in subtropical and tropical regions of the world, developing countries have the additional burden of water-borne diseases such as cholera and schistosomiasis which are not a problem—or in the case of cholera no longer a problem—in developed countries in temperate climates. For these reasons contamination of water by sewage is a greater health hazard in developing countries of the world—the very countries in which sanitation and water supplies are often at a primitive level, particularly in urban areas.

In addition to the transmission of the above diseases, the failure of control of water stores in tropical urban areas can lead to serious increases in diseases such as filariasis and schistosomiasis. This is due to the unrestricted breeding of the animal vectors of the disease in water—mosquitoes in the case of filariasis and snails in the case of schistosomiasis (page 226).

Food taken from polluted waters can also be a health hazard. Foods such as fish and shellfish may be contaminated either by pathogenic bacteria and viruses (see typhoid fever, page 141) or heavy metals (see mercury poisoning by contaminated fish, page 139).

Bathing in polluted waters can also be a danger to health, particularly in areas of the world with a high incidence of such diseases as typhoid fever and cholera. Even in the British Isles no surface water is safe from possible contamination by sewage (see Typhoid fever) or rats (see Leptospirosis). Only waters which have been disinfected by chlorination are really safe for bathing. In tropical and subtropical areas of the world, water may also contain the infective forms of various parasitic worms, e.g. hook worms, schistosomes.

We will now look in detail at some typical water-borne diseases—at typhoid fever, leptospirosis and cholera.

It may seem strange that we are going to pay so much attention to diseases such as typhoid and cholera. Cholera is now unknown in Great Britain; it has disappeared not only from our islands but also from our textbooks of medicine and hygiene. Typhoid fever is an uncommon malady in Great Britain, and when it does occur it is more often than not an imported disease—acquired on some holiday, e.g. in Southern Europe or North Africa. Cholera has been eradicated only from our Western textbooks and the minds of our clinicians. In many parts of the world it now reaches proportions typical of bygone ages. This disabling and often fatal illness has recently spread in pandemic-like form to involve large numbers of countries that have

been long free of the disease. The disease *could* return to our shores if our sanitation and water supplies were grossly disturbed by natural disaster or by war. Although typhoid is at the moment an uncommon illness in Great Britain, in terms of world incidence it is a fairly common disease; in 1963 there were an estimated two million cases of typhoid. It is only the constant vigilance of our sanitation and water authorities which prevents typhoid from becoming epidemic in Great Britain. It is a disease that smoulders perpetually ready to be fanned into flames.

Typhoid and paratyphoid fevers

Typhoid has been one of mankind's greatest scourges. Before 1875 the disease was widespread in Britain, but the Public Health Act of that year was followed by improvements in sanitation and water supplies which led to a dramatic fall in the prevalence of the disease. Typhoid is typically a disease of armies and overcrowded communities weakened by the effects of poverty, starvation, natural disasters and war. In the Boer war in South Africa the British army had over 57 000 cases of typhoid and over 8000 deaths, in a troop population of 550 000. Only 7500 died of wounds received in battle. During the insanitary trench warfare of the First World War (1914–18) the incidence of typhoid was negligible—thanks to the effect of vaccination. In recent years about 1–200 cases of typhoid have been notified each year in England and Wales but at least half of these were acquired abroad, usually on holiday visits. Typhoid fever is always with us in the form of actual cases of the disease and, more important for the spread of the disease, in the form of chronic carriers of the infecting organisms. The disease is still a major problem in tropical and subtropical countries—and in many parts of Southern and Eastern Europe.

Both typhoid and paratyphoid infections are derived ultimately from the faeces of a case of the disease or from a chronic carrier of the organisms. The organisms do not infect animals other than man. Small numbers of organisms can cause typhoid so that the disease is commonly spread by water (or food contaminated by water) in which dilution of the organisms in a bulk of water does not prevent transmission of the disease. The development of a paratyphoid infection needs a larger 'dose' of infecting organisms and the disease is typically transmitted by food in which the organisms can multiply.

There are many ways in which water can

become contaminated by *Salmonella typhi*. In a densely populated country such as England, no water—lake, stream or pond—is permanently safe from contamination by human excreta and thus is not safe from contamination by *S. typhi*. Water supplies may be contaminated by seepage of sewage into a reservoir or surface contamination of a shallow well, leakage from defective sewers underground, discharge of sewage into a river etc. The organisms can live for about a week in sewage and they can survive for longer periods when the sewage has been diluted by water. There were typical water-borne outbreaks of typhoid in Zermatt (Switzerland) in 1963 and in Croydon (1937). The Croydon outbreak was caused by a carrier of *S. typhi* who excreted the organisms in his urine. He worked in the town's wells and the urine-contaminated water supply caused an explosive outbreak of typhoid with 310 cases and 43 deaths. Carriers of *S. typhi* often excrete the organisms only intermittently so that by the time the outbreak of typhoid fever has occurred there may be no organisms in the water supply. Every effort must be made to detect carriers responsible for outbreaks of the disease. If necessary the sewers must be swabbed for bacteriological culture, starting first in the main sewers and then tracing the source of the contamination up the tributaries until the offending residence has been identified.

Serious epidemics of typhoid have also been traced to food, in particular milk. Milk may be contaminated directly by a carrier or indirectly by means of contaminated water which has been used to clean equipment. Milk or milk products were the vehicle of several recent epidemics in Great Britain, e.g. in Epping, 1931 (260 cases with 8 deaths), Bournemouth, 1938 (718 cases with 70 deaths). In 1964 there was an outbreak in Aberdeen which was thought to be caused by contaminated corned beef. Corned beef was thought to have been infected in the country of processing by untreated river water used for cooling tins of corned beef after sterilization. Obviously only incompletely sealed tins could be contaminated in this way. Shellfish are a notorious food for transmitting typhoid and other diseases. Oysters are filter feeders and large volumes of sea water pass through these molluscs in the course of feeding. If the water around oyster beds is contaminated by sewage (e.g. by pouring untreated sewage into the sea or sewage effluents into rivers) then many organisms become concentrated in the animals. These pathogenic organisms, although they do not affect the oyster, will readily transmit infection to man. Bathing, particularly in sewage-contaminated fresh water is also a recognized way of acquiring typhoid. When the disposal of sewage is primitive and human excreta are exposed to the air, then flies may become important transmitters of typhoid as well as other human diseases.

We have already seen that paratyphoid fever is usually a food-borne disease. The foods which are most commonly involved are cream, synthetic cream, ice cream, cakes and desiccated coconut.

Features of the typhoid in man

After a dose of the infecting organisms has been swallowed, the organisms migrate through the wall of the bowel and spread to lymphatic glands, where they multiply. During this stage symptoms are usually absent—this is the incubation period of the disease. After about ten days the organisms begin to enter the blood stream from the lymphatic glands. The patient begins to feel ill, with headache and various muscular aches and pains. A fever develops which rises in a 'stair-case' fashion, reaching its peak after a week. The abdomen is uncomfortable and tender and there is usually constipation. A faint rash may appear.

In the second week of the illness, the patient's condition rapidly deteriorates. Constipation gives way to diarrhoea. Mental confusion appears and the patient becomes apathetic with a pinched looking face, flushed cheeks and dilated pupils. The illness reaches its peak in the third week. The patient may now progressively deteriorate and die. If the patient is going to recover the temperature gradually falls, mental confusion gives way to clearing of consciousness, the appetite returns and the abdominal discomfort disappears. This classical progress of the disease is now rarely seen in civilized communities because appropriate treatment with drugs cuts short the illness.

Nearly every organ of the body may become involved during the course of typhoid fever so that there may be bronchitis, pneumonia, meningitis and abscesses of bone and soft tissues. Infection of patches of lymphoid tissue in the wall of the small bowel results in the formation of many ulcers of the bowel wall. These ulcers may perforate so that contents of the small bowel may pour into the abdominal cavity, or blood vessels in the base of the ulcer may be eroded, causing haemorrhage into the bowel.

Because typhoid is no longer a common disease in Great Britain, and because of the variety of symptoms which may occur, it is a disease which may not readily be suspected or diagnosed, particularly when it is in its early stages. Anyone who has a fever without obvious cause may be suspected of having the disease, particularly if there is a history of recent travel abroad. Every effort is made to isolate the bacteria from the blood of the patient to make a certain diagnosis. A sample of blood is taken from the patient and is cultured in a nutrient broth in the laboratory. The disease may also be diagnosed by evidence that the patient is manufacturing antibodies against *S. typhi*. Again, blood samples are taken from the patient and serum is prepared from the blood. The serum is then tested in the laboratory for its effect upon suspensions of *S. typhi*. The results of this test are particularly significant if repeated blood samples show a rising concentration of antibodies.

Even with modern drugs the management of cases of typhoid fever call for the highest standards of nursing care. The patient must be isolated and his room and belongings disinfected. His faeces and urine must be carefully collected and thoroughly disinfected before being poured into the sewage system. Before the use of antibiotics about 15–20 per cent of cases of typhoid died, often due to perforation of the bowel wall or loss of blood into the bowel from an ulcer. Using modern drugs such as the antibiotics chloramphenicol or a special type of penicillin (ampicillin), the mortality rate has fallen to below 5 per cent.

The prevention of typhoid fever

The most important measure to prevent typhoid is an adequate purification of water supplies by filtration and/or chlorination, and the safeguarding of piped water supplies against subsequent contamination. The provision of safe water must also be accompanied by the safe disposal of sewage. Food must also be free of contamination by *S. typhi* and *paratyphi*. All milk, cream and liquid egg should be pasteurized. Cooks and anyone handling food should be scrupulous in their personal hygiene. Great care should be taken with food which is eaten raw; oysters should not be gathered from sewage-contaminated water, and watercress should not be grown in polluted water.

The symptomless carrier of the organisms presents a special problem. After an attack of typhoid most patients excrete organisms in the faeces for several weeks. A few cases (about 3 per cent) go on excreting organisms for

several months, and some have been known to excrete the organisms for over forty years. In Great Britain the number of carriers of *S. typhi* is probably under two per 100 000 of the population, but in parts of the world where typhoid is a much commoner disease, the carrier rate is much higher. Some carriers excrete the organisms in the faeces, others in the urine, particularly if the kidneys are otherwise diseased. Following infection by *S. paratyphi* the carrier rate is lower. Under the Public Health (Infectious Diseases) Regulations 1953 carriers may be prohibited from working in any occupation where food or drink has to be handled. Carriers are, of course, carefully instructed in the importance of their personal hygiene. This education of the chronic carrier is obviously very effective in the prevention of the spread of typhoid, for outbreaks of the disease are seldom traced to *known* carriers. Drugs, in particular ampicillin, have been used to try to eradicate the organisms in carriers. The organisms in the faecal carrier appear to come mainly from the gall bladder, and surgical removal of this organ from the chronic faecal carrier can clear up the infection in over 70 per cent of cases.

Another line of defence against typhoid is the active immunization of individuals by injecting them with a suspension of killed bacteria. Each cubic centimetre of heat killed phenolized vaccine contains:

S. typhi	1000 million organisms
S. paratyphi A	500 million organisms
S. paratyphi B	500 million organisms

Two injections are needed with a four week interval between them. This vaccine is called T.A.B. and is used (combined with tetanus toxoid) routinely in the British armed forces. Unfortunately there can be reactions, sometimes severe, to vaccination with T.A.B. In most cases these reactions are local—pain and swelling at the site of injection—but there may be generalized reactions associated with fever (see also page 57).

Vaccination must be regarded as a last line of defence. It is a poor substitute for adquate control of sanitation and water supplies, and is only recommended for people living in or travelling to areas of the world where sanitation is poor. These areas include not only Africa, India and other Asian countries but also parts of southern and eastern Europe. Vaccination also has a place in the management of an epidemic of the disease. The value of vaccination has been fully demonstrated in several research

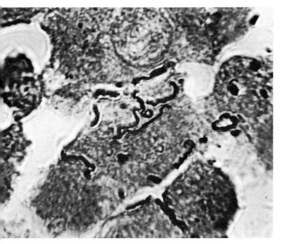

Figure 13.6   Leptospira in kidney tissue
×2500. (*By courtesy of WMMS.*)

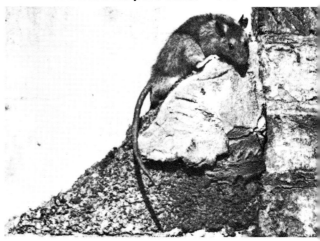

Figure 13.7   *Rattus rattus* can transmit many
diseases to man. Rat urine may transmit
leptospirosis. (*From Dr R. A. Davis, Ministry of
Agriculture and Fisheries. By courtesy of
WMMS.*)

programmes. The incidence of the disease is greatly reduced, and even if an immunized person contracts typhoid the disease is generally milder with a much lower mortality.

Leptospirosis

This term covers a wide range of animal and human infections by micro-organisms of the genus Leptospira. These organisms all have the structure of a coiled filament (Figure 13.6). In Great Britain there are two diseases caused by Leptospira, Weil's disease and canicola fever.

Weil's disease

The Leptospira which cause Weil's disease are transmitted indirectly to man from small rodents (rats and field mice) which harbour the organisms in their kidneys and urine (Figure 13.7). Usually Weil's disease is an occupational illness of men who work in conditions where the skin is likely to be in contact with water which has been contaminated by rat urine. Thus most cases occur in agricultural workers, sewer workers, coal miners, fish cleaners etc. There are, however, many reported instances of infection transmitted by bathing in rat-infested pools and from drinking water from wells contaminated by rat urine.

The disease is a severe one and the liver and kidneys may be seriously damaged, sufficiently so to cause death. Treatment should be carried out in a hospital which is capable of treating failure of the kidneys, if necessary by an artificial kidney machine.

Canicola fever

Human beings are usually infected by contact with dog urine, although infection can occur by bathing in contaminated fresh water.

Prevention of leptospirosis

The prevention of Weil's disease and canicola fever depends upon the following:

1. Rats should be destroyed and buildings made rodent-proof.
2. Food should be protected from rodent contamination.
3. Individuals who are at special risk should wear protective clothing to prevent contaminated water from coming into contact with the skin. If a worker damages part of the skin under conditions likely to lead to infection or is bitten by a rat, then treatment with penicillin will prevent the illness. Penicillin is also used to treat established infections, although it is only effective if it is given very early in the course of the disease.
4. Bathing in rat-infested water should be prohibited.
5. Dog owners should be made aware of the dangers of contracting the illness from their pets. Dogs suffering from canicola fever should be adequately treated with drugs, e.g. streptomycin, to prevent them from becoming chronic carriers of Leptospira. Any sick dog should be isolated until it is known that the animal is not suffering from canicola fever. Both dogs and humans

can be immunized against the disease by means of a vaccine and this can be used for men who, because of their work, are at special risk of contracting the infection.

Cholera

The organisms which cause the human disease cholera is a vibrio. Vibrios are comma-shaped motile bacteria found in many situations. One species, *Vibrio cholerae*, causes a serious and often fatal disease of man, multiplying in the intestine, dying and liberating a powerful endotoxin which sets up a violent inflammation of the mucous membrane of the intestine without involving other tissues. *V. cholerae* flourishes only in the human intestine although it can survive for long periods outside the body. Cholera is thus a purely human disease. The main source of infection is water contaminated by faeces containing the organisms.

The disease was once endemic in England and Europe, but has now disappeared following the introduction of effective sanitation and the treatment of water.* In recent years outbreaks of cholera have been reported from most of Asia. This spread of cholera in a pandemic form has involved a large number of countries which were once free of the disease. In some Asian countries, e.g. the Philippines, cholera has now become endemic, although in other countries, e.g. Hong Kong and Korea, the disease seems to have disappeared following the initial outbreaks. India is the country most highly infected with cholera and it has several endemic areas. Hardly a week passes without the disease being reported from some part of India.

Transmission of cholera

In order to develop cholera an individual has to ingest an appreciable number of vibrios. Traditionally it has been thought that the cholera case is the principle source of infection in a community. A typical case of cholera produces about ten to twenty litres of diarrhoea, each cubic centimetre of which contains up to a thousand million vibrios. If the patient is not restricted to a hospital then he is potentially capable of contaminating a wide area with vibrios. The mild case of cholera may create a greater hazard

because he is not restricted and is free to move around. Children, who often have mild attacks, are particularly likely to defaecate at random and contaminate soil, vegetation and water.

Even more than the actual case of cholera, the symptomless 'carrier' of vibrios is of the greatest importance in the spread of infections. Many individuals when infected with vibrios do not develop the typical symptoms of cholera. These cases occur up to five or ten times as often as individuals who develop frank cholera. Although the faeces of carriers contain much smaller numbers of organisms than those of the frank case of cholera (100–100 000 per gramme) the large number of carriers and their free movement make them a real threat to public health. These cases usually stop excreting vibrios after a week, but there are chronic carriers of vibrios who may excrete the organisms for an indefinite period.

Before cholera can become endemic in an area, the sewage and waste disposal practices of a community must be sufficiently inadequate to permit excreted vibrios to persist in the immediate environment. Poor water hygiene is particularly important. Cholera is typically a disease of the poor and underprivileged, the underfed and the overcrowded.

The spread of cholera across national frontiers is not essentially different from the spread between communities in a country. During the one or two weeks in which mild cases of cholera excrete vibrios, wide spreading of the bacteria is possible. Chronic carriers are an even greater danger.

Features of cholera

The principle feature of the disease is severe diarrhoea due to the irritation of the bowel by vibrio endotoxin. The diarrhoea is so profuse and liquid that it is given the name of 'rice-water'. These rice-water stools have to be carefully collected, not only so that they can be disposed of in a sanitary fashion but also to obtain a measurement of the fluid lost by the patient. Loss of water with contained mineral salts is a prime cause of death—about 50 per cent in untreated cases. Salts and fluid may have to be infused into a vein in the collapsed patient.

Various anti-microbial drugs, such as tetracyclines and chloramphenicol, shorten the duration of the diarrhoea and the excretion of vibrios. They reduce the fluid requirements of the patient and the duration of the stay in hospital.

---

*In 1971 cholera spread to Russia, Middle East, parts of Africa and Southern Europe. One case was reported from Britain.

The prevention of cholera

The following measures are required:

1. vaccination,
2. public health measures in endemic areas,
3. sanitation,
4. health education,
5. prevention of international spread.

Vaccination Present cholera vaccines can give some protection to individuals living in endemic areas. They have been found to prevent 40–80 per cent of vaccinated individuals from developing cholera. However, protection is generally lost in three to six months after vaccination, although individuals who have once been vaccinated react rapidly to a second vaccination; this second vaccination can be looked on as providing immediate protection against cholera, and this may be useful during the management of an epidemic.

Because vaccination cannot provide certain protection against cholera, it must be regarded as a supporting measure to other controls.

Public health measures In areas where cholera is endemic, the appearance of an outbreak of cholera must be detected early. In order to diagnose cholera, all diarrhoeal diseases—and these are many—must be suspected of being cholera and must be examined bacteriologically. Ideally there should be treatment centres for diarrhoeal diseases in which not only can accurate diagnosis be made but effective treatment given.

The outbreak of cholera should be reported to regional, national and international health services to give some advance warning of the spread of the disease.

Health education The public must be educated in the most effective way in the prevention of enteric diseases. Particular emphasis should be given to food hygiene, handwashing after defaecation, particularly by food handlers, and the dangers of water and methods of disinfection of water. However, this may be pious advice to a population in which food is scarce and where individuals have to walk miles for a small daily ration of water.

Sanitation The proper disposal of human excreta can control the spread of vibrios from cholera cases and from carriers of the organisms. Attention must also be paid to the control of the quality of water, fly control and food handling. In areas of the world where cholera is endemic or epidemic, there are no water-borne sewerage systems in urban areas and most villages are still without a centralized water supply system.

Prevention of international spread It is very difficult to prevent the spread of cholera across national boundaries. Vaccination of a traveller is no guarantee that he is not suffering from a mild form of cholera or that he is not a symptomless carrier of vibrios. Severe quarantine regulations imposed on travellers from countries which have reported epidemics may have disastrous effects. Severe restrictions on travellers and exporters of foodstuffs encourages countries to conceal an outbreak of cholera and deprives cholera-free countries of advance warning of possible invasion of the disease.

14. Diseases transmitted by foodstuffs

A VERY large number of diseases can be transmitted to man by way of the food he eats and the water he drinks. The organisms transmitted by way of food or water may be bacteria, viruses, parasitic worms or protozoa. The importance of water in the spread of disease will be dealt with in some detail in a separate section (Chapter 13) as will parasitic worms and protozoa (Chapters 19, 20). Here we are mainly concerned with some of the commoner diseases that can be transmitted by food and the importance of proper handling, preparation, storage and cooking of food in the prevention of these diseases.

Salmonella food poisoning (salmonellosis)

Salmonellosis is the most frequently reported food-borne disease of man. When foodstuffs are examined for bacterial contamination, the bacteria called Salmonellae are found more frequently than any other bacteria.

Food habits and the way in which food is prepared play a very important part in the spread of the tiny Gram-negative bacteria which are responsible for the disease. There are, in fact, many varieties of Salmonella organisms. *Salmonella typhi* is the organism responsible for typhoid fever in man; typically it is a waterborne disease and we have dealt with it in a separate section (Chapter 13). *Salmonella paratyphi* produces paratyphoid fever, a disease very similar to typhoid fever, but usually less severe. The 'dose' of bacteria needed to produce these two diseases is very different. Only a few organisms are needed to cause typhoid fever but a large number of organisms is needed to cause paratyphoid fever, and this latter disease is usually caused by eating some food, e.g. milk, cream, ice cream, in which the bacteria have multiplied. Thus typhoid is typically a waterborne infection while paratyphoid is usually a food-borne infection. We do not, however, usually include paratyphoid fever in the class of 'food poisoning'. Symptoms of typhoid and paratyphoid fevers do not usually occur until one or two weeks after infection. 'Food poison-

ing' describes illnesses which come on suddenly —in hours or a few days after infection. These illnesses are caused by Salmonella organisms other than *S. typhi* and *S. paratyphi*. Similarly we do not include 'bacillary dysentery' under the heading of food poisoning. This infection of the bowel, in which there is colicky abdominal pain and diarrhoea with blood and mucus, comes on two or three days after swallowing an infecting dose of bacteria of a species called Shigella. The disease is spread by faecal contamination, usually from hands, of lavatory equipment, towels, toys, dishes etc. Food *can* be infected by a carrier of the bacteria or by the action of flies. However, in temperate parts of the world bacillary dysentery behaves like a contact disease and food is not a very important method of transmission.

Even in countries with advanced standards of medicine and public health, it is difficult to get a realistic estimate of the incidence of Salmonella food poisoning in a population; not every case of food poisoning is treated by a doctor, and even then the case may be merely labelled 'diarrhoea and vomiting' and a bacteriological study (culture of vomit, faeces and suspected foodstuffs) may not be made. In many cases the illness may be so brief that a doctor is not called. Salmonellosis is indeed a notifiable disease, but for the reasons given above the incidence of the disease is probably ten to a hundred times higher than the figures which are given in official reports.

Features of salmonellosis

Symptoms of Salmonella food poisoning usually appear within twelve to twenty-four hours of eating the contaminated food. They usually appear suddenly, with feverishness followed by diarrhoea and vomiting. The temperature ranges from 100–103 °F (37.7–39.4 °C) and may remain high for several days. Although most cases of Salmonella food poisoning appear as an attack of gastro-enteritis, occasionally the bacteria may enter the blood stream and settle down in the nervous system or bones.

The diagnosis of salmonellosis is suggested by the combination of fever, vomiting and diarrhoea

—for other kinds of food poisoning do not usually show all these three features. For a firm diagnosis, however, the responsible organisms must be isolated from a specimen of the faeces.

Although tests in the laboratory with various antibiotics show that these are effective against Salmonella organisms, the results of giving such antibiotics as tetracyclines, ampicillin etc. to human cases are very disappointing. The mainstay of treatment is to replace the fluid and salts which are lost in vomit and diarrhoea and to use drugs to soothe the irritable and overactive bowels.

Some individuals who have suffered an attack of salmonellosis may excrete the organisms in their faeces for some time. Most of these 'carriers' stop excreting the organisms in three to four months, but some continue to excrete the organisms for two or three years.

In England and Wales two to five per thousand of the general population are 'carriers'. There is no really satisfactory way of testing whether 'carriers' have stopped excreting Salmonellae, for the appearance of organisms in the faeces is intermittent, and even after six consecutive stool cultures have been shown to contain no Salmonellae, the individual may yet again excrete the organisms in the faeces. Because of this problem, the testing of faecal samples from patients convalescing from salmonellosis is really an educational measure, impressing upon the patient the importance of personal hygiene—principally the importance of washing the hands thoroughly after using the lavatory. However, those patients engaged in the food industries should not be allowed to return to work until they have had six consecutive stool cultures with no Salmonellae in them over a period of three weeks.

The sources of Salmonella organisms—The Salmonella cycle and Salmonella in animals (Figure 14.1)

Salmonellosis is not only a disease of man it also attacks many food animals (calves, horses, poultry, pigs) from which man can be infected. In a well-run abattoir sick animals are usually detected and eliminated by the meat inspection service, so that meat from clinically ill animals is not very important in the spread of salmonellosis to man. In many countries, including Great Britain, poultry do not undergo inspection.

Although obviously ill animals can be detected and excluded in slaughter houses and meat factories, many apparently healthy animals excrete Salmonellae in their faeces—the so-called 'carriers' of the disease. This means that Salmonella infections can spread among animals which are transported over long distances and then held in large numbers in pens for fattening or slaughter. Modern large-scale slaughter processes readily lead to cross-contamination from diseased to healthy carcasses.

Salmonella organisms may also be excreted in the faeces of animals, including rats and mice, which may contaminate animal or human foodstuffs as they feed. Flies can also transfer the organisms to foodstuffs. Thus environmental hygiene (e.g. fly and rodent control) is very important in the prevention of salmonellosis. It is, however, very difficult to obtain complete control of environmental contamination on farms. We may have to accept a degree of food contamination by Salmonella organisms—up to ten per cent of samples of sausages are contaminated by them!—and concentrate on more readily manageable kinds of control, namely proper food preparation, cooking and storage.

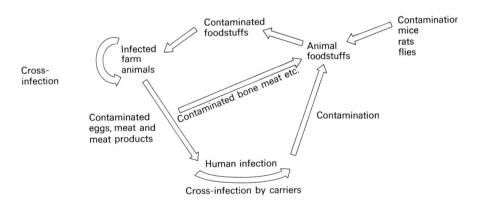

Figure 14.1   Drawing of the Salmonella cycle.

Table 12 Food transmitting Salmonella infections in 733 outbreaks and family cases in England and Wales, 1949–63, in which the offending food was identified

Vehicle	Description	Presence of Salmonellae	Outbreaks Number	Percentage of total
Meat	Fresh	2		
	Gravy, soup, stock	8		
	'Meat'	25	347	47.3
	Canned	30		
	Processed and made up	182		
Eggs	Dried egg	3		
	Hen egg	5	181	24.7
	Liquid and frozen	22		
	Duck	151		
Sweetmeats	Trifles, ice cream custard, cream confectionary	119	119	16.2
Milk	Cheese	4		
	Canned	3	40	5.4
	Dried	5		
	Fresh	28		
Fish	Shellfish	5		
	Canned	7	27	3.7
	'Fish'	7		
	Processed	8		
Fruit	Fresh	9	10	1.4
	Canned	1		
Vegetables	Canned	2		
	Dried	3	9	1.2
	Fresh	4		

Data modified from *Food-borne infections and intoxications* ed. by Hans Riemann, Academic Press, 1969.

Contamination of food (see Table 12)

In most countries the main source of salmonellosis is meat. Pork is often highly contaminated because of the large number of healthy 'carriers' among pigs. Contaminated meat creates a very serious health problem where meat and meat products are eaten raw or insufficiently cooked. Even when poultry meat is thoroughly heated, Salmonellae from raw meat in the same kitchen can contaminate processed products such as chicken salads and chicken sandwiches. Thus refrigeration and hygienic handling of meat at *all* stages of processing, from the slaughter house to the kitchen, are of the greatest importance for the prevention of food-borne diseases.

Hen's eggs are seldom contaminated by Salmonella inside the fowl, but the outside of the shells are often contaminated by Salmonellae and these can penetrate the eggs when the shell is cracked. The processing of eggs for the catering trade, i.e. the preparation of liquid egg, can result in the contamination of large quantities of processed egg from a few infected shells. Bulk liquid egg should be pasteurized and then refrigerated. Dried eggs are also very likely to be contaminated; they should be used immediately after they have been reconstituted with water, and should not be allowed to stand at room temperature when Salmonellae could multiply rapidly.

Duck eggs are notorious for being contaminated by Salmonella and have been responsible for many outbreaks of salmonellosis. Not only are duck eggs frequently contaminated, but the Salmonellae are present inside the egg and are very difficult to kill by cooking. Fortunately the public seems to be generally aware of the dangers of duck eggs and their importance in causing salmonellosis has fallen in recent years. Duck eggs should not be used in lightly cooked dishes, but they can be made safe by adequate boiling.

Milk and milk products present little risk as sources of human salmonellosis, owing to the fact that pasteurization is carried out routinely in many countries and probably also because few cows are infected. However, contamination can occur *after* pasteurization. It is therefore necessary to handle milk products, such as raw milk, powdered milk, cream and milk dishes hygienically.

Fish, oysters and other shellfish can transmit Salmonellae, and this risk is increased if the fish or shellfish have been in contact with sewage-polluted water.

Vegetable products are also potentially dangerous if contaminated water or sewage is used in their cultivation. Further, in many hot countries vegetables are 'freshened' by sprinkling with water which may not be of drinkable quality. In view of the increasing world trade in vegetables and vegetable products, this problem may be of greater importance than is now generally realized. One vegetable product—desiccated coconut—is a well recognized source of human salmonellosis and should always be pasteurized before human consumption.

that they should be repasteurized or irradiated (see page 163) in this country. It has been clearly shown that foods treated in this way do not cause salmonellosis in animals, whereas such infections frequently result from the use of untreated foods.

The handling of a particular food contaminated with Salmonella, e.g. eggs, poultry or meat, desiccated coconut, can readily lead to cross-contamination of other foodstuffs in butchers' shops, bakeries, retail dairy shops etc. The mass-production methods used in canteens, hotels and various catering establishments increase the risk of cross-contamination, which has been responsible for major outbreaks of salmonellosis. Common sources of such contamination include the following: boards used for cutting of both raw and cooked meats, dish towels, unwashed hands, and dirty kitchen utensils. Water dripping

Figure 14.2   This photograph shows a butcher eviscerating a hen (i.e. removing the bowel, liver, and heart) on a wooden board close to a joint of meat and very near to a cooked veal, ham, and egg pie on a marble working surface. The risks here are many. Poultry, because they are likely to contain salmonellae in the bowel, should be eviscerated in a special part of the shop where there is no chance of contaminating other food, particularly cooked meats which will be eaten without being heated. The hands should be thoroughly washed after such a process. Many butcher's shops have only a wet rag for this purpose and this particular shop had no separate hand washing facilities.

The nature of a working surface is important for food hygiene. Here we see a pitted wooden surface in use, for a foodstuff that may be highly contaminated.

Cross-contamination of foodstuffs (Figures 14.2–14.4)

We have already mentioned the cross-contamination that can occur in slaughter houses where, because of contamination of processing equipment such as work tables, cutting tools etc., one infected carcass can contaminate enormous amounts of meat. By-products of slaughter houses such as bone meal, blood, feather meal, are also readily contaminated, not only from infected carcasses but also by the activities of rodents, flies and man himself. Some animal foodstuffs containing this processed material are often imported from areas where sanitary conditions are not adequate, and this leads to the re-introduction of Salmonella into man via the cycle of food → animal → food → man (see below). If animal foodstuffs are contaminated on importation into this country, it is necessary

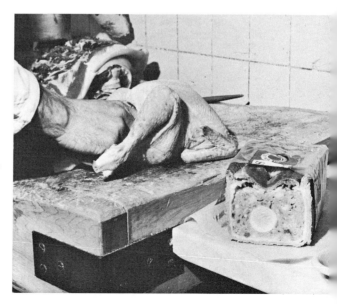

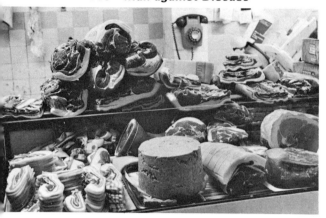

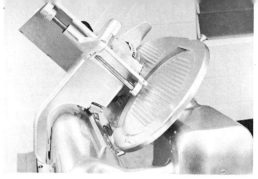

Figure 14.3 Several risks of cross-contamination.

This photograph was taken in the same shop as Figure 14.2. The chaotic cooling compartment contains a mixture of cooked foods (cooked ham, tongue, pressed beef) and uncooked meat (bacon and ham). Behind the cabinet and to the right of the freezer there is a slicing machine that is used for both cooked and uncooked meats. The working surfaces are mainly of worn wood and there is no separate hand washing basin in the shop.

Figure 14.4 (above right)   This photograph shows a well cleaned stainless steel meat-slicer. In this shop the slicer is used only for

from thawing frozen foods—particularly poultry and meat—can contaminate the kitchen. If these dangers are not recognized and avoided, large numbers of individuals may become infected when food is prepared on a commercial scale, but on a smaller scale the same sources of contamination are a danger in family kitchens where housewives are often not familiar with these potential dangers to health. It is important that *every* person handling food should be aware of the dangers of salmonellosis and the measures that should be taken to avoid food contamination.

The control of salmonellosis

The following is a list of the important measures to be taken in the control of salmonellosis.

1. The storage of animal feeding stuffs in vermin-proof rooms. Destruction of rats and mice. Bacteriological control of animal feeding stuffs.
2. Slaughtering of animals as soon as possible after arrival at abattoirs.
3. Disinfection of equipment in slaughter houses and butchers' shops to reduce the risk of spreading infection from one carcass to another.

cooked meats. These machines may, however, be a real risk to health. In 1964 there was an outbreak of typhoid fever in Aberdeen that almost certainly came from a single contaminated can of corned beef. However, not all of the numerous victims of this outbreak ate the corned beef. It is very likely that in this and similar outbreaks a variety of meats were contaminated from a slicing machine used to slice the meat from the infected tin, or indeed from any surface on which the infected meat was laid. Since this disaster in Aberdeen there has been great interest in the use and cleaning of slicers, knives etc. that can spread bacteria from one kind of food to another. There has been considerable research into the most efficient way of cleaning these machines. The best method has been found to be a two-stage treatment, first the removal of grease and many bacteria by means of a detergent and second, a treatment with a disinfectant (e.g. a hypochlorite solution, strength of 200 parts per million). This kind of treatment reduces but cannot abolish cross-contamination between foods, for it is obviously quite impracticable to clean and sterilize such an instrument after each use! A sharp knife that can be cleaned after each cutting operation is obviously safer, at least as far as cross-contamination of food is concerned.

Figure 14.5 (below)   The handling of food *after* refrigeration is also important in relation to food hygiene. The photograph shows a 20 lb deep-frozen turkey. Many outbreaks of food poisoning, mainly of the salmonella type, have resulted from cooking deep-frozen birds that have not been fully thawed before cooking. Hens, ducks, and turkeys are commonly contaminated by salmonellae. Many of these bacteria survive deep-freezing and if the birds are not fully thawed before cooking then parts of the carcass will not be adequately cooked and will contain living salmonellae. Furthermore these surviving salmonellae can multiply in a slowly cooling carcass, so increasing the likelihood that the food will cause salmonella food poisoning.

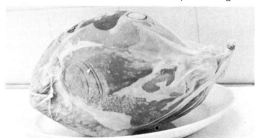

4. Evisceration of poultry away from carcass meat or cooked meat.
5. Refrigeration of meat at all stages of processing from abattoir to kitchen.
6. The thorough cooking of meat.
7. Storage of cooked meat products away from raw meat.
8. Avoidance of duck eggs for lightly cooked dishes.
9. Pasteurization of bulk liquid egg followed by refrigeration.
10. The education of all who handle food in the risks of food poisoning.
11. The exclusion of human 'carriers' of Salmonella from employment in the food industries.
12. The thorough thawing of frozen foods before cooking (e.g. frozen poultry). Figure 14.5.

Clostridial food poisoning

Clostridium welchii is a Gram-positive anaerobic sporing bacillus. Various strains of the organism have been named according to the kind of toxins they produce. One strain produces a toxin which is responsible for food poisoning.

These bacteria are widely distributed in nature. They are present in soil, sewage, water and in the bowel of man and animals. There are thus many opportunities for food, particularly meat, to become contaminated. Raw meat and poultry are frequently contaminated before they reach the kitchen. Once food reaches the kitchen it can be contaminated by dust or by unwashed hands. The spores of the food poisoning clostridia can survive four to five hours of boiling. If cooked meat is allowed to cool under suitable anaerobic conditions, e.g. in a rolled joint or a stew, then spores which have survived the cooking or which have later come from dust, may germinate and produce large numbers of vegetative bacilli within a few hours. Anyone consuming such meat would develop acute food poisoning.

Many outbreaks of clostridial food poisoning have been traced to the eating of meat, either cold or warmed up, after it has been allowed to cool slowly in the form of large masses such as roasts. Rolled roasts (Figure 14.6) are particularly dangerous since outer surfaces which may be contaminated are rolled into the centre where anaerobic conditions are good and where heat penetration and heat loss is poor, thus allowing the bacilli to grow rapidly in warm moist conditions inside the food.

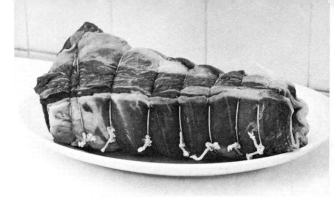

Figure 14.6 This photograph shows a 12 lb rolled joint of uncooked beef. If there are any pathogenic bacteria on the surface of the meat used in the preparation of this 'joint' they are introduced into the interior of the joint during the rolling procedure. Foodstuffs gain and lose heat slowly, which means that the interior of this relatively large joint may not be sufficiently heated during cooking (particularly if it is cooked for people who like 'rare', i.e. semi-cooked, beef) and may cool slowly afterwards, thus allowing surviving bacteria to multiply within the slowly cooling mass of meat. These problems are exaggerated when large joints of meat have to be cooked. The food poisoning bacteria that are most likely to be involved in this case are heat-resistant strains of *Clostridium welchii*, the growth of which are encouraged by the anaerobic conditions inside the joint. If this meat is not to be eaten hot, i.e. before any surviving bacteria have had time to multiply, then it should be rapidly cooled, under cover, in a cold room, and not left standing in a warm kitchen. As soon as possible it should be refrigerated.

This kind of food poisoning would not occur if meat were eaten immediately after cooking. Roasts should not weigh more than 2–3 kg so that heat can penetrate into the centre of the roast. Roasting and pressure cooking are the safest methods of cooking, because these procedures kill spores. When meat is removed from the oven, then if it is not to be eaten immediately it should be placed in such a position that cool air can circulate underneath and around it; it should then be refrigerated not later than one and a half hours after cooking. Unfortunately hot meat cannot be placed directly in the refrigerator for this leads to condensation of water over the surfaces and contents of the refrigerator.

Features of clostridial food poisoning in man

Clostridial food poisoning has a longer incubation period (twelve to twenty hours) than staphylococcal food poisoning and the illness is less severe. Fever and vomiting are unusual and colicky abdominal pain and diarrhoea are the main features. Usually Clostridia can be isolated from the suspected food and may also be found in the patient's stools for two weeks after the attack. The disease is less prolonged than Salmonella food poisoning and the victim usually recovers completely in twelve to twenty-four hours.

The control of clostridial food poisoning

We can now summarize the factors necessary for the prevention of clostridial food poisoning.

1. Joints of meat, particularly rolled joints, should be small so that cooking can destroy the spores. Roasting and pressure cooking are more likely to destroy spores than boiling.
2. Meat should be eaten shortly after it is cooked. If it is not eaten straight away it should be cooked quickly and stored in a refrigerator.
3. Meat should be covered to prevent contamination by dust.

Staphylococcal food poisoning

When certain strains of *Staphylococcus aureus* grow and multiply in food, they produce a toxin which can cause acute vomiting and diarrhoea in man. To cause illness in man, the toxin must be present in sufficient quantity; substantial multiplication of the staphylococci is necessary to produce illness. Conditions which are favourable to such multiplication include:

1. A relatively high temperature. Multiplication occurs slowly at 10 °C but increases progressively with temperature, reaching a maximum at about 35 °C.
2. A fairly high pH. No multiplication occurs in acid products (i.e. with a pH below 4.5).
3. The presence of substances such as carbohydrate or protein needed for bacterial growth.

Occasionally the staphylococci come from animals. Staphylococci from cows with mastitis (inflammation of the udder) have been responsible for outbreaks of food poisoning involving milk or cheese. Most of the contaminating staphylococci usually come from food handlers —from the nose, throat or skin (e.g. infected wounds or boils on the hand and forearms). Food handlers should be watched for evidence of infection by staphylococci, and persons showing them should be prevented from coming into contact with food.

The toxin responsible for staphylococcal food poisoning is resistant to heat and may withstand boiling (100 °C) for thirty minutes. The foods usually causing outbreaks of staphylococcal food poisoning are the partially preserved or manufactured meat dishes such as pressed meat, cold ham, brawn, corned beef and pies. In addition, custards, cheese and milk may be responsible.

Features of the disease in man

The illness begins very shortly after eating food containing the toxin, usually within one to six hours. There is an abrupt onset of vomiting, followed by diarrhoea. Usually the illness is brief, with complete recovery in six to twenty-four hours, but death can occur in weak individuals from loss of water and salts in the diarrhoea and vomiting, which can lead to collapse of the circulatory system. Fever is not a feature of the illness.

There is no specific treatment of the disease, and the most important thing is to replace fluid and salts, either by mouth or by intravenous infusion.

Figure 14.7 This photograph shows a piece of cooked ham being shown to a customer before being sliced on a machine. The man handling this cooked meat has a plastered finger. The plaster could cover a clean uninfected cut but it might well hide an infection teeming with pathogenic staphylococci which could readily contaminate the cooked meat. If this were the case the meat would give rise to food poisoning if the food were stored at room temperature for several hours, enabling the staphylococci to multiply and release their toxins.

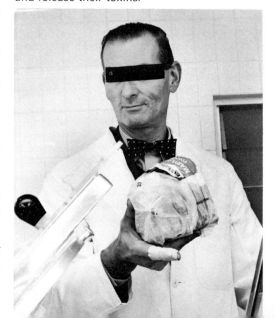

The control of staphylococcal food poisoning

1. Pasteurization of milk and milk products.
2. Rapid refrigeration of food to prevent multiplication of staphylococci.
3. The reduction of food handling to a minimum.
4. The education of food handlers in personal hygiene.
5. The exclusion of food handlers with septic skin lesions (Figure 14.7).

Botulism

Food poisoning due to Salmonellae, Clostridia and staphylococci is usually an illness of relatively short duration from which most individuals make a full recovery. A fatal outcome of the disease occurs only in the very young, the very elderly or in those who are already ill and debilitated from some other disease. The food poisoning which is called botulism is by no means such a benign illness. Although it is a rare disease, it is one with a high mortality—over 50 per cent of reported cases—and it has created concern wherever outbreaks have occurred. Human botulism is due to eating of food in which *Clostridium botulinum* (a Gram-positive, sporing, soil bacterium) has grown and produced its toxin.

Conditions leading to botulism

Usually botulism poisoning can only occur if certain requirements are met.

1. The food must be contaminated with *Cl. botulinum* spores. Since the organism is so very widely distributed in nature it can be readily assumed that *all* raw food is contaminated.
2. The food must be treated in such a way that the normal contaminating micro-organisms are destroyed, leaving only the spore forms to survive without competition. This condition is met where food is processed by mild heating, salting and pickling.
3. The composition of the food must be suitable for the growth of the organisms and toxin production. The pH of the food should be above 5.0, i.e. the food must not be acid.
4. The food must be held at a suitable temperature for a sufficient time to allow growth and toxin formation.
5. The food must not be cooked before it is eaten. Boiling, even for a few minutes, is sufficient to inactivate the toxin.
6. The bacillus is an obligatory anaerobe, that is it can live and multiply only when air is excluded. Modern methods of food preservation by canning, potting, pickling and smoking provide the necessary anaerobic conditions. Any foodstuff in a hermetically sealed can or bottle *must* be in anaerobic conditions. The interior of a smoked ham or fish may similarly be anaerobic because the process of smoking coagulates the proteins in the outermost layer of the meat or fish to make a relatively air-tight seal. Modern food preservers and canners are well aware of the dangers of botulism and take strict precautions to prevent contamination of foodstuffs and ensure conditions in which any contaminating clostridial spores do not germinate and produce toxin.

Foodstuffs which meet the above requirements include under-processed home-bottled vegetables (i.e. they have not been cooked sufficiently to kill spores), lightly salted cured meats, fish pickled without enough acid and lightly salted, smoked and partly dried fish.

The control of botulism

Botulism can thus be prevented by any of the following measures:

1. Destruction of spores by adequate heating.
2. Inhibition of growth of clostridia by:
   (a) reduction of pH, i.e. acid conditions, e.g. addition of vinegar,
   (b) reduction of water content of food which prevents *all* bacterial growth including *Cl. botulinum* e.g. by thorough drying, salting or addition of sugar,
   (c) refrigeration or freezing to prevent bacterial growth,
   (d) the addition of inhibitors of clostridial growth, e.g. nitrites.

Features of botulism in man

As a rule *all* individuals who eat affected food develop the disease, usually within twenty-four hours. Prominent features of the illness are vomiting, constipation, paralysis of muscles, e.g. eye and throat muscles, and intense thirst. We have already said that this is a rare disease with a high mortality. Because of its rarity, it may not be suspected by the doctor who is caring for a case. If the disease is suspected then it can be confirmed by demonstrating the presence of the toxin in the suspected food—mice are useful for this purpose because they are very susceptible to the toxin. The organisms can also be isolated from suspected food or from vomit or faeces of the patient. Treatment of the disease is difficult, but for some types of the illness an anti-toxin can be given to the patient to neutralize the toxin, and this treatment has dramatically reduced the mortality of one kind of botulism which occurs in Japan. In Great Britain the last outbreak of botulism was in 1922 among a party of holiday makers in Scotland. Eight people ate sandwiches made of potted wild duck pâté prepared locally, and all died.

Transmission of viruses and Rickettsiae by foodstuffs

Until recently there has been a lack of reliable laboratory techniques for the isolation and growth of many viruses. For this reason there has been little investigation of the role of food in the spread of virus diseases.

Some food products can transmit some viral and rickettsial disease to man. Some entero-viruses such as polio virus and Echo viruses can be transmitted by water and uncooked veget-ables. Tick-borne encephalitis virus and the Q fever organism (a rickettsia) have been shown to be excreted in the milk of sheep, goats and cattle. Many individuals have been infected with tick-borne encephalitis after eating untreated products made from goat's milk. There is conclusive evidence for the transmission of infectious hepatitis virus (producing a kind of infective jaundice) to man through oysters, clams and other foods that are eaten raw.

The transmission of animal parasites by foodstuffs

Metazoan animal parasites, e.g. parasitic worms, are not usually dealt with in accounts of food hygiene and microbiology. They do, however, cause important food-borne infections. Some examples of these parasites will in fact be looked at in more detail in another section of the book (Chapters 18–20) and here we will just list some of the food-borne animal parasites.

We can conveniently divide food-borne parasites into two groups: first, parasites originally present in the food, and second, parasites introduced later by contamination. The first group includes parasites which are already present in the tissues of the food animal where they persist in a form that is infective to man. Effective transmission of these parasites depends upon eating food which is either raw or which has not been cooked enough to destroy the parasites. In this group we can include the following parasites and foodstuffs which may be infective.

Parasite	Foodstuff
Beef tape worm	Beef
(*Taenia saginata*)	
Pork tapeworm	Pork
(*Taenia solium*)	
Fish tapeworm	Fish
(*Diphyllobothrium latum*)	
Flukes, e.g.	
Paragonimus westermani	Crabs
Clonorchis sinensis	Fish
Heterophyes heterophyes	Fish
Nematode worms	
Trichinella spiralis	Pork

In the second group we can include parasites which are not initially present in the food, but the food later becomes contaminated from soil, water, animals and food handlers. In this class we can include such parasites as the round worm (*Ascaris lumbricoides*), flukes, e.g. liver fluke (*Fasciola hepatica*), oriental fluke (*Fasciolopsis buski*), dwarf tapeworm (*Hymenolepis nana*). The protozoan parasite responsible for amoebic dysentery (*Entamoeba histolytica*) is transmitted in the same way.

Control of animal parasites in food

The best method for the control of infections by food-borne animal parasites is the elimination of such parasites from food animals and from the environment. At the moment this is not a realistic aim, and control must depend on the processing of infected food and on the prevention of contamination of food. A further important measure is the health education of the public, who should be informed of the dangers of eating raw or under-cooked food that is likely to be infected. If all pork, beef and fish were adequately cooked then tapeworm infections and trichiniasis (page 233) would disappear.

Food poisoning in different countries

Food, cooking and eating habits vary widely from country to country, and this is reflected in the number and kinds of food poisoning that occur in different countries. In Great Britain, Salmonella

Table 13 Data for food poisoning incidents of all kinds in 1966

Organisms	All cases		General outbreaks	
	No.	%	No.	%
Salmonellae	4214	65	95	60
Staphylococci	262	4	8	6
Clostridium welchii	1947	30	47	33
Other organisms	10	–	1	1
Chemicals	1	–	–	–
All agents	6434	100	141	100
Causes not discovered	2350		40	
Total	8784		181	

food poisoning forms the bulk of cases, followed by clostridial food poisoning. Cases due to staphylococcal contamination of food are in the minority (see Table 13). In the U.S.A. the situation is reversed, and staphylococcal food poisoning is the major identifiable cause of food poisoning. This state of affairs in the U.S.A. may be related to the enormous number of commercially prepared, served and catered meals that are consumed by the American people in public eating places. In Japan, food poisoning in the summer is common. Here, sea fish and fish products are important in the outbreaks, for it is the custom to eat raw fish. The culprit has been unknown for a long time but recent studies suggest that a group of salt-tolerant vibrios are responsible for the bulk of food poisoning (see Table 14). These salt tolerant organisms—*Vibrio parahaemolyticus*—are Gram-negative straight or slightly curved rods. They may be responsible for over 70 per cent of cases of bacterial gastro-enteritis in Japan. Food poisoning in England and Wales is reviewed yearly by the Epidemiological Research Laboratory of the Public Health Laboratory Service. It is a notifiable disease, and the annual figures are based on reports made by pathologists in public health and hospital laboratories to the Public Health Laboratory service and on returns submitted by Medical Officers of Health to the Ministry of Health.

Examples of outbreaks of food poisoning

The following examples of actual outbreaks of food poisoning are meant to illustrate the sort of foods and the kind of errors in handling that can give rise to food poisoning. The descriptions of the outbreaks are based upon weekly epidemiological reports published in the *British Medical Journal*; these reports originate from the Public Health Laboratory Service. I am indebted to both the Director of the Public Health Laboratory Service and to the Editor of the British Medical Journal for their permission to use extracts from the epidemiological reports.

Clostridial food poisoning ('*Clostridium welchii* food poisoning', page 566 *British Medical Journal*, 1970, **4**, 507–68, No. 5734)

Two outbreaks of clostridial food poisoning were reported in the *British Medical Journal*. The first outbreak was in a hospital and was caused by contaminated pease-pudding. In this hospital for mentally subnormal patients, a total of 186 individuals became ill with diarrhoea. In some cases there was also abdominal pain and vomiting. All cases recovered rapidly. Each patient had eaten a lunch containing ham and pease-pudding. Other patients in the same hospital who had eaten a different lunch were not affected. Heat-resistant strains of *Cl. welchii* were found in the remains of the pease-pudding, also in the faeces of eighteen out of twenty patients who had been ill.

The vegetable dish (pease-pudding) had been prepared the day before it was served. Bacon

Table 14 Food poisoning in Japan in 1963

Organism	Cases (Total no.: 21 830) Percentage of total	Outbreaks (Total no.: 717) Percentage of total
Vibrio parahaemolyticus	59.4	73.1
Staphylococci	12.8	13.7
Coliforms	12.5	3.8
Salmonella	4.8	5.4
Others	12.5	4.0

bones and onion had been added to the peas to give flavour. After cooking, the pease pudding was allowed to cool slowly in bulk in a metal trough. The following day it had only been warmed before serving.

The second outbreak of *Cl. welchii* food poisoning occurred in individuals receiving food from a 'meals-on-wheels' service. Thirty-one people were ill after a meal which included minced beef that had been reheated. Three of those affected had to be admitted to hospital.

The mince was bought in frozen packs weighing 3 kg. Six of these packs were cooked for two hours in one pan of chicken stock. The mince was not defrosted before being placed in the pan. After cooking, the mince was allowed to cool in a poorly ventilated room at a temperature of 21°C. After five hours at this temperature the pan of cooked mince was then refrigerated. At 8 a.m. the following morning, some of the mince was reheated for a period of twenty minutes before being distributed with cooked vegetables in 134 foiled containers. By the time the food had been packed into the containers and ready to go into heated cabinets for distribution it was found to be cold. The cabinets were, however, not designed to warm up food but to keep already heated food at a safe temperature (i.e. to maintain hot food at a temperature of 63°C which is regarded as the minimum safe temperature for storage of such food—Food Hygiene Regulations 1970). At the end of the distribution round the food was at 29°C.

Discussion

These two outbreaks demonstrate well some of the pitfalls in the cooking of food and the storage of cooked food. In the case of the pease-pudding the food had been cooled too slowly so that living spores of *Cl. welchii* that had survived the cooking were able to germinate and multiply rapidly in the slowly cooling food. On the following day the pudding was not heated sufficiently to kill the bacteria. In the second outbreak in which minced beef was involved, a variety of factors contributed to the outbreak. In the first place frozen food, particularly large packs, should be thawed before cooking. Second, cooking is most thorough in small pans with regular stirring of the food to ensure thorough cooking. The third error in this case was the slow cooling of the mass of minced beef, which permitted surviving spores of *Cl. welchii* to germinate and multiply before the mince was finally refrigerated. Finally there was a failure on the following day to main-

tain the food at 63°C, so that the bacteria survived and were eaten.

The prevention of this type of poisoning, from food prepared on a large scale by institutional cookery, is difficult and should be based on the assumption that in all cases spores are already present in the food at the time of cooking. Heating is the most important method of eliminating clostridia and other types of food poisoning micro-organisms from food. If all foods were boiled (heated to 100°C) shortly before consumption, food-borne diseases would never occur, with the exception of staphylococcal food poisoning (the toxin here is heat-resistant) and toxins of plant, animal or fungal origin. If food has to be stored before eating, it should be rapidly cooled and stored at less than 4°C or it should be maintained above 63°C.

Staphylococcal food poisoning
('Staphylococcal food poisoning', page 122, *British Medical Journal*, 1970, **4**, 63–124, No. 5727)

Two outbreaks were described in the *British Medical Journal* and involved sixty-three cases in June 1970. One outbreak affected twenty-three people in five different families living in four different towns. All these people developed an illness during one weekend in June. They suffered mainly from vomiting and abdominal pain but in some there was also diarrhoea. These symptoms came on three to six hours after eating cakes containing a vanilla filling. The cakes had been made by one bakery and delivered to several market stalls which, incidentally, had no means of keeping the cakes cool on a hot June day.

The 'cream' filling for the cakes had been made on Friday evening, kept in the refrigerator overnight, and then piped onto the cakes on Saturday morning. The cakes were then delivered to the various markets. Four samples of the cake were found to contain between eighteen and twenty million staphylococci per gramme. These staphylococci produced a toxin that was responsible for the symptoms of food poisoning. Similar staphylococci were also found in the bakery from a metal mixing bowl and from patches of damaged skin from two bakers who had been concerned in preparation of the cakes.

Another outbreak occurred at a wedding reception where forty of the 139 people at the reception developed vomiting and diarrhoea within two hours of eating a meal that included ham and turkey. The meat had been cut the previous night by someone who had several small septic spots on her left hand that had been used to hold the meat. The cut meat had not been refrigerated but had been stored at room temperature until the next day. Similar strains of staphylococci were isolated from many of those who suffered the food poisoning, from samples of ham and turkey and from the nose and septic spots of the person who had cut the meat.

Discussion

The lessons to be learnt from these outbreaks are clear. Anyone with septic skin lesions should not handle food. If staphylococci do reach food, they can be prevented from multiplying and producing their toxin by refrigeration. In both of these outbreaks food was left for hours at air temperature, and in the case of the cream cakes this amounted to incubation on a hot June day. Staphylococcal toxin is heat-resistant and it will persist in food that is cooked after the staphylococci have multiplied and produced their toxin.

Salmonella food poisoning

Food poisoning by Salmonella organisms is the commonest confirmed cause of this illness in Great Britain. The following two accounts of Salmonella food poisoning are adapted from reports that appeared on page 185 of the *British Medical Journal*, 1970, 4, p. 125–88, No. 5728.

On a Thursday in April a teacher and the housekeeper at a boys' school became ill with vomiting and diarrhoea and the following day three of the boys started to suffer a similar illness. By the following Monday thirty-nine of the 155 boys at the school were absent. After a species of Salmonella had been isolated from one of these boys and other cases notified by general practitioners in the area, investigations of the outbreak were started. Eventually Salmonella organisms were isolated from forty-one boys and four members of the staff who had been ill. It was not possible to identify the particular article of food that had been responsible for the outbreak, but it was assumed that boiled beef eaten at lunch on the day before the first case fell ill was the most likely source of infection. The meals for the school were prepared at the home of a caterer and taken to the school by car, where the food was reheated in the school kitchen. Swabs taken at the caterer's home and from various articles in the school kitchen produced no Salmonellae. The caterer, however, was found to be a symptomless excretor of Salmonellae, and her son, who had had an attack of diarrhoea,

was still excreting Salmonellae two weeks after his illness. Members of the catering staff who were excreting Salmonellae were stopped from work until three samples of faeces were shown to be free of the bacteria, and until all members of their families stopped excreting the bacteria. There was no hand-washing basin in the kitchen toilet and no separate hand-washing facilities in the kitchen, and it was suggested that these deficiencies should be rectified. Hand-washing notices in the kitchen toilet were also introduced.

Another outbreak occurred in August at a sea-side resort. Salmonellae organisms were isolated from a swab of the rectum of an individual who developed an acute attack of diarrhoea six days after arrival at the resort. By the end of the month a further seventeen cases were reported, including one symptomless carrier of the bacteria. These visitors were staying at four different boarding houses and one holiday flat. Some residents of the town also began to develop symptoms of food poisoning. One of these cases suffered from abdominal pain which led to the removal of a normal appendix; he was later found to be excreting Salmonellae. He had become ill a day after eating two meat pies. In the factory producing the pies five out of twenty-five employees were found to be excreting the organisms, and four of these were suffering from diarrhoea. No Salmonellae were isolated from slicing machines and samples of meat from the factory, but these studies were made at the end of August, towards the end of the outbreak. The real culprit of this incident went undiscovered but it was thought possible that it was a foreman butcher whose illness began in the first week in August.

The following account of an outbreak of salmonellosis is adapted from an account appearing on page 777 of the *British Medical Journal*, 1970, 3, 719–78, No. 5725. This outbreak was caused by a common source of salmonellosis—poultry. Infection took place at a wedding reception. Thirty of the fifty-nine people at the reception became ill with vomiting, diarrhoea and abdominal pain within a day of the reception. A species of Salmonella was isolated from twenty-five of those who were ill and also from some individuals who were free of symptoms. The probable cause of the outbreak was infected cooked chicken. Fifteen chickens were served at the wedding reception and these had been cooked in batches and then placed in a refrigerator. In the same refrigerator there were also uncooked chickens and raw fish. Presumably the outbreak was due to the method of storage of cooked and raw birds.

Discussion

Several discussion points arise from these descriptions of outbreaks of salmonellosis but the only one we will pursue is the question of hand-washing by those who prepare food, and in particular hand-washing after a visit to the toilet. Many different kinds of pathogenic organisms—bacteria, viruses and the infective stages of parasitic worms—can be transmitted to food by the hands. From the accounts of staphylococcal food poisoning we have seen how staphylococci from septic spots can be transmitted to foodstuffs. Many otherwise healthy people carry pathogenic staphylococci, chiefly in the nose and on the perineum. The figure for nasal carriers is about 30–50 per cent of the population and this rises to 60–80 per cent for those who work in hospitals. With this level of carriers it is little wonder that staphylococci may contaminate many foodstuffs, particularly those foods that are handled during processing and preparation.

Faecal contamination of hands is important for the spread of a variety of food-borne infections. Investigations of normal faeces has shown that *Clostridium welchii* can be isolated from 100 per cent of faecal specimens if repeated examinations are made. Many of these clostridia are heat sensitive and are not responsible for food poisoning. However, 2–30 per cent of individuals excrete heat-resistant strains in their faeces. The higher percentages are found in individuals who work in institutions. These individuals are what we call symptomless carriers; although they excrete the organisms in the faeces they do not suffer from the symptoms of food poisoning. After an attack of food poisoning, however, the faeces may contain vastly increased numbers of these bacteria.

Clostridia may reach food from many other sources than faecal contamination. The food may be contaminated at source, e.g. meat in the abattoir, or it may become contaminated from flies or kitchen dust. When we come to salmonellosis, however, we find that the most important source of contamination is the intestine of many different vertebrates, including man. When man suffers from Salmonella poisoning, large numbers of Salmonellae are excreted in the faeces— about 10^9 organisms per gramme. This level of excretion is kept up for several weeks and then gradually falls until they disappear from the faeces. An individual who has had an attack of Salmonella food poisoning is thus a potential danger for weeks after the symptoms have disappeared. An even more insidious problem is the number of completely symptomless carriers of Salmonellae that are invariably found in any outbreak of the disease.

It has been estimated that the size of the dose of Salmonella organisms needed to cause symptoms of this form of food poisoning varies from 10^5 to 10^9 bacteria, depending upon the strain of Salmonella. Since the number of Salmonellae in the faeces of an excretor may approach 10 000 million (10^{10}) per gramme of faeces, an infective dose of bacteria can be caused by a very small amount of faeces (10^{-5}g). This amount could readily be transmitted from unwashed hands.

Fungal contamination of food

Fungal spoilage of food crops

The spores of moulds are very widely distributed in the world, and any foodstuff can become contaminated with a wide variety of fungi. Everyone is familiar with the growth of moulds on stale bread, jams etc. Many food crops are prone to mould damage—grains, fruits, vegetables and oil seeds. A conservative estimate of the annual world losses of food due to the activity of micro-organisms has been put at two per cent, but this average loss rises steeply in tropical and subtropical regions where it may soar to as much as 45 per cent of annual production, and the bulk of these losses are due to moulds.

Mycotoxicoses—aflatoxicosis

In addition to damaging foods and making them inedible, the growth of fungi produces another problem by the release of toxins which can affect man and other animals. Diseases caused by these toxins are called mycotoxicoses. The first mycotoxicosis to be discovered was ergotism (St Anthony's fire). This poisoning results from eating rye and other grains that have been contaminated by the fungus called ergot (*Claviceps purpurea*). The substances that cause the disorders in man were isolated and identified in the 1930s and include several alkaloids, all derivatives of lysergic acid. Epidemics of ergotism are now rare; the last outbreak in the U.S.A. was in 1825 although serious epidemics occurred in Russia in 1926–7 and in England in 1928. This particular danger to human food has largely been eliminated but the growth of the fungus on some pasture grasses still causes problems for grazing animals in some parts of the world.

Aflatoxicosis is the most recent kind of poisoning by fungal toxins to have been identified. It was first recognized in 1960 when there were serious outbreaks of disease and death in turkey flocks in the south and east of England. In the first outbreak losses of turkeys were as high as 100 000 birds and the disease was, for want of a better name, called 'Turkey-X' disease. Within a short time, however, a similar disease was found in chickens, ducklings, pigs and young cattle. It was fairly soon recognized that the disease was due to some toxic substance in foodstuffs. The common factor in the various foods was a peanut meal that came from Brazil. Later it was found that samples of peanuts from many countries was contaminated by a toxin that could be extracted from the food and which could cause disease and death in various animals. Furthermore, similar toxins were found in other seeds—oil seeds, grains of various sorts and pulses (peas, beans, etc.). The offending fungus was found in peanuts; it was a fungus called *Aspergillus flavus* and the toxin was thus appropriately named aflatoxin. Several different aflatoxins are now recognized.

When aflatoxins are given in large doses to animals, they are lethal, mainly because of the severe liver damage that results. In smaller doses over longer periods, they cause visible changes in various tissues, including the development of tumours. The first evidence that aflatoxins could produce malignant tumours was seen in 1961 when investigators reported that the inclusion of a toxic peanut meal into a purified rat diet (one part of peanut meal in five parts of food) resulted in the appearance of liver tumours in nine of eleven survivors after six months on the special diet.

Other mycotoxicoses and their significance for human health

In farm animals, many other diseases are caused by the presence of fungal toxins in foodstuffs. These diseases have considerable significance for agriculture and economics. Some of the diseases are also significant for human health, although the full measure of their effect on man is unknown. There is a suspicion that the eating of mouldy food may be one of the factors in the development of cancer of the liver; this cancer is rare in Europe and America (less than 2.5 per cent of all cancers) but relatively common in tropical areas of the Orient and in Central Africa (14 per cent of all cancers). These suspicions apart, there are two mycotoxicoses

that may seriously affect human populations directly. One of these is ergotism (page 158) and the other is a disease called alimentary toxic aleukia (ATA) which has been reported only from the U.S.S.R. There have been frequent and serious outbreaks of this disease in the U.S.S.R. It is a serious and often fatal disease which affects the ability of the bone marrow to produce blood cells of one or more types, and those affected may die of very severe anaemia (deficiency of red cells), haemorrhages (deficiency of platelets) or overwhelming infections (deficiencies of white blood cells). The bone marrow is damaged by eating grains, particularly millet, when these have been left unharvested in the fields over the winter.

Control of the various mycotoxicoses involves changes in agricultural practice and technology —changes in harvesting methods, post-harvest drying, storage and transport. Various precautions are being taken to prevent the contamination of human food by toxins. Thus it has been found that mechanical or electronic sorting of peanuts based on such features as discolouration or size of the nuts can eliminate those that contain aflatoxins.

Food processing in relation to food hygiene

The purposes of food processing are many and include the following:

1. to change the form of the product to make it easier to market and more attractive to the consumer;
2. to inhibit or eliminate factors that will cause deterioration of the food;
3. to kill any pathogenic micro-organisms which may be present;
4. to improve the nutritional value of the food.

Whatever the purpose of processing may be, it can fail to eliminate certain pathogenic micro-organisms; indeed these may be actually introduced during the processing. Thus all food processing has very important implications for food hygiene. New kinds of food are continually appearing on the market, e.g. frozen raw or cooked foods, pre-cooked and ready-to-eat meals. These introduce new ways of handling foods and the need for continual education of the public.

We will consider food processing under the following headings:

1. thermal processing, including pasteurization;

2. freezing;
3. dehydration;
4. use of microbe inhibitors;
5. control of water content;
6. radiation processing.

Thermal processing

Foods which are subjected to thermal processing are exposed to different amounts of heat for different periods of time and they inevitably vary widely in their keeping properties. We will look at three classes of foodstuffs processed by heat:

1. indefinitely stable products, e.g. some canned foods,
2. products of limited stability,
3. perishable products, including pasteurized and pre-cooked products.

Indefinitely stable products

A stable food is one which is processed in such a way that the number or activity of micro-organisms is reduced to such a level that few if any can be detected in the treated food. No spoilage of microbial origin will occur no matter how long the food is stored—provided, of course, that it is not re-contaminated, e.g. by puncture of a can. Foodstuffs of this kind include canned meats, vegetables or fruits, and vegetables and pickles stored in hermetically sealed containers. If the foodstuff has a pH over 4.5 (e.g. meats) then the thermal processing must be adequate to destroy the spores of *Clostridium botulinum*. Provided this requirement is met then the food is indefinitely stable and safe—unless contamination occurs as a result of imperfect sealing of the container. Less thorough heat processing is needed for acid fruits, vegetables and pickles with a pH below 4.5. *Cl. botulinum* spores cannot grow in a strongly acid medium. To make such foodstuffs indefinitely stable, they need only be processed in such a way to prevent the growth of organisms which might cause spoilage.

Products of limited stability

The texture and flavour of some foods are altered by the degree of heat processing which is necessary to destroy spores of *Cl. botulinum*. Hams, for example, are sometimes marketed in hermetically sealed cans after a mild heat treatment. Such products are not, however, indefinitely stable at room temperatures and they must be refrigerated. Sometimes they contain toxigenic staphylococci and they may present

a health danger if they are not properly handled. These products should be subjected to strict marketing control.

Perishable products

Pasteurization

Milk usually contains a wide variety of micro-organisms which will cause spoilage within a short period of time unless the milk is pasteurized and refrigerated. We have dealt with milk as a health hazard and the pasteurization process in more detail in Chapter 12. Here we will say that pasteurization is a mild form of heat treatment which reduces the number of micro-organisms present to such a degree that when properly packaged, handled and refrigerated it will remain in a satisfactory microbiological condition for a much longer time.

In addition to the micro-organisms which cause spoilage of the milk (i.e. 'souring', 'curdling') milk may contain pathogenic micro-organisms of many kinds, e.g. bovine tuberculosis, Brucella, streptococci, staphylococci etc. This fact must be taken into account in determining the temperature and other conditions of the pasteurization process. Furthermore, milk and milk products must be protected from recontamination after they have been pasteurized, for they may form an excellent culture medium for organisms such as *Salmonella paratyphi*.

Fruit juices are also processed by pasteurization. Fruit juices present fewer problems than milk. They are acid (i.e. have a low pH and do not encourage the growth of pathogenic micro-organisms or toxin producers. The main problem is the spoilage which results from the growth of yeasts and fungi. A much lower pasteurization temperature can be used for fruit juices compared to milk. Heat treatment which destroys the yeasts is usually sufficient.

Pre-cooked products

These include an enormous number of different food products which may contain a variety of ingredients, each of which may introduce different kinds of micro-organisms to the finished foodstuff. It must always be borne in mind that Salmonella organisms may be present (e.g. from meat, eggs, coconut) and that heat treatment must be adequate to kill these pathogens. This treatment does not, however, destroy spore-forming micro-organisms, e.g. *Cl. botulinum*, which may be present in vegetable and cereal ingredients. The products must be frozen or refrigerated after cooking. Recontamination of such foodstuffs, e.g. in packing, storage or after thawing, may be very dangerous since the foods usually have a high pH (i.e. are not acid), with perfect nutritive conditions for micro-organisms which can grow and multiply rapidly if the food is allowed to stand at room temperature.

Freezing

In many countries a great variety of food is marketed in the frozen form—meat, poultry, fish, shellfish, fruit, vegetables. Many of these foods are frozen in the raw state so that control of microbial content by hygienic handling is all that can be relied upon to render them safe. The freezing process does not necessarily kill micro-organisms, and spore-bearing organisms are particularly resistant to freezing. There may be a gradual reduction in the number of bacteria present after prolonged freezing, but even prolonged storage does not ensure the elimination of pathogens.

Some frozen foods are so widely distributed—sometimes across the world—that it is essential that they should present no health hazard. This can only be achieved by hygienic preparation, handling, storage and adequate and safe packaging to prevent recontamination of the foodstuff.

When frozen foods are removed from the freezer, bacterial growth and multiplication will occur as soon as the temperature of the food rises. They should be eaten soon after thawing. If the frozen food is to be cooked before being eaten (fowl, joints of meat) it is very important that the thawing process should be complete before the food is cooked. Frozen poultry can be particularly dangerous if it is cooked before thawing is complete; the cooked poultry may be removed from the oven before the frozen interior of the carcass has been exposed to an adequate temperature for an adequate period to kill pathogens such as Salmonella organisms. Frozen poultry should carry a label to this effect, but unfortunately many do not. The refreezing of thawed foodstuffs is a particularly dangerous habit because of the increase in the number of bacteria which has occurred during the thawing process, when new microbes may also reach the food by contamination from handling, air, dust.

Some frozen foods—shellfish, dairy products, sauces etc. may be eaten without cooking. These foods need special packaging to prevent contamination during storage. Other frozen foods, e.g. ready-to-bake meat pies and fruit pies, are cooked before eating, and these should be adequately cooked so that they present no risk to health.

Dehydration

There are many kinds of dehydrated food on the market and each present their own particular micro-biological problem. These foods are very useful to the food industry because they are light in weight and they keep well. Dehydrated food is stable because the water which is needed for bacterial growth and reproduction has been removed from the food. Food may be dehydrated in various ways:

1. spray drying,
2. hot-air drying,
3. open-air drying,
4. freeze-drying.

In spray drying, liquid foods such as skimmed milk and eggs are rapidly sprayed into a fast moving stream of hot air which removes moisture from the food, leaving a powder containing little moisture. The drying process cannot be relied upon to kill micro-organisms; although the temperature in the drying chamber is high, the small food particles are cooled by the evaporation of their water so that the particles never reach a high enough temperature to kill micro-organisms. Spray-dried foods tend to re-absorb water from the atmosphere, i.e. they are hygroscopic. This means that they have to be packed in air-tight tins or plastic bags. This kind of packaging has the added advantage of preventing microbial contamination of the dried food.

Some meats, fruit and vegetables are dried on trays in hot air tunnels. This process reduces the number of microbes in the food but it cannot be guaranteed to produce a hygienic product—indeed, if the trays are overloaded the drying process is slowed and bacterial multiplication occurs in the warm moist food. The food must thus enter the drier in a clean condition and should have been prepared and handled in a hygienic fashion. To prevent changes in colour and flavour, many fruits are treated with sulphur dioxide; this, together with the low pH of most fruits, gives some protection against bacterial contamination. Meat and vegetables, with a higher pH, have no such protection and great care should be taken to prevent bacterial contamination of these foods.

In some countries large amounts of food such as fish, meat and fruit may be dried in the open air. In this situation foods are exposed to contamination of many kinds—air, dust, insects, birds, rodents—and little can be done to control the bacterial content of such foodstuffs. The only safeguard is thorough cooking of the food by the consumer.

are now dried by the process of ; these include meat, poultry, fish, it and vegetables. The food to be s way may be either raw or cooked. : freeze-drying process food is frozen ially in the form of small pieces or slices. The frozen food is then placed in a vacuum dehydrator and subjected to a high vacuum, i.e. air is pumped out of the chamber and the food subjected to negative pressure. Moisture evaporates from the surface of the frozen food by sublimation, i.e. it passes from the solid state (ice) into water vapour without liquefying. After completion of the process the food is a spongy mass with a water content of only 2–5 per cent. This method of drying preserves the natural texture and appearance of the food to a much greater degree than does conventional hot-air drying.

Like other forms of drying, freeze-drying kills few bacteria. The food product contains essentially the same micro-organisms that were present before drying. For this reason strict sanitary standards must be maintained, particularly since freeze-drying entails considerable handling of the food by workers. Like all dried foods, protective packaging is needed with freeze-dried products to prevent the absorption of water which will obviously encourage bacterial growth.

Use of microbe inhibitors

Many different kinds of foodstuffs can be preserved by the presence or addition of substances which slow down the growth of some micro-organisms. These do not kill the micro-organisms, which thus remain on the food product.

Natural inhibitors

(a) Lactic acid, present in fermented shredded cabbage—sauerkraut, cucumber fermented in brine, fermented salt herrings followed by canning in acid sauce without heat treatment.

(b) Acetic acid, added hot to pickles and some meat and fish products.

(c) Fatty acids, produced in the fermentation of many types of cheese. Note that food poisoning organisms and other pathogens that enter the cheese after it has been pasteurized can survive the remaining processing.

(d) Alcohol, e.g. produced during alcoholic fermentation in wine production. Pro-

ducts processed by alcoholic fermentation must be sealed to exclude oxygen. Sugar, which is necessary for the growth of yeast, is removed by the fermentation process and converted into alcohol. The alcohol inhibits only the growth of organisms which may cause spoilage.

Additives

(a) Salt—dry salted meat and fish can be kept without deterioration for long periods since the high salt content inhibits both bacterial growth and enzymatic action in the tissues which leads to putrefaction. Note that pathogens may persist in brine-cured products.

(b) Smoke. Some meat products—ham, bacon etc.—are smoked after being cured in salt. The smoke dries the surface of the meat and also contains substances which retard the growth of micro-organisms. Many kinds of fish—eel, salmon, trout etc.—are exposed to a smoking process which slightly cooks them, dries their surface and deposits substances which act as surface preservatives. Such products are usually not salted or only slightly so, and they have occasionally given rise to food poisoning, sometimes with the fatal *Cl. botulinum*. Note that smoking, curing and brine-preserving do not guarantee the absence of pathogens.

(c) Chemical inhibitors—sodium benzoate, trichloroacetic acid etc. These substances are used to control certain kinds of spoilage organisms but they are not effective against a wide range of micro-organisms.

(d) Antibiotics. Some countries, but not Great Britain, permit the use of antibiotics to inhibit the growth of spoilage organisms in some foods.

Control of water content by the addition of sugar

We have seen that some foods can be processed to improve their keeping life by various types of drying. Sugar also acts as a preservative when it is present in high concentrations. Concentrated sugar syrups do not undergo spoilage because they have only a low water activity. Water activity is a way of expressing *available* moisture content, and it is the vapour pressure of the solution divided by the vapour pressure of water. Because of the large amount of sugar which is present, the water is not available for the activity of micro-organisms and this inhibits the germination of bacterial spores and the growth of vegetative cells. Thus honey and jams do not spoil readily. Fruits may be preserved in concentrated sugar solutions or by crystallized sugar (glacé fruits). Sugar also preserves condensed milk (produced by pasteurization of milk followed by concentration (removal of water) and the addition of sugar. If pathogens are present in such a product then it means that contamination or leakage of the container has occurred.

Radiation processing

The use of ionizing radiation for the processing of food has been studied in many countries over the last eighteen years. These studies have shown that irradiation of food can not only control the micro-organisms that cause spoilage of food, but also those that can endanger health. In addition irradiation can control animal parasites in food and also insects that live and multiply in the foodstuffs. *Small* doses of radiation can kill most of the non-sporing organisms that cause spoilage of food and those that are potential pathogens. These small doses of radiation produce their effects without altering the appearance or the taste of food. Either raw or cooked foods can be treated in this way. To destroy *all* micro-organisms, including spore-formers, larger doses of radiation are needed; this treatment produces food that is stable for indefinite periods provided that the food is protected from subsequent contamination by micro-organisms.

Advantage of radiation

The advantages of radiation processing are obvious. The 'shelf-life' of many types of raw or cooked foods (fruit, meat, fish and eggs) can be prolonged without changing the appearance or the taste of foods. Furthermore this can be carried out with the food already in sealed containers so that after irradiation the food is safe from recontamination with bacteria.

Disadvantage of radiation

Irradiated food is still a novelty, and there is too little experience of the effects of this food on human health for us to know all the disadvantages of this method of food processing. One certain disadvantage is that the dose of radiation that kills most of the non-sporing micro-organisms does not destroy the enzymes natur-

ally present in the foodstuff. The activity of many of these enzymes produces a gradual deterioration in the quality of the foodstuff—its appearance, texture, flavour and so on. Although food altered in this way may well be safe to eat, it is not attractive to the consumer. Irradiated food may thus have to be refrigerated to slow down this action of enzymes. Higher doses of radiation *can* inactivate the enzymes, but the higher doses *may* affect the flavour of the food. The flavour of beef is changed markedly at high radiation doses, although that of chicken or pork is unaltered. Thus the dose of radiation used has to be chosen bearing in mind the kind of food and the aims of processing.

Another disadvantage of radiation is that viruses are resistant to this kind of processing and can only be destroyed by doses far greater than those that kill bacteria. If viruses are present then some other type of processing is needed. If, however, it is not important to maintain the fresh nature of the food then a combination of radiation and mild heat treatment (e.g. 60 °C) can destroy bacteria and inactivate some enzymes and some viruses.

The acceptance of irradiation processing

In many countries radiation processing has received an unenthusiastic reception and the early hopes that radiation would give an easy, cheap and safe way of preserving food have yet to be realized. The U.S. Food and Drug Administration (FDA) recently turned down an application by the American army for approval of irradiation sterilization of canned ham. Studies by the FDA of the army's test results showed that in experimental animals the eating of irradiated food led to a higher infant mortality, adverse effects on body weight and on the number of red cells in the blood, and also an increased number of animals with cataracts or tumours. In America irradiated food comes under the 1958 amendment to the Food, Drug and Cosmetic Act. Under this law, food irradiation must be proved safe and it also must be shown to be a significant advance over existing methods of food preservation. The action of the FDA has delayed the construction of massive food irradiation plants in America. These will have to wait for further investigations on the safety of irradiated food—although the FDA *has* approved irradiation treatment of bacon, wheat (for insect disinfestation) and potatoes (to prevent sprouting).

In Britain the working party on the irradiation of food which reported in 1964 (Ministry of

Health 1964) recommended that irradiation of food for human consumption should generally be prohibited, and that special exemptions from this general prohibition must be applied for. In 1967 regulations made it an offence to irradiate food except in *very* small doses (not more than 10 rad). In May 1967 the Advisory Committee on the irradiation of food was set up to examine applications for exemptions from the general prohibition, and in 1969 a special exemption was made for the irradiation of food for patients who need a sterile diet as part of their treatment. Some types of patients are particularly likely to succumb to overwhelming infection because of a general reduction in their resistance to infection. This may be the result of the disease from which they are suffering (e.g. a marked fall in the number of white cells in the blood) or a result of drugs which interfere with resistance.

These patients are more likely to survive if they are housed in a pre-sterilized room and by restricting human contact to a minimum. They also need sterilized food. Food treated by irradiation has proved to be very satisfactory; these foods are not only sterile but they lose little of their palatability. Complete meals are prepared, packaged, frozen and then irradiated by passing the frozen packages on a conveyor belt around a source of radiation (cobalt 60). After irradiation, most foods are stored frozen until required.

It must be emphasized that these new regulations apply only to food for patients needing a sterile diet as an essential part of their treatment. Because of the serious nature of the illnesses they suffer from and because of the relatively short period of treatment the relaxation of the law would appear to be justified, and it has been welcomed by the few special hospital units that treat various kinds of patient in a sterile environment.

There are two forthcoming applications for exemptions from the general prohibition. One application is for the use of irradiation to eliminate Salmonellae from frozen horse meat that is imported for use in pet foods. At the moment the frozen blocks of meat have to be thawed and then heated to kill the bacteria. Irradiation would greatly simplify the processing of this food. A second application is for the

Table 15 Uses of radiation processing

Country	Food	Purpose of irradiation
U.S.S.R.	Potatoes	Sprout inhibition
	Grain	Insect disinfestation
	Dried fruits	Insect disinfestation
	Fresh fruit and vegetables	Radurization (i.e. pasteurization by radiation treatment) producing extension of market life
	Semi-prepared raw beef, pork and rabbit products in plastic bags	Radurization
	Eviscerated poultry in plastic bags	Radurization
	Cooked meat products in plastic bags	Radurization
	Onions	Sprout inhibition
Netherlands	Asparagus	Radurization
	Cacao beans	Disinfestation
	Strawberries	Radurization
	Mushrooms	Radurization
	Potatoes	Sprout inhibition
Israel	Potatoes	Sprout inhibition
	Onions	Sprout inhibition

Note. Many of the above irradiated foods are being produced in experimental batches only, to test consumer responses or to study the economic advantages of irradiation.

irradiation of white fish, sufficient to extend the 'shelf life' of the food for a few days; this would greatly assist in the distribution of this highly perishable food. However, it appears that much more basic research will have to be carried out on the effects of irradiated food in animals before irradiation has a chance of rivalling the time-honoured techniques of canning, drying, refrigeration and so on, at least in countries such as Great Britain and the U.S.A. Some countries have been much less conservative in their attitude towards irradiation, particularly the U.S.S.R., the Netherlands and Israel. Listed in Table 15 are the uses of irradiation in these countries, and the list illustrates the versatility of the applications of irradiation.

Poisonous animals and plants

Introduction

No account of the dangers of food for human health would be complete without some mention of the many animals and plants that produce acute poisoning if they are eaten by man. These poisons are present in the living animal or plant and are not the by-product of some strain of bacteria or fungus that has contaminated the raw or cooked food. Man has always faced this problem of distinguishing the animals and plants that are poisonous from those that can be safely eaten. The distinction between safe and poisonous foods is often straightforward in that some organisms are always poisonous, but sometimes the position is uncertain, for other organisms are at some times safe and at other times poisonous.

It is difficult to assess the extent of illness or death in the world due to eating poisonous animals or plants, and much of this uncertainty comes from poor reporting of cases. No part of the world is, however, free from poisonous animals or plants. The education of all children should include the development of a cautious attitude to unfamiliar plants and animals, and even to the unusual parts of familiar food plants. One source estimates 12 000 plant poisonings a year in children in the U.S.A. alone, and between 1940 and 1960 there were 72 deaths from these poisonings.

Poisonous plants

The nature of poisonous plants varies widely from country to country, and here we will mention only the common poisonous plants of Great Britain. These include laburnum, deadly

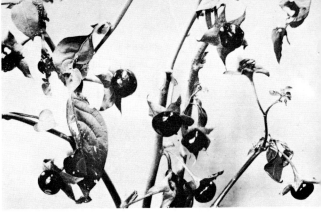

Figure 14.8 (above)   Deadly nightshade. (*Photograph from Natural History Photographic Agency.*)

Figure 14.9 (below)   *Amanita phalloides*, the 'Death-cap' or 'Destroying angel'. It has a shining greenish yellow or olive surface, yet this is the species most frequently mistaken for an edible mushroom, often with fatal results. The two are not at all alike at maturity but the 'button' stage—when both are white —are rather similar. (*Photograph from Natural History Photographic Agency.*)

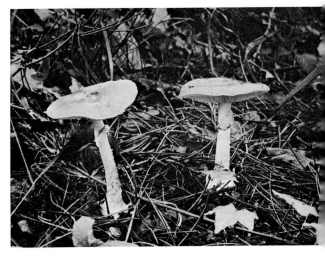

Figure 14.10 (below)   The fly agaric *Amanita muscaria*. (*Photograph by S. C. Bisserot, Bruce Coleman Ltd.*)

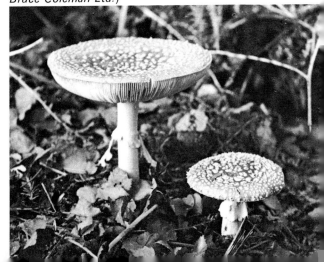

nightshade (Figure 14.8), hemlock, monkshood, holly berries, yew berries, Daphne berries, sweet pea, iris rootstocks, jasmine, mistletoe, wisteria and various mushrooms. The task of distinguishing poisonous from non-poisonous mushrooms is one for the expert, and it should be a general rule that only cultivated mushrooms bought from a reputable shop should be eaten. We can mention two particularly poisonous mushrooms. *Amanita phalloides* is aptly called the death angel and is one of the most poisonous of plants (Figure 14.9). If this mushroom is eaten, death occurs in 50–90 per cent of all cases, usually two to eight days after eating the plants. There is an antiserum that is said to be effective if it is given soon after the symptoms appear. In France, where mushroom shows are held annually, poisoning by the death angel is not uncommon and the law requires that anti-phalloidian serum should be available to all doctors. This serum is not generally available in Great Britain and, like the anti-venom for adder bites, its safety and protective effects are in doubt. Another highly poisonous mushroom is the fly agaric, *Amanita muscaria* (Figure 14.10). Poisoning by this mushroom is now rare, probably because it is unlike other poisonous mushrooms in that its appearance is so striking that it is easily identifiable; the cap is large (7–20 cm across) and is bright yellow to orange-red. On the continent of Europe the collection of edible fungi is a fairly common pastime and accounts for the number of reports of poisoning. It takes very little of a mushroom to produce poisoning, and the symptoms of abdominal pain, vomiting, visual disturbances and perhaps eventual coma will occur even when the mushrooms have been cooked. Even so-called experts can collect and eat poisonous mushrooms. The more conservative British palate ensures relative freedom from this sort of poisoning and cases are more likely to be children.

Several common edible plants have parts that are poisonous. In the case of the rhubarb the stalk is edible but the leaf is toxic and can produce fatal poisoning. Apples as usually eaten are safe but the consumption of large numbers of apple seeds can be fatal because they contain cyanogens and liberate the highly poisonous hydrocyanic acid (prussic acid) in the body. Even the common potato can sometimes be poisonous. The sprouts of the potato and the green tissues of potatoes that have been exposed to light can contain enough of a toxin called solanine to produce severe poisoning and even death.

Poisonous animals

Throughout the world poisonous animals produce more illness and death than do poisonous plants. The exact size of the problem is unknown but in Great Britain it is small. Few people in these islands eat sea anemones, starfish, sea urchins, sea cucumbers, octopus, squid, moray eels, lampreys, puffers, fugi fish etc. that may cause poisoning in other countries, nor do they eat sled dogs, seals and polar bears (Figure 14.11) which may contain so much vitamin A, particularly in the liver, as to be highly toxic. The main risk in Britain comes from molluscs—mussels, scallops, oysters and so on. Indeed, since about two million metric tons of sea molluscs are eaten annually in the world, poisoning by molluscs is the most important fraction of poisoning by animals. We have already seen how molluscs, particularly if they are filter feeders and so can concentrate bacteria from sea water in their bodies, can transmit such diseases as typhoid fever (see page 140). The most common kind of poisoning from eating molluscs is due to the presence in their bodies of minute unicellular plants (dinoflagellates) that form part of the 'soup' of living creatures in surface waters that we call plankton. In some seasons certain dinoflagellates multiply so extensively that the sea is coloured by the multitude of their minute coloured bodies, the so-called poisonous red tide. Different dinoflagellates produce different kinds of toxins; in some cases a single mollusc can concentrate enough of these creatures in its body to produce a fatal toxic dose, and numerous cases of death from this source have been reported from many countries. 'Red tide' and poisonous molluscs occasionally occur on the coasts of Great Britain; innumerable numbers of fish and large numbers of birds died off the coast of Northumberland and Durham in the summer of 1968, and about seventy people in the Newcastle and Durham area suffered from a kind of gastro-enteritis in which some patients showed symptoms of damage to the nervous system. In the Farne islands only about a hundred shags could be counted in a population that normally numbers at least 2000 birds; some of the dying birds had lost their powers of muscular coordination and sat on their breasts rather than their feet. The human cases of poisoning was traced to mussels, and indeed pigeons that fluttered down to the mussel beds to feed died rapidly of a potent toxin. This outbreak of human and animal poisoning was attributed to poisonous dinoflagellates (Figure 14.12). Among the various dinoflagellates that

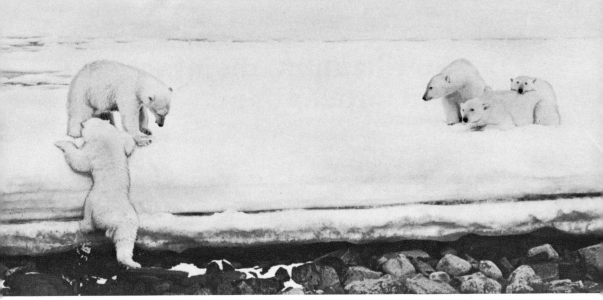

Figure 14.11   Polar bear meat, in particular the liver, may be highly toxic because of the unusually large amounts of vitamin A that it contains. (*Photograph by Suen Gillsaten, Bruce Coleman Ltd.*)

may cause these outbreaks of poisoning one species produces an extremely powerful toxin—paralytic shellfish poison (PSP)—which is said to be more potent than botulinum toxin (page 153). The symptoms of this kind of mollusc poisoning are tingling or burning of parts of the face which spreads to other parts of the body. Numbness in these parts develops later and there may be dizziness, aching joints, excessive salivation, intense thirst and difficulty in swallowing or in moving various muscles. If muscular paralysis increases then death may result. In some parts of the world outbreaks of 'red tide' may contain so many poisonous dinoflagellates that spray from the tide can cause irritation of the lungs. These toxins are usually heat-stable substances and are not destroyed by cooking. As in most types of poisoning, first treatment consists in trying to remove all the swallowed shellfish by making the patient vomit or by washing out the stomach. Alkaline fluids such as baking soda may be of use because the toxin is unstable in alkaline solution. In this and many other poisonings no specific antidote is available, and symptoms have to be treated as they occur; this may include artificial respiration if paralysis is severe.

Poisoning by fish is very uncommon in Great Britain because we eat familiar fish that are almost always safe (this, of course, may well not be true in the future if the increasingly polluted seas enable familiar fish to concentrate such poisons as pesticides and mercury (see page 139). In the tropics, however, many fish become poisonous by feeding on poisonous organisms.

More than 300 different species of fish have been reported to cause poisoning; puffer fish seem to have the most potent toxin since mortality after eating this fish may be as high as 50 per cent.

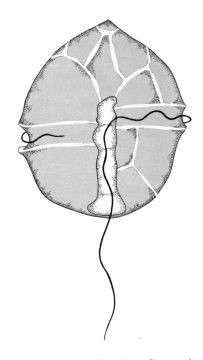

Figure 14.12   A dinoflagellate *Gonyaulax tamarensis* which was responsible for a recent outbreak of poisonous red tide in Britain. The organism is only 36 μm in length. (*Based on a drawing by Dr P. A. Ayres, Ministry of Agriculture and Fisheries Laboratory, Burnham-on-Crouch.*)

15. Sterilization, disinfectants, and antiseptics

In various parts of the book we have discussed the destruction of living micro-organisms in or on a variety of materials by an almost equally varied range of techniques. Here we will generally review the aims and techniques of destroying micro-organisms.

Pasteur and Lister

The development of techniques to destroy micro-organisms—bacteria, fungi and viruses—had naturally to await the recognition of these organisms as causes of disease and decay (see Chapter 1). The influence of Pasteur was thus profound. Before the studies of Pasteur, the state of surgery was depressing both to surgeons and patient alike. The introduction of general anaesthetics such as chloroform in the early part of the nineteenth century permitted rapid advancements in the techniques of surgery; operations that were previously quite impossible because of the pain they caused now became practicable. However, the deeper the surgeon went into the human body, the greater was the risk of wound infection. At this period every surgical operation was followed by a period of fever and pain, and commonly by such diseases as tetanus (page 69), erysipelas (page 73), septicaemia of various sorts and gangrene. This was the state of affairs when Joseph Lister took up his post of Regius Professor of Systematic Surgery in the University of Glasgow in 1860.

Lister was soon to come under the influence of Pasteur's findings. He began to reject the vague ideas of 'poisonous miasmas' as a cause of wound infection, and he developed techniques to rid the hospital environment of those unseen living organisms that Pasteur had indicated were the cause of infectious disease. Of course, Pasteur had already paved the way by showing that micro-organisms could be killed by various methods such as heat, by filtration, or by the use of certain chemicals. Lister developed chemical methods for the destruction of micro-organisms, and he chose for this purpose crude carbolic acid. His experiments with carbolic acid applied to wounds, surgical instruments, ligatures, and even to the surgeon's hands and the air in the operating room, soon produced a marked fall in the number of post-operative infections in his ward. In spite of strong opposition to his views and techniques, his methods were adopted by more and more surgeons. Lister himself soon realized that he could now enter joints, a field which had previously been closed to surgical attack because of the disastrous consequences of infection of joints and bones.

The surgeons who followed Lister tried to reduce their dependence on antiseptics, and their aim was to exclude micro-organisms from the area exposed by the surgeon's knife rather than killing the organisms after they have been introduced. This was the replacement of antiseptic surgery by aseptic surgery, achieved by the use of sterilized rubber gloves, the steam sterilization of dressings, gowns, caps and masks, better methods of sterilizing catgut and of killing micro-organisms on the patient's skin before it was cut open by the scalpel.

The meaning of the terms antiseptic, disinfectant and sterilization

The techniques for destroying micro-organisms thus first arose from the needs of surgery, but they were soon applied to the prevention of cross-infection between patients and to increase the safety of food, milk and water etc. We must now clearly define these terms antiseptics, disinfectants and sterilization.

Sterilization describes the destruction or removal of *all* micro-organisms. This process, e.g. in the preparation of dressings, instruments, drugs, ligatures and the like, can seldom be achieved by the use of chemicals. The only reliable method of sterilization is by physical means such as heat, filtration or gamma irradiation. These physical methods are described briefly on pages 169–172.

Disinfectants and antiseptics are chemical substances that destroy micro-organisms, although in the ways that they are used they do not usually destroy *all* micro-organisms; they are used to destroy *most* harmful micro-organisms. The term antiseptic is used for a chemical that is used on a living surface such as skin, whereas the term disinfectant is used for a chemical that is used on an inanimate surface such as cutlery, crockery, drains, working surfaces etc.

Sterilization techniques

We have seen that sterilization is the removal of all life of any form from an object or material. There are many kinds of material that require sterilization. Liquids that require sterilization include:

1. culture media for micro-biological work,
2. water for sterile processes,
3. liquids to be injected into the body,
4. some creams e.g. those for use on the eye.

Solids requiring sterilization are micro-biological equipment, clothing and instruments for operating theatres, walls, floors, ceilings etc. 'sterile' rooms and operating theatres; drugs and vaccines.

Also the air for 'sterile' rooms, operating theatres etc. must be sterilized. The method of sterilization depends on the material to be sterilized. The various techniques use heat, filtration, radiation and gases.

The use of heat for sterilization

Heat is very widely used for sterilization. The material may be heated in a dry oven or heated by means of steam (e.g. in an autoclave, see below). If the material to be sterilized is in a liquid, e.g. canned foods, then heat is applied to raise the temperature of the liquid. Non-perishable objects such as surgical instruments and dressing can be heat sterilized. Living vaccines and some drugs would be made useless by heat treatment and another technique, such as filtration, is needed. Plastics which may be damaged by heat can be sterilized by exposure to gamma radiation.

The heat treatment of foods

The use of heat is one of the oldest ways of processing food. Food is heated to make it edible, palatable and safe. We are here concerned with the effects of this form of processing on the safety of food. Heating is the most important method of killing bacteria, viruses, parasites (e.g. the bladder-worm stage of tapeworms in meat) and some toxins. If all foods were boiled or heated to 100 °C, shortly before eating them, then food-borne diseases would never occur, with the exception of staphylococcal food poisoning (staphylococcal toxin is stable to heat)—and the poisoning due to toxins found in some plants, fungi and animals that are heat-resistant.

The degree of heat treatment that is used in commercial food processing depends upon the kind of food, the kind of micro-organisms which commonly occur in the food, and the temperature at which the food will be stored after heat treatment. It is difficult to give a precise answer to the question of the minimum temperature needed to kill commonly occurring pathogenic bacteria in food. The answer depends on the

Table 16 The resistance of non-sporing bacteria to heat

Food	Temperature (°C)	Duration of exposure (seconds)	Organism	Destruction
Milk	60	1800	*Mycobacterium tuberculosis*	Incomplete
	62.8	1800	*Mycobacterium tuberculosis*	Complete
	71.7	15	*Mycobacterium tuberculosis*	Complete
Cured ham	55	3600	*Brucella abortus*	Complete
	63	18	*Brucella abortus*	Complete
Milk	60	198	*Staphylococcus aureus*	90 per cent
Custard	60	462	*Staphylococcus aureus*	90 per cent
Beef soup	60	150	*Staphylococcus aureus*	90 per cent
Liquid egg	55	600	Salmonella	90 per cent

type of bacteria, whether or not they are in the vegetative form or in the stage of resistant spores, and upon the duration of exposure to heat. When bacterial cells or spores are exposed to heat the number killed depends both on the cooking temperature and on the duration of exposure to heat. Table 16 gives data which illustrates the effect of both absolute temperature, the nature of food, and the duration of exposure to heat, on various pathogens.

Those who heat-process foods on a commercial basis need to have very exact information of the effect of heat on bacteria. Fortunately it is possible to predict the survival of bacteria and spores after a particular kind of heat treatment. When bacteria are exposed to heat, the proportion that survive at any particular time during the processing can be plotted against the period of heat treatment to give what is called a 'survival curve' (Figure 15.1). This curve is often exponential, and if one plots the logarithm of survivors against time in arithmetic units a straight line is obtained. From this type of graph it is possible to express the *heat resistance* as the number of minutes it takes to kill 90 per cent of the spores or vegetative cells at a definite temperature; this is called the D value. In the case of bacterial spores the reference temperature is usually 121.1 °C: the highest heat resistance values (D 250) is for some kinds of *Cl. botulinum* spores, these have a D 250 of 0.204 minutes, i.e. at 250 °C, 90 per cent of the spores are killed after 0.204 minutes. The survival time increases dramatically when the heating temperature decreases, usually by a factor of ten for a fall in temperature of 10 °C, i.e. the D value of *Clostridium botulinum* spores is 0.204 min at 121.1 °C, 2.04 at 111.1 °C, 20.4 at 101.1 °C, 204 at 91.1 °C.

This kind of information is very important in planning heat treatment of canned foods which may be stored for long periods before the food is eaten. Because of the variability in the heat resistance of spores, probably no heat treatment will kill *all* spores in *all* cans, but the use of these calculations can help to plan heat treatments that reduce the number of living spores to a very low level. Because vegetative bacteria are so heat-sensitive compared to spores, no system has been developed for the calculation of minimum safe-heat processing (pasteurization of milk is an exception, see page 126). In recent years, however, the discovery of heat-resistant strains of Salmonellae have led to the laying down of standards of pasteurization for liquid egg.

Not all kinds of tinned foods are subjected to the kind of heat treatment that is necessary to

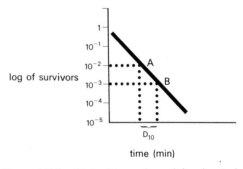

Figure 15.1 Plot of log. of surviving bacteria against time in arithmetic units at a constant temperature.
A and B represent two points on the survival curve corresponding with surviving fractions of 10^{-2} and 10^{-3} of the original count.
The interval on the time scale D depends only on the slope of the line and is independent of the actual values of the surviving fractions.
D value, D_{10} value or the decimal reduction time (DRT) is the time needed to inactivate 90 per cent of the cells present at any moment. The time needed to reduce the population to $\frac{1}{10}$ of its number will be the interval during which the straight line crosses one complete logarithmic cycle, i.e. between points A and B.

kill *Cl. botulinum* spores. The acidity of some foods (fruits, fruit juices etc.) inhibits the growth of all known food poisoning organisms except fungi, and tinned foods of this kind are heat-processed only to ensure 'shelf life'.

Autoclaves

The autoclave is the best known and most widely used piece of equipment that is used for heat sterilization. There are many types of autoclaves but the essentials of the apparatus are very similar and are shown in Figure 15.2. The wall of the autoclave is a steel shell in which there is a door for loading and unloading the apparatus. Around the steel shell there is a steam jacket. The main shell and the jacket are fed with steam independently and each is fitted with a temperature indicator. After the material to be sterilized has been placed in the autoclave and the door closed then air is pumped out of the instrument, creating a vacuum. The air may be displaced by a flow of steam or it may be pumped out. Steam is now introduced into the autoclave under pressure. The time of exposure of the materials to the steam depends upon the temperature and the pressure in the autoclave. Unless the material being sterilized is very heat-sensitive or has a high heat capacity, the temperatures and times in Table 17 are regarded as being adequate (after J. J. Perkins, 1956).

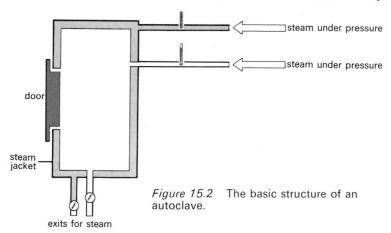

Figure 15.2 The basic structure of an autoclave.

Table 17 Sterilization times at various temperatures

Temperature (°C)	Time (minutes)
116	30
118	18
121	12
125	8
132	2

pressure 138–172 kNm (20–25 p.s.i.g.)

Autoclaving will destroy vegetative bacteria, spores and viruses. Moist heat, as in the autoclave, will sterilize at much lower temperatures than dry heat because latent heat is liberated when steam condenses on the material being sterilized. Many spores are highly resistant to dry heat, and relatively high temperatures must be used to kill them.

The efficiency of autoclaves must be tested periodically. Various methods are available which include the use of cards impregnated with a heat-sensitive material that changes colour in proportion to the temperature at the time of heating. Another method is to use a test paper impregnated with spores of a heat-resistant bacteria.

Sterilization by filtration

Air or heat-sensitive liquids can be sterilized by filtration through materials that hold back micro-organisms in the mesh of the filter. There are many types of filter materials used, e.g. beds of fibrous material (paper, cotton, wool, glass etc.), ceramic candles, and membranes of various types. Membrane filters (usually of mixed cellulose esters) are available in a wide range of pore sizes. It is usually necessary to filter under pressure. Examples of material that are sterilized by this technique include solutions for injection, and antibiotics such as penicillin or streptomycin that are filtered to produce sterile solutions before the final crystallization or freeze-drying operation (see page 162) under aseptic conditions.

Radiation sterilization

The effects of electromagnetic radiation on micro-organisms increase with the frequency of the radiation. Visible light has little effect on bacteria, nothing more than a warming effect. With shorter wave-lengths, such as ultra-violet radiation, mutation and finally death can result if the dosage is high enough. X-rays and gamma rays are much more effective in destroying micro-organisms and can be used very effectively for sterilization. This technique is now used for medical and surgical instruments, particularly of the 'disposable' type made of plastic which cannot withstand heat treatment. Food can also be sterilized by radiation (see page 163).

Three main types of radiation are used for sterilization on a large scale—gamma radiation, accelerated electron beams and ultra-violet radiation. Gamma radiation from radio-isotopes is a powerful penetrating radiation that enables simple and readily controlled sterilization of certain materials, e.g. bandages, disposable hypodermic syringes, scalpels, sutures etc. Cobalt 60 is one of the best sources of gamma radiation, and the usual sterilizing dose is about 2.4 Mega rad (1 Mega rad equals 10^6 rad; 1 rad is the quantity of radiation which results in the absorption of 100 ergs/g). Accelerated electron beams (e.g. from the Van de Graaf accelerator or microwave linear accelerator) are used for various industrial sterilization units. Ultra-violet irradiation, because of its poor penetrating powers, is rarely used as a sterilizing agent; its main value is in disinfection—in reducing the number of living micro-organisms present.

Gases

Toxic gases such as chlorine, ozone, formaldehyde, sulphur dioxide, ethylene oxide can be used for the sterilization of heat-sensitive materials, but with the exception of ethylene oxide these gases are used mainly as disinfectants. Ethylene oxide is one of the few gases which has been used commercially for true sterilization. This gas damages relatively few materials; it is mainly used in the pharmaceutical industry for the sterilization of rubber and plastic bottles.

Disinfectants and antiseptics

The techniques we have been discussing—heat, radiation, filtration, gases—can also be used to produce a *relative* fall in the population of micro-organisms, i.e. they can be used as disinfectants. However, we are going to restrict our description of disinfectants and antiseptics to various liquid preparations. The efficiency of the various techniques of sterilization can usually be easily and accurately measured by physical means, and there are standard specifications for the use of such pieces of equipment as autoclaves. When we come to the use of chemicals acting as disinfectants or antiseptics, the situation is very different. Individual chemicals differ in various properties, in the kind of organisms that they readily destroy, in their inactivation by the presence of such things as organic matter, hard water, detergents etc., and in the effect of temperature and exposure time on their action. There is no one ideal disinfectant or antiseptic, and for each situation one has to make a deliberate choice of the most suitable chemical. Furthermore, despite nearly a century of endeavour there are no generally accepted tests for assessing the effects of a disinfectant or antiseptic.

Factors affecting the action of disinfectants and antiseptics

1. The nature of the micro-organisms. The resistances of different micro-organisms to any given disinfectant vary considerably. Of all micro-organisms, vegetative cells are the most easily destroyed. Tubercle bacilli, because of their waxy coat, are more resistant. Some viruses are as susceptible as vegetative bacteria, but others such

as polio virus are more resistant. The most resistant forms to chemicals are the spores of bacteria and fungi which are not destroyed by cold chemical disinfectants as they are normally used.

2. Obvious factors that effect the action of a disinfectant are temperature and concentration of the chemical. In addition, the presence of materials such as organic matter (e.g. protein) may considerably reduce the effectiveness of some disinfectants. Disinfectants seem to act on the surface of micro-organisms, and anything that prevents the intimate contact of disinfectant with the surface, e.g. a deposit of protein or wax, can reduce the efficiency of the disinfectants.

Testing of disinfectants

One of the most widely used methods of testing the effectiveness of a disinfectant or antiseptic is to compare its effectiveness with that of phenol under carefully controlled conditions, using a specific organism—usually *Salmonella typhi* (page 140) for the test. In making the test, five solutions of the disinfectant are made up, containing different concentrations, and five solutions of phenol are prepared, also of different concentrations. Equal volumes of the various disinfectant and phenol dilutions are inoculated with equal volumes of a broth culture of *S. typhi*. The mixtures are incubated and loopfulls of the mixture are removed at intervals of $2\frac{1}{2}$, 5, $7\frac{1}{2}$, and 10 minutes from each tube and checked for the presence of living *S. typhi*. In calculating what is called the phenol coefficient, one is interested in the disinfectant and phenol concentrations for which there is growth of *S. typhi* after $2\frac{1}{2}$ and 5 minutes but none after $7\frac{1}{2}$ or 10 minutes. The phenol coefficient is given by the following formula:

$$\text{Phenol coefficient} = \frac{\text{concentration of phenol needed}}{\text{conc. of test disinfectant needed}}$$

Thus if a concentration of one part in five hundred of a disinfectant is needed to give the same effect as a concentration of one in one hundred of phenol, then

$$\text{phenol coefficient} = \frac{1/100}{1/500} = \frac{500}{100} = 5.0$$

There are various other ways of testing the activity of a particular disinfectant, but it is important to note that these estimates may be misleading because the conditions under which the disinfectants are to be used may be quite unlike the test conditions.

Individual disinfectants and antiseptics

A wide range of disinfectants and antiseptics is commercially available. No one is suitable for all purposes and a careful choice has to be made depending upon the conditions under which the chemical is to be used and the kind of micro-organisms which have to be eradicated. Below is a classification of the chemicals available.

Alcohols

Ethyl and isopropyl alcohol are often used as antiseptics (e.g. for preparation of the skin before an injection) or as disinfectants (for storing boiled syringes). These substances, when diluted to 70 per cent with sterile water, destroy vegetative bacterial cells including tubercle bacilli and some viruses, but not the spores of fungi and bacteria. However, these materials are fairly expensive and also inflammable, and because of the lack of commercial interest, and thus absence of advertizing, they are not widely used.

Hypochlorites

Hypochlorites are readily available in the form of calcium hypochlorite (chloride of lime) and sodium hypochlorite (e.g. Domestos, Lever Bros. Ltd. and Milton). The disinfectant action depends on the formation of hypochlorous acid (HOCl); this in turn liberates oxygen in a highly active state, which rapidly kills fungi, yeasts, bacteria and viruses. However, spores are more resistant, and in order to kill them a longer contact time or a higher concentration of the disinfectant is needed.

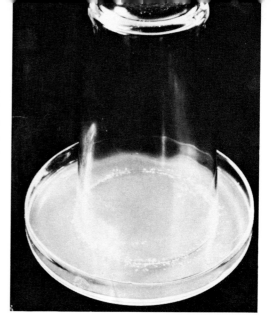

Figure 15.3 Improperly washed drinking glass placed on an agar plate. Note the bacterial colonies growing around the rim of the glass. (*By courtesy of The Domestos Hygiene Advisory Service.*)

The efficiency of hypochlorite is due to the fact that even slight oxidation of the protein in the living cell causes cell death. These cheap and useful disinfectants have a long history. Hypochlorite was first used by Ignaz Semmelweiss (1818–65) who was convinced that puerperal fever, which was rampant in the obstetrical ward in the Allgemeines Krankenhaus of Vienna, was due to infection carried on the hands of doctors into the medical wards from the dissecting rooms. The washing of hands in chlorinated lime before examining the patients reduced the incident of puerperal fever from 11.4 to 1.27 per cent.

Table 18 The concentration of Domestos and the contact time needed to completely kill various bacteria at 20°C

Type of bacteria	Contact time (minutes)	Effective p.p.m. available chlorine	Concentration oz/gal Domestos
Vegetative bacteria (*Staphylococcus aureus, Pseudomonas pyocynae* and *Escherichia coli*)	5	125	$\frac{1}{5}$
	30	30	$\frac{1}{20}$
Tubercle bacilli	10	125	$\frac{1}{5}$
	30	65	$\frac{1}{10}$
	240	35	$\frac{1}{20}$
Bacterial spores *C. tetani*	5	500	$\frac{4}{5}$
	30	250	$\frac{2}{5}$

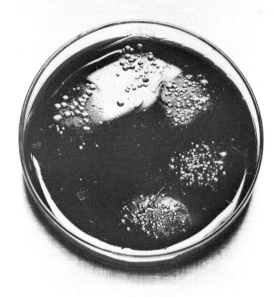

Figure 15.4 An agar plate cultured after unwashed fingers were pressed on to the agar. Note the many bacterial colonies. (*By courtesy of the Domestos Hygiene Advisory Service.*)

Hypochlorites are now widely used both in the home (disinfection of babies' feeding bottles, working surfaces, equipment, toilets) and garden and in industry (e.g. laundries, dairies and other food industries). They are both effective and cheap; their chief disadvantage is that they are powerful bleaching agents.

Table 18 is a statement supplied by the Domestos Hygiene Advisory Service on the effectiveness of this hypochlorite preparation against various bacteria. Figures 15.2, 15.3 show the bacterial contamination of various kitchen articles and the effects of Domestos. Table 18 (page 173) illustrates the sensitivity of different types and forms of bacteria to the action of hypochlorite. Note that if organic matter is present then higher concentrations of hypochlorite are needed, because the chemical reacts with the organic matter making less available for the action against bacteria. Thus if soil is added to the solution (one part dry weight in one hundred cubic centimetres of solution) the concentration needed to kill tubercle bacilli after 10 minutes' exposure rises from 125 p.p.m. (1/5th oz. Domestos per gallon) to 2000 p.p.m. (3 oz per gallon).

Iodine and iodophors

Iodine itself is now rarely used except as an antiseptic (dissolved with potassium iodide in 90 per cent ethyl alcohol) supplied to superficial cuts and scratches. Its use is limited because of its staining effects, although it is strongly and rapidly bactericidal, killing both vegetative forms and spores.

New forms of iodine are now available in which the iodine is complexed with other compounds to produce non-irritating, non-staining chemicals called iodophors. The iodophors are dissolved in detergents of various sorts so that the mixture can act as both a detergent and a disinfectant (or antiseptic). Iodophors are also relatively non-toxic at the dilutions which are used for disinfection. They can be used as an antiseptic (on skin or mucous membranes) or as a disinfectant for operating rooms, wards and nurseries. Furniture and equipment can also be wiped with a cloth rung out of freshly made iodophor.

Phenolics and substituted phenolics

Phenol was the first of the disinfectants and antiseptics, and its germicidal activity was dramatically demonstrated by the work of

Figure 15.5 (a) A disc of agar was placed on the surface of an uncleaned wooden preparation board and then cultured. Note the many bacterial colonies.
(b) A disc of agar from a board washed with detergent only.
(c) A disc of agar from a board washed with detergent and then Domestos. No bacterial colonies are present. (*By courtesy of the Domestos Hygiene Advisory Service.*)

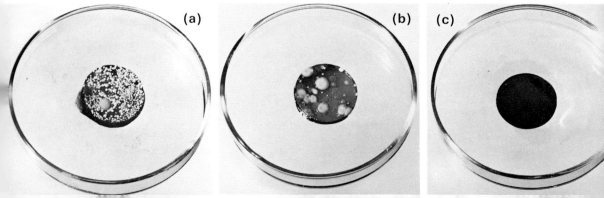

(a)　　　　　(b)　　(c)

Table 19 Bacterial counts from surgeons' hands

Preparation used	Before surgery		After surgery	
	Palm	Upper surface	Palm	Upper surface
5 min scrub plus 95 per cent alcohol rinse	77	128	105	132
pHisoHex (3 per cent hexachlorophene plus detergent)	33	41	8	6
2 per cent hexachlorophene soap	90	131	102	101
1.3 per cent chlorxylenol cream	137	150	150	137
1 per cent chlorhexidine	81	114	125	125

Lister in 1867. As an antiseptic it is rarely used nowadays, for less irritating and poisonous substances are available. Crude carbolic acid is sometimes still used for the disinfection of excrement.

Several synthetic phenols (e.g. 'amphyl') are available for use in medicine and in sanitation. These are good disinfectants with a wide range of activity against micro-organisms. They are also used in combination with detergents for hospital cleaning purposes. They are relatively non-toxic to skin and mucous membranes.

One chlorinated phenol—hexachlorophene—has found wide use as a skin antiseptic. This substance markedly inhibits the multiplication of bacteria, but considerable time is needed to kill them. The antiseptic can be used in various forms, e.g. in a lotion combined with a detergent or incorporated into tablets of soap. It should be emphasized that the reduction in the bacterial flora of the skin occurs only after several days of the use of hexachlorophene soap. After a single scrub with such a soap the reduction in the bacterial count is no greater than with a non-medicated soap. When the soap is used repeatedly, the chemical accumulates on the skin and reaches its maximum concentration in two to four days. If now a non-medicated soap is used, the hexachlorophene film is removed and regrowth of the normal bacterial flora begins promptly. There are several hexachlorophene lotions or soaps available. Wide application has been found in medical practice, e.g. 'scrubbing up' before surgical operations, the cleansing of burns and wounds, and in maternity hospitals for nurses, midwives, and the hygiene of infants. Skin infections and rashes such as acne, impetigo (page 73) and nappy rash are also improved by

the anti-bacterial and detergent action of lotions such as 'pHisoHex' which contains three per cent hexachlorophene in an emollient emulsion containing a detergent.

Recent reports from America have shown that hexachlorophene can cause brain damage in rats. Hexachlorophene is now no longer recommended for treating large areas of skin—particularly in infants—to avoid absorption which would lead to high enough blood levels of the drug which could cause brain damage. Further studies of the toxicity of hexachlorophene are being carried out.

The action of hexachlorophene on the bacterial 'count' from surgeons' hands before and after operations is shown in Table 19.

Hexachlorophene is also important in the food industry, where it can reduce the bacterial hazards in food handling, particularly from pathogenic staphylococci. Note that hexachlorophene has much less activity against Gram-negative organisms such as coliforms and Salmonellae. Its main use is in the eradication of pathogenic staphylococci that are so important in infections in surgical wards, operating theatres, maternity units and nurseries (see page 75).

Detergents

Water alone is an inefficient cleanser, surprisingly enough because it is not very efficient at 'wetting' things. If you pour water into a glass then immediately empty the glass and inspect the inside surface, you will note that this is very unevenly wetted. Instead of a uniform film of water one finds that the water has shrunk away from many areas, leaving them dry. This behaviour is due to the surface tension of water.

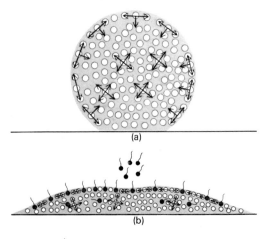

(a)

(b)

Figure 15.6 (a) A drop of water with the intermolecular forces indicated and (b) the effect of the addition of detergent to the drop.

If we consider a drop of water on a glass plate (Figure 15.6(a)), the innumerable molecules in the drop are strongly attracted to one another. In the middle of the drop these attractive forces operate in all directions and neutralize the effects of one another. At the surface of the drop there are no forces operating from outside; all the forces are in an inward direction and tend to maintain the drop of water in the shape with the smallest surface area. The inward force which attracts the molecules is balanced by a tension in the surface film between the molecules which prevents further shrinking of the drop. This is the 'surface tension' of the drop. To make the water droplet spread evenly over a large area, this surface tension has to be broken. Detergents, be they soapy or non-soapy, carry out this function by the insertion of detergent molecules between the surface molecules of water. This breaks the attractive bonds between the water molecules and reduces the surface tension, thus allowing the drop to collapse (Figure 15.6(b)). In Figure 15.6(b) the structure of the detergent is shown as being like a tadpole with a hydrophilic (water-loving) head and a hydrophobic (water-hating) tail. The hydrophilic heads push between the surface water molecules. Because of the effect of this insertion of detergent molecules into the surface film, detergents increase the 'wettability' of water. Furthermore, when surfaces are covered by grease the water-hating tails of the detergent molecules stick into the grease, the heads remaining in the water; mild agitation can now separate the grease from the surface. Once greasy particles have been dislodged from a surface

they tend to become coated with molecules of detergent. This coating of detergent molecules helps to keep the grease dispersed and prevents its reattachment to the surface, partly because the particles now carry electrical charges which make particles and surfaces repel one another.

The main value of detergents in disinfection is this ability to make surfaces wettable and so bring disinfectant molecules onto the surface. The additional effect of removing grease is also of great value. This cleansing action of detergents is often vital before the application of a disinfectant. Cleansing with a detergent not only removes bacteria with grease and dust but it allows the penetration and disinfectants to be used afterwards.

Some chemicals do in fact combine the two properties of detergency and disinfection (or antisepsis). These are what are called quaternary ammonium salts which are found in such proprietary antiseptics as 'Cetrimide' or 'Cetavlon'. These chemicals have a wide spectrum of activity against micro-organisms, although they are less active against Gram-negative than Gram-positive bacteria. Tubercle bacilli, bacterial spores and fungi are relatively unaffected by these antiseptics. In the recommended dilutions they are relatively non-toxic to skin and mucous membranes. This safety, combined with the lack of odour and colour, makes them suitable for cleansing and disinfection of dishes, glassware and other eating utensils and also equipment in dairy and food-producing plants. Like most disinfectants these substances are inactivated by organic matter. Furthermore, different classes of detergents, such as soaps, interfere with their action on micro-organisms.

Chlorxylenol ('Dettol')

Chlorxylenol, marketed under various names, the best known of which is 'Dettol', gained fame as an antiseptic for use in obstetrics, in the prevention of sepsis during and after childbirth. Its activity is restricted to vegetative bacterial cells. Its powerful odour precludes its use as a disinfectant for crockery, cutlery etc.

The uses and abuses of disinfectants and antiseptics

In the preceding pages we have discussed the use of various chemicals as antiseptics or disinfectants and probably no group of chemicals in medicine is used more widely than these. It must be pointed out, however, that the layman often uses these easily available chemicals in a ritual way that may have no beneficial effect, or indeed in a way that can have harmful effects. No doubt part of this behaviour is the result of the pressure of advertizing which can make individuals routinely apply these substances to every nook and cranny of their homes and perhaps also to every surface and to every cavity of their body—in the form of mouth washes, gargles, nasal washes and douches for internal 'female hygiene'. Much of this activity is unnecessary. In the case of repeated spraying and douching of the eyes, nose or female genital tract, even the bland antiseptics can have harmful effects when used over long periods. It is obviously important to choose a particular antiseptic or disinfectant for use in a rational way.

Below is a classification of the antiseptics and disinfectants suitable for various tasks.

1. Suppression of bacterial flora on skin of surgeons, midwives, food handlers: e.g. hexachlorophene.
2. Disinfection of large areas: hypochlorites (e.g. Domestos, Milton), quaternary ammonium salts (e.g. Cetavlon, Cetrimide) and synthetic phenolics.
3. Disinfection of small articles: 70 per cent ethyl alcohol, iodophors, quaternary ammonium salts, synthetic phenolics, hypochlorites.
4. Antiseptics for use on skin or mucous membranes: alcohol, hexachlorophene, chlorxylenol (Dettol), iodophors, quaternary ammonium salts.

16. Arthropods and disease

Introduction

THE arthropods form a very large group of animals which show certain special features such as segmented bodies, paired limbs (of which at least one pair function as jaws), a stout jointed *exo*-skeleton, and a nervous system very similar to that of worms, placed ventrally in the body. This large group of animals is split into various sub-groups including Crustacea (crabs, crayfish, lobsters etc.), Insecta (cockroaches, grasshoppers, bees, wasps, houseflies, fleas, mosquitoes) and Arachnida (spiders, scorpions, mites and ticks).

Table 20 is a list of some insects and arachnids which may cause disease in man.

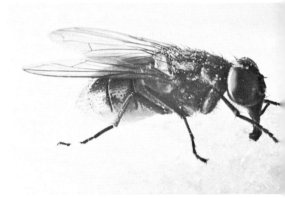

Figure 16.1 A housefly feeding on a lump of sugar. Note the long mouthpart—the proboscis —applied to the surface of the sugar. (*By courtesy of WMMS.*)

Table 20 Diseases transmitted by arthropods

Arthropods	Disease
Insect	
Houseflies and blow-flies (Figure 16.1)	Bacillary dysentery and other intestinal infections Poliomyelitis
Mosquito (Figure 16.2)	Yellow fever, malaria, dengue, filariasis, viral encephalitis
Tsetse fly (Figure 16.3)	Sleeping sickness (trypanosomiasis)
Fleas (Figure 16.4)	Bubonic plague, typhus
Lice (Figure 16.5)	Typhus, French fever, relapsing fever
Sandflies	Leishmaniasis, sandfly fever
Arachnids	
Ticks (Figure 16.6)	Tickborne typhus-like fevers e.g. Rocky mountain spotted fever, South African tick fever, Q. fever, tularaemia, viral encephalitis, tick paralysis
Mites (Figure 16.7)	Mite typhus (scrub typhus)

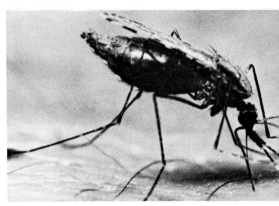

Figure 16.2 A malaria-carrying mosquito puncturing the skin of its victim. (*WHO photo.*)

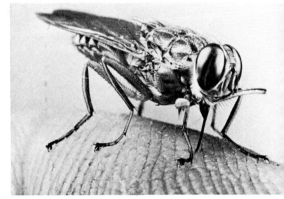

Figure 16.3 A tsetse fly puncturing human skin. (*WHO photo.*)

Some of these arthropods spend the whole of their life on man, e.g. the mites which cause the human disease called scabies. At the other extreme, insects such as mosquitoes or tsetse flies only visit man at intervals to obtain a meal of blood. The disorders caused by arthropods can be relatively mild and arise mainly from the effect of bites in which irritating saliva or other secretions are injected into the wound, e.g. bed bugs (Figure 16.8), mites, horse flies. In the act of biting the arthropod may, however, transfer bacteria, viruses or parasitic protozoa etc. which may cause serious and perhaps fatal illnesses. Moreover some arthropods, e.g. houseflies, may cause disease in man even although they do not come into direct contact with him; these insects may transfer bacteria to food which when eaten may result in dysentery and other intestinal infections. We can now look at some examples of these arthropod parasites, at the diseases they may transfer and at the ways in which the arthropods can be controlled. It will soon become obvious that the life cycles of the different arthropods vary greatly and that a detailed understanding of the life cycles is necessary for an intelligent attack on the animals.

The structure and life cycle of insects

The housefly belongs to the sub-group (class) Insecta of the large group or phylum Arthropoda. Insects show the features of arthropod structure which we have already mentioned (page 178). They all show a further feature, that in the adult stage of the animal the body is divided into three distinct regions:

1. *the head*, which carries a single pair of antennae which are jointed, sensitive structures. The mouthparts consist of a pair of mandibles (jaws) and two pairs of maxillae.

2. *the thorax*, which is the middle region and carries three pairs of legs and one or two pairs of wings. Some primitive insects have not developed wings and in some other highly specialized insects the wings have disappeared in the course of evolution, e.g. fleas.

3. *the abdomen*, which carries neither legs nor wings. Insects also show a special mode of breathing—air is circulated to all parts of the body in a branching network of tubes called tracheae. These air tubes open to the surface of the body by way of small pores or spiracles, and air is pumped in and out of the body through the spiracles by the action of movement of the body.

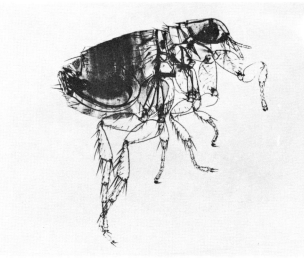

Figure 16.4   Photomicrograph of a flea. (*By courtesy of WMMS.*)

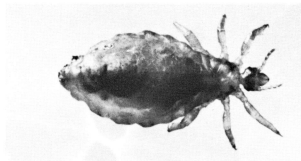

Figure 16.5   Photomicrograph of a louse. (*WHO photo.*)

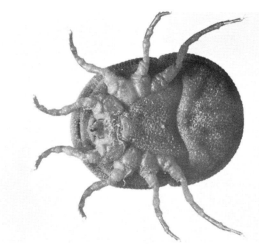

Figure 16.6   Photomicrograph of a tick. (*WHO photo.*)

The life history of insects varies somewhat from one species to another. In all of them the life cycle begins with the laying of fertilized eggs. From the fertilized egg may hatch an animal which in many ways is a miniature replica of the adult except that its sexual organs are immature and it does not bear wings. This miniature adult

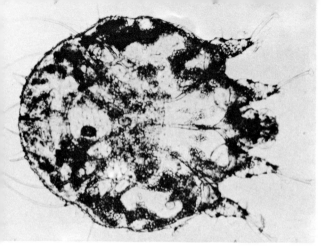

Figure 16.7 High power photomicrograph of the mite (female) which causes scabies. (*By courtesy of Dr J. O'D. Alexander and reproduced by permission of the Editor of The Practitioner.*)

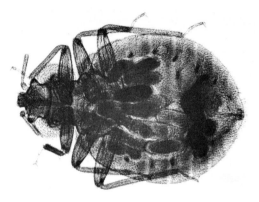

Figure 16.8 Photomicrograph of a bed bug. The long biting mouthparts are not easily visible because they are folded under the body (view from under surface). (*Photograph by Brian Bracegirdle, B.Sc., M.I.Biol., F.R.P.S.*)

is called a nymph. Growth of the nymph is not a continuous process but occurs at distinct phases in the life of the nymph called moults. At the moult the hard exo-skeleton is shed, exposing a soft pliable new exo-skeleton. Some growth in size occurs before this soft skin becomes transformed into the rigid cuticle. At each moult the nymph assumes more of the structure of the adult—its wings grow and the sexual organs develop. We can summarize the life cycle of such an insect in the following way:

egg→nymph→nymph→nymph→adult (imago)

This gradual transition to the adult form is called metamorphosis—gradual or incomplete metamorphosis. Insects such as the cockroach and the bed bug show this kind of development.

In other insects such as the housefly, blow-fly, flea, mosquito, bee, wasp and butterfly, the life history is very different. In these insects the fertilized egg hatches to reveal an individual which is quite unlike the adult insect in appearance, behaviour and feeding habits. This individual is given various names—the larva, caterpillar, grub and other names, depending on the kinds of insects—but whatever the name we use, all of these creatures show similar features. Here we will use the term larva. The main purpose of the life of the larva is to eat. Growth in size occurs mainly at the stages of moulting, and the number of moults varies from one species of insect to another. Inside the larva are tiny rudiments of the organs of the adult insect. These remain dormant until the next stage in the life history—the pupa.

When growth of the larva is complete it becomes transformed into the pupa, which often has a hard envelope. Whereas the larva is characterized by mobility and feeding, the pupa is characterized by immobility. Inside the pupa the organs of the larva are destroyed to provide the raw material for the growth and development of the adult organs. The tiny rudiments of adult organs which were present in the larva now grow, and the adult slowly develops inside the pupal skin. At the appropriate time the pupal skin is ruptured and the adult insect emerges. We call this kind of life cycle complete metamorphosis, and we can represent it in the following way:

egg→larva→larva→larva→pupa→adult (imago)

The common housefly—*Musca domestica* (Figures 16.1, 16.9)

This species of insect is very familiar and is certainly the most widely distributed of all insects. Almost everywhere in the world where man is able to live, the housefly has followed and has adapted to breeding on various articles of food and on the excreta of man and domestic animals. Houseflies show typical insect structures. They are about 6 mm in length and greyish in colour, with four narrow black stripes on the thorax. The body and legs are covered with fine hairs. There are sticky pads on the tips of the legs which enable the fly to walk on ceilings (Figure 16.9). The mouth parts are specialized to enable the animal to spread saliva on the food and then after an interval to suck up the partly digested food. When the animal secretes saliva on to exposed human food this becomes contaminated, from the stomach of the fly, with the products of the last meal—which may have been the contents of a dustbin, or human or animal faeces. In the act of walking over food micro-organisms may also be deposited

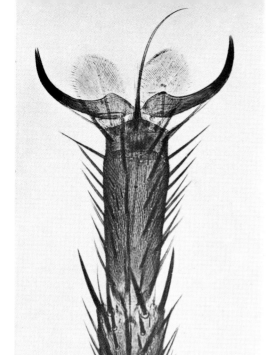

Figure 16.9 Photomicrograph of the leg of a housefly. (*By courtesy of WMMS.*)

from the hairy legs and body and from the sticky pads on the feet.

Life cycle

The eggs of the housefly are laid on virtually any kind of animal or vegetable material provided it is fairly moist and will offer a source of food for the larvae. Thus the eggs may be laid on vegetable refuse in dustbins, or on human or animal faeces. Egg laying does not occur throughout the year, and in Great Britain breeding normally finishes in October until early summer (June). The insects overwinter in the larval or pupal stages, although occasionally a few adult flies live through the winter, particularly if the weather is relatively mild.

The eggs are glistening white and are laid in batches of about 150. Each egg is about 1 mm long. A single female fly may produce up to a total of 900 eggs during a period of 4–12 days. The incubation period of the eggs depends on temperature and ranges from eight hours to three days.

The larva is a white legless creature, conical in shape, tapering towards the mouth end. It has two pairs of breathing pores (spiracles), one on segment two and the other on segment ten. With adequate food and a high temperature the larva may be fully developed in three days. Then the larva leaves its moist feeding place and seeks a cooler, drier place to pupate.

Pupation usually occurs in the soil where the larva may burrow several centimetres deep. The pupa is barrel-shaped with rounded ends and a dark brown or black colour. Within the pupa the adult insect develops, and the speed of development (3–28 days) again depends upon temperature.

Diseases transmitted by houseflies

Houseflies do not transmit infection directly to man, but because of their feeding habits they may contaminate human food with the organisms responsible for several diseases. Because they transfer organisms from human faeces to food, they are especially implicated in the spread of infections of the bowel—paratyphoid and typhoid fevers, summer diarrhoea of babies, 'food poisoning' caused by bacteria of the Salmonella group, and poliomyelitis. But the list of pathogens i.e. organisms, which can be carried by houseflies in various parts of the world is in fact much longer than this, and includes the organisms responsible for amoebic dysentery, hook worm, tapeworm, whipworm, blood fluke, and cholera.

Eradication and control of houseflies

There are three fundamental ways of preventing contamination of human food by flies:

1. covering of food,
2. destruction of breeding sites of flies,
3. destruction of adult flies.

Food should never be left uncovered and this is particularly important during the summer months. Flies will not only feed on and contaminate food, but will also lay eggs on suitable foodstuffs. Flies must not be permitted to breed near houses; regular emptying of dustbins or removal of garbage is essential. If there are any delays in dealing with household garbage, DDT powder should be applied to it. Flies also breed in the garden in manure and compost heaps, and these should be covered with a layer of soil to prevent egg laying. DDT does not kill larvae, so that each new batch of adults hatching from a manure heap must be brought into contact with DDT. Repeated spraying is essential. The eradication of breeding places also assumes a civilized standard of sanitation, for flies will breed on human excreta.

In the house, flies can be killed by spraying of a 'knock down' type of insecticide. Places in which flies regularly alight—lamp shades and bulbs, window frames, can be treated with an

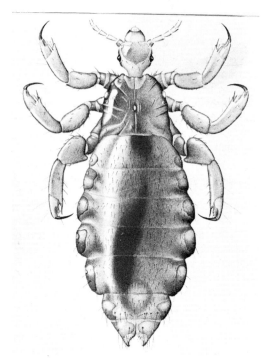

Figure 16.10   H.P. drawing of *Pediculus humans* var. *corporis*, the body louse. (*By courtesy of WMMS.*)

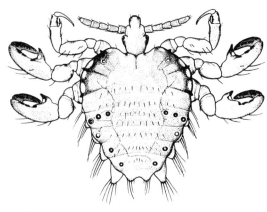

Figure 16.11   H.P. drawing of *Phthirus pubis*, the crab louse or pubic louse. (*By courtesy of WMMS.*)

insecticide with a persistent action—e.g. DDT. Various kinds of traps are also available—e.g. tanglefoot traps (resin and castor oil on paper strip), DDT paper trap and poison traps.

Lice

There are two kinds of lice, biting lice and sucking lice. Biting lice are mainly pests of birds and occasionally mammals, e.g. the dog-biting louse. There are about 2600 different species of biting lice in the world but none of them feed on man. The sucking lice are all parasitic on mammals. They have mouth parts which are specially adapted for piercing the skin and sucking blood. There are two species of lice which attack man:

1. *Pediculus humanus*—the human louse which occurs in two forms:
   (a) the head louse—*P. humanus* var. *capitis*
   (b) the body louse—*P. humanus* var. *corporis* (Figure 16.10).
2. *Phthirus pubis*—the crab louse or pubic louse (Figure 16.11).

Life cycle

Like other insects, lice reproduce their kind by means of egg laying. After a few days the eggs hatch into nymphs which moult three times while growing into the adult louse. The eggs of head and pubic lice are attached to the shafts of hairs by means of a sheath of a cement-like substance with a small platform of cement for the egg. These cemented eggs are called nits (Figure 16.12). The head and pubic louse lives on the clothing, where it lays its eggs among the fibres of cloth. It only moves on to the skin for the purposes of feeding. All three kinds of lice are transferred from person to person by direct contact—or in the case of the body louse by infected clothing or bedding.

Pediculosis capitis

The frequency of this disease has dropped in recent years. Most of those affected are girls and women because of their longer hair in which the louse finds more shelter. The only symptom of the disease is intense itching of the scalp which results in scratching of the skin. This scratching may result in eczema of the scalp and impetigo— blisters or ulcers infected with staphylococci (see page 73). The disease is diagnosed by

Figure 16.12   Nits of head lice on scalp hairs. (*By courtesy of Dr J. O'D. Alexander and reproduced by permission of the Editor of The Practitioner.*)

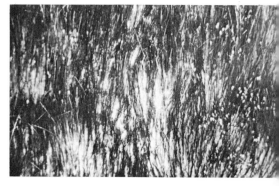

finding nits on the hairs and, less commonly, adult lice, about 4 mm long, greyish and actively crawling among and along the hairs. Nymphs are more difficult to see. The nits are tiny globules about 1 mm long, firmly attached to the hairs. The unwary can confuse them with dandruff or fragments of hair lacquer on the hair shafts.

Pediculosis corporis

This is now an uncommon disease in Britain and is almost entirely restricted to tramps (vagabond's disease) who neglect to bathe and change their clothes. The main symptom is itching, and the skin shows evidence of extensive scratching. Lice are virtually never found on the skin, but the clothing may contain hundreds of small glistening nits—like small grains of sand—in the seams of underclothing and around buttonholes and buttons (Figure 16.13).

Pediculosis pubis (Figure 16.11)

This disease is often venereal in origin, i.e. it is transmitted during sexual relationships, and thus it may accompany other diseases such as gonorrhoea, syphilis and sometimes scabies.

Again the main symptom is itching, mainly in the pubic region. The louse only lives in hairy regions and it lies flat to the skin, clinging on to a hair shaft. It can easily be missed on examination—it resembles a small crust of blood. If there are large numbers of lice in the pubic region then some may migrate to other regions, e.g. armpits and even eyelashes, eyebrows, beard and moustache. The scalp hair does not become infected.

Treatment

There are several substances available for the prevention or treatment of pediculosis:

1. *Dicophane (DDT)*. This kills lice very effectively. In 1943 a typhus epidemic (spread by lice—see page 184) was quelled by treating large numbers of civilians with a ten per cent dicophane dusting powder. Using a 'dusting gun' which is inserted into openings in the clothing, it is possible to kill lice without the need for undressing. Some strains of body lice are now resistant to DDT so that the use of this drug entails some risk of failure of treatment. During the Korean war, for example, it was found that dicophane powder did not prevent the spread of body lice among army prisoners of war. However, dicophane-resistant strains of

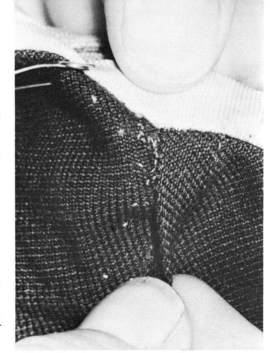

Figure 16.13 Nits around the seam of a skirt. Note the small recently hatched louse near the white waistband. (*By courtesy of Dr J. O'D. Alexander and reproduced by permission of the Editor of The Practitioner.*)

the head louse and crab louse have not yet appeared.

A great advantage of dicophane is that its effect persists for some time; clothing impregnated with the powder will kill lice for several weeks. This is important because larvae hatch up to ten days after the eggs are deposited.

2. *Gamma benzene hexachloride* (Gamma BHC). This substance has a rather more rapid action than dicophane but it does not have such a persistent effect. Strains of lice which are resistant to Gamma BHC are not yet a problem, but they may appear later. A variety of preparations of Gamma BHC are available and include dusting powder, lotion, cream and shampoo.

3. *Paraffin oil* (kerosene) is sometimes used for treating head lice.

Methods of treatment

Pediculosis capitis

Dicophane application (15 cm³) or Gamma BHC application or lotion (15 cm³) is rubbed into the hair after wetting. If the head is unwashed for the next seven to ten days, any lice which hatch after the treatment will be killed. This may not always be convenient, particularly for women, in which case the alternative is to wash the hair after twenty-four hours and then re-apply the lotion after a week. It is advisable also to treat family contacts of a patient with pediculosis capitis. Since older girls and adults may object to applying the lotion to the hair, a single washing of hair with a shampoo such as two per cent Gamma BHC is reasonably effective. In the patient with pediculosis capitis it is unnecessary to comb out the nits—except for reasons of appearance. It is important that hats and false hair pieces should be disinfected by heat or powdered over with Gamma BHC or dicophane powder and left on one side for several weeks. It is only necessary to cut the hair in very severe cases.

Sometimes paraffin oil is used for pediculosis capitis. This destroys both lice and nits. About one tablespoon of paraffin oil is rubbed into the hair, which is then wrapped in a wet towel and shampooed two hours later. This procedure *must* be carried out in a room where there is no fire, naked flame or smoking.

Pediculosis corporis

In this condition the body and underclothing are powdered with dicophane dusting powder or Gamma BHC dusting powder.

Special attention should be paid to the clothes, since it is here that the lice live when they are not feeding and it is here that the eggs are laid. Heavily infected clothes and bedding should be destroyed. Lightly infected clothing can be disinfested by steam or by ironing. Alternatively they can be dusted with dicophane or Gamma BHC powder and stored for two to three weeks. In the case of vagrants, it is important to have their lodging houses inspected and disinfested.

Pediculosis pubis

This condition can be readily cleared by dicophane or Gamma BHC powder or application. One treatment followed by another after one week is usually adequate. Since the armpits are also infected in some cases, it is best to treat these at the same time. Shaving of hair is not necessary.

In all three kinds of pediculosis contacts should be traced and also treated.

Pediculosis is a disease which should be preventable under normal circumstances. Regular inspection of individuals living under crowded conditions—schools, hospitals for the mentally ill and chronic sick, armed services etc.—is an important aspect of prevention. Regular bathing, shampooing of the hair and clean clothing are also very important. In peacetime the occasional outbreak of pediculosis does not cause what one could regard as a serious, much less a fatal, illness. Infection with lice is, however, highly irritating, and because of scratching and secondary infection with pathogenic bacteria this may give rise to impetigo or eczema.

When there is overcrowding associated with poor personal hygiene and malnutrition, as for example, in prison camps and concentration camps, lice can be responsible for spreading three serious illnesses from one individual to another and so cause epidemics. These diseases are typhus, relapsing fever and trench fever. The organisms responsible for these illnesses are acquired by the lice during the act of sucking blood from an infected human. The organisms multiply in the louse which can then infect other humans.

Typhus

Typhus is caused by organisms called Rickettsiae—minute bacterium-like bodies. Epidemic typhus is a purely human disease, spread from case to case by infected lice. The bite of a louse is not infective but the Rickettsiae in their faeces are introduced into the skin by means of scratching. Dried faeces can also be inhaled, particularly when infected clothes are handled. Hospital staff are at special risk because of their contact with both infected lice and contaminated clothing. They should wear protective clothing which includes an efficient face mask to reduce the risk of inhaling dried faeces, and goggles to prevent the eyes from being contaminated. A louse-free typhus patient is not infective. Spread of infection can thus be stopped by disinfesting the population with an insecticide. The severity of the disease can be greatly reduced by active immunization with an efficient vaccine, although immunity is short-lived and needs re-inforcing every three months during an epidemic. In the established disease the use of antibiotics such as chloramphenicol or tetracycline produces rapid cure.

There is another form of typhus called endemic typhus, which is caused by a different species of Rickettsiae. Endemic typhus occurs sporadically in many parts of the world. Rats form a reservoir of the infecting organisms, which seems to cause little harm to the rat. The infection is transmitted from rat to rat by means of the rat flea or the rat louse. Although the rat louse does not feed on man, the rat flea will sometimes do so. Thus individuals who work or live in close contact with rats may develop endemic typhus. This disease is controlled by means of the public health measures directed at destroying rats.

Scabies

The human disease called scabies is caused by infection with a mite *Sarcoptes scabiei*, which lives in the epidermis of the skin (Figure 16.7). One needs a proper understanding of the life cycle of the parasite and the clinical picture of the disease in order to eradicate infection. The mite reaches the skin from another infected individual, usually a bed mate or at least a member of the same household, but occasionally a fellow pupil or occupant of the same dormitory, and nurses caring for scabetic patients may contract the infection. There is only one kind of mite which is infective, and that is a female bearing fertilized eggs. When she reaches the skin, the gravid female begins to burrow into the epidermis, laying eggs as she burrows. Burrowing occurs at a rate of about 0.5–5 mm a day. This superficial burrow in the skin is diagnostic of the disease. It is a grey-black linear mark on the skin surface 1–10 mm long (Figure 16.14). At the end of this burrow are minute scales which show where the mite entered. At the other end of the burrow is a tiny red spot 1–2 mm across, and the mite can be found at this point. It can be extracted by rupturing the roof of the burrow with a needle; the mite adheres to the needle point. During her life the female lays about fifty eggs. These hatch in three to four days after laying and the nymphs enter adjacent hair follicles. After two moults they reach adult size (0.2–0.4 mm length); this takes about six days. The only mites which burrow into the epidermis are the gravid females. Nymphs, males and barren females do not burrow. In fact, few of the females ever become gravid and a single patient rarely carries more than ten to twenty gravid females.

Scabies is a skin disease of long history; the Mosaic laws of cleanliness (Leviticus) suggested that the Israelites suffered from scabies, and Aristotle was aware of the disease. In more recent times it has been a common disease in countries such as Scandinavia and Scotland. The disease can be an important source of economic loss in a community; in 1942 there were 72 000 army cases in Britain—which in terms of time off from active duty during treatment is equivalent to a battalion of 800 men being invalided for a whole year. At this time the civilian rate of infection was considerably higher.

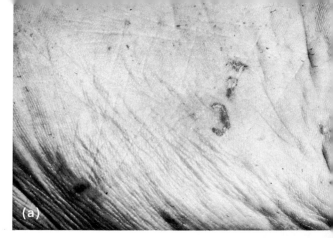
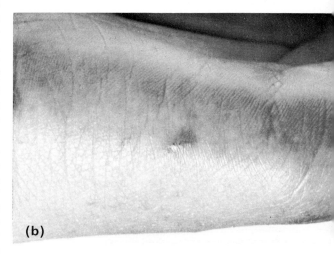

Figure 16.14 (a) Scabies burrow on the sole of the foot and (b) scabies burrow on the border of the hand. (*By courtesy of Dr J. O'D. Alexander and reproduced by permission of the Editor of The Practitioner.*)

The clinical features of scabies

At first the presence of burrowing mites in the skin produces no symptoms, but after about a month the patient becomes sensitive to secretions of the mite (? saliva). When this occurs itching begins, and it may be localized to the site of burrows, commonly on the hands and feet. Later, a generalized itch develops. Associated with this itch are small red spots which are due to the nymphs wandering about the skin, feeding in various hair follicles. The only certain way of diagnosing the disease is to find burrows from which a mite can be isolated. Later in the disease the effects of continued scratching and secondary infection—producing impetigo, boils etc. (see Figure 16.15)—make diagnosis less easy. The disease should be suspected in any itching condition of the skin and then cases will not be overlooked.

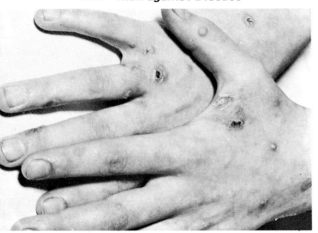

Figure 16.15 Scabies of the hands with infected spots caused by scratching. (*By courtesy of J. O.'D. Alexander and reproduced by permission of the Editor of The Practitioner.*)

Treatment of scabies

There are several preparations available for the treatment of scabies, but whichever drug is chosen a correct use is necessary for success in treatment. The preparations available include the following:

1. ten per cent sulphur ointment,
2. twenty-five per cent emulsion of benzyl benzoate,
3. one per cent lotion of gamma benzene ointment.

The patient first takes a bath and the preparation is applied, the ointment being rubbed into the skin while lotions are painted on to the skin. The principles of treatment are as follows:

1. All members of a household, whether affected or not, must be treated. This may extend also to frequent visitors to the house.
2. The whole body surface below the collar line must be treated. If this is not clearly explained to the patient then only itching areas may be treated, which results in failure of treatment.
3. The lotion or ointment should be used for only three applications at 12–24-hour intervals.
4. Underclothes, night attire and sheets should be steam-disinfested or laundered and put aside for a week, after which they will no longer be infective.
5. Patients and contacts should be inspected after a week to check the success of treatment.

When properly applied, anti-scabetic preparations rarely fail to cure. The commonest cause of failure is the misapplication of the preparation. Similarly failure to treat all contacts, clothing and bedding results in re-infection.

Fleas

Fleas are brownish jumping insects which have no wings. They are considerably flattened from side to side and this enables them to move easily between hairs. They spend most of their time on their host but lay their eggs away from the host—in dust, the cracks between boards, kennels, birds' nests etc. The eggs hatch in three to fourteen days according to the temperature. From the egg hatches a dirty white larva, sparsely covered with long fine hairs. This larva remains on the ground, feeding on organic matter, and it reaches its full size after about two weeks. It then seeks a dark place and here spins a cocoon in which it pupates for about two weeks. In the pupa most of the tissues of the larva are broken down and become the raw material for the construction of the adult flea, which usually emerges after about two weeks and seeks its host. However, the flea can remain dormant in the cocoon for months, and then emerge rapidly when there is mechanical vibration nearby such as might be caused by the passing footsteps of a new host—man.

Man is the natural host of only one species of flea—*Pulex irritans*. The effect of infection with the flea consists mainly of local irritation from the bite of the animal. Both female and male fleas suck blood. They first cut the skin by sword-shaped mandibles (jaws) and then they insert the sucking apparatus. Saliva of the flea runs into the wound to prevent blood from clotting, then blood is sucked out by a pump which is in the 'throat' of the flea. The irritation of flea bites is best treated by some simple remedy such as a lotion of two per cent phenol in water.

Fleas can be eradicated by treating infected personal clothes, bedding and the dwelling house. Clothing and bedding can be disinfected by DDT powder. Carpets and upholstery should be similarly treated—or discarded and destroyed if possible. Hard floors can be washed and brushed but if infection in the household is heavy then an insecticide such as kerosene (inflammable) or naphthalene should be applied to the floors and skirting boards. Obviously a great improvement in the standards of personal and general hygiene are necessary both to treat infection with fleas and to prevent re-infection.

If a person has to enter a flea-infested dwelling then an insect repellant (e.g. dimethyl phthalate) can be applied to parts of the clothing (socks, neckband, trouser turn-ups) and to the skin—provided that the mouth, eyes, nose and ears are avoided.

The human flea is not usually the carrier of pathogenic organisms—except those which may produce local infection at the site of the bite. Fleas which normally live and feed on other mammals may also attack man. The rat flea, *Xenopsylla cheopis*, is the most important one in this respect since it can be responsible for spreading two dangerous diseases to man, bubonic plague and endemic typhus (page 184).

Bubonic plague

Plague is a disease of rodents (rats, gerbils, ground squirrels etc.) which is spread from one animal to another by means of blood sucking insects, especially fleas. These insects may also bite man and so infect him. During the history of man, millions of human beings (and rats) have died of the disease. Although the disease is virtually non-existent in civilized communities with good standards of public health, rat plague is still endemic in some parts of the world, e.g. India, and is responsible for outbreaks of the disease in man. Search for plague-infected rats is an important part of public health work in ports and in endemic areas.

In India, plague is commonest in the grey rat and is spread by fleas. The blood of a rat with plague contains enormous numbers of bacilli some of which are taken up by fleas when they take a meal of blood. When the rat dies of plague the fleas leave the body to seek a new host, carrying with them the organisms responsible for plague. When plague is rampant among the grey rat (*Rattus norvegicus*) it then spreads to the black rat (*R. rattus*) which lives in houses. When these animals die of plague the fleas may easily find their way on to man. The bite of an infected flea leads to bubonic plague similar to the disease in rats. The disease is so-called because the organisms spread from the bite to the neighbouring lymph glands, which become swollen—bubos. From the bubos the organisms enter the blood stream, but in the human disease there are fewer organisms in the blood so that fleas which bite human cases do not usually transmit the infection. However, the disease in man can spread to the lungs to produce a pneumonia and this is a highly infective condition, for the organisms are coughed out in droplets of secretion. Pneumonic plague, as it is called, is invariably fatal. It is probably the most infectious of all human diseases caused by bacteria, and readily gives rise to epidemics. When the lungs are not involved in human plague, the mortality is still over 50 per cent unless antibiotics such as streptomycin are used in the treatment.

Prevention of plague depends largely on the public health measures which are aimed at reducing the population of rats and preventing their entry into human dwellings. DDT and other insecticides can be used to kill wandering fleas, and houses in which rats or men have died of plague are compulsorily evacuated until all fleas have been destroyed. There is also a vaccine available to increase the resistance of individuals to the organisms.

The bed bug (*Cimex lectularius*)

There are, of course, many species of bugs (Hemiptera) but this is the only one which affects man. Bed bugs are round, flat insects of a reddish brown colour—hence the name 'mahogany flats'. They have well developed legs and can move well, but they are almost wingless.

They are likely to be found in any dwelling where there is a low standard of hygiene. Usually it is the bedroom which is infected, for it is here that the bugs find their sleeping prey. During the day the bugs hide in crevices in walls, woodwork, under loose wallpaper, and in furniture of all sorts. From these places the bugs emerge at night to obtain a meal of blood from sleeping humans. The bite of a bug consists of a central red area where the blood has been sucked, surrounded by a wheal which may itch intensely and last a week or two before it disappears. No known diseases are transmitted in the act of biting, although the bites may become secondarily infected by scratching.

Bed bugs usually gain access to a house by means of infested bedroom furniture, suitcases, clothes which have been hung against an infested wall etc. Their flat bodies also allow them to enter adjacent rooms in terraced houses through cracks in ill-fitting joints and poorly constructed brickwork. It is important to note that a bug which has recently been fed may survive up to nine months without another meal—hence the danger of secondhand bedroom furniture.

Life cycle

Female bugs lay large numbers of eggs. One female at $25\,^{\circ}$C and with frequent feeding, e.g.

two meals a week, will lay about 350 eggs. These are dirty white in colour, about 1 mm long and are laid in clusters on bedding, mattresses etc. They are covered with a glue-like substance which cements them in position. The incubation period depends on temperature, the eggs hatching quickly at high temperatures (e.g. in five days at 28 °C). From the egg hatches a nymph very similar in appearance to the adult except that it is much smaller and is more transparent because the cuticle is thin. The nymph moults five times before the adult stage is reached. Between each moult a meal of blood is taken.

The length of the life cycle is very dependent upon room temperature. At normal room temperatures (18–20 °C) with adequate opportunity for feeding an adult bug may live for nine to eighteen months. At higher temperatures the length of the adult life is shorter.

Control of bed bugs

Before the arrival of modern insecticides, fumigation with the very poisonous gas hydrogen cyanide was the only effective way of dealing with a serious infestation of bed bugs in a house. This kind of treatment needed experts to carry it out and, moreover, the residents had to be found other accommodation for at least one night. Further, since the eggs are relatively resistant to fumigation, this had to be repeated about ten days later when the eggs present at the first treatment had hatched. In addition to fumigation with hydrocyanic acid gas, sulphur can be burnt to produce the irritating gas sulphur dioxide. Again, this involves moving out residents.

The development of insecticides which have a persistent action has meant that fumigation is not necessary in most cases, although large pieces of stuffed furniture are still best dealt with in this way since they are difficult to treat by spraying with insecticide. If insecticides are used then a solution of five per cent DDT in kerosene is employed (caution, inflammable). This must be used liberally—about 30 g per square metre. Walls, underneath loose wallpaper, pictures, furniture, skirting boards, mattresses and bed frames should all be treated. The floor should not be washed after spraying.

Household insect pests and the law

There are Acts of Parliament which to some extent protect society against people who permit their houses to become 'verminous'. In this context a 'verminous' building is one infested with bed bugs and/or fleas, and a 'verminous' person is one infested with lice or scabies mites.

Under the Public Health Act (1936) a Medical Officer of Health or a Public Health Inspector (Sanitary Inspector) may report the presence of verminous buildings or persons to the Local Authority. The Local Authority has the power to act in various ways to eradicate this nuisance. They may serve notice to the owner of a verminous house to have it disinfested at his own expense, and they may destroy or clean verminous articles in a house (provision is made for compensation for destruction of articles).

A verminous person may be forced by an Order of Court to be disinfested. Under the Education Act of 1944 a County Medical Officer of Health has the right to inspect school children in schools of Local Education authorities for verminous conditions. When children are discovered who have a verminous condition then the parents or guardians are required to disinfest the child within twenty-four hours. Further, under the Scabies Order 1941 the Local Authority has the power to inspect houses which they may believe are inhabited by verminous persons. Any person living in such a house may be required to attend a medical examination and, if necessary, undergo treatment or disinfestation.

Summary

A glance at Table 20 will show that we have only been able to deal with some of the commoner arthropod vectors of disease, and in particular those which occur in Great Britain. However, some general principles of arthropods as vectors of disease can be drawn from this study.

1. Arthropods can cause problems in two distinct ways.
   (a) The presence of feeding arthropods on human skin causes irritation, often intense itching, and the penetration of the skin barrier by arthropod mouth parts and by scratching paves the way for infection by bacteria. This secondary infection may take the form of localized spots or boils or a more generalized skin infection called impetigo (page 73).
   (b) Arthropods may cause more serious diseases because they may have had a previous meal on an infected human or animal or on infected refuse or human excreta.

2. Personal hygiene and public health measures

are very important in the prevention of arthropod-transmitted diseases. It may seem strange that we have looked in some detail at arthropod-transmitted diseases such as bubonic plague and typhus, diseases which are no longer endemic in Europe, certainly not in Great Britain. However, this has not always been so. In the fourteenth century the 'Black Death', another name for bubonic plague, destroyed about 25 million people in Europe alone, roughly three-quarters of the population. The plague then raged inter- mittently in Europe for the next three centuries, and the Great Plague of London in 1665 killed about one-fifth of the popula- tion. Our freedom from plague in modern times is not due to the fact that we are immune to the disease or that we no longer have the animal vectors of the disease, for rats and their fleas abound in Europe. Our freedom is due to our greatly improved standards of housing, sanitation, personal and communal hygiene and the rigid control over all ships which reach our shores from ports abroad where plague is endemic. Plague is still endemic in some parts of the world, and if our standards of hygiene were to fall, e.g. by a national disaster, then plague might again reach our shores and become epidemic. Epidemics of typhus have occurred in more recent history, during the First and Second World Wars. It has now been eradicated from most European countries, but like the plague it could readily return in epidemic form in the presence of national distress and famine. From where would these two diseases come? They would come from countries with a low standard of personal and public hygiene where the diseases are still endemic, just as the Black Death was introduced into Constantinople and then the rest of Europe from Asia in the fourteenth century.

3. A knowledge of the life history of the arthro- pod. A last generalization we can draw from our limited study of arthropods is the importance of understanding the habits and life cycle of the arthropod in order that we may successfully eradicate them. We need to know where houseflies lay their eggs, where bed bugs hide in the day time, how lice and mites are spread from one human being to another, and so on.

17. Zoonoses, especially diseases transmitted by pets and laboratory animals

Introduction

THE recent appearance (1970) of rabies in a dog in England raises in a dramatic fashion not only the questions of restrictions on the importation or the quarantine of animals imported into this country, but also the whole spectrum of the risks involved when man comes into close contact with animals, as pet owner, laboratory worker or farmer. The dramatic photographs of the muzzling of dogs in Camberley and the shooting of wild animals in an area where the rabid dog ran wild for an hour or so should impress on all the seriousness with which health authorities regard the possible spread of rabies in England, a country which has been free of the disease for many years. Rabies belongs to a group of diseases called the zoonoses, i.e. diseases which can be transmitted to man from other vertebrate animals. More than 150 zoonoses are now recognized, and of these many diseases those which are transmitted by way of domestic animals are of particular importance because of man's close contact with such animals. In this chapter we will be considering mainly two groups at risk, pet owners and those handling laboratory animals (school children, technicians, research workers etc.).

We have in fact seen many examples of zoonoses in other chapters of the book. We have seen that cows may transmit, among other diseases, brucellosis (page 128) and bovine tuberculosis (page 126). Rats may transmit leptospirosis (page 143), plague (page 187) and salmonellosis (page 146). Some zoonoses are transmitted directly from animal to man, as when a veterinary surgeon contracts brucellosis from handling an infected cow, or when an infected dog transmits rabies in the act of biting man. Other zoonoses are transmitted indirectly from animals to man by arthropods such as mosquitoes and ticks (e.g. yellow fever, malaria, trypanosomiasis).

Often zoonoses are occupational diseases faced by agricultural, industrial and laboratory workers. Anthrax (page 3) occurs more frequently in those who are in contact with infected animals or animal products, i.e. in raisers of livestock, carpet weavers and workers with animal hair in the textile industry. Leptospirosis is more common in those occupations which bring man into contact with rats or with water contaminated by rat urine—e.g. workers in sewers, ditches and water-logged agricultural land. Q fever occurs more frequently in workers in abattoirs, jungle yellow fever and tick-borne zoonoses in woodcutters, salmonellosis in food processers, bovine tuberculosis in farmers, ornithosis in workers in poultry-processing plants, rabies in veterinarians, field naturalists and dog-control employees.

We do not know the exact economic importance of zoonoses but it is certainly considerable. It includes death, acute and chronic illnesses in man and loss of life and reduction in productivity of livestock. Developing countries of the world suffer much greater losses than do technically advanced nations; this is in the main due to lack of adequate public health and veterinary services. Apart from the enormous burden of human suffering and death, it is estimated that in Latin American countries alone zoonoses such as brucellosis, bovine tuberculosis, rabies and hydatid disease cause economic losses amounting to hundreds of millions of dollars annually. Some zoonoses are of such economic importance that national campaigns have been established to eradicate the diseases from animals. Thus in some economically advanced countries, zoonoses such as plague, rabies, bovine tuberculosis and brucellosis have been eradicated. However, in some countries eradication of zoonoses may well not be possible, either because of the prohibitive cost or because inaccessible wild animals form a reservoir of the disease, e.g. bats which act as a reservoir of rabies or monkeys of yellow fever. Even if eradication is not a practicable measure, it is necessary to make a continuous effort against these diseases to prevent the eruption of epidemics which can take a high toll of human life or cause serious economic losses.

We will now turn to deal specifically with diseases which can be acquired from animals kept in the home as pets. No longer do the dog, cat, rabbit, budgerigar and tortoise satisfy the needs of pet keepers, and a vast range of species is becoming popular in the home—parrots, lovebirds, cockatoos, snakes, lizards, monkeys, bush babies—to mention but a few. In view of the increase in the keeping of pets, the rapidly expanding list of species which are becoming available and acceptable as pets, and the closeness with which humans handle their pets, it is indeed surprising that diseases acquired from pets are still rather uncommon. However, such diseases do occur and sometimes cause serious illness and even death. Because of their relative infrequency it would perhaps be unreasonable to urge that the keeping of pets should be declared a serious hazard to health; but it is important that those who keep pets or who buy them for their children should be aware of the possible risks and the steps which can be taken to eradicate some zoonoses from the animals they keep. If any pets were to be banned then it should be monkeys; these are difficult to keep in the home and they can transmit a large number of diseases to man. One of these diseases, herpes B virus infection, although uncommon, is one of the worst infectious diseases from which man can suffer.

Rabies

Rabies is an invariably fatal disease which mainly affects carnivorous animals—dogs, cats, foxes, skunks, jackals, wolves, coyotes, mongooses etc. It also occurs in cattle, and in Latin American countries this is a serious economic problem. The disease is caused by a virus, and the bite of an infected animal can transmit the disease to other animals, including man. The incubation period of the disease is very variable, and ranges from ten days to seven months depending upon the amount of virus which has entered the body. The virus spreads from the site of the bite along the nerves to reach the brain. In the absence of medical care death is inevitable and often occurs during a convulsion caused by infection of the brain by the virus. The disease is sometimes called hydrophobia because the throat often contracts painfully on swallowing water or even at the mere sight of water.

The recognition of the relationship between the disease in man and the bite of a dog occurred in the nineteenth century. In England alone there were 1113 reported human cases between 1848 and 1898. The first Rabies Order was passed in 1886 and was followed by the muzzling of dogs in infected areas and restriction of

their movements. These measures gradually reduced the number of rabid dogs, until by 1902 the disease was eliminated from this country. In 1918 the disease was re-introduced into Great Britain, probably by way of the illegal importation of a dog that subsequently developed rabies. The disease persisted until 1922, and during the intervening period 319 animals were diagnosed as rabid and 144 persons bitten by these animals had to have courses of vaccine. This terrible disease was again eradicated from Great Britain. Wild carnivores (which can form a reservoir of the disease) are relatively rare in this small island and strict quarantine regulations on imported dogs and cats can prevent the re-introduction of the disease. Since 1922 about 100 000 animals have been subjected to quarantine, during which time twenty-seven developed rabies and were destroyed. The general belief was that the incubation period of rabies was about three months; if dogs and cats could be quarantined for six months, avoiding direct contact of one animal with another, it seemed that the introduction of rabies could be completely prevented.

On 11 October 1969, a dog which had been imported from Germany in April and released from quarantine after six months was noticed by its owner to develop a weakness of the hind legs, followed by aggressiveness. The dog later escaped, killed a cat, and ran at large for nearly an hour. The owner was the only person bitten by the dog. The dog was returned to quarantine where it later died and a diagnosis of rabies was confirmed. Fortunately the owner had previously been immunized against rabies. This episode was followed by the total destruction of wildlife in an area of 1200 hectares in which the dog may have been at large (to prevent the disease establishing itself in wildlife). A further episode occurred when a dog imported from Pakistan developed rabies three months after release from quarantine. As a result of these incidents the period of compulsory animal quarantine was extended to twelve months, and all new imports of dogs and cats were suspended pending the results of a government-sponsored enquiry into the rabies situation. Further, there was a restriction on the importation of many species of 'exotic' animals known to be possible carriers of the disease.

These kind of measures are not practicable for countries which have the additional burden of an abundant and varied wildlife capable of harbouring the disease. In these countries the incidence of rabies can be reduced by vaccinating as many dogs and cats as is practicable,

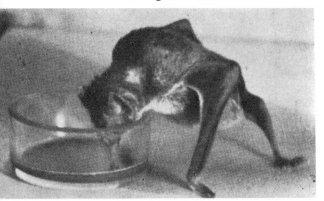

Figure 17.1 A blood-lapping bat feeding in captivity from a glass container. (*By courtesy of WMMS.*)

and by keeping down the numbers of wild carnivores which can harbour the disease. There are various kinds of vaccines available for the prevention of rabies in dogs and cats. Some vaccines are composed of living rabies virus which has been modified by repeated sub-culture in chick embryos or rabbit brain. Other vaccines use inactivated virus which has been cultured in duck embryos or rabbit brain. Some of these vaccines can also be used to protect men who are at special risk of contracting rabies— veterinary surgeons, dog-handlers and field naturalists. Vaccine is also used to protect cattle in Latin America, where rabies can be trans-mitted by vampire bats. These feed only on blood and they have become abundant in tropical regions of the world where cattle ranches pro-vide easy meals of blood. The vampire bat (Figure 17.1) also transmits rabies to man, and since 1935 there have been about 160 cases in man due to bites by vampire bats.

If a man is bitten by an animal suspected of having rabies, various lines of treatment are possible. An important step is to confine and observe the animal responsible for the bite to determine whether in fact it has rabies or will develop rabies. Treatment must not, however, be delayed for the results of such observations. First-aid treatment of the wound is important and the wound must be carefully washed; some disinfectants are known to kill the rabies virus and these can be used to irrigate the wound. Passive immunity is then conferred on the bitten man by injecting antibodies against the rabies virus. These antibodies are prepared by injecting animals (e.g. horses) with rabies vaccine and, after an interval, removing blood to prepare serum which contains the antibodies. If neces-sary the serum containing these antibodies can be injected in the region of the bite to neutralize

the virus. Following passive immunization active immunization is obtained by injecting a suitable rabies vaccine which stimulates the individual to produce his own antibodies against the virus.

Psittacosis and ornithosis

Psittacosis and ornithosis are diseases caused by similar micro-organisms. The term psittacosis describes the disease when it occurs in psittacine birds, i.e. those of the parrot family—parrots, parrakeets, love-birds, budgerigars etc. Orni-thosis describes the disease when it occurs in other kinds of birds, i.e., poultry and pigeons. The micro-organism responsible is somewhat unusual and is intermediate in size between viruses and bacteria. The organisms are classified in a group called the Bedsonia; psittacosis and ornithosis are very common diseases of birds and have been described in over 130 species. Many birds seem to carry the organism without showing signs of disease, i.e. they are carriers; it is estimated that 90 per cent of the pigeons in Trafalgar Square are carriers of the organisms. Young budgerigars and parrots usually suffer only a mild illness when infected, and they dis-charge the virus in their droppings and nasal secretions. Adult birds are not always infective, but the sitting females tend to shed virus in the droppings and infect the young in the nest. Man is chiefly infected by inhalation of dust contain-ing dried droppings and secretions. In the past, parrot-like birds have been recognized as an important source of the disease in man. Most infections have occurred in persons having close contact with the birds—breeders, sales persons, pet owners etc. More recently it has been recognized that ducks, turkeys and pigeons are also an important source of infection, and cause disease in farmers and poultry processers. Plucking birds is especially dangerous, but no disease has been traced to eating poultry.

In man the disease may produce a mild feverish illness which is mistaken for influenza, but it can appear as a severe pneumonia. The disease should always be suspected when those who keep pet birds or poultry develop influenza-like illnesses or pneumonia. Fortunately the antibiotic tetracycline is very effective in treating the illness; penicillin is of no value.

There is no effective vaccine which can be given to birds to prevent infection and thus transmission to man, but the disease can be eradicated from birds by means of tetracycline given in pellet food. This kind of treatment is strongly recommended for all those who keep flocks of birds for breeding; when these have been made free of the disease, re-infection must be prevented by having clean, well ventilated, uncrowded premises and by treating any new additions to the flock with tetracyclines. Anyone who keeps one or more birds can abolish the risk of transmission of psittacosis or ornithosis by this kind of treatment. If details of treatment are required they can be obtained from the World Health Organization, Technical Report Series, No. 378, a joint FAO/WHO Expert Committee on Zoonoses, obtainable from H.M. Stationery Offices.

Of course, the control of ornithosis in poultry is more difficult and expensive. It is important that wild parrot-like birds should be treated with tetracycline before and during shipment to various countries. The incidence of psittacosis in wild birds is usually only 5 per cent or less, but if they are held together in large numbers in transit or in quarantine—in accordance with government regulations—the incidence of the disease may be as high as 30–40 per cent. Thus if these birds are not treated before or during shipment, they may arrive in the acute phase of psittacosis, shedding large numbers of virus particles, and are a real hazard to health, both to other birds and to man. If birds have been treated with tetracyclines, they should not on arrival be mixed with untreated birds from which they can contract the disease.

Herpes virus infections and monkeys

In man, infection with a virus called *Herpes simplex* is one of the commonest of all virus infections. It usually produces a very mild illness with sores in and around the mouth—'cold sores'—although it may invade the eye or the nervous system to produce a much more serious illness. In monkeys a similar virus, Herpes B virus or *Herpes simiae*, produces a similar mild illness in the monkey. In man infection by this same virus produces a rapidly fatal disease. In the twenty to twenty-five cases which have been reported in man, all but two ended fatally shortly after the onset of the disease. Rhesus monkeys and cynomolgus monkeys from South-East Asia are frequently infected in the wild. When these monkeys are gathered together in compounds to be shipped abroad, infection spreads rapidly among them. In some cases 80 per cent of monkeys arriving in laboratories have shown evidence of infection. The most dangerous species—rhesus and cynomolgus

monkeys, should be placed in individual cages on arrival and kept in quarantine for six to eight weeks. Any monkeys showing blisters or sores in the mouth or on the tongue and lips should be killed and the body incinerated. Of course, handlers of monkeys should observe strict hygienic precautions.

Because of the risks of contracting Herpes B virus infections, the laboratory use of rhesus and cynomolgus monkeys has decreased. African green monkeys are becoming more popular. But even these are not without risk. In 1967 there were seven deaths in Germany in laboratory staff handling green monkeys for the manufacture of poliomyelitis vaccine. The nature of their illness has not been clearly established, and these green monkeys could have easily found their way into pet shops and into homes. There is no available vaccine which can be used to protect those who handle monkeys, nor is there any effective treatment for infections by Herpes B virus. It has been suggested that persons in contact with monkeys should carry a card with the name of a medical specialist to be consulted in the event of any infection that seems to involve the nervous system.

Other monkeys or primates—squirrel monkeys, marmosets and owl monkeys—may transmit another virus, Herpes virus T or M, to man to cause a serious illness which involves infection of the nervous system.

Other diseases transmitted by monkeys

Monkeys can in fact transmit a wide variety of illnesses to man, although most of them are much less serious than that caused by Herpes B virus. These diseases include poliomyelitis, infectious hepatitis, salmonellosis, malaria and tuberculosis.

Leptospirosis (canicola fever) and dogs

In discussing water-borne diseases, we have already discussed leptospirosis and its transmission by rats and dogs (page 143). We can here remind dog owners of the risk they run of contracting canicola fever from infectious dogs. Any sick dog should be suspected of having the disease until shown otherwise and the animal should be isolated. Dogs shown to have the disease should be adequately treated with an antibiotic, streptomycin. If they are not efficiently treated then the animal may go on excreting organisms in the urine for up to three years

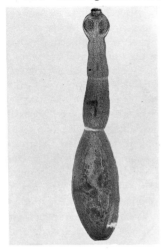

Figure 17.2 Photo-
micrograph of the hydatid
tapeworm. (*By courtesy
of WMMS, photograph by
Prof. Hans Vogel, Hamburg.*)

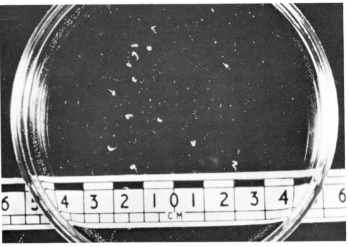

Figure 17.3 A collection of hydatid tapeworms obtained
from one dog. (*Photograph by A. I. Wright, B.V.Sc.,
M.R.C.V.S., Department of Veterinary Medicine, University
of Bristol.*)

after they have recovered from the acute illness.
Dogs can be successfully immunized against
canicola fever; this will prevent the development
of an acute attack of the illness but we do not yet
know if this prevents the excretion of the
organism in the urine of the dog. Dog urine
should always be avoided if possible; of course,
untrained puppies can be a great hazard.

Hydatid disease and dogs

A small tapeworm, the hydatid tapeworm
(*Echinococcus granulosus*) sometimes lives in the
bowel of the dog and other carnivores such as
the fox and the cat. The tapeworm consists only
of three or four segments and a small head
bedecked with hooks and suckers with which it
attaches itself to the wall of the bowel. The
whole adult worm is less than 10 mm in length
(Figures 17.2, 17.3). The life history of the
tapeworm is shown in Figure 17.4. The ripe
segments, full of eggs, pass out in the faeces.
They do not develop further until they are eaten
by an animal which can act as an intermediate
host (see page 201) for the parasite; possible
intermediate hosts are many and include man,
sheep, pigs, and cattle. Inside the intermediate
host the eggs change into a hooked embryo which
migrates through the wall of the bowel to settle
down in various tissues of the body. In the tissues
the embryos develop into a type of bladder-worm
called a hydatid cyst (Figures 17.5(a) and (b)).
These cysts are much larger than the bladder-
worms of other tapeworms. They are full of
fluid and contain numerous heads, so that when

a cyst is eaten by a dog or other final host it can
give rise to numerous adult worms. The cysts
may develop in any organ of the body, but they
most commonly appear in the liver. Many cysts
do not grow larger than an orange but some go
on growing year after year and come to contain
quarts or gallons of fluid. The cysts cause illness
by creating pressure in the organs where they
develop—and this is particularly dangerous if
they develop in the brain.

In civilized communities man becomes infected and develops hydatid disease by swallowing eggs which are liberated from tapeworms in
the dog. Stroking and kissing of dogs may
transfer eggs from the coat of the dog to the
mouth. Dog faeces may also contaminate food,
and this is most dangerous if it is food that will
not be cooked, e.g. salads. Of course, the life
cycle of the parasite is not normally completed
by dog eating man (and his hydatid cysts), but
in many countries dogs have access to the offal
from dead sheep and cattle, which are other
intermediate hosts for the parasite.

Hydatid disease is an important public health
problem in every continent. Wherever man,
dogs, sheep or cattle congregate together, the
disease tends to be common. At the end of the
last century some 70 000 people in Iceland kept
about 20 000 dogs and over a third of the
population had hydatid disease! In Great
Britain the disease is commonest in the sheep
farming districts of Wales. It has now been
eradicated from Iceland. Routine post mortem
examinations showed that 15–22 per cent of the
inhabitants who were born between 1841–81

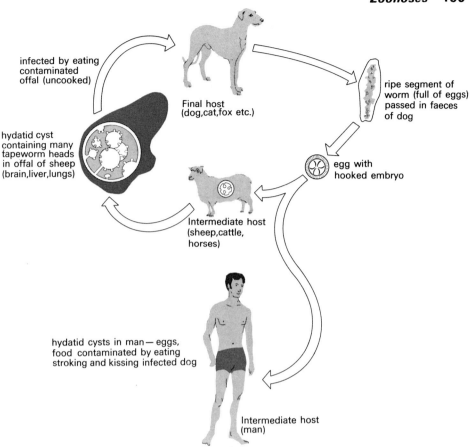

infected by eating
contaminated
offal (uncooked)

Final host
(dog,cat,fox etc.)

ripe segment of
worm (full of eggs)
passed in faeces
of dog

hydatid cyst
containing many
tapeworm heads
in offal of sheep
(brain,liver,lungs)

egg with
hooked embryo

Intermediate host
(sheep,cattle,
horses)

hydatid cysts in man — eggs,
food contaminated by eating
stroking and kissing infected dog

Intermediate host
(man)

Figure 17.4 The life cycle of the hydatid tapeworm.

carried hydatid cysts. The last human infection was seen in 1960 and the last infection in sheep in 1953. Examinations of 350 dogs since 1950 have not shown a single infection. Thus the disease can obviously be eradicated. Iceland used an educational campaign against the disease for twenty-seven years. From 1890 dogs were banned from cities, and elsewhere their numbers were restricted. All dogs were treated annually with a drug to kill the tapeworms, and the practice of slaughtering sheep in the home was radically reduced because special slaughter

Figure 17.5 (a) (left) Hydatid cyst in lung. Petri dish contains hydatid 'sand' — numerous microscopic heads of worms. (b) (right) Hydatid cyst in liver. (*Photograph by A. I. Wright, B.V.Sc., M.R.C.V.S., Department of Veterinary Medicine, University of Bristol.*)

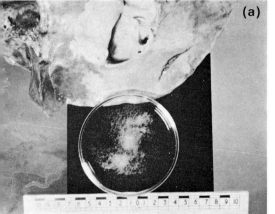

(a)

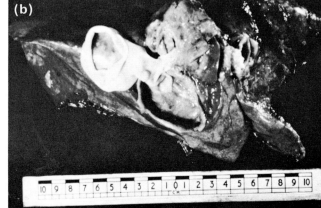

(b)

houses were constructed throughout the country. There were also important changes in sheep husbandry, in particular a reduction in the age of sheep for slaughter, from four to five years to four to five months. This shorter period is not sufficient for hydatid cysts in the sheep to become mature enough to be infective for dogs. New Zealand passed a Hydatids Eradication Act in 1959. Fines of up to 560 U.S.A. dollars can be levied for anyone feeding raw viscera (which might contain hydatid cysts) to dogs. All dogs are registered and are given a dose of a drug (arecoline hydrobromine) at a central dosing site three times a year. The stools which are collected from the dogs are then sent to a national hydatids testing station where they are examined for tapeworms, and any dog found to be infected with the tapeworm is given a further test with the drug. Before the campaign in New Zealand the infection rate in dogs in the country was up to 37.3 per cent, but after twelve years it fell to 8 per cent. There was a parallel fall in the number of cases of hydatid disease in men which needed surgical treatment. During the period 1946–51 there were twenty-seven cases of surgical hydatid disease per 100 000 of the population; this fell to seventeen cases per 100 000 in the period 1958–63.

Dogs, cats and toxocariasis

Dogs and cats may harbour a worm in their intestine (Figure 17.6) which can attack man at a certain stage in its life history to produce results which can be as serious as those of hydatid disease. This worm is a round worm, 10–15 cm in length and it has a life history similar to that of Ascaris (page 230). When eggs of this worm are swallowed by man they hatch in the intestine and burrow their way through the wall of the bowel to enter the blood stream, which distributes them to the various tissues of the body. These small worms in human tissues do not undergo the same course of development that they do in their normal hosts, cats and dogs, as they do not eventually re-enter the bowel and mature into egg-laying worms; instead they have a short life of weeks or months, but in this short life their presence excites considerable surrounding inflammation, the seriousness of which depends on the position of the worm larvae in the body. Their presence can cause enlargement of the liver, asthma, bronchitis and so on, but their most serious effects occur if they settle down in the eye, where the inflammation they cause may be so extensive as to suggest a

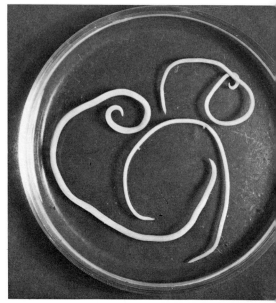

Figure 17.6   Toxacara canis. (By courtesy of WMMS.)

malignant tumour of the eye and lead to its unnecessary removal.

The worm is a common parasite of cats and dogs. The number of animals infected with it varies between 2 and 40 per cent from one part of the country to another and in different parts of the world; thus the reservoir of toxocaral infection is high. Recent work suggests that at least 2 per cent of humans are or have been infected by the parasite. The disease was virtually unrecognized ten years ago; however, now that we know the potential magnitude of the problem, the public health aspects of the disease need urgent attention, and there is obviously a great need for an increased awareness of the potential dangers of dogs and cats to human health. Infection in the dog is difficult to prevent because it is so often acquired before birth, but the worms are readily killed by a number of available drugs. A problem of increasing concern is the widespread fouling of public places such as gardens, playgrounds, parks and streets with dog faeces. They provide an ever-increasing source of infection for man, particularly for children.

Salmonellosis

We have already dealt in some detail with infection by bacteria of the Salmonella group. These bacteria typically cause food-borne infections, but the disease can also be spread directly by way of contaminated articles or by animals. Practically every species of animal that has been examined show that some individuals carry Salmonella organisms. Surveys of dogs has shown a carrier rate of 1–30 per cent depending on the area. Up to 12 per cent of cats may also carry the organisms, depending upon the area and the conditions in which they live. Chicks, ducklings, pet budgerigars, canaries and exotic species of birds have also caused Salmonella infections in man, particularly children. Recently it has been shown that tortoises, snakes and lizards may also transmit the disease to man. The unhygienic conditions under which these animals are kept in some pet shops and households make them an even greater hazard to health.

Fungus infections

We have already looked at some fungi which can parasitize man. One kind of fungus infection involves the skin and hair only, i.e. the fungi cause superficial infections known as dermatophytoses. Some of the fungi which affect human skin and hair are caused by human-type organisms which do not infect other animals, but a considerable percentage of 'ringworm' in man is caused by 'animal-type' fungi, with animals serving as reservoirs and vectors of infection. In cities and towns the cat and the dog are the commonest source of animal ringworm in man. In country areas the source of animal ringworm is more commonly cattle and horses. Any case of animal-type ringworm in man must be investigated to find the source of infection. When the offending animal has been identified it must be placed under proper veterinary care. For small animals—cats and dogs—there is a safe antibiotic called griseofulvin which is given by mouth to eliminate fungi from skin and fur. Because of the expense of the drug it is not suitable for larger animals such as cattle and horses; for these, non-toxic anti-fungal dips, shampoos and sprays are available.

Conclusion

It has not been the intention in this chapter to frighten those who keep pets or to dissuade them from keeping pets, but the potential dangers from pets should be recognized by all who keep them. Apart from attention to basic hygiene in the home or in quarters maintained for pets, there are specific measures which must be considered by pet owners; these include regular worming of dogs and cats and the elimination of psittacosis from birds.

The maintenance of animals in schools

Introduction

In these days many different species of animals are maintained in schools—rodents, birds, amphibia, reptiles, fish, arthropods etc. These are kept for a variety of educational motives, ranging from the aesthetic to the more down-to-earth studies of animal genetics, behaviour, embryology and the like. Some schools may keep rather exotic animals including primates of various kinds and members of the parrot family. Yet other schools may maintain larger animals such as hens, pigs, goats etc. Listed in Table 21 are some possible zoonoses which *may* be transmitted by laboratory animals commonly kept in Great Britain. Excluded from this list are monkeys; we have already seen that there are very sound reasons for avoiding these animals as pets in the home, and these same reasons apply even more forcibly to their exclusion from schools.

Table 21 Zoonoses transmitted by laboratory animals in Great Britain.

Zoonosis	Laboratory animals which may transmit the disease
Salmonellosis	Rodents and other mammals, birds, tortoises, terrapins and other reptiles
Q. fever	Sheep, goats, birds
Brucellosis	Goats, sheep, pigs
Psittacosis (Ornithosis)	Parrot-like and other birds—finches, pigeons etc.
Newcastle disease	Chickens
Leptospirosis	Rodents
Pseudotuberculosis	Rodents, fowls
Rat-bite fever	Rodents
Ringworm	Small mammals, poultry
Anthrax	Swine, ruminants

Table 21 refers specifically to Great Britain; it would be considerably longer if it included animals abroad, particularly animals captured from the wild. Nor does the list include the disease tetanus (page 69), which is normally acquired by contamination of wounds by soil or other matter containing tetanus bacilli or spores. The disease can, however, be transmitted to man by *any* animal bite, since faeces, soil etc. contaminating the cage of an animal may well contain tetanus organisms which can be introduced into man by the bite of the animal.

It should be obvious from the above account that due care is necessary in the purchase, maintenance and handling of laboratory animals. The following summarizes briefly the responsible handling of laboratory animals.

1. *Source of animals.* Animals should be obtained from a reputable source. A local pet shop may well not be the best source of animals, particularly if animals are maintained under conditions of overcrowding when cross-infection between animals becomes likely. The Laboratory Animals Centre, Medical Research Council, Woodmansterne Rd., Carshalton, Surrey, runs a system of accredited breeders, and can provide a current list. Some suppliers can provide animals guaranteed to be free from certain (or even all) pathogens. Not all types of animals can be obtained from these accredited breeders. Supplies of zebra finches, canaries etc. may have to be obtained from reputable specialist breeders.

2. *Maintenance of animals.* For maintenance of animals reference should be made to specialist literature. Obviously strict principles of hygiene should apply to the housing of animals, including periodic sterilization of cages and feeding appliances. Overcrowding *must* be avoided. Sick animals must be isolated. They should not be handled by students, and if expert veterinary advice is not available they should be painlessly destroyed, particularly in the case of small animals.

3. *Handling of animals.* Whatever species of animal is involved, due care in handling is vital. Faecal and urinary contamination of working surfaces should be avoided, or if unavoidable, should be followed by appropriate cleaning and disinfection. Hand washing is a *must* after handling any species.

4. *Treatment of bites and other injuries.* These should be treated by a responsible medical adviser. In schools the only treatment that should be attempted is thorough washing of a wound with soap and water, pressure to arrest bleeding and a clean (preferably sterile) dry dressing. The risk of tetanus following an animal bite can and *must* be avoided by appropriate treatment (page 70).

Allergy to animals

It is possible that pupils are or may become allergic to animals kept in school laboratories. Subjects who are most likely to present this problem are those already suffering from 'allergic-type' diseases such as asthma or eczema. The risk is very small and arises most commonly in those working with locusts over a long period of time. The earliest symptoms of allergy are similar to those of hay-fever (an allergic condition itself—allergy to pollens)—nasal stuffiness, running nose and sneezing which may be followed by asthma and skin rashes of various sorts. It is probably best not to maintain locusts in a room used for teaching one class throughout the week nor to keep them in a small preparation room where technicians are in hourly proximity to them. The Anti-locust Research Centre, College House, Wrights Lane, London, W8 is prepared to advise on this problem.

18. Parasites and man

Introduction

IN THIS and subsequent chapters we will be looking at animals which parasitize man. In this context parasitism describes the relationship between two animals. One, the parasite, lives upon or inside the other animal (man), appropriately called the host. The host (man) provides the parasite with food and shelter and receives nothing in return. In fact the host is injured in the relationship, sometimes only slightly but sometimes severely; indeed, the activities of a parasite can kill the host. A parasite which does this is poorly adapted to its way of life, as it has thus 'killed the goose that lays the golden egg'; more successful parasites establish a relationship with the host whereby the host supplies the necessary food and shelter without becoming mortally damaged in the process. Indeed the host may not only develop tolerance to the presence of the parasite, it may actually resist the invasion of the body by other parasites.

Here we are going to consider only animal parasites of man. The activities of bacteria, fungi and viruses are considered in separate sections of the book. Most animal parasites are invertebrates (animals without backbones). Only very few vertebrate animals have taken to the parasitic way of life; these include blood sucking bats and the hag fishes which bury their cylindrical heads into the bodies of their hosts and consume their tissues.

We can distinguish two types of invertebrate animals which parasitize man. One type lives predominantly on the surface of the body—on skin and hair—and these are called ectoparasites. Most of these animals belong to that large group (phylum) of animals called arthropods. Not only do they feed on the surface of the human body, but in the act of feeding they may also inject into human tissues a variety of other organisms which may cause serious, sometimes fatal, diseases—e.g. malaria, sleeping sickness etc. Thus these ectoparasites whose activities in themselves are relatively harmless may introduce into man bacteria, viruses and parasitic protozoa which may cause much more serious disease. These arthropod ectoparasites are thus called *vectors* of disease and they are considered in a separate chapter, Arthropods and disease, page 178.

We are concerned here with a second group of animals which parasitize man, the endoparasites which live within the body, in the alimentary canal or the blood stream or in various body tissues. We will be looking at two kinds of endoparasites—the vast group of 'worms' and the minute unicellular protozoa which cause diseases such as malaria, amoebic dysentery and sleeping sickness.

The world problem

Today, in 1970 there are hundreds of millions of people suffering in various degrees from the effects of infection by one or more kinds of parasite. Probably the most weakening and widespread chronic parasitic diseases are schistosomiasis (Bilharzia), ankylostomiasis (hook worm infestation) and malaria. Schistosomiasis may not kill but it weakens hundreds of millions of people in many parts of the world; losses caused by this disease are not easily measured in terms of money, but they are enormous. Of all parasitic diseases, however, malaria probably causes the most devastation, both personal and economic. It brings sickness to about 250 million people every year and death to about two and a half million of them.

Table 22 lists just some of the parasitic diseases of man caused by 'worms'. Yet other parasitic diseases are caused by those minute unicellular creatures of the phylum Protozoa—malaria, amoebic dysentery and sleeping sickness. In addition there are diseases in variety caused by infestation by fungi; these range from fairly innocuous infections of the skin to the more lethal kinds in which internal tissues are attacked by fungi and 'yeast-like' organisms (see Chapter 9).

There are many obstacles in the way of attempts to control these parasitic diseases. Many of the parasites which attack man have very complicated life cycles; they may spend part of their life cycle in one or indeed several other host animals or in the soil. Many failures in past attempts to control parasitic diseases have been due to a lack of understanding of the complex life history of the parasites. A full knowledge of the whole life cycle of the parasite is vital to any attempt to control it; for this reason we will be looking in some detail at examples of life histories and the ways in which this knowledge has contributed to the control of some parasitic diseases. A lack of information is, however, by no means the only reason that many parasitic diseases flourish uncontrolled in many parts of the world. Most of the developing countries which bear the brunt of these diseases lack finances, medical and laboratory resources and trained personnel.

The World Health Organization is helping considerably in the eradication of parasitic diseases from the world. First, it has investigated many diseases in order to assess the public health importance of the major parasitic infections in various countries. This information is vital in order that a proper priority can be assigned to particular control schemes. It has also assisted countries by giving technical advice, providing help with the training of personnel and by sponsoring research, both in the laboratory and in the field.

Some features of animal endoparasites

Endoparasites have a very special kind of life, living as they do in the bowel, bathed in the blood or embedded in the tissues of some other animals, in total darkness, constant temperature, and unable to move directly to another potential victim. This kind of life is invariably associated with the development of special structures or behaviour and with the loss of unnecessary ones. Here we will briefly consider these peculiarities of structure and behaviour, but the following chapters will provide numerous examples of adaptations to the parasitic way of life.

1. Features associated with feeding and attachment to the host animal

Parasites living in the gut are surrounded by a moving column of predigested foodstuffs. If they obtain their nourishment from this bath of food then they may have no alimentary canal and digestive organs of their own. However, they need some means of attachment to the host, otherwise they would pass along the alimentary canal and be ejected with the faeces. The forms of attachment vary from one species to another and usually take the form of hooks or suckers.

Yet other parasites of the bowel may have sufficient muscular power to maintain their position in the bowel.

If the intestinal parasite feeds on the tissues of the intestinal wall rather than on the bath of food in the lumen, the parasite may have special features which assist it to burrow into the tissues. Hook worms, for example, have teeth and a muscular pharynx which sucks out the blood from the bleeding eroded tissues of the bowel wall.

2. Modifications of the organs of locomotion

Many endoparasites, once they are established in their host, lead inactive lives. Tapeworms live with their tiny head fixed to the wall of the intestine and their long body floating in the intestinal juices. Organs of locomotion are inappropriate and the musculature is ill-developed. Although the adult forms of many endoparasites may be inactive, the 'larval' forms may well have special organs to allow them to move and seek new hosts. The 'larval' forms of some parasites may thus carry cilia or flagellae enabling them to swim to their hosts. Some adult parasites do have special organs of locomotion related to their way of life; thus the minute protozoan called Trichomonas which lives in the viscid secretions of the human vagina carries locomotor organs in the form of flagellae.

3. Modifications in the reproductive process

It is in their capacity to reproduce their kind that endoparasites show dramatic adaptations to their way of life. The endoparasite usually lives and dies in the host, yet somehow it has to achieve the task of infecting other hosts. This it does in an enormous variety of ways depending upon the particular species of parasite. Thus the round worm living in the intestine of man produces eggs which pass out with the faeces; these eggs will produce new worms only if they are eaten by man. Of course, many of the eggs will never reach another man and will eventually die. This latter fate is particularly likely to happen in countries with developed systems of sewage disposal, i.e. where the chance of faecal contamination of food or water is low. The parasite is well adapted to this situation. *Each adult female round worm (Ascaris lumbricoides)* may liberate some 200 000 eggs a day into the bowel of man. In the pages that follow we will see many examples of the enormous reproductive potential of endoparasites.

The life cycle of parasites may be much more complicated than the straightforward pattern that we see in the case of the round worm, i.e. egg → man → worm in gut → eggs → man. The parasite may exist in different forms in several kinds of animal, and in each kind of animal it inhabits some form of reproductive process is involved. Thus in man the malarial parasite reproduces itself asexually by repeated fission. This in itself produces vast numbers of parasites, some of which mature into sexual forms (gametocytes) which develop no further unless they are sucked up in the blood meal of a biting mosquito. This parasite 'uses' the mosquito to spread its kind from man to man. Inside the body of the mosquito the ingested gametocytes undergo a process of sexual reproduction followed by a further phase of asexual multiplication, so that the body of the mosquito becomes permeated by vast numbers of a form of the parasite which is able to infect man when the mosquito punctures human skin for its next meal of blood.

The human liver fluke reproduces its kind by liberating large numbers of eggs into the bile passages, and these ultimately reach the outside of the body in the faeces. These eggs are, however, not infective for man. They release a minute motile form of the parasite which penetrates and parasitizes a kind of water snail. In the snail the parasite grows and reproduces, producing large numbers of minute motile forms which are capable of infecting man. Each of these forms—the cercariae—is potentially capable of developing into an adult fluke in the human liver, provided of course man eats food contaminated by a cercaria. These additional hosts for the parasite, the snail in the case of the human liver fluke or the mosquito in the case of the malaria parasite, are called *intermediate hosts* of the parasite. In the case of the malaria parasite the intermediate host is directly responsible for transmitting the disease from man to man, and this kind of intermediate host is thus acting as a *vector* of the disease. Usually the intermediate hosts are less severely harmed than the *final host* (man), but even the intermediate host *may* be killed by the infection. Thus the snails that are the intermediate host for the liver fluke or the blood flukes may be killed by unusually heavy infections with the parasite.

19. Protozoan parasites of man. Malaria

Malaria

Ross and Grassi establish mosquitoes as infecting agents

THE minute intracellular organisms which infect the red blood cells of man and cause malaria were seen as long ago as 1880 by a French army surgeon called Laveran. The way in which these parasites are transferred from one human being to another was discovered later in the nineteenth century by two other workers, Ronald Ross (Figure 19.1), an officer in the medical service in India, and Giovanni Grassi (Figure 19.2), an Italian doctor and zoologist. Ronald Ross was the friend of an English doctor, Patrick Manson, who was obsessed by the idea that mosquitoes transmitted malaria. At this time in the nineteenth century it was known that mosquitoes fed on the blood of man and other animals and Manson thought that if mosquitoes sucked the blood of a sufferer from malaria, the parasites taken up in the meal of blood might transform themselves into some infective form which could be released into water when the mosquitoes died. If man were to drink this infected water then he would develop malaria. Manson told Ross of these ideas, and on his return to India Ross put them to the test.

After some considerable efforts Ross trapped mosquitoes and persuaded them to bite Indians who were suffering from malaria. He then proceeded to kill the mosquitoes and mash them up in water, which he fed to patients who were not suffering from malaria. By these experiments he was quite unable to transmit malaria from one person to another. His work on human malaria did not in fact progress much, although he did make the exciting discovery that a mosquito developed tiny cysts in the wall of its stomach after it had bitten a patient suffering from malaria. These cysts grew and became full of tiny dots. The dots, he thought, might be the malarial parasites developing in the mosquito.

Ross's greatest achievement came when he began to study malaria in birds. On St Patrick's day in 1898, Ross released ten grey mosquitoes into a cage containing three larks whose blood

Figure 19.1   Ronald Ross. (*WHO photo.*)

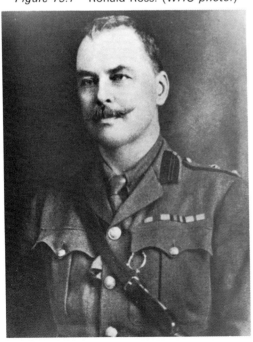

Figure 19.2   Giovanni Grassi. (*WHO photo.*)

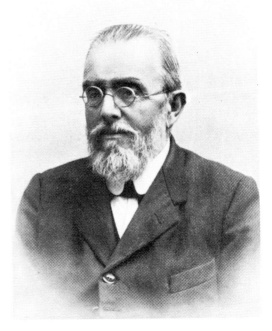

teemed with malarial parasites. After the insects had fed on the larks' blood he trapped them again. After several days he killed some of the grey mosquitoes and discovered tiny swellings in the wall of their stomach—just as he had found cysts in the stomach of the brown mosquito after it had fed on human sufferers from malaria. But how could the parasites in the wall of the mosquito's stomach reach healthy birds to infect them?

The answer to this question came when he dissected other mosquitoes that had fed on birds with malaria. He was dissecting one of these insects, that had made a meal of blood seven days before from a bird with malaria, when he saw the swelling in the stomach burst and liberate hundreds of minute spindle-shaped threads which swarmed through the body of the mosquito. On another occasion he saw these hordes of spindle-shaped threads invade the salivary gland of the mosquito. The answer was clear. It was the bite of the mosquito that transmitted malaria. These minute threads in the salivary glands were transmitted in the saliva via the piercing mouthparts of the mosquito to another bird when the mosquito made its next meal of blood. Ross's ideas were confirmed when he found that he was able to transmit malaria to healthy birds by letting certain mosquitoes bite them—these were mosquitoes that had bitten a malarious bird several days previously, mosquitoes whose salivary glands swarmed with the minute threads from the cysts on the stomach. This was a great step forward in the understanding of the life history of the malaria parasite. It was obvious that the parasite lived for only part of its life cycle in the bird in which it caused malaria; there was also a hidden phase of the life cycle in the body of the mosquito where the parasite multiplied and eventually invaded the salivary glands, ready to be transmitted to other birds. For this work Ross was awarded a Nobel prize worth more than £7000.

Ross had discovered how malaria was transmitted to birds, but it was Giovanni Battista Grassi who showed that human malaria is transmitted in the same fashion, by the bite of an infected mosquito. In the late nineteenth century malaria was rampant in certain areas of Italy. There were extensive lowland areas which were impossible to cultivate because the workers became ill with this terrible sickness. Grassi started his investigations by looking at the distribution of various kinds of mosquitoes. In some parts of Italy there were mosquitoes but no malaria, but malaria never occurred in a place where there were no mosquitoes. He found that in malarious areas there was always one special kind of mosquito present, one that the locals called 'zanzarone'. This was a mosquito with four dark spots on its wings. Its official name was *Anopheles claviger*. Grassi became convinced that if human malaria was transmitted by mosquitoes then this must be the culprit. His ideas were put to the test in the Hospital of the Holy Spirit, high on a hill in Rome where 'zanzarone' never came and where no one ever contracted malaria. Grassi collected various kinds of mosquito and allowed them to bite a willing patient in the Hospital of the Holy Spirit. Nothing happened to this unlucky patient until Grassi brought a bottle containing several female 'zanzarone'. Ten days after the patient was bitten by these mosquitoes he began to shiver, then his temperature soared and his blood teemed with malaria parasites. He repeated these experiments many times with other individuals. As soon as he was sure that he had transmitted malaria to an individual, he gave them a dose of quinine to kill the parasites. Only a fly which had bitten a patient with malaria was able to pass on the disease to other men. He collected anopheline mosquitoes from areas where malaria was endemic and allowed the females to lay their eggs in water. When these eggs had hatched and transformed themselves by way of the larval and pupal stages into adult mosquitoes he exposed himself—and his friends —to their bite; but none of them contracted malaria. Thus he was able to show that mosquitoes did not pass on the malaria parasites to their offspring.

These discoveries made little impact in Italy until he made his large-scale experiment in one of the worst malarial regions of Italy, along the railroad running across the plain of Capaccio. In this plain, every summer brought devastation and illness to farmers, railroad workers and their families. Many people left the plain each year, leaving their jobs and farms to go to the hills that were free of malaria. In the summer of 1900, Grassi went to the plain of Capaccio to carry out his experiment on over a hundred railroad workers and their families. His aim was to prevent them from being bitten by anopheline mosquitoes. Since mosquitoes bite mainly at dusk, he persuaded the families to stay inside their screened houses after dusk. Around these protected houses were the unscreened neighbouring station houses containing over four hundred individuals. These unscreened individuals were destined to be the control for his experiment. In that dreadful year of 1900 almost every person, man, woman and child fell ill with malaria in the unscreened houses. In the screened houses only five persons went down with malaria. Thus Grassi provided clear proof that it is the bite of the mosquito that transmits malaria to man and that the disease could be prevented by avoiding the bite of the mosquito.

No doubt Grassi thought that the conquest of malaria in Italy was in sight, but it was over sixty years later before malaria was eradicated from Italy, and there are still many millions in the world who suffer from this disease. In most parts of Africa, for example, malaria is still the most important public health problem, affecting more than half the children under three years of age and almost the whole population over this age. Before we examine more closely the ways in which malaria may be eradicated from the world and the intense efforts which are now being made to achieve this objective, we will take a closer look at this parasite, its life history and its effect on individuals and communities.

The life cycle of malarial parasites

Malaria and the mosquito

In discussing malaria we have to consider two distinct parasites, the malarial parasite itself, a microscopic protozoan which multiplies within the cells of man, and the mosquito which is an ectoparasite of man, coming for occasional feeds of blood, and in this act being potentially capable of transmitting malaria. The several kinds of malaria which occur in man can be transmitted only by mosquitoes which belong to the genus Anopheles, and indeed only by certain species of this genus. Only the female mosquito sucks blood and thus only the female can transmit malaria. The male obtains his food by sucking fruit juices. In order to transmit malaria from one human being to another the female mosquito must take at least two bites, and with a fairly long interval between these bites. The first bite must be of a human suffering from malaria. When the insect sucks up human blood into its stomach it also takes up malarial parasites which are present within the red blood cells. We will be looking at the life cycle of the malarial parasite in more detail in a later section. Here we can say that within the body of the mosquito, certain stages of the malarial parasite undergo a process of sexual reproduction to produce those minute infective threads—called sporozoites—which migrate to the salivary glands of the mosquito. These phases of multiplication of the malarial parasite in the mosquito

take at least twelve days to complete, and it is after this period, that the mosquito can infect a man with malaria. When the mosquito thrusts its biting mouthparts into human skin, there is an initial outpouring of saliva to clear the sucking parts and prevent blood from clotting in the mouthparts and blocking them; the sporozoites are poured into the wound made by the mouthparts with the saliva.

We have seen that the transmission of malaria from man to man depends upon the feeding habits of female anopheline mosquitoes. The distribution of malaria in the world is thus determined by the distribution of the various species of anopheline mosquitoes in which malarial parasites undergo their phase of sexual reproduction. Whenever anopheline mosquitoes are unable to breed, malaria is absent. They cannot breed at altitudes above 3000 m and they cannot breed in deserts. Reference to Figure 19.3 will show that malaria is not found north of latitude 60°N or south of latitude 30°S; but these areas represent only a small part of the world. This distribution of malaria depends mainly on the fact that the sexual phase of the parasite requires a certain temperature. Thus in England, malaria was, at one time not an uncommon disease in East Anglia and the south-east coast as far west as the Isle of Wight. Serious epidemics were not seen, because even in the summer the temperature was rarely high enough for long enough to permit the parasites to undergo sexual reproduction in the mosquito to produce sporozoites. The species of malarial parasite which is most likely to be transmitted in Britain is one called *Plasmodium vivax*. The sexual cycle of this species of malaria can be completed at lower temperatures than the other species of malarial parasite. The four species of malarial parasites in man are *Plasmodium vivax*, *P. falciparum*, *P. malariae*, and *P. ovale*. *P. vivax* is the most widely distributed and is the most important kind of malaria in temperate latitudes, for reasons we have mentioned above. In 1946 there was even a case as far north as Northern Ireland, where a case of vivax malaria was caused by mosquitoes which had been infected in that country. *P. falciparum* is less common in temperate latitudes and is more common in subtropical and tropical areas. It is present in most tropical countries and in Southern Europe.

The efficiency with which a particular species of anopheline mosquito can transmit malaria depends upon several factors, but mainly upon the length of life of the mosquito and its feeding habits. If the average life of a mosquito is short,

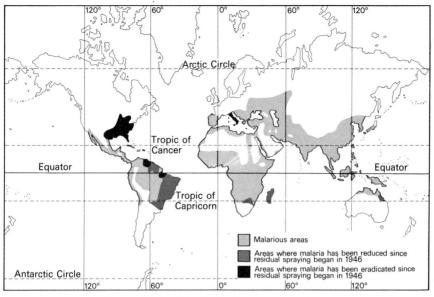

Figure 19.3   World distribution of malaria

particularly if it is less than the twelve or so days which are necessary for the sexual reproduction of the malarial parasite within the insect, then it is an inefficient transmitter (vector) of malaria. If, in its feeding habits, it prefers animals other than man, it is also an inefficient vector of malaria. Probably the most efficient transmitter of malaria is *Anopheles gambiae*, the main vector of malaria in tropical Africa. *A. gambiae* is both long-lived and a man-biter by preference. Because of this efficient transmitter, almost all adults in much of Africa suffer from malaria. It is a great killer of infants and children. Those who survive develop a considerable immunity to the disease. Tragedy follows the introduction of this species of mosquito into parts of the world where a large fraction of the population have little or no immunity to malaria. When *A. gambiae* invaded Mauritius in the 1860s, malaria killed about one-fifth of the population in two years. In 1930 *A. gambiae* somehow reached Brazil from Africa, perhaps in aircraft or on a fast French destroyer. These mosquitoes found water on the South American coast where they were able to breed; they established themselves here and then gradually invaded the interior of the country. Malaria was already present in Brazil but was transmitted by much less efficient vectors than *A. gambiae*. This new, efficient vector mosquito rapidly converted malaria in man from isolated sporadic cases to an epidemic illness involving hundreds of thousands of cases. Between April and October of the year 1938 about 100 000 people were

infected and about 20 000 died. The economics of Brazil was disrupted. Enormous efforts to destroy *A. gambiae* cleared the entire infected area, so that by 1940 this species of mosquito had disappeared from Brazil. A similar conquest of *A. gambiae* followed a few years later in Egypt, after the species had invaded this country.

If *A. gambiae* were to be accidentally introduced into the developing countries of the East, the results would be only a little less damaging than atomic warfare. Outside tropical Africa, malaria is usually transmitted by much less efficient vectors. The species of mosquito involved have shorter lives and are not so specifically feeders on man. When the vector is inefficient, malaria tends to be a seasonal epidemic illness. During the winter or the dry season—when breeding of mosquitoes declines —people lose part of their immunity to malaria. When the mosquito population increases, e.g. during the wet season, transmission of malaria is resumed in the susceptible population and the numbers of those involved may reach epidemic proportions, affecting adults and children alike.

Figures 19.4, 19.5 show parts of the life cycle of the mosquito. Note that the larval and pupal stages of the life of this insect occur in water. For some species of mosquito this may be fresh water, for others it is brackish water. Without water, mosquitoes cannot breed. There have been attempts to control mosquitoes by drainage of breeding grounds or destruction of larval and pupal stages in water. However, there

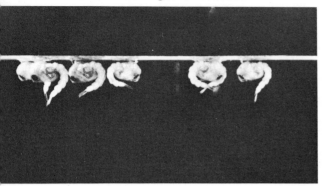

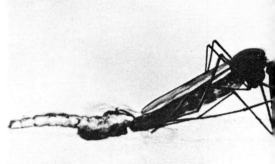

Figure 19.4 (above left)   Life cycle of the mosquito. The eggs are laid in water and hatch into larvae. These live, feed, and grow under the surface film of water and ultimately transform into pupae in which the body of the adult fly develops. This photograph shows pupae hanging from the surface film of water with their breathing tubes projecting into the air. (*WHO photo*.)

Figure 19.5 (above right)   The adult mosquito emerging from the skin of the pupa. (*WHO photo*.)

are considerable difficulties in controlling mosquitoes in this way; it is virtually impossible to drain or treat every stretch of stagnant water, large and small. We look later at more successful ways of controlling mosquitoes and thus controlling malaria.

The malaria parasite in man

We have seen that malaria is transmitted to man by a mosquito during its act of blood sucking. The infective form of malaria is a minute spindle-shaped cell called the sporozoite (Figure 19.6). Thousands of these organisms may be injected into a man during a single act of feeding. After a few hours the sporozoites disappear from the blood stream and from examining the circulating blood one would be unable to find any evidence that the person was infected. It was not until the 1940s that investigators discovered that the sporozoites settle down in various cells of the body outside the blood, particularly in the liver (Figures 19.7, 19.8). Each sporozoite enters a body cell and begins to feed on its substances. When the sporozoite has completed its growth we describe it as a schizont because this creature will now undergo multiple division or schizogony to produce many minute infecting organisms called merozoites. Infections by *Plasmodium falciparium* may produce 40 000 merozoites in the human liver during the course of about six days. Other species produce much smaller numbers of merozoites e.g. *P. vivax* produces about 1000. This phase of multiplication in the liver is called the exo-erythrocytic phase, i.e. outside the red cells. In *P. vivax* infections some of these merozoites invade further liver cells to

undergo another phase of multiplication; this has a special significance for the treatment of vivax malaria in man. Many of the merozoites of *P. vivax* and all merozoites of other malarial species now leave the liver and attack the red blood cells. After a merozoite has entered the red blood cell it gradually utilizes the cell contents for its own development and growth. The tiny merozoite becomes transformed into a small amoeba which eventually almost fills the red cell on which it has fed. When fully grown it undergoes a similar asexual process of multiplication to that which occurred in the liver. The average number of merozoites produced by the parasite in each red blood cell is sixteen. When the asexual reproduction (schizogony) is complete the red cell bursts, liberating into the circulating blood the merozoites and the remnants of the red cell contents. These merozoites now enter new red blood cells so that eventually thousands, sometimes millions, of parasites are present in the blood. We noted that the exo-erythrocytic multiplication of *P. falciparum* produces about 40 000 merozoites. Each of these can infect a red blood cell and each eventually produces twelve merozoites which then invade other red cells. If this process is not arrested there may be 10–20 per cent of the red cells infected with parasites—with over 500 000 parasites in each cubic centimetre of blood. No wonder *P. falciparum* malaria is called malignant malaria!

Eventually some of the merozoites do not develop into individuals (schizonts) which multiply to produce further merozoites; instead they develop into male and female forms of the parasite called gametocytes. These gametocytes

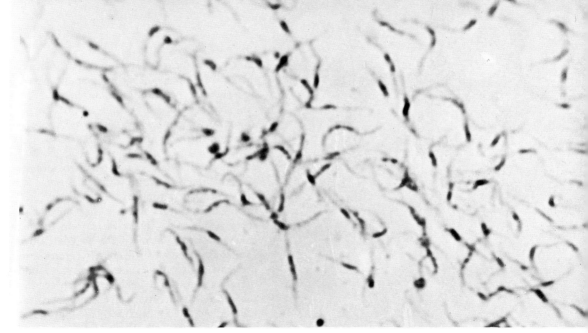

Figure 19.6   H.P. photomicrograph of malarial sporozoites in mosquito saliva.

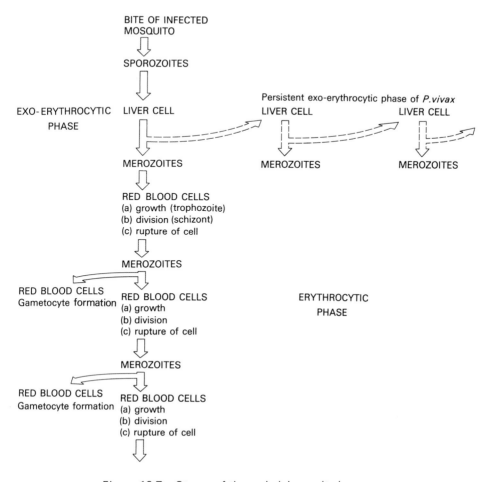

Figure 19.7   Stages of the malarial parasite in man.

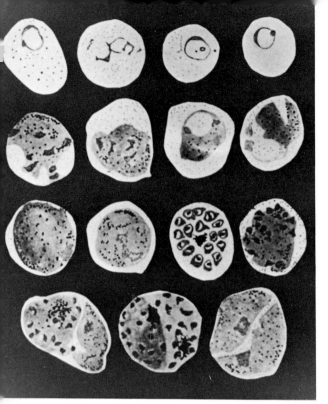

Figure 19.8 Malarial parasites in red blood cells.

Column 1 shows young trophozoites in red blood cells. The young trophozoite has a small body with a deeply staining nucleus. The stained cytoplasm surrounds an unstained central vacuole giving the appearance of a 'signet ring'. The infected red cell gradually enlarges and accumulates spots of pigment — the Schüfner dots.

Column 2 shows older trophozoites. In these the cytoplasm becomes actively amoeboid, throwing out numerous pseudopodia. The outline of the parasite thus tends to be irregular in stained blood films.

Column 3 shows developing and mature schizonts. The parasite continues to grow and the cytoplasm becomes more compact. The nucleus begins to divide and eventually the fully developed schizont contains 12–24 merozoites. These are released when the red cell ruptures and the merozoites enter new red cells to restart the cycle.

Column 4 shows red cells containing gametocytes. For reasons that are not understood some of the merozoites that enter red cells develop not into schizonts but into gametocytes which undergo no further development unless they are taken into the stomach of a mosquito. The male (microgametocyte) and female (macrogametocyte) differ very little from one another in the red cell. The main difference lies in the nucleus, which is compact or diffuse according to the sex. In the cells there is plentiful pigment scattered throughout the body of the parasite. (WHO drawing.)

undergo no further development in man, and they will eventually die if they are not sucked up by a suitable species of mosquito in which they can develop further (Figure 19.9). In the mosquito, the gametocytes survive the process of digestion in the stomach and transform themselves into male and female sex cells. The nucleus of the male gametocyte divides into several segments, each of which goes into a long thin process of cytoplasm on the surface of the male gametocyte. These are the equivalent of spermatozoa. They break away from the male gametocyte and swim to the female gametocytes, which they fertilize. After fertilization the female sex cell becomes transformed into a motile organism, the ookinete, which swims in the stomach contents. It eventually penetrates the wall of the stomach, where it grows and eventually divides repeatedly to produce sporozoites in a cyst (Figure 19.10). This swelling in the stomach wall is called the oocyst. It eventually ruptures to liberate the sporozoites into the blood space around the gut. Now they make their way to the salivary glands of the mosquito. The number of sporozoites produced in the mosquito is enormous, depending upon the number of oocysts which develop in the stomach wall. There may be up to fifty oocysts in the stomach, each of which may produce 10 000 sporozoites.

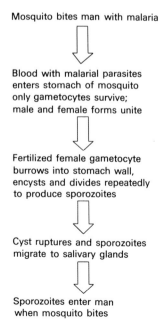

Mosquito bites man with malaria

⇩

Blood with malarial parasites enters stomach of mosquito only gametocytes survive; male and female forms unite

⇩

Fertilized female gametocyte burrows into stomach wall, encysts and divides repeatedly to produce sporozoites

⇩

Cyst ruptures and sporozoites migrate to salivary glands

⇩

Sporozoites enter man when mosquito bites

Figure 19.9 The malarial parasite in the mosquito.

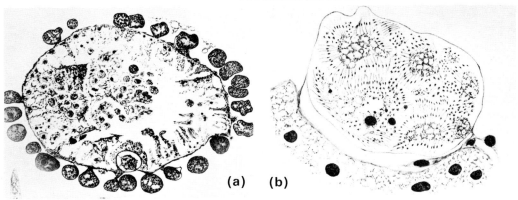

Figure 19.10   (a) (left) Section of the stomach of a mosquito bearing numerous oocysts. (b) (right) H.P. drawing of an oocyst showing the development of sporozoites. (*By courtesy of WMMS.*)

The effect of malaria on man and human communities

The effect of infection with the malaria parasite depends on whether or not an individual has had previous contact with the parasite and has developed some immunity. In those individuals who have been exposed to the infection since birth and have survived attacks of malaria, a considerable degree of tolerance may develop; there may be a considerable number of parasites in the blood with few symptoms. In the individual who has had no previous infection, or no recent infection, serious illness may develop rapidly. About ten days after infection with the parasites fever develops, increasing gradually over the course of a few days or appearing suddenly with a body temperature as high as 105–107 °F (40.6–41.7 °C). The duration of the fever varies considerably; it may be short or it may last for as long as twelve hours. The fever is associated with such symptoms as headache, nausea, generalized aching and pain over the spleen—which is often enlarged and tender (Figure 19.11). After a variable period of fever, sweating starts and the body temperature falls to normal or below. The symptoms of malaria occur when enough cycles of multiplication of the parasite have occurred to produce enough rupturing red cells—releasing parasites and cell debris in amounts sufficient to cause a fever. The onset of fever coincides with the rupture of large numbers of parasitized red cells. The period of schizogony in the red cell varies from one species of malaria to another; textbooks usually describe the fever of malaria as occurring at regular intervals, on every third day in *Plasmodium vivax*, *P. falciparum*, and *P. ovale* malarias and every fourth day in *P. malariae* malaria. These

regular bouts of fever occur only when there is a single infection by one species of malaria parasite, and not always then, for the merozoites are often liberated from the liver in 'broods' which produce successive attacks on the red cells so that schizogony in the parasitized red cells is not often in phase. The situation is even more complicated by successive infections from mosquitoes. Fever may thus be continuous, irregular or occur once or twice a day.

In infections by *P. falciparum*—so called malignant malaria—the fever, which is apt to become more or less continuous, is overshadowed by other symptoms. We have already noted the enormous multiplication of the parasite which occurs in the liver in *P. falciparum* malaria. The blood becomes very heavily para-

Figure 19.11   The French Cameroons showing examination of the spleen, which is usually enlarged in both acute and chronic malaria. (*WHO photo by Pierre Pittet.*)

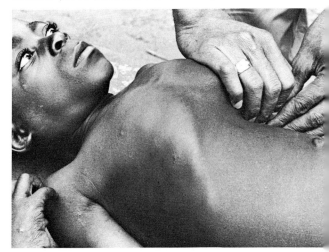

sitized. The red blood cells which are parasitized become sticky and tend to adhere to the walls of blood vessels. This process is particularly likely to occur in the blood vessels of the brain, lungs, kidney and bowel. The small blood vessels of these organs may become virtually blocked by enormous numbers of parasitized red cells. There may be convulsions and coma from brain involvement, kidney failure and pneumonia. *P. falciparum* malaria can be a fatal disease within a day or two unless it is vigorously treated.

Fortunately infections by other species of malaria produce a less serious disease in terms of mortality rate, but they can have drastic effects on the economic life of a community. Epidemic malaria tends to occur twice yearly, in the autumn and the spring. The spring is the season of planting, the autumn that of harvest, the worst periods of the year to have agricultural workers incapacitated by malaria; nor can modern industry operate efficiently when large numbers of workers are intermittently off work with malaria. Further the control of the disease can have dramatic effects on the economic life of a community. Various estimates have been made of the cost of malaria in different countries. It was estimated that in 1908 malaria cost the U.S.A. 100 million dollars a year and that in 1938 the cost had risen to 500 million dollars. Now, when malaria is rare in the U.S.A., it still has marked economic effects because the imports of goods coming from malarious areas (e.g. wood, cocoa, coffee etc.) cost the U.S.A. 5 per cent more than they would cost if the malarious areas had not to spend so much money on the control of malaria. During periods of war, malaria has presented such problems to commanders of armies that top priority has been given to the control of this disease.

In recent wars, malaria has devastated armies in Macedonia (1916), in India, Burma, the South Pacific and the Mediterranean regions during the Second World War, and more recently in Korea and Vietnam. Of the British forces in Macedonia in 1916, a quarter of the fighting force of 123 000 men had to enter hospital to be treated for malaria. During the Second World War, in the South Pacific over 60 per cent of the forces were casualties of malaria between September 1943 and February 1944. Adequate funds for malaria research and control always become available when military danger is imminent, and radical improvements in malaria control have thereby arisen from the needs of war.

The eradication of malaria

In 1955 the 8th World Health Assembly decided 'on the implementation of a programme having as its ultimate objective the worldwide eradication of malaria'. Vast sums of money had to be found to further this aim—for training of personnel, research into basic aspects of malaria, advisory services, provision of equipment—insecticides, sprayers, transport etc.

The ways in which malaria can be controlled and eventually eradicated are various, and include not only the eradication of the disease in individuals suffering from malaria but also the destruction of the vectors of the disease, i.e. the mosquitoes. We will consider the methods that can be employed under the following headings:

1. drainage of the breeding grounds of mosquitoes,
2. destruction of mosquito larvae,
3. destruction of adult mosquitoes by using insecticides,
4. destruction of malarial parasites in man.

Drainage of breeding grounds

This was one of the earliest methods used to attack the mosquito. Drainage was used in ancient Rome to try to clear the Pontine marshes, but this was not successfully done until 1930. Then efficient drainage of the Pontine marshes converted an uninhabitable area into one of 8000 hectares of farmlands. In other parts of the world drainage has been used with success in the control of mosquitoes, but the process is expensive and incomplete; it is virtually impossible to drain all the small ditches and ponds in which mosquitoes find breeding places.

Destruction of larvae

Various substances such as Paris green or petroleum oils can be added to water to destroy mosquito larvae. The larvae and pupae of mosquitoes obtain the oxygen necessary for their life by means of small tubes which they thrust through the surface of the water (Figure 19.4). A layer of oil on the surface of the water blocks these breathing tubes and suffocates the insects. This method can be very successful. It was used in the campaign against *Anopheles gambiae* in Brazil (page 205), but it is expensive and laborious and more suited to the eradication of mosquitoes from a small area. Nowadays the method of choice is to attack the adult mosquito.

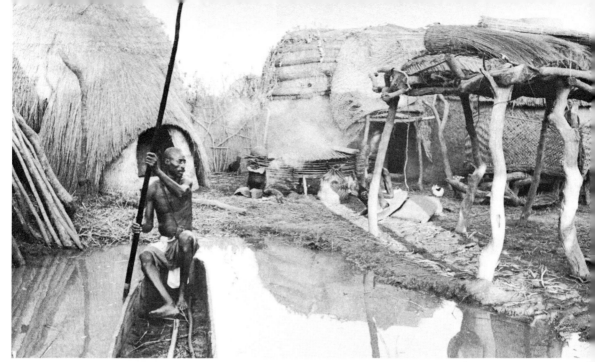

Figure 19.12 A banana village in the French Cameroons, built into a swamp—an ideal breeding place for mosquitoes. (*WHO photo by Pierre Pittet.*)

Destruction of adult mosquitoes with insecticide (Figure 19.3–19.6)

The basic concept of modern malaria eradication is not to try to exterminate mosquitoes completely but rather to kill mosquitoes entering dwelling houses by spraying indoor surfaces of dwellings with a persistent insecticide. Of the four species of malaria, the two important ones, *P. vivax* and *P. falciparum*, eventually die out in untreated patients in about three years. If dwellings are sprayed with persistent insecticide for three years, the cycle of transmission of man-mosquito-man can be broken. After this period the mosquitoes can be left to breed freely, for there will be no human infective cases left from whom they can transmit malaria.

Four different insecticides have been used against the adult mosquito—petroleum extract of pyrethrum, DDT, benzene hexachloride (BHC) and dieldren. The last three are persistent insecticides; when these insecticides are sprayed on the interior surfaces of dwellings, they leave a deposit which retains its lethal properties for a considerable time. This is the procedure in what is called the 'attack phase' of malaria eradication. During this phase human cases of malaria must be detected and adequately treated with drugs, and this includes detecting and treating any cases imported into an area.

The undertaking of an eradication programme involves considerable planning and organization. In many countries a national malaria eradication service had to be set up so that the whole malarious areas of the country could be surveyed and mapped, and every house recorded. A large number of professional staff is involved, including doctors, nurses, entomologists (Figure 19.17), surveyors etc. and an army of spraymen for the attack phase. The eradication phase may have to be preceded by a 'pre-eradication' programme to investigate the malaria situation, to decide the most suitable means of attack and to expand and develop the health services.

After the eradication phase comes the consolidation phase, in which continual surveillance is necessary to detect and treat any case of malaria and to check that transmission of the disease by the mosquito has ceased. After this comes the maintenance phase. Malaria is now eradicated, but constant vigilance is necessary to prevent its re-introduction from malarious countries.

Some countries of the world, notably tropical Africa, could not, for various reasons, undertake eradication programmes. Pre-eradication programmes, however, have been set up to gradually build up the organization necessary for launching a full-scale eradication programme. Malaria has already been reported as eradicated in areas with a population of nearly 300 million—in some Caribbean islands, Chile, Cyprus, France, Italy, the Netherlands, Singapore, five republics of the U.S.S.R. and the U.S.A. The progress of malaria eradication has varied from region to

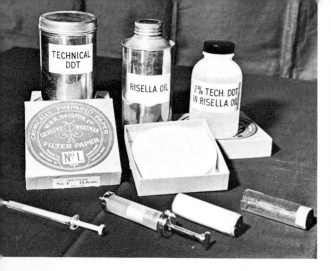

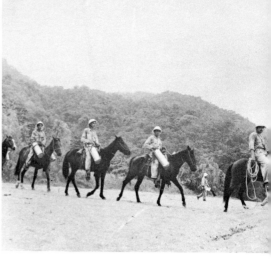

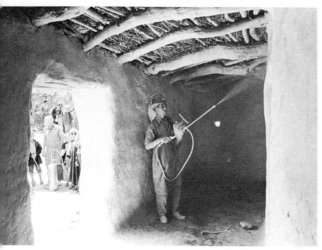

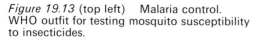

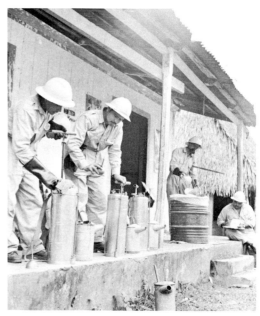

Figure 19.13 (top left)   Malaria control. WHO outfit for testing mosquito susceptibility to insecticides.

Figure 19.14 (top right)   Mexico against malaria. A spray team sets out for a day's spraying operation. (*WHO photo by Eric Schwab*.)

Figure 19.15 (bottom left)   Spraying DDT in a Moroccan village. (*WHO photo by Philip Boucas*.)

Figure 19.16 (bottom right)   Mexico against malaria. With safety equipment for self-protection, the spraymen prepare the insecticide (dieldren) for an onslaught against the mosquito hideouts. (*WHO photo by Eric Schwab*.)

region. In most parts of Africa, malaria eradication is still the most important public health programme, and the attainment of the eradication of malaria from all parts of the world is still distant. Problems have arisen when there is an unequal development of eradication programmes in neighbouring countries. National boundaries have to be respected by man but they are not respected by mosquitoes; malaria is a disease which travels widely and rapidly.

Various factors militate against the aim of malaria eradication, including political, financial and organizational stumbling blocks, and war. There is also the problem of the development of resistance to insecticides by mosquitoes. Until recently DDT has been the most effective insecticide against mosquitoes and other arthropod pests, but strains of mosquitoes, plague-transmitting fleas and human body lice have appeared which are resistant to DDT. In 1951 the first DDT-resistant strains of vector mosquitoes was reported from the U.S.A., Greece and Panama. In some parts of the world, particularly in Mexico and Central America, DDT spraying no longer prevents the transmission of malaria. Benzene hexachloride (BHC), dieldren and other substances are already being used against arthropods that are resistant to DDT.

The malarial parasite itself has also evolved

resistance to drugs which have been the basis of the treatment of malaria in man for years—but more of this below.

Destruction of malarial parasites in man

Control of an acute attack of malaria

There is a large number of different drugs which have been used in the prevention and treatment of malaria in man. Unfortunately there is no single drug which we can use to kill all the various forms of the parasite—sporozoites, exo-erythrocytic stages in the liver, schizonts in the red blood cells, and the gametocytes. In treating a patient who is acutely ill with malaria, the prime aim is to stop the schizogony in the red blood cells, thus preventing the rhythmical break-down of large numbers of red cells and the liberation of merozoites and waste products into the circulation. Various drugs have been used for this purpose, e.g. chloroquine, quinacrine and quinine. Quinine is the oldest drug used in the treatment of malaria; it comes from the bark of the cinchona tree which grows in South America and the Far East. By 1640 the drug had already been introduced by the Spaniards into Europe and was widely used in the treatment of various fevers, and at a later date more specifically for the treatment of fever caused by malaria. Although the drug can be synthesized, the procedure is complex and expensive and it is still obtained from cinchona bark. With the introduction of powerful synthetic antimalarial drugs, the use of quinine gradually declined.

Destruction of the exo-erythrocytic phase of P. vivax malaria

When drugs such as chloroquine, quinacrine or quinine are used to treat an acute attack of malaria, they often produce a complete cure of the disease. An exception to this is in the case of infections caused by *P. vivax*. We have already seen that in infections by this species the merozoites liberated from the liver cells do not all enter the red blood cells. Some re-enter other liver cells to produce further broods of merozoites which behave in the same way. We say that this species has a persistent exo-erythrocytic phase. The parasites in the liver are not affected by the drugs which are used to control an acute attack of malaria, so that the disease can recur when a new generation of merozoites has been released from the liver cells. We say that the disease relapses. We do have drugs which can kill the exo-erythrocytic stages of vivax malaria but they are too toxic for general use. Their use

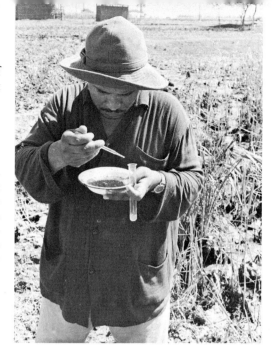

Figure 19.17   Malaria eradication. The entomologist, a member of the team fighting malaria. (*WHO photo by Philip Boucas.*)

is only justified when a patient is going to leave an area which is endemic for *P. vivax* malaria, i.e. when the patient is unlikely to be infected again.

The prevention of malaria

The drugs which are used to treat acute attacks of malaria can also be used to *prevent* an attack of malaria—if they are taken regularly, in adequate doses, in an area where infection is likely. The drugs do not actually kill sporozoites introduced by mosquitoes or prevent them from settling down and multiplying in the liver, but they do block the schizogenous cycles in the red blood cells. They are described as suppressive drugs. In some parts of the world attempts have been made to reduce the number of parasites in the blood of the general population—and so reduce the transmission rate—by adding a suitable drug to salt (Figures 19.18, 19.19).

Drug resistance of malarial parasites and the development of new drugs

The drugs used in the control of malaria changed little between 1900 and 1940, and at the start of the Second World War quinine and quinacrine (atabrine) were used to prevent and treat malaria, and pyrethrum—a non-persistent insecticide—was used to control mosquitoes. During the Second World War there was a movement of

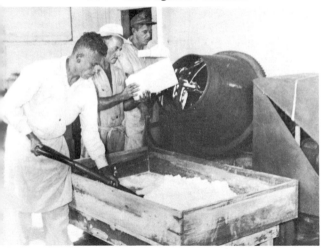

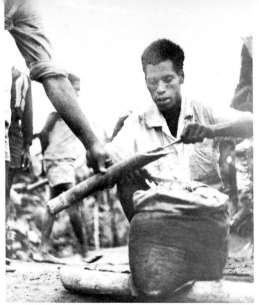

Figure 19.18   Prevention of malaria. An antimalarial drug is mixed with salt. (*WHO photo.*)

Figure 19.19   Prevention of malaria in New Guinea. Antimalarial salt being distributed. (*WHO photo.*)

large numbers of forces into malarious areas—Polynesia, Far East and Mediterranean regions. The only commercial sources of quinine were in the South Pacific, and these were soon taken over by the Japanese. The Germans had anticipated the need for an alternative to quinine, and before the war they had developed the drug called quinacrine. This drug was produced in large amounts in America in the early part of the Second World War. Attempts were also made to increase the supplies of quinine, and the cinchona plantations of South America were revitalized. However, quinacrine had certain disadvantages and there was obviously the need for a better drug. Intense research went into satisfying this need. In two years over 1600 chemical compounds were tested for their activity against the malarial parasite in birds. Since there are differences between the parasites causing malaria in birds and man, potentially useful drugs had to be tested further in human volunteers infected artificially or naturally by the four species of human malaria. Only about eighty of the 1600 drugs were in fact tested in this way in human volunteers. This research programme produced such drugs as chloroquine, chlorguanide (paludrine) and pyrimethamine (daraprim). These were new and effective drugs, but they still had the limitations of the older drugs in that no single drug could destroy all the various forms of the malarial parasites in the human body. Some could be used effectively in the treatment of an acute attack of malaria or in the prevention of malaria, but others had to be used to destroy the phases in the liver and so produce a permanent cure of *P. vivax* malaria.

Yet another drug had to be used if one wanted to destroy gametocytes and so prevent transmission to mosquitoes and block the transmission cycle. In spite of this kind of limitation there now existed effective drugs for all stages of the parasite in man. Moreover the introduction of the persistent insecticide DDT, revolutionized the control of mosquitoes. It would seem that at the end of the Second World War the control of malaria was solved. We have already noted the gradual evolution of strains of mosquitoes resistant to DDT. The same fate befell the various drugs used to control malaria in man—they became less and less useful.

The World Health Organization reported that from 1948–50, resistance of malaria parasites to chlorguanide was detected in Malaysia. From 1950–59, resistance to various antimalarial drugs, including quinine, was noted in other parts of the world. In 1960 the first cases of *P. falciparum* malaria resistant to chloroquine were found (South America). In 1961 troops of the Commonwealth and the U.S.A. contracted chloroquine-resistant falciparum malaria in Vietnam, Thailand, Cambodia and Malaysia. It became a serious threat to the U.S. forces in Vietnam. Malaria is a disease which travels far and fast; resistant strains of *P. falciparum* malaria potentially threatened the rest of Asia. Further intensive studies followed, and the Walter Reed Army Institute of Research tested more than 11000 chemicals for antimalarial activity.

The new antimalarial drugs which appeared have come from the recognition that protozoa are extremely sensitive to a deficiency of the vitamin called folic acid—which is also a vital food component for man and many animals. Combinations of drugs which interfere with various stages of the metabolism of folic acid in the malarial parasite were found to have dramatic effects in chloroquine-resistant *P. falciparum* malaria in man. The results were so good that a cure could be obtained with a single dose of the combinations of drugs. These drugs cannot be used to prevent malaria because the prolonged taking of the drugs would interfere with the folic acid metabolism of man himself and produce serious side-effects, but in 'one-shot' treatment the drugs kill the parasites without affecting human tissues. These combinations of drugs (e.g. a sulphonamide and trimethoprim) although they destroy the schizonts in the red blood cells, do not affect the gametocytes. Anyone leaving an area where mosquitoes are transmitting chloroquine-resistant *P. falciparum* malaria (e.g. U.S. troops returning to the U.S.A. from Vietnam) is treated with another drug (e.g. primaquine) to destroy the gametocytes and so prevent them from infecting mosquitoes in their homeland with this problem-strain of malaria. No doubt there will be even further battles with malaria parasites when in their devious ways they 'discover' ways of avoiding destruction by the drugs in use today.

Conclusions

We have looked in some detail at the history of man's battle against the malarial parasite. We have seen that Plasmodium spp. show considerable adaptation to the parasitic way of life. Not only are two kinds of animal involved in the life cycle of the parasite, with the mosquito playing the role of transmitter of the parasite from man to man, but the parasite itself shows enormous powers of multiplication, both in man and in the mosquito. It should be quite apparent that a detailed knowledge of the life history of the parasite and the mosquito vector is necessary for an efficient attack on the parasite. We have a wide armament of substances which we can use to destroy both the mosquito and the malarial parasites in man, but these must be used with a thorough knowledge of their limitations. In particular, no single drug will destroy all the various forms of the parasite in man; one has to choose an appropriate drug according to one's aim—whether this is to prevent an attack of malaria, treat an acute attack of malaria, destroy the exo-erythrocytic stages of *P. vivax* malaria and so produce a permanent cure, or to destroy gametocytes. The solution of the world malaria

problem is still distant. We still have fully to deploy the arms we already possess against the parasite, and we may yet have to devise new ways of attack if pesticide resistance by mosquitoes and drug resistance by the malaria parasite continues to evolve.

Amoebiasis—a disease caused by *Entamoeba histolytica*

This amoeba is just one of several species of amoebae that may inhabit the large bowel (colon) of man. Like the malarial parasite and the trypanosome, the amoeba belongs to the phylum Protozoa. Entamoeba is a member of the class Rhizopoda of the phylum Protozoa; these organisms have no fixed shape, for they continually put out extensions of the body material—the pseudopodia—into which the rest of the body then moves. These pseudopodia may also

Figure 19.20   (a) (top) Photomicrograph of *Amoeba proteus*, a free-living organism living in water. Note the pseudopodia.
(b) (bottom) *Entamoeba histolytica* from the bowel wall containing ingested red cells.
(*By courtesy of WMMS.*)

(a)

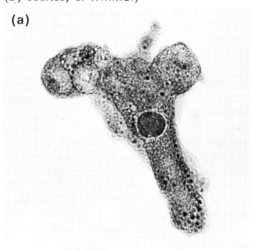

(b)

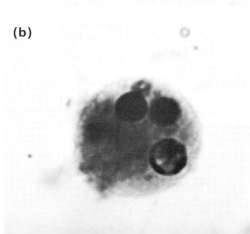

enclose and take into the body food material; the food becomes enclosed in the body in a food vacuole where it is digested (Figure 19.20). The feeding motile amoeba which lives in the colon is a microscopic creature measuring only about 20 micrometers across (1 micrometer = $\frac{1}{1000}$ mm).

In many individuals *Entamoeba histolytica*, like the other species of amoeba that inhabit the bowel, causes no illness; it lives as a harmless commensal of the large bowel, feeding on bacteria and other foodstuffs in the bowel. Individuals carrying these harmless commensals are called symptomless carriers of the disease amoebiasis. For reasons that are not understood this harmless commensal form of the organism can become a dangerous parasite. This is particularly likely to occur in tropical and sub-tropical regions of the world. The amoeba now attaches itself to the lining of the large bowel and begins to invade the wall of the bowel, feeding on the tissues and red blood cells. This causes ulceration of the bowel wall.

Multiplication of amoebae occurs by simple binary fission; the nucleus first divides and then the cytoplasm separates into two portions, each of which then takes half of the original nucleus. Large numbers of amoebae may be produced by this process. The invasion and ulceration of the bowel wall may result in an acute attack of dysentery. The patient with acute amoebic dysentery is distressed with abdominal pain, frequent loose stools containing blood and mucus, nausea, vomiting and fever. Amoebic dysentery can be a fatal illness, particularly when it occurs in the young, the elderly, the under-nourished or in those already weakened by other illnesses. Losses of water and salts are important factors in determining the seriousness of the illness, but death can be rapid if the amoebic ulcers of the bowel erode a large blood vessel, leading to massive haemorrhage. The bowel may also be perforated by the ulceration.

Another potentially serious complication of amoebic infection of the bowel is the release of amoebae into the circulating blood. These amoebae are transported to various organs in the blood stream and may settle down and multiply in various tissues; the liver is a favourite site of infection, but the lungs and brain may also be involved. Local inflammation occurs and amoebic abscesses may develop. These are particularly dangerous when they occur in the brain.

Acute attacks of amoebic dysentery may be followed by a more chronic infection of the bowel, with periodic flare-ups of the disease in the form of attacks of dysentery.

Distribution of the parasite

Amoebiasis is a disease of world-wide distribution; no longer is it regarded as a tropical disease. In some regions in temperate climates the incidence of the disease may be as high as in the tropics if sanitary conditions are poor. Certainly the disease is rare in Britain, and when it does occur it is, like typhoid, most likely to be imported from some continental or North African holiday resort. Certain areas of the U.S.A. have an incidence as high as 20 per cent. It is in fact difficult to obtain a true estimate of the incidence of the disease, particularly in undeveloped areas of the world, because many infectious diseases of the bowel cause dysentery with blood and mucus in the stools. The disease can be diagnosed with certainty only by demonstrating *Entamoeba histolytica* in the stools; any amoebae that are found must be carefully distinguished from the harmless commensal species of amoebae which may inhabit the bowel.

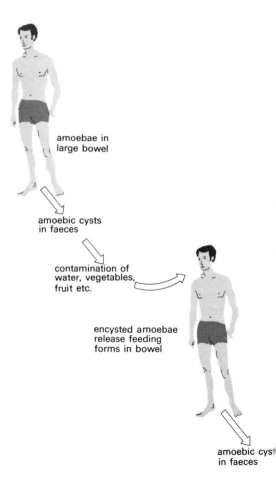

amoebae in large bowel

amoebic cysts in faeces

contamination of water, vegetables, fruit etc.

encysted amoebae release feeding forms in bowel

amoebic cyst in faeces

Figure 19.21   The life cycle of the dysentery amoeba.

Life cycle of *Amoeba histolytica* and the control of the disease (Figure 19.21)

The life cycle of this amoeba is a fairly simple one. In the lumen of the bowel or in the wall of the ulcerated intestine, individual amoebae multiply by binary fission. Large numbers of amoebae may be present, and living motile amoebae may be found in the stools. In the outside world these motile forms cannot survive. Survival is ensured by the development of a protected phase in the life of the parasite—the encysted amoeba, which contains four nuclei. No further change will occur in these spherical cysts unless they are swallowed by man; then the cysts pass down the alimentary canal in contaminated food until they reach the small intestine, where the cyst walls are dissolved, liberating amoebae containing four nuclei. The nuclei undergo further division and the cytoplasm divides, resulting in eight small amoebae.

Treatment of amoebiasis

There is a variety of drugs which are available to treat amoebiasis—emetine, chloroquine, arsenicals, antibiotics and so on. Not all members of this armoury of drugs can destroy amoebae both in the intestine and in other tissues (liver, lung, brain). To some extent the choice of drugs depends upon the sites of infection, and members of this group, although they will rapidly terminate an acute attack of dysentery, are valueless for clearing the symptomless passer of amoebic cysts.

Prevention and eradication of amoebiasis

Man can contract amoebiasis only by eating amoebic cysts excreted by another case of amoebiasis. The essence of control of amoebiasis is the safe disposal of faeces (containing encysted amoebae), a safe water supply (uncontaminated by faeces), hygienic handling and adequate cooking of foodstuffs. Uncooked foodstuffs, e.g. salads, in undeveloped regions of the world (i.e. with poor sanitation and unsafe water supplies) are obviously potentially highly dangerous. Cases of frank dysentery should be followed up to ensure that the organisms are eradicated from the bowel. Symptomless excretors of amoebic cysts are a danger to any community, especially if they handle food with unwashed hands. Flies also play their part in the transmission of amoebic cysts from faeces to food, and fly control is thus a necessary component of measures aimed at reducing the frequency of the disease.

Trypanosomiasis

The African form of the disease

African trypanosomiasis, like malaria, is caused by a minute protozoan parasite that lives in human blood. Unlike the malarial parasite which lives in the red blood cells, the trypanosome lives in the fluid part of blood, i.e. plasma. This protozoan causes a disease which is particularly lethal to man (called sleeping sickness) and domestic stock—cattle, horses etc., (called nagana). It is a disease which is widespread through the African continent from the southern borders of the Sahara to a latitude 20 °S, making agriculture and stock-raising virtually impossible over more than 10 million square kilometres of fertile land. It is one of the major factors restricting the economic development of Africa today.

The parasite and its life history

The structure of the parasite is shown in Figure 19.22. It shows an elongated, flattened body with a projection called the flagellum. Along its length the flagellum is bound to the rest of the body of the trypanosome by means of a ribbon of protoplasm called the undulating membrane. When the trypanosome is moving about in the blood the flagellum and undulating membrane produce wave-like movements. There are in fact three different species of trypanosome, *T. gambiense* and *T. rhodesiense* cause the sleeping sickness of Africa, and they are transmitted from man to man by tsetse flies, while *T. cruzi* causes

Figure 19.22   Trypanosoma rhodesiense in a smear of blood. (*By courtesy of WMMS.*)

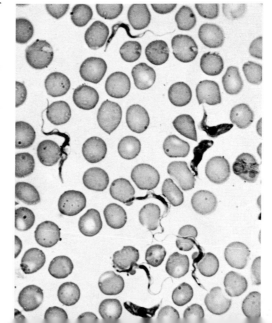

a different disease of man in the Americas, and it is transmitted by means of blood sucking bugs.

In Africa trypanosomes are transmitted to man and domestic stock by tsetse flies of several species (Figure 16.3). The domestic animals form a reservoir of the disease for man, i.e. trypanosomiasis is a zoonosis (page 190). Trypanosomes are taken up by the tsetse fly as it takes a meal of blood from man or animal. Inside the tsetse flies the trypanosomes undergo various changes during their passage through the food canal. These changes include multiplication by longitudinal division of the animal, and enormous numbers of trypanosomes may be produced in this way. These eventually migrate to the proboscis of the fly and up the duct of the salivary gland. Here they undergo yet further multiplication. The whole cycle in the tsetse fly takes fifteen to thirty-five days. There are so many trypanosomes in the tsetse fly that it probably can transmit the disease for the rest of its life—which may be a few months. This kind of transmission in which the trypanosomes undergo a cycle of development in the tsetse fly is not vital. A simpler form of transmission—by

Figure 19.23   A victim of sleeping sickness from the Cameroons. (*WHO photo.*)

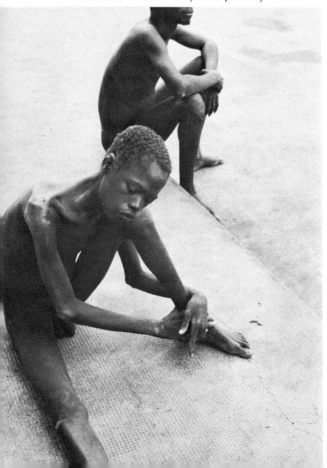

any blood sucking insect—is possible. Thus if a fly is disturbed when taking a blood meal from a man suffering from trypanosomiasis it may then alight on another man, its proboscis still wet with blood containing living trypanosomes, and directly transmit the disease to the man by plunging its mouthparts into his skin.

Sleeping sickness in man (Figure 19.23)

The diseases caused by *T. gambiense* and *T. rhodesiense* differ somewhat. *T. rhodesiense* produces a rapidly developing disease which may be fatal within a year if it is untreated. The disease produced by *T. gambiense* follows a slower course and may last for several years. In both forms of the disease the lymphatic and nervous systems are involved. At the site of a bite of an infected tsetse fly, a painless lump appears and the lymph glands in the groin and neck become enlarged. Within two or three weeks after infection, the parasites can be detected in these glands by plunging a needle into the gland and drawing off fluid for examination under the microscope. In addition to enlargement of the lymph glands, there is fever and enlargement of the liver and spleen. Later the parasite involves the central nervous system, and at this stage it can be found in the fluid that bathes the spinal cord and brain. During this phase of the disease the patient develops mental apathy, muscular spasms, uncoordinated movements and sleepiness. Sleepiness may be so pronounced that the patient falls asleep even when standing or eating. Nutrition becomes impaired and weight loss may be extreme. Death occurs in coma.

Treatment of sleeping sickness

There are a variety of drugs available for the treatment of the African form of trypanosomiasis—sleeping sickness. The earliest stages of the disease are the easiest to treat; one can in fact prevent the development of the disease by a single intramuscular injection of a drug called pentamidine every few months. Unfortunately the drugs which are needed for late cases of the disease are very toxic and need to be given under close medical supervision. There is still a need for a safe drug which is easy to administer, relatively non-toxic to the patient, and which can be used for all stages of the disease.

Prevention of sleeping sickness

The tsetse flies which can transmit trypanosomiasis live in certain restricted areas—'fly belts' —that are as large as 13.5 million square kilometres. A great deal of information is still needed on the biology of various species of tsetse flies. Eradication of the flies is not a practicable possibility in a continent as economically poor as Africa. Attempts have been made to control some flies in some areas; some species seek the shade and humidity of the vegetation along rivers and lakes, and the clearing of this vegetation can control these kinds of tsetse flies. Other species of fly live in open country feeding on the blood of wild game, and these are obviously more difficult to control.

Man can reduce the likelihood of being bitten by tsetse flies, but the methods are laborious and expensive. These measures include fly screens on doors and windows of houses, vehicles, river boats etc., the use of insect repellant creams, spraying of cattle with DDT, spraying insecticides over places inhabited by the flies by aeroplanes, and moving human settlements to areas cleared of flies, e.g. by destruction of vegetation along lakes and rivers. These methods have been successful in restricted areas of Africa, e.g. along the shores of Lake Victoria and the rivers of Kenya and the southern Sudan. Wild game can also be controlled or killed to remove animals such as the wild pig and antelope which act as reservoirs of the disease in man.

The conquest of trypanosomiasis in Africa is in the distant future. Many more studies are needed on the geographical distribution of trypanosomes and their responses to drugs; on the biology and control of the important species of tsetse flies; on the biology and importance of wild animals which act as a reservoir of the disease; and research into the development of vaccines and drugs to prevent or treat the infection of man and animals.

American trypanosomiasis

American trypanosomiasis or Chaga's disease is caused by *Trypanosoma cruzi*, and the parasite is transmitted to man by the bite of certain reduviid bugs (Figure 19.24). The disease is limited in its distribution to the Americas—

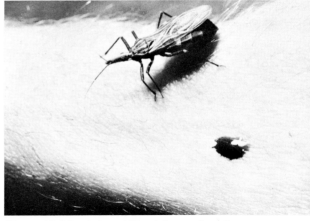

Figure 19.24 A bug (*Rhodnius prolexus*) on human skin with a faecal drop after feeding. This insect is the transmitter of Chaga's disease. (*By courtesy of WMMS, photograph by Dr W. Petana, Liverpool School of Tropical Medicine.*)

South and Central America and certain southern states of the U.S.A. It is a zoonosis (page 190) and many domestic and wild animals can act as a reservoir of the disease. It has been estimated that at least 7 million people are infected by *T. cruzi* and some 35 million are exposed to the risk of infection; acute cases of the disease in children carries a mortality of 10 per cent. Much work remains to be done on the diagnosis, prevention and treatment of the disease as at the moment there is no effective drug for the treatment of the disease.

Other protozoan parasites of man

We have looked in some detail at three important diseases of man caused by protozoan parasites. Space does not permit us to consider other protozoan species that may infect man, e.g. *Leishmania* species, *Toxoplasma* or *Giardia intestinalis*, but sources of information can be found in the list of references. In the section of venereal diseases we will be looking at one protozoan parasite of the genital tract, *Trichomonas vaginalis*, which is sometimes transmitted during sexual intercourse.

20. Parasitic worms

Introduction

AN ENORMOUS variety of worms can and do infect man. There is a rich variety of structures, feeding habits, life histories and the degrees of injury that they inflict upon their hosts. Parasitic worms fall into two main groups, the Platyhelminthes or flat worms (tapeworms and flukes) and the Nematoda or round worms, and we will be looking at various representatives of these two groups (phyla) of worms. Table 22 lists some parasitic tapeworms, flukes and round worms and their importance for world health. This list is not exhaustive and details of many other parasitic worms can be found in the literature listed in the references. The following is a list of the parasitic worms which we will be looking at in this chapter.

Tapeworms (Cestoda)
  Pork tapeworm (*Taenia solium*)
  Beef tapeworm (*Taenia saginata*)
  Fish tapeworm (*Diphyllobothrium latum*)
  Dwarf tapeworm (*Hymenolepis nana*)

Flukes (Trematoda)
  Liver fluke (*Fasciola hepatica*)
  Blood flukes (Schistosoma species)

Round worms (Nematoda)
  The large round worm (*Ascaris lumbricoides*)
  Hook worms
  The trichina worm (*Trichinella spiralis*)
  Filarial worms
  Pin worms (*Enterobius vermicularis*)

Table 22 Calculated numbers of human worm infections in millions calculated on a 1963 world population of 3165 million

Worm	Number of infected cases in Europe (excluding U.S.S.R.)	Total world cases
Trichinella spiralis	4.4	39.4
Taenia saginata (beef tapeworm)	0.9	60.6
Taenia solium (pork tapeworm)		3.9
Dyphyllobothrium (fish tapeworm)	3.2	13.4
Schistosoma species		203.8
Hymenolepis nana (dwarf tapeworm)	1.8	29.4
Onchocerca volvulus (blinding filaria)		39.4
Wuchereria bancrofti (Bancroft's filarial worm)		295.5
Enterobius vermicularis (pin worm)	69.9	291.2
Hook worm	1.6	715.6
Ascaris lumbricoides (round worm)	36.1	986.4

Data from 'Major Communicable diseases', W. Harding Le Riche, in *Health of Mankind*, Ciba Foundation Symposium 100, Ed. G. Wolstenholme and M. O'Connor, J. and A. Churchill Ltd., London.

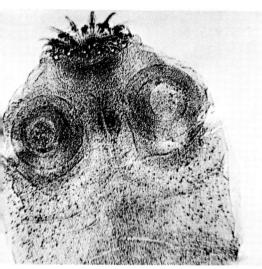

Figure 20.1   Photomicrograph of the scolex of *Taenia solium* showing suckers and hooks. (*By courtesy of WMMS.*)

Tapeworms

In general, all tapeworms shows a similar structure and type of life cycle. We will look at only one representative in any detail, the pork tapeworm, and point out how other species differ. The pork tapeworm is by no means the commonest tapeworm; it is very rare in Great Britain but a knowledge of this species seems to be required by many examining boards in Great Britain.

The pork tapeworm (*Taenia solium*)

Unlike the bodies of flukes, which are 'one-piece', the body of a tapeworm consists of a small head (scolex) at the anterior end followed by a series of segments (proglottids). These segments arise by a process of budding from the region behind the scolex. The scolex is minute compared with the segments, but it bears organs which attach the worm to the wall of the bowel. The scolex of *Taenia solium* bears hooks and suckers (Figure 20.1). There is no mouth, indeed there is no alimentary canal, for the tapeworm absorbs pre-digested food over the entire body surface.

Budding of segments from the neck of the worm is a continuous process. Each new tiny segment pushes the succeeding segment further away from the head. The individual segments grow and mature as they move away from the head. The adult worm may be 2–3 m long, 0.5 cm wide and 0.1 cm in thickness. Each segment is an individual as far as reproduction is concerned; as the segments enlarge the male and female organs develop. Figure 20.2 shows the structure of a single mature segment of the pork tapeworm containing the various male and female sex organs. The sex organs consist of an external female genital opening lying close to the male external genital organ, from which the penis or cirrus protrudes to introduce sperms into the female vagina. Eggs that are liberated from the ovary are fertilized by the sperms and receive yolk and shells from the yolk glands and shell glands. The eggs then pass into the uterus, where they accumulate. The sex organs ultimately degenerate, leaving an egg-packed uterus that virtually fills the entire segment.

The egg-loaded segments (gravid proglottids) are at the end of the chain of segments that constitute the body of the worm. Each ripe segment can deliver to the outside world some 30 000–40 000 eggs. At intervals the tapeworm detaches several ripe segments and these pass out with the faeces; man soon becomes aware of

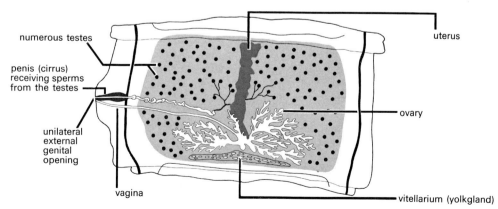

Figure 20.2   A single segment of the pork tapeworm *T. solium* showing the reproductive organs.

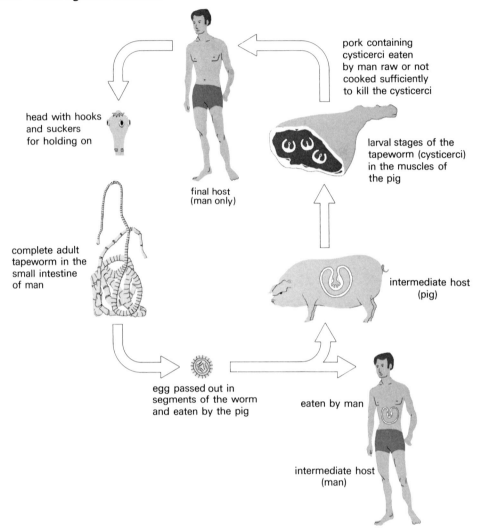

head with hooks
and suckers
for holding on

final host
(man only)

pork containing
cysticerci eaten
by man raw or not
cooked sufficiently
to kill the cysticerci

larval stages of the
tapeworm (cysticerci)
in the muscles of
the pig

complete adult
tapeworm in the
small intestine
of man

intermediate host
(pig)

egg passed out in
segments of the worm
and eaten by the pig

eaten by man

intermediate host
(man)

Figure 20.3   Life history of the pork tapeworm.

the parasite he is harbouring in his bowel by the presence of these creamy-white segments in the faeces. The ripe segments of the pork tapeworm are virtually inactive, but the beef tapeworm discharges single segments which are highly active and may crawl about their host, their squirming movements squeezing out the eggs. Active or not, the ripe segments soon degenerate in the outside world. Each of the thousands of eggs is surrounded by a protective shell and contains an embryo (hexacanth embryo) already bearing armoury in the form of six hooks to enable it to burrow into the wall of the bowel of its next host.

These eggs do not develop further unless they are eaten by the *intermediate* hosts of the parasite

(Figure 20.3). In the case of the pork tapeworm, the intermediate host is the pig. When the eggs are swallowed by a pig they release their embryo into the gut of the animal. The embryo becomes an active creature and burrows its way into the bowel wall with its armoury of six hooks. Ultimately these embryos reach the blood stream and are distributed around the body. They settle down in various tissues, usually muscle, and develop into a small bladder or cyst. This becomes filled with fluid and develops a tiny tapeworm head, at first turned inside out so that the suckers lie inside it. This is the larval phase in the intermediate host—the cysticercus, or bladder-worm. The bladder-worms remain dormant in the tissues of the pig and ultimately

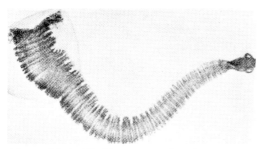

Figure 20.4 Bladder-worm of pork tapeworm hatching. (*By courtesy of WMMS.*)

die unless the pig is killed for human consumption and the meat cooked so briefly that the bladder-worms are not killed. The number of bladder-worms in pork obviously depends upon the number of eggs eaten by the pig. Some infestations may be heavy, with thousands of bladder-worms in each kilogramme of meat.

Once the living bladder-worms are released into the human intestine they become active. The bladder is digested away and the head fastens itself to the wall of the intestine and proceeds to bud off segments (Figure 20.4). Within ten weeks or so it begins to release ripe segments loaded with eggs.

The effect of the tapeworm on man

The symptoms caused by the presence of a pork tapeworm in the bowel of man are usually few; there may be vague abdominal discomfort, but quite often the first evidence of infection is the appearance of the creamy-white segments in the faeces. The adult worm in fact appears to cause little damage to man. However, there is one feature of the life history of this creature, which is unique to the pork tapeworm, which makes treatment of the infection a matter of urgency. Man can act not only as the final host for the parasite (i.e. the host in which the adult worm develops) but he may also act as the intermediate host; this means that eggs liberated from a man bearing the worm may infect other men, or indeed he may be re-infected himself. These develop in just the same way as if they were eaten by a pig, i.e. they develop into bladder-worms. Human cysticercosis, as the infection is called, may be contracted from any food which has been contaminated by water or faeces containing the eggs of the tapeworm. Inadequate processing and disposal of sewage, especially on sewage farms (page 122) may play an important role in the spread of this infection. Raw sewage may be placed on cattle pastures or discharged into inland waterways or the sea.

The distribution and control of the pork tapeworm

This worm is less widely distributed than the beef tapeworm and infection is rare in Great Britain, the U.S.A. and Canada. The disease occurs mainly in Europe, Africa, S. America and parts of Asia.

The pork tapeworm, like the beef tapeworm, is an obligatory parasite of man (i.e. it cannot live in other animals). Both species can be eradicated from man by the use of appropriate drugs. This should in turn reduce the frequency of cysticercosis in pigs. The treatment of human infections should also be accompanied by an improvement in the meat hygiene services, and by public education which points out the dangers of eating undercooked pork. General public health measures should include the provision of adequate sewage-treatment plants and the prohibition of the discharge of raw sewage into inland waters or the sea.

The beef tapeworm (*Taenia saginata*)

The beef tapeworm has a structure and life history similar to that of the pork tapeworm. The intermediate hosts for this tapeworm are cattle, and man contracts the disease by eating undercooked beef. Because of the eating habits in Great Britain, i.e. 'rare' beef, the beef tapeworm is the commonest tapeworm in these islands, but its distribution is world-wide. It is very common in some areas of Europe and in some populations

Figure 20.5 Beef carcass cut to show a bladder-worm. (*Photograph by A. I. Wright, Department of Veterinary Medicine, University of Bristol.*)

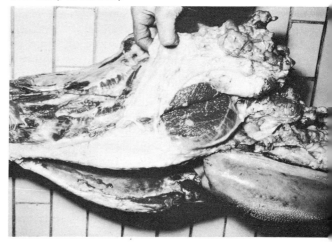

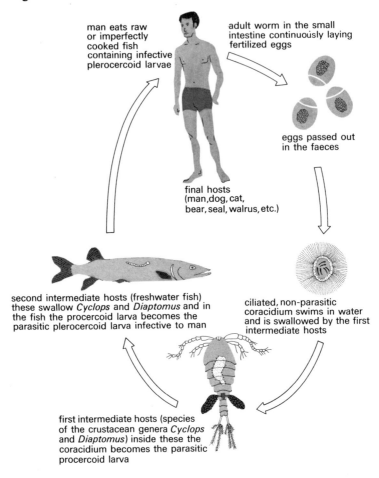

man eats raw or imperfectly cooked fish containing infective plerocercoid larvae

adult worm in the small intestine continuously laying fertilized eggs

eggs passed out in the faeces

final hosts (man, dog, cat, bear, seal, walrus, etc.)

second intermediate hosts (freshwater fish) these swallow *Cyclops* and *Diaptomus* and in the fish the procercoid larva becomes the parasitic plerocercoid larva infective to man

ciliated, non-parasitic coracidium swims in water and is swallowed by the first intermediate hosts

first intermediate hosts (species of the crustacean genera *Cyclops* and *Diaptomus*) inside these the coracidium becomes the parasitic procercoid larva

Figure 20.6   Life history of the fish tapeworm.

of East Africa virtually all individuals carry the worm. Since the distribution of the adult worm is cosmopolitan, it follows that the distribution of bladder-worms in cattle is also cosmopolitan. In European countries up to 1.25 per cent of slaughtered cattle show bladder-worms in the flesh, but this figure is probably an under-estimate; when the carcasses of cattle are inspected for the presence of bladder-worms, only certain parts are examined—incisions are made in muscles that are 'the sites of predilection' (Figure 20.5). Bladder-worms *can*, however, occur anywhere in the carcass. In some East African countries as many as 30–80 per cent of slaughtered cattle show bladder-worms.

The disease is treated and controlled in exactly the same way as described for the pork tapeworm. Fortunately man cannot be the intermediate host for the beef tapeworm, so that human cysticercosis does not arise in infections with this species.

The fish tapeworm (*Diphyllobothrium latum*, Figure 20.6, 20.7)

This tapeworm is called the fish tapeworm because man becomes infected by eating fresh water fish which contain the infective larval phase of the worm. It is a much commoner tapeworm in Europe than either the beef or pork tapeworm, particularly in countries bordering the Baltic sea, in the lake districts of Switzerland and in Ireland. It is present also in Africa, Asia and N. America.

The adult worm is the largest tapeworm of man and it may reach up to 10 metres in length; multiple infections can also occur. The worm is named *Diphyllobothrium latum* because of the character of the scolex; it attaches itself to the wall of the intestine not by means of hooks and suckers like the pork tapeworm, but by means of two slit shaped suckers called bothria, one on each side of the spoon-shaped head (Figure

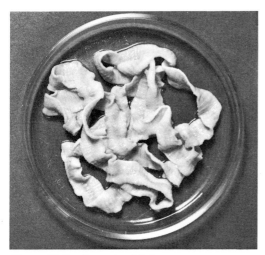

Figure 20.7 Length of fish tapeworm expelled after treatment. (*By courtesy of WMMS.*)

20.8). Two intermediate hosts are involved in the life history of this worm. The eggs which are liberated from the worm in the bowel hatch in water to release a ciliated structure (the coracidium) which may be swallowed by the first intermediate host; these are Crustacea called copepods—minute water creatures. Inside the tiny crustacean the coracidium becomes an elongated larva about 0.05 cm long, the procercoid larva. These develop no further unless the crustacean is eaten by a fresh water fish—trout, pike, perch, salmon, eel etc. Inside the fish the larva enters the organs of the fish and develops into the next larval phase—the plerocercoid larva—an elongated creature about 10 mm long. Humans are infected by eating raw or under-cooked fish containing the plerocercoid larvae.

A special feature of infection by the fish tapeworm is the development of a special kind of anaemia. This is caused by a deficiency of vitamin B_{12} which is presumably removed from food by the tapeworm.

The dwarf tapeworm (*Hymenolepis nana*)

This is the smallest tapeworm of man, measuring only 7–100 mm in length, but very many— thousands—may be present in one individual. It is a common tapeworm in warm countries, and is the commonest in the southern states of the U.S.A. It can cause severe illness, particularly in children; there may be abdominal pains, diarrhoea or even convulsions. This tapeworm needs *no* intermediate host. The eggs are directly

infective to man, and when the eggs are swallowed in food or water they develop into mature worms in the human intestine. The worm can, however, also live in mice and the larval stage can exist in the flour beetle (*Tribolium confusum*).

Hydatid tapeworm (see page 194)

Treatment of tapeworms in man

Fortunately there are a variety of safe drugs which can be used to eradicate tapeworms from man, and these include drugs that are also used in the treatment of malaria—mepacrine or chloroquine. Since single large doses of these drugs often cause vomiting, and thus loss of the drug, the drugs may be poured directly into the duodenum through a swallowed rubber tube. The position of the tip of the swallowed tube is first checked by X-rays to ensure that it is in the duodenum. Then a dose of the drug is poured down the tube. After a suitable interval a purgative (laxative) is given and all faeces passed are collected and examined. In dealing with infections caused by the beef or pork tapeworm, when only a single worm is usually present it is very important to look for the presence of a scolex. The worm may break in the bowel under the influence of the drug and purgative, leaving the scolex embedded in the wall of the intestine; the scolex and neck then bud off new segments and the infection persists, so that the absence of a scolex in the faeces means that a cure cannot be guaranteed. In the case of the fish tapeworm there may be more than one worm in the bowel so that the presence of a single scolex in the faeces is not a guarantee of cure.

Flukes (trematodes) of man

A variety of flukes may infect man and, according to their species, live in the blood vessels, lungs, liver and bile ducts or in the bowel. We are going to look at two representatives of parasitic flukes,

Figure 20.8 Scolex of fish tapeworm. (*By courtesy of WMMS.*)

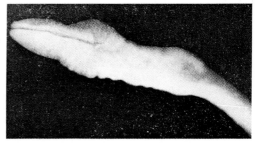

first the blood flukes, which are the most widespread of all fluke infections, and second the liver fluke, which is the only representative in Great Britain.

The blood flukes (Schistosoma species)

Schistosomiasis, as infection by these flukes is called, attacks and debilitates over 200 million people in the world. It has been known for many years that this parasite can profoundly debilitate those infected by it. In 1960 the Ross Institute of Tropical Hygiene, London, with the support of the World Health Organization, made some studies of the frequency of schistosomiasis in the United Republic of Tanzania and came up with some unexpected findings. They found that 20 per cent of the child population were severely affected. Adults were less frequently affected, and only some 10 per cent showed serious disease. These figures suggested that schistosomiasis is a cause of an unsuspected and considerable mortality in children. Many tropical and subtropical areas of the world are plagued by this disease—Africa, Southern Europe, South America, and the Middle and Far East.

There are three different species of schistosomes. One species (*S. haematobium*) inhabits the blood vessels near the bladder and kidneys; these are the organs most severely damaged by the parasite. Man is virtually the only final host for this species. *S. mansoni* chiefly affects the blood vessels of the large bowel, and again man is the only final host for the species. The third species, *S. japonicum* lives in the blood vessels of the small intestine; this species occurs only in China, Japan and other parts of the Far East. Man is not the only final host for this species, which can live in many domestic animals (cattle, water buffalo, sheep, goats, dogs, cats), and these can be a source of infection to man. All these parasites have, however, a similar type of life cycle, and we will consider them together.

Life cycle

The adult male and female flukes live in the blood vessels of the abdomen and pelvis of man (Figure 20.9). The male is smaller (10 mm long, 1 mm diameter) than the female (20 mm long, 0.25 mm diameter) and when he is fertilizing the female he is held in a groove in the body of the female. The fertilized eggs are laid in the blood vessels. The main injury to man is caused by the eggs working their way into adjacent organs (bowel, bladder, etc.) in order to reach the outside of the body. The eggs

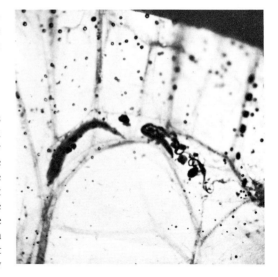

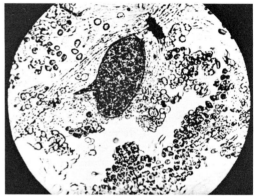

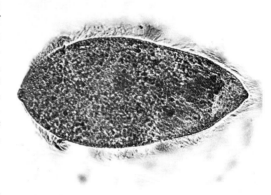

Figure 20.9 (top)   Schistosomes in the small blood vessels of the bowel in an experimental animal ×3. (*By courtesy of WMMS.*)

Figure 20.10 (middle)   Egg of blood fluke ×150 bearing spike. (*By courtesy of WMMS.*)

Figure 20.11 (bottom)   H.P. photomicrograph of the miracidium of a blood fluke, bearing cilia. (*By courtesy of WMMS.*)

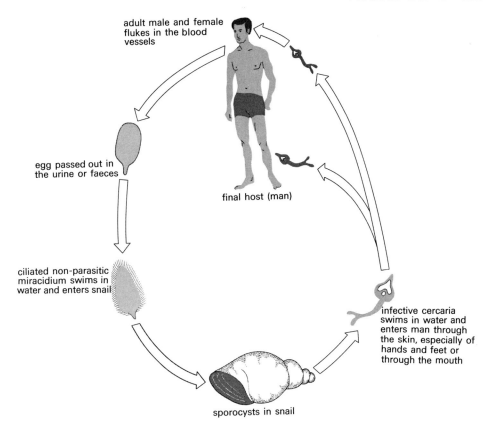

adult male and female
flukes in the blood
vessels

egg passed out in
the urine or faeces

final host (man)

ciliated non-parasitic
miracidium swims in
water and enters snail

infective cercaria
swims in water and
enters man through
the skin, especially of
hands and feet or
through the mouth

sporocysts in snail

Figure 20.12   Life cycle of the blood fluke.

achieve this task in various ways, assisted by the presence of spines on the surface of the egg (Figure 20.10). The eggs thus gradually work their way through the walls of the blood vessels into the bladder or bowel and are excreted by the host in the urine or faeces. The presence of multitudes of these spinous eggs in human tissues causes various effects, including severe inflammation, abscesses, scarring, and bleeding and pain on passing urine. Not all the eggs reach the outside of the body; some of them drain with the blood into the larger blood vessels of the abdomen and reach the liver and spleen, which may be severely damaged by the presence of the eggs.

When the eggs reach the exterior of the body, they hatch to release a tiny motile form—the miracidium (Figure 20.11). This lives only for a few hours and dies unless it reaches one of the intermediate hosts of the parasites—various species of aquatic snails. If the miracidium does reach a snail, it bores its way into the creature

and grows to form a structure called a sporocyst. Each sporocyst produces hundreds of further daughter sporocysts, and each of these produces many tiny motile cercariae which leave the snail in search of the final host, man. This multiplication in the body of the snail is an important feature of the life cycle, for it greatly increases the chances of ultimately infecting man. It has been estimated that the invasion of a snail by a single miracidium results in the production of hundreds of thousands of cercariae, liberated by the snail over a period of time.

The tiny cercariae have a forked tail and are strong swimmers (Figure 20.13). If man comes into contact with water containing these creatures, they bore into the skin or membranes of the mouth and reach the blood stream. They are then transported around the body in the blood and they settle down in the vessels of the abdomen or pelvis; here they mature into adult male and female worms (life story shown in Figure 20.12).

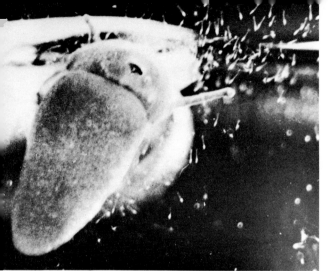

Figure 20.13 Photograph of a snail releasing large numbers of cercaria into the water. (By courtesy of WMMS.)

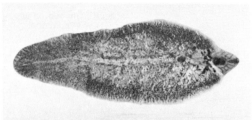

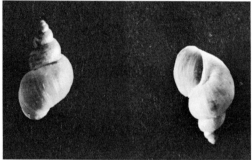

Figure 20.14 (top) Liver fluke stained to show internal organs. (By courtesy of WMMS.)

Figure 20.15 (bottom) Shell of L. truncatula, the intermediate host of the liver fluke. (By courtesy of WMMS.)

Treatment and prevention of schistosomiasis

Success in treating an individual infected with blood flukes depends upon early diagnosis and prompt treatment. The longer the flukes lay eggs, the more the tissues become damaged, and this damage may be irreparable. The oldest drugs for this disease are the organic anti-monials, but they are toxic and need to be given under close medical supervision—a severe dis-advantage in underdeveloped countries. Trials of new and possibly safer drugs are being assisted by the World Health Organization.

Unfortunately the disease is increasingly man-made. The disease was unknown in some areas, e.g. parts of Egypt, until the introduction of perennial irrigation with its effect on the snail population. In Southern Rhodesia the Umshandige Irrigation Scheme, which cost £3 000 000, had to be abandoned in 1949 mainly because infections with blood flukes reached such vast numbers of people. It is obvious that irrigation engineers must cooperate with experts on snails and experts on the distribution of blood flukes in order to incorporate appropriate snail-controls in methods of irrigation. A variety of chemicals can be added to water to kill snails (so-called molluscicides), and work continues in various areas in the development and testing of new molluscicides.

The liver fluke (Fasciola hepatica)

Fasciola hepatica is the common liver fluke of cattle, sheep, rabbits and other mammals, including man. The adult flukes live mainly in the bile ducts of the final host. They are fairly large, flat leaf-life creatures 1–3 cm long

(Figure 20.14). The life history of the liver fluke is very similar to that already described for the blood fluke; both types of fluke use snails as intermediate hosts. Large numbers of eggs are released by the liver flukes and these reach the exterior of the body in the faeces. The eggs release the tiny motile miracidia which swim in water seeking a suitable snail. In Great Britain the intermediate host is a species of snail called *Limnaea truncatula* (Figure 20.15). In this snail occur sporocyst formation and a further stage of multiplication in the form of structures called rediae. But ultimately, as in the case of the life cycle of the blood flukes, the snails release large numbers of tiny motile cercariae which can infect the primary host. The motile cercaria ultimately settles down on water plants or grass, casts off its tail and forms a protective membrane around itself. This encysted cercaria waits until it is eaten by a browsing animal. Man is infected usually by eating contaminated watercress, although occasionally by eating wind-fall fruit or other vegetables on which cercariae have encysted. The encysted cercariae become active in the alimentary canal, penetrate the wall of the intestine and ultimately reach the liver and bile ducts where they mature into the adult flukes (life cycle of liver fluke, Figure 20.16).

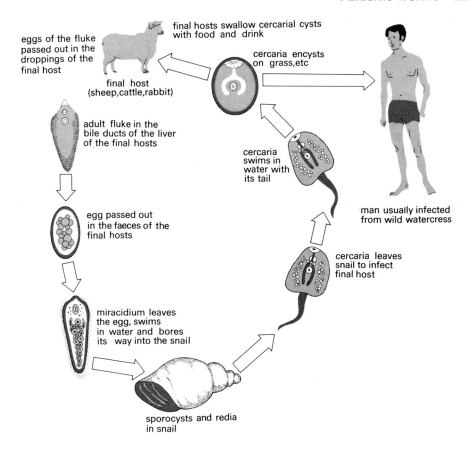

Figure 20.16 Life cycle of the liver fluke.

Symptoms and control of fascioliasis in man

Human infections with the liver fluke are reported from time to time in Great Britain. These are often isolated cases or small epidemics. The largest recent epidemic was reported in 1970 ('Fascioliasis—A large outbreak' by Hardman *et al.*, *British Medical Journal*, 29 August 1970). Forty-four cases of infection were diagnosed near Chepstow, Monmouthshire. The epidemic may well have been larger than this number since some of the diagnosed cases had no symptoms and were investigated because members of the same family with symptoms were found to be suffering from the disease. In the same edition of the British Medical Journal a further but smaller outbreak (five cases) was reported from Shropshire. A further three outbreaks were reported in 1969. In all cases infection was due to eating *wild* watercress, i.e.

watercress growing in ditches near to sheep or cattle.

Some cases of fascioliasis have no symptoms. Many cases, however, have intermittent fever, feel unwell and have night sweats, weight loss and pain under the right rib margin (i.e. over the liver). Eggs can be demonstrated in the faeces. Treatment is not simple and the patient has to be in hospital, particularly when toxic drugs such as emetine have to be used. Treatment is continued until the symptoms disappear and fluke eggs are no longer present in the faeces.

Obviously strict control on the growth and sale of watercress is necessary—indeed watercress is *cultivated* in water which is uncontaminated by the faeces of sheep or cattle. The danger lies in the collection of wild watercress which *may* be infective. Fascioliasis is a common disease of sheep or cattle, and wild watercress growing near these animals is *always* suspect.

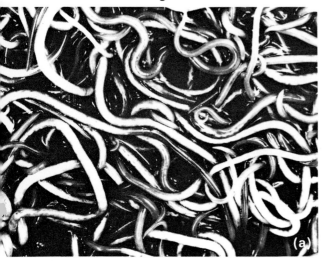 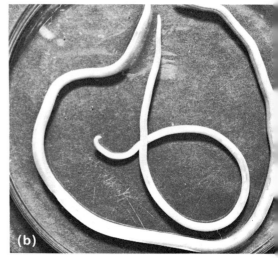

Figure 20.17 (a) A mass of ascarids evacuated after treatment of a patient with piperazine, and (b) adult male and female round worms. (*By courtesy of WMMS.*)

Nematode parasites of man

The nematodes are unsegmented worms with an elongated body which is pointed at both ends. Like the trematodes, but unlike the cestodes, they possess an alimentary canal and digestive glands. The sexes are usually separate, i.e. they are not hermaphrodite. In this phylum of animals there are many free living forms, e.g. in the soil and in water, but others are parasites of animals or plants. In this chapter we will be taking a look at four common and important nematodes parasitic in man.

The large round worm of man (*Ascaris lumbricoides*, Figure 20.17)

This species, which lives in the small intestine of man, is one of the largest of the round worms, being up to 30 cm in length and up to 4 mm in diameter. When removed from the body these worms are a glistening white or pink in colour. Large numbers of them may be present in the bowel—so many that they may become entangled to form a mass which can obstruct the lumen of the bowel. The adult female liberates eggs into the bowel and these are passed out in the faeces. Vast numbers of eggs are produced—hundreds of thousands each day. Some workers estimated the output of round worm eggs in the Chinese population and arrived at a figure of many thousands of tons of eggs produced annually! These eggs have resistant shells which enable them to survive for long periods in the outside world, particularly when they are kept moist, and they may well resist sewage treatment. There is no intermediate host in the life cycle of this round worm. The eggs are directly infective to man—provided that sufficient time has elapsed for an infective larva to develop within the egg.

When the egg, with its contained infective larva, is swallowed by man, the shell is digested to release the larva. This at once bores its way through the wall of the intestine into the blood stream. Many of the larvae settle down in the blood vessels of the lungs, where they mature further before breaking out of the vessels into the air spaces of the lungs. This action inflicts at least temporary damage to the lungs, causing inflammation, cough, breathlessness etc. The larvae do not, however, stay in the lung. They wriggle their way up the air passages and find their way to the back of the throat, where they are swallowed and pass into the stomach and intestine. They can now settle in the intestine and mature into adult male and female worms; after two or three months the females begin to release their store of eggs. The life of the adult worms is, however, relatively short, and if man is not re-infected the worms would die out in a year or so.

The effects of the parasite of man

We have already seen two types of injury caused by these parasites. Their very number in the bowel can cause intestinal obstruction, and during their life cycle they regularly damage the lungs. In warm countries of the world the infection is one of the major causes of ill health in children, and is responsible for many deaths. It causes severe malnutrition and recurring illness by means that are not fully understood.

Mechanical damage by the parasites is common enough and easily understood. Excess mechanical activity of the parasites is particularly likely to occur if ineffective drugs are given to the patient which 'stir up' the parasite but do not kill it. The irritated worms may perforate the bowel wall, migrate up the bile duct and cause obstruction or liver damage, or—as previously mentioned—mass into a tangle of worms which obstruct the bowel.

Distribution and control of the large round worm

This worm infects man all over the world and it is one of the commonest parasites of man (see Table 22). It is fortunately rare in Great Britain but it is common enough on the continent of Europe.

We will consider two aspects of control; treatment of the infection in the individual patient and measures aimed at prevention of infection. There are a variety of safe and effective drugs which can kill round worms. These drugs, such as piperazine, have made the mass treatment of populations safe, effective and feasible. The public and personal health measures which are necessary to prevent transmission of the disease are identical to those already described for many diseases caused by agents excreted in the faeces. Inadequate sanitation, poor water supplies, contamination of water and food by faeces, all contribute to the spread of the parasite. Unfortunately the disease flourishes among the overcrowded and underprivileged, those very communities with primitive public health and medical services. Probably the best attack in such areas is mass treatment of populations with piperazine. Pilot trials sponsored by the World Health Organization in Ceylon and China (Taiwan) showed that mass treatment with piperazine, even in the absence of improved sanitation, could effectively reduce transmission of the parasite to a low level.

Human hook worms (several species, Figure 20.18)

These parasitic nematodes of the intestine do not browse around the intestinal contents for their food like the large round worm. Instead they feed off blood in the wall of the intestine. These small nematodes (7–13 mm long according to species and sex) have a bell-shaped structure around the mouth, and inside the mouth there are 'teeth' which erode the lining

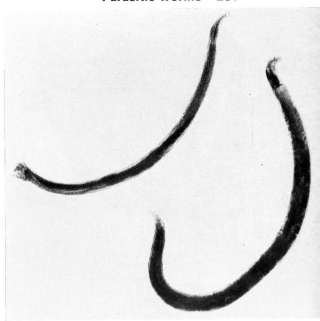

Figure 20.18 Male and female hook worms ×14. *(By courtesy of WMMS.)*

of the bowel until the animal reaches and penetrates a blood vessel. A special secretion of the worm prevents the blood from clotting and large amounts of blood passes through the alimentary canal of the worm, far more than is needed for its own food supply. Large numbers of these blood sucking worms may be present in the intestine of one individual.

Life history of hook worms (Figure 20.19)

The adult females in the intestine release fertilized eggs which pass out in the faeces. In the outside world the larva inside the egg undergoes a process of development to produce an infective larva. This is an active creature about 0.5 mm in length. Unlike the eggs of the large round worm of man, which has to passively wait to be swallowed by man, the infective larvae of hook worms can actually penetrate human skin, although they can also successfully infect man if they are swallowed in food. The larvae which penetrate the skin or are swallowed in food ultimately enter the circulation of blood. Like the larvae of the large round worm they leave the circulation in the lungs, from which they migrate up the air passages and ultimately reach the intestine.

The infective larvae survive best in warm moist soil, so that hook worm infections are commonest in warm countries of the world.

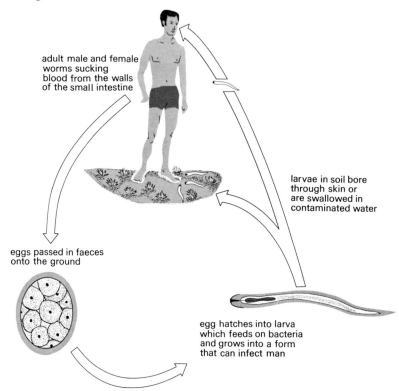

adult male and female worms sucking blood from the walls of the small intestine

larvae in soil bore through skin or are swallowed in contaminated water

eggs passed in faeces onto the ground

egg hatches into larva which feeds on bacteria and grows into a form that can infect man

Figure 20.19   Life cycle of the hook worm.

They do occur in Europe, particularly Southern Europe. Indeed hook worms were a scourge of the miners who constructed the St Gotthard tunnel in Switzerland. When the miners returned to their native lands of Holland, Belgium, Germany, France and England they infected mines in their own countries—and hook worms flourished until sanitation control of mines and miners eradicated them. In Great Britain the disease is rare except in immigrants from warm countries.

Effects of the parasite on man

Two kinds of disturbance are caused by hook worms, first by the presence of adult worms in the intestine, and second, by the invasion of the skin by infective larvae. Invasion of the skin often occurs on the feet and ankles, particularly if the individual walks barefoot over soil or vegetation contaminated by infective larvae. The penetrating hook worm larvae cause an intense itching and inflammation called 'ground itch', but the more serious consequence of infection by hook worms is the result of the blood sucking activities of the adult worms in the intestine. Anaemia is a common complica-

tion of the infection, particularly in children and women. In tropical countries infection by hook worms is the commonest cause of iron-deficiency anaemia.

Control of infections by hook worms

Various drugs are effective in treating the individual case of the disease (drugs such as tetrachlorethylene, hexyl resorcinol, bephenium), but none are as safe (i.e. free from side-effects) or as effective as is piperazine for the treatment of round worm infections. Mass treatment of populations is thus not likely to be a suitable weapon until safe and effective drugs become available. Two precautions are needed in the treatment of hook worm infections. First, the general state of the patient may be so poor that anaemia may have to be corrected by tablets of iron salts taken by mouth or occasionally by transfusions of blood; this may have to be done before embarking on drug therapy to kill the worms. Second, mixed infections with hook worms and round worms is fairly common. However, not all drugs used for hook worms are effective against the round worms, and use of these drugs for hook worms stir up the round worms into dangerous mechanical activity. Careful selection of drugs is thus necessary.

Proper disposal of human faeces can prevent transmission of the disease, as it did in the case of the miners of Europe. Proper sanitation is still a major problem in developing of primitive communities where untreated human faeces are often used as manure for the land and where agricultural workers spend their days barefoot on soil contaminated by hook worm eggs.

The trichina worm (*Trichinella spiralis,* Figure 20.20–20.21)

Infection by this worm produces a serious disease of man called trichiniasis. Man becomes infected by eating raw or undercooked meat containing encysted larvae of the worms. The most important source of infection is the pig, but many other animals, e.g. wild boar, bear, seals etc., may harbour the larvae in their muscles

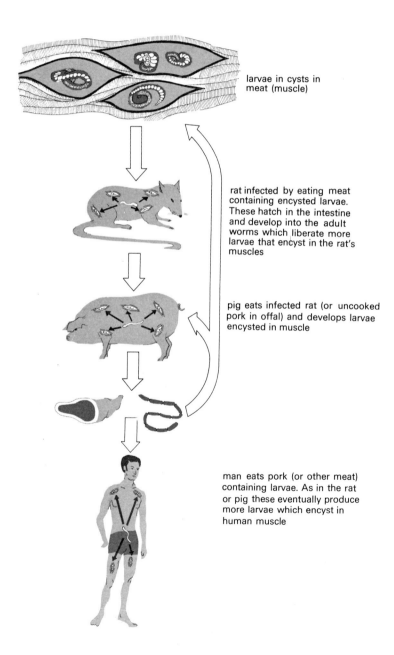

larvae in cysts in meat (muscle)

rat infected by eating meat containing encysted larvae. These hatch in the intestine and develop into the adult worms which liberate more larvae that encyst in the rat's muscles

pig eats infected rat (or uncooked pork in offal) and develops larvae encysted in muscle

man eats pork (or other meat) containing larvae. As in the rat or pig these eventually produce more larvae which encyst in human muscle

Figure 20.20   Life cycle of the trichina worm.

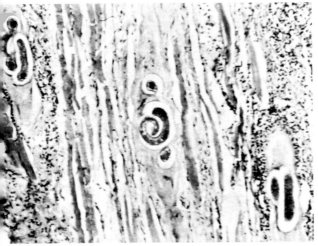

Figure 20.21 Section of calf muscle of a fatal case of trichiniasis showing larvae in muscle. (*WMMS photograph by Prof. G. S. Nelson, London School of Hygiene and Tropical Medicine.*)

Human infection today is thus a 'blind alley' for these worms. However, this was not the case in the days when men were killed and eaten by wild carnivores—or by other men! At this time in history the larvae from human muscle would develop into adult worms in the intestine of the carnivore; these worms would liberate larvae to settle down in the muscles of the body, waiting for the carnivore to be attacked and eaten by another carnivore—and so the cycle would go on. We have seen that undercooked or raw meat from the pig is the main source of human infection today. How do pigs become infected by the Trichina worm so that their muscles come to harbour Trichina larvae? Infection results when pigs are fed on garbage containing infected pork or when they have access to wild animals such as rats which may also carry the infection.

Distribution, diagnosis, treatment, and eradication of trichiniasis

Formerly trichiniasis has been regarded as a disease of northern, temperate countries but recently outbreaks of the disease have occurred in many other parts of the world, in Africa, South America, the Far East, and New Zealand. It is also a serious problem in the arctic, where eskimoes become infected by eating the flesh of bears and marine mammals. The disease is by no means an easy one to diagnose, for the symptoms themselves may be vague. For a firm diagnosis the larvae should be demonstrated by removing a small piece of muscle under local anaesthesia, e.g. from the deltoid region of the arm, for microscopic examination.

There is really no effective drug which can kill the larvae in human muscle, and the best that can be done is to use those drugs called corticosteroids (e.g. cortisone, hydrocortisone) which suppress inflammation in tissues, whatever the cause. These drugs may be urgently needed if the muscles of the tongue or larynx are involved, when the swelling could readily interfere with breathing.

Probably no drugs can be expected to replace good standards of animal husbandry and meat hygiene. All pork products that are eaten raw or incompletely cooked should be held at 3°C or lower for thirty days; this will destroy the larvae. Of course, adequate cooking will do the same. In addition all garbage or meat scraps which are fed to pigs should be heat-treated to kill any Trichina larvae which may be present. If proper heating cannot be provided then raw meat scraps, offal and garbage should not be

and be a source of infection in some human communities. In the human intestine the larvae mature into adult male and female worms. These are small, the male being only 1.5 mm long and the female about 33 mm long. At this stage of the infection severe damage to the host does not occur, and the main symptoms are diarrhoea and other features of disturbed intestinal function. In any case the mature worms in the intestine only live for a matter of three months.

More serious consequences of the infection arise when the fertilized female worms burrow into the wall of the small intestine, where each female releases over a thousand larvae, each some 0.1 mm in length. These ultimately reach the heart by entering small blood vessels or lymph channels; they then circulate throughout the body and enter various tissues. The larvae that enter voluntary muscles undergo further development; they grow and curl into a spiral form (about 1 mm long) and become male or female larvae. The invasion of muscle by these larvae produces a variety of symptoms—fever, pain and stiffness of muscles (which may be regarded by the patient as 'rheumatism'). The muscles around the respiratory tract are favourite sites of attack by the larvae—muscles that include the diaphragm, intercostal muscles, and the muscles of the tongue and larynx; swelling of the latter muscles can cause serious difficulties in breathing.

The larvae do not develop further in human muscles; after a matter of months the cysts begin to calcify and the enclosed larvae die.

fed to pigs. The disease in pigs could obviously be eradicated by these measures.

Pin worms or thread worms (*Enterobius vermicularis*, Figure 20.22)

These small nematode worms are world-wide in their distribution; they are a common parasite, especially in children, but they rarely cause more than irritation around the anus. The adult male and female worms live in the colon, although occasionally they travel up the bowel to the small intestine or higher. The worms are tiny. The male is only 2–5 mm in length and is rarely seen; the white spindle shaped worms some 10 mm in length that appear in the faeces are the ripe females full of eggs. When the female worm is full of fertilized eggs she migrates down the alimentary tract and makes her exit via the anus. As she moves around the anus depositing her eggs she causes irritation, and this is sometimes intense. This itching is the main symptom of infection. Scratching results in the deposition of eggs under the finger nails, and re-infection occurs if the fingers are put into the mouth. The life history is similar to that of the round worm in that no intermediate host is involved and the eggs are directly infective to man. The eggs of the pin worm are not as resistant as those of the round worm but this is partly compensated for by their stickiness which keeps them on their host. However, the eggs do dry and blow about in the air and are inhaled or settle down in dust or on food, bedclothes etc. The swallowed eggs hatch in the bowel and directly mature into adult male and female worms.

Figure 20.22 Pin worms ×3.5. (*By courtesy of WMMS.*)

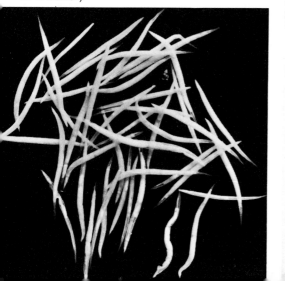

The whole life history of the parasite from the swallowing of eggs to the appearance of adult worms in the bowel is short, a matter of about five weeks. Individuals who re-infect themselves often suffer from anal irritation every five weeks or so as each new batch of mature female worms emerge from the anus.

Treatment and control of pin worms

Various safe drugs can be used to clear the bowel of this fairly harmless parasite, drugs such as gentian violet, hexyl resorcinol and piperazine. It is important to bear in mind that infection is always a household one. All members of the household should be treated at the same time. The use of drugs should be accompanied by a general increase in the standard of hygiene in the home, and this should include hand-washing after toilet, cutting of nails etc. The eggs of pin worms can live for about three weeks in the home, on clothes, in dust etc., so that patients may be cleared of worms only to be re-infected by eggs laid several weeks previously. It is thus best to give two courses of treatment, an initial course which will eradicate all worms from the bowel and a second course about three weeks later in case the patient has been re-infected from eggs in the home.

Filariasis—infection with Bancroft's filarial worm (*Wuchereria bancrofti*)

This animal and a related form called *Brugia*

Figure 20.23 H.P. photomicrograph of micofilaria of *Wuchereria bancrofti* in a blood film. Compare the size of the larva with that of the white blood cells shown. (*By courtesy of WMMS.*)

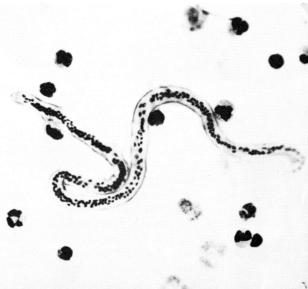

malayi are round worms which invade and live in the lymphatic channels of man—those valved tubes through which some of the tissue fluid is drained and ultimately returned to the blood system. The adult worms are creamy thread-like worms 40–100 mm in length and about 0.1 mm in diameter. In the lymph glands and lymph channels, the female worms lay not eggs, but tiny living larvae about 200 microns in length, known as microfilariae. These minute creatures drain with the lymph into the circulating blood, and tend to accumulate in the blood near the surface of the body—the peripheral blood. The microfilariae may not be present at all times in the peripheral blood. In some strains of the worm the number of microfilariae fluctuate in a rhythmic manner, the rhythm being repeated every twenty-four hours.

The microfilariae cannot develop further in man. They have to be taken up by a mosquito when it takes a meal of blood. A large number of different kinds of mosquito can act as vectors for filarial worms. Inside the mosquito the microfilariae undergo further development to become larvae which can infect man. During the act of sucking human blood, these infective larvae break through a thin membrane covering part of the lower lip of the mosquito and get onto the human skin. They then enter the body through the puncture wound made by the mosquito or they crawl into some other wound. Having entered the body, they make their way to lymph nodes and glands and gradually grow into the adult worms.

The effects of filaria on man

Adult worms

Some months after being infected with larvae the infected person may experience pain in parts of the body where the worms have developed. Lymphatic glands tend to become swollen and tender and the genital organs are often affected. There are also less specific symptoms such as headache, backache and loss of appetite. The presence of adult worms in the lymphatic channels has several effects. First, they cause inflammation of the channels and surrounding tissues. Second, the channels are stretched and their valves no longer function efficiently; there is a back-flow of lymph which is made worse because of man's erect posture, and the channels become dilated and tortuous. Since the lymph channels are an important route for the drainage of tissue fluid—the clear salty fluid which bathes all cells—these changes in the channels interfere

with drainage of fluid; fluid tends to accumulate in the tissues, particularly in the legs and genital organs. Over the course of years enormous and grotesque swelling of the legs and external genitals may occur—a condition called elephantiasis—'legs like elephants'.

Microfilariae

The presence of microfilariae in the blood produces remarkably few effects on human tissues, but in some individuals the larvae produce fibrosis in the lungs.

Distribution of filariasis and the size of the problem

Filariasis is of great concern to many countries, and rapid urbanization in the developing countries has aggravated the problem by creating favourable conditions for the breeding of mosquito vectors of the disease. The disease is present in most of the subtropical and tropical parts of the world—in parts of Europe, parts of Africa, India, Malaya, China, Korea, Japan and South America. In these countries it is distributed mainly along the coasts. In India there are over 120 million people living in endemic areas, and it has been estimated that over 5 million people are affected.

Treatment of filariasis

As in the treatment of malaria, the control of filariasis in a country involves destruction of the vectors of the disease (mosquitoes) and the adult parasites in man. It is important to deal with the adult worms in man because they have a long life span during which they release microfilariae into the circulating blood. A drug called diethylcarbamazine has been widely used in the treatment of filariasis. The main effect of this drug is to remove most of the microfilariae from the blood and so prevent transmission to mosquitoes and ultimately to other men; probably some adult worms are also destroyed by the drug. The main obstacle to the use of diethylcarbamazine is in persuading people to take the drug. Many individuals are free of symptoms for long periods although they have microfilariae in their blood, and they see no reason for taking the drug. Side-effects of the drug, particularly after the first dose, are also a deterrent. The problem has been overcome in some countries; in Japan, for example, low doses of the drug have been included in children's orange juice or miso soup, and the drug has been given to all of the population of small communities, e.g. dormitories of industrial workers. Another way to obtain mass treatment is to include the drug in cooking salt. This method of treating mass populations has been widely used for administering iodine (to prevent goitres in parts of the world where the iodine content of food and water is low) and also for the administration of chloroquine to control malaria.

A second method for the control of filariasis is the control of the vector. Unfortunately there are many possible vectors each with different habits. The control methods one can use depend upon the vector(s) in a particular area. In some parts of the world the spraying of houses with DDT or dieldren has interrupted transmission of the disease. Unfortunately the main urban vector of filariasis (*Culex pipiens fatigans*) is not very susceptible to DDT and develops resistance to the insecticide. In addition to destruction of the adult mosquito, the larvae can also be attacked in their breeding places in water.

Unfortunately vector control is slow to produce changes in the number of individuals suffering from filariasis. The number of mosquitoes must be reduced to a low level for a long time, until the adult filarial worms die out in the bodies of men. This prolonged control favours the development of insecticide resistance by the mosquitoes. A combined control method—use of drugs in man and also mosquito control—will give a more rapid control of transmission of the disease, but each method alone can nearly achieve interruption of transmission. Thus in parts of Japan the microfilariae rate (an expression of the prevalence of microfilariae, which is the percentage obtained by dividing the number of microfilariae carriers by the total number of persons examined for microfilariae) fell from 5 per cent to less than 1 per cent within five years of the use of diethylcarbamazine. In Mauritius, where one species of mosquito vector was eradicated and another reduced by spraying insecticide, the microfilariae rate fell from 28 per cent to 1.2 per cent over a period of twelve years.

Onchocerus volvulus

This is another filarial worm. Unlike Bancroft's filarial worm, it lives not in the lymphatic system but in the connective tissues, particularly those of the skin. The parasite is widely distributed in the world, in Central Africa and parts of the Americas. In its life history it resembles Bancroft's filarial worm, although the vectors are not mosquitoes but are black flies that live near quickly flowing streams (Figure 20.24).

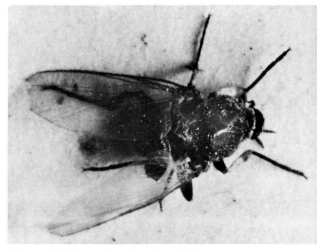

Figure 20.24 A simulium fly which can transmit *Onchocerus volvulus*, the blinding filaria. (*WHO photo.*)

The infective larvae are introduced into the skin by the bite of the flies, and in the skin they migrate through the tissues, causing intense irritation and inflammation. As a result the worm becomes embedded in fibrous tissue which form lumps under the skin up to 5 cm in diameter (Figures 20.25, 20.26). These lumps are slow-growing and may take several years to reach full size, but although disfiguring, they are not a serious effect of invasion by the worm. The most dangerous effects of the parasite are caused by the liberation of the microfilariae; these can cause inflammation and thickening in the skin, inflammation and enlargement of the lymphatic glands which may result in obstruction to the flow of lymph and the development of elephantiasis, and inflammation in the eye which may so

Figure 20.25 Lumps in the scalp caused by *Onchocerus volvulus*. (*By courtesy of WMMS.*)

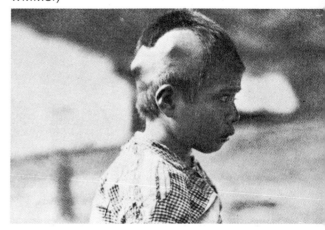

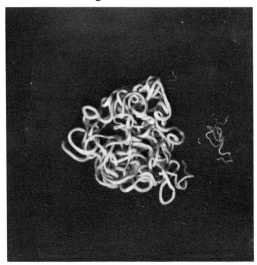

Figure 20.26   Onchocerus volvulus. A mass of adult worms extracted from a nodule. *(By courtesy of WMMS.)*

severely damage the eye as to result in blindness.

The second World Health Organization con-ference on onchoceriasis (Brazzaville, 1961) recognized that onchoceriasis with its associated blindness was a major endemic disease affecting the development of large parts of the African continent and parts of the Americas (Figure 20.27). The problem of onchoceriasis has been aggravated by many projects of water development. In some well defined regions, e.g. Kenya, control of the disease has been achieved by control of the vector, but there have been difficulties in other regions. It is vital to have detailed information on the life habits of the black flies which transmit the disease—resting places of adult flies, flight range of the flies, feeding habits etc., and the World Health Organization has set up a programme study on the flies. One survey in 1961, in four areas of Kenya, where the disease was once endemic before the vector was eradicated, has shown that in the absence of re-infection the adult worms in man can live as long as twelve to eighteen years. Obviously this is a disease which has yet to be conquered.

Figure 20.27   Onchoceriasis, or river blindness, is so widespread in Central America and Central Africa that infection rates of 80–100 per cent are reported in some areas. In districts heavily infected there are villages where all the adults are blind. This WHO photo shows children leading the blind adults.

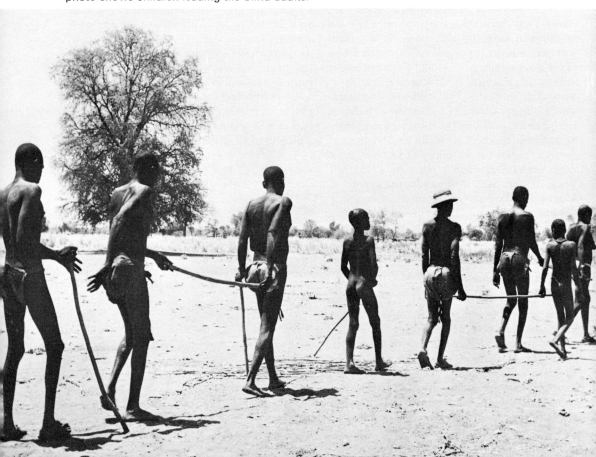

21. Genetics, human health, and medicine

Introduction

AN UNDERSTANDING of the influence of heredity on human health requires some appreciation of how the factors that guide the development and functions of our bodies are passed on from one generation to another, and how changes in man's genetic nature arise. The following introduction to the subject is not a concise course in genetics, but is intended to make the later discussions comprehensible to someone who has received no formal training in heredity.

Chromosomes

The union of two minute cells of scarcely measurable weight, a sperm and an egg, is the starting point in the development of each human being. Each human fertilized egg contains forty-six minute rod-shaped structures called chromosomes, and it is these microscopic structures that bear the hereditary factors that are called *genes*. The sperm and the egg make equal contributions to the hereditary material of the fertilized egg and each supplies twenty-three chromosomes. For each chromosome supplied by the sperm the egg provides a chromosome that matches it in size and shape to produce what is called an *homologous pair* of chromosomes. The fertilized egg thus contains twenty-three pairs of homologous chromosomes. (There is one exception to this state of affairs, for the two chromosomes that are concerned mainly with the determination of the sex of an individual are not identical with one another, at least in the male.) These homologous chromosomes do not occur as pairs in the nucleus of the cell but they are scattered at random within the nucleus. Only at a certain stage in the development of a few of the body's cells—the germ cells—do these chromosomes come together so that they are arranged in homologous pairs for a brief moment in time. Later we will look in some detail at this brief but supremely important event.

Heredity and environment

The fertilized egg of man thus comes to contain forty-six chromosomes. In these chromosomes is carried in an unbelievably compressed form the information needed to develop, maintain and repair an entire organism. Of course, neither the fertilized egg nor the fully developed human being exist in a vacuum. They exist in complex and fluctuating environments and the net product, the adult human, is the result of a long series of interactions of the information in the chromosomes with the environment. Not all the information that is carried by the chromosomes will find expression in the form or function of the adult human being. Part of the failure of the expression of some of the genetic material is due to its presence in what is called a recessive form, which can be suppressed by the presence of genetic material present in a dominant form. Another reason why some genetic information may fail to be expressed is the absence of the appropriate environment that is needed for expression. As I write this section of the book the month is December and my skin is pale. My body carries the information and machinery to produce pigment that will darken the skin but at the moment the appropriate environment, sunlight, is missing. A colleague of mine sitting across the library table is an African. On one of his chromosomes he carries a factor (gene) which makes his red blood cells different from mine. His red cells contain less of a certain enzyme— glucose-6-phosphate dehydrogenase—that is necessary for the normal metabolism of the cells. This and other enzymes protect the cell from damage by oxidizing agents. My colleague, however, appears healthy; he is in fact compensating for a shorter life span of his red blood cells by producing more red blood cells from the bone marrow. Thus the presence of this different gene on one of his chromosomes does not alter the number of his red blood cells compared to mine. However, if we change the environment and give him a drug such as a sulphonamide that tends to damage red blood cells then the situation will change dramatically. His unprotected red blood cells will be damaged and destroyed and an acute anaemia will develop.

These rather crude examples are meant to illustrate that what we are is the product of a long series of interactions between our inheritance and environment, an interaction that continues throughout life. It is often extremely difficult to untwine these interacting forces to try to establish which is the more important factor in determining a particular character or disorder. Some disorders of health may be caused by genetic factors in one individual and by environmental factors in another individual. Deaf and dumb children are not uncommon; in some of them the condition is determined by genetic factors and in others it is caused by one of a variety of environmental factors that include infection by German measles whilst the foetus is in the uterus, inflammation of the brain or its covering membranes, or infections of the middle ear. A genetic cause of a disorder can often be demonstrated by a study of the 'family tree' of affected individuals, which may show the pattern of inheritance of the disorder.

The study of twins has also given valuable information of the interaction of heredity and environment. Human twins are of two kinds, identical (monozygotic) and non-dentical (dizygotic). Non-identical twins develop from two separate fertilized eggs, and they resemble one another no more than do brothers and sisters born at different times. Identical twins arise in a different way. They come from the same fertilized egg; the first division of the fertilized egg produces two cells which, in the case of twinning, separate so that each cell will produce an individual. The two individuals are of the same genetic constitution; they have the same genes and they are of the same sex. Twins are usually brought up in similar environments, but if they happen to be brought up in different places then this provides a rare opportunity to study the interplay of genetic and environmental factors in the development not only of physical and mental diseases but also of such features as intelligence, aptitudes, physical development and the like.

Chromosomes and cell division

We left our study of chromosomes at the stage of the fertilized egg, which contains twenty-three pairs of homologous chromosomes. The fertilized egg begins to undergo the first of many cell divisions—it divides to produce two cells. Each of these cells divides, so producing four cells, and so on until vast populations arise that later differentiate into the various tissues and organs of the body. Each cell divides in such a way that each daughter cell has the same chromosome composition; each comes to have a replica of the chromosomes of the fertilized egg. All normal cells of all normal human beings have forty-six chromosomes, twenty-three pairs of homologous pairs per cell. Moreover the shape and length of each homologous pair is similar in all human beings. In spite of this superficial similarity of the chromosomes, the information that they carry varies from one man to another— some men are short, some tall, some are negroes, some white, some are dull-witted, some intellectually brilliant and so on.

The cell divisions that populate the body with cells from the fertilized egg are called *mitotic* divisions. For the purposes of description the course of a mitosis is divided into various stages called prophase, metaphase, anaphase and telophase, although in reality the process is a continuous event. These stages are illustrated in Figure 21.1. In a resting cell the chromosomes are very difficult, nay impossible, to observe under the microscope. When a cell begins the process of division, the chromosomes become both visible and increasingly easy to stain. The chromosomes that appear have already split into two strands, called chromatids, lying side by side. The staining substance of the chromosomes is not continuous from end to end; at one point at least there is a non-staining gap, or centromere constriction. The position of this constriction is constant for each chromosome. The centromere at this stage holds the two chromatids of the chromosome together. The chromosomes now shorten and thicken and move to the nuclear membrane, which later disappears. Inside the cell there now appears a delicate web of material called the spindle. At the beginning of the stage called metaphase, the chromosomes become attached to the spindle by means of the centromere construction, at a point mid-way between the two ends (poles) of the cell.

At a certain stage (anaphase), the centromere of each chromosome divides into two; it no longer holds together the two chromatids of the chromosome and these begin to repel one another, each half of the chromosome moving to opposite poles of the cell. The function of anaphase is the separation of two groups of like genetical constitution. Telophase is the term which describes the period in which the two groups of chromatids each become surrounded by their own nuclear membrane. The cytoplasm of the parent cell now divides into two equal parts, each investing one of the new daughter

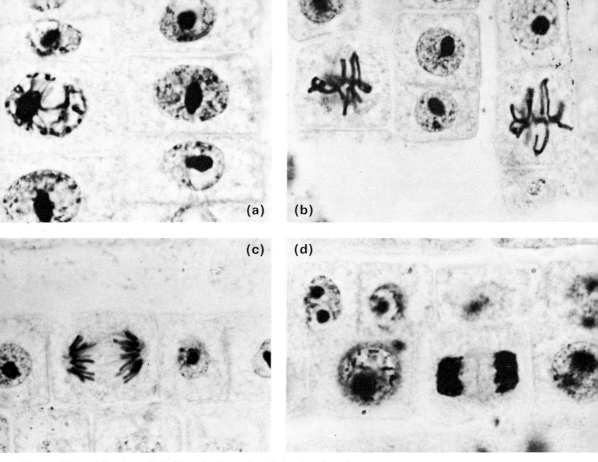

Figure 21.1 Mitotic cell division in the cells of the tip of a plant root.
(a) (top left) Prophase; only one cell is in prophase. The chromosomes are clearly visible. (b) (top right) Two cells are at the stage of metaphase. (c) (bottom left) Anaphase. (d) (bottom right) Telophase. (*Photographs by Gene Cox of Micro Colour International.*)

nuclei. During the resting phase each chromatid manufactures an identical partner, i.e. the chromatid becomes a chromosome.

Thus this kind of cell division ensures that each cell of the body comes to contain a replica of the genetic material of the fertilized egg. The division is not very relevant to our study of heredity except in so far as mitosis is the proto-type of another type of cell division—called meiosis or reduction division—that occurs only during the formation of the germ cells, the sperms and eggs. In this kind of cell division the chromosomes manoeuvre in such a way that each daughter cell comes to contain only half the number of chromosomes, one of each pair of homologous chromosomes. This number is called the haploid number and contrasts with the diploid number of chromosomes that is found in the fertilized egg and in all the non-germinal cells of the body. If each gamete, egg or sperm, brought with it the full diploid number of chromosomes then the fertilized egg would contain ninety-two chromosomes, and this number would be doubled in each generation.

In man, and in most other organisms, it is important to maintain the normal number and structure of chromosomes. We will see later how the presence of even quite small changes in chromosome number or composition can pro-duce radical changes in the offspring, changes that are seldom to the advantage of the individual possessing them.

This, then, is the important function of the special kind of cell division called meiotic or reduction division. Before we go on to look at how the halving of the chromosome number is achieved, we will consider briefly the significance of the number of chromosomes per cell in different organisms. All the non-germ cells of the body of a mammal, indeed the cells of all vertebrates, contain the diploid number of chromosomes. In some organisms, however, the body cells contain the haploid number of chromosomes, and the diploid number is only achieved at fertilization of the egg; the diploid state does not, however, last long, and a reduc-tion division ensures that the animal or plant tissues are populated by cells containing the haploid number of chromosomes. There are some real disadvantages in this state of affairs. If there is any spontaneous change (mutation) in one of the genes on a chromosome then the effect of this change will be shown in the characteristics (phenotype) of the organism. This is so despite the fact that most mutations are recessive ones. The recessive mutant gene finds expression in a haploid organism because only one chromosome of a homologous pair is present in the organism; thus the normal dominant gene present on the homologous partner cannot suppress the expression of the effects of the recessive mutant gene. In the diploid organism the genes occur always in pairs, one on each member of a homologous pair of chromosomes, and there is always the strong possibility that a mutant recessive gene is accompanied by a dominant gene at a corresponding position on the homologous chromosomes. Hence a diploid organism may carry many recessive genes without these finding

expression in the structure or function of the organisms. Diploid organisms will thus tend to show fewer variants than haploid organisms; they will not suffer from the effects of deleterious recessive mutations (and most mutations are deleterious, see page 260) unless a double dose of the mutant is present, one on each pair of homologous chromosomes.

Meiotic or reduction division

We can now look at the special type of cell division that ensures that offspring have the normal number of chromosomes appropriate to a species. Meiotic division occurs during the development of an egg or sperm. For the purposes of description we can divide meiosis into the same stages which we used for mitosis, i.e. prophase, metaphase, anaphase and telophase. Meiotic division differs from mitotic division in various ways, but the basic distinction can be

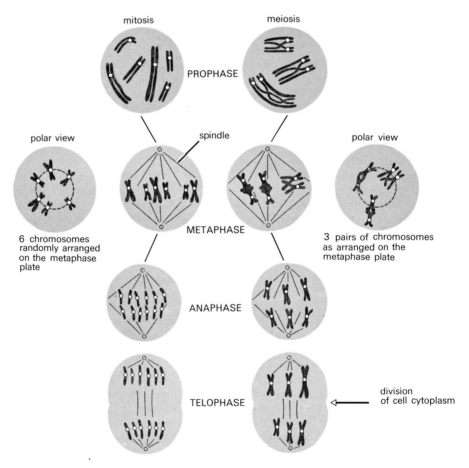

Figure 21.2 Diagrammatic representation of mitotic and meiotic cell division. All cells are seen from the side except for those labelled polar view which are seen from the ends of the cells. For the sake of simplicity the nuclear membranes are not included.

seen by looking at the stage of metaphase when the chromosomes are attached to the spindle. Figure 21.2 shows a drawing of a cell in mitotic metaphase as seen from the end of the cell, i.e. what we call a polar view. Six chromosomes are arranged on the metaphase plate, each chromosome being split into two chromatids which will later separate from one another. A very important point to note is that the chromosomes are not grouped in homologous pairs; they are distributed at random on the metaphase plate. Figure 21.2 also shows the same view of a cell at meiotic metaphase. Here there are three bodies on the metaphase plate; each of these bodies consists of a pair of homologous chromosomes so that during anaphase it is homologous chromosomes that separate from one another, not the chromatids of a single chromosome as in mitosis. Each daughter cell will come to have three chromosomes instead of three pairs of homologous chromosomes.

The pairs of homologous chromosomes at the metaphase plate in meiosis have an unusual shape because they have become bound very closely together during the stage of prophase.

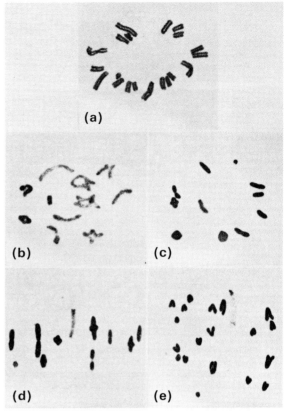

(a)

(b)   (c)

(d)   (e)

Figure 21.4   Photomicrograph of cells from a grasshopper testis showing some stages of meiotic cell division. (*Photographs by courtesy Dr K. R. Lewis.*)
(a) Polar view of metaphase plate of a cell engaged in *mitotic* division for comparison with (b)–(e) which are of stages of *meiosis*. Twenty chromosomes are arranged on the metaphase plate and each chromosome is split into two chromatids. Homologous chromosomes are *not* paired.
(b) Meiosis—prophase. All chromosomes except the sex chromosomes (in this species the male is XO and the female XX, i.e. there is no Y chromosome) are in bivalents, i.e. pairs of homologous chromosomes. Seven bivalents have one chiasma and two have chiasmata.
(c) Meosis—metaphase. (Polar view.) The X chromosome is in the centre. The chromosomes are condensed and chiasmata are not readily seen. Compare with (a).
(d) Meiosis—metaphase. (Side view of metaphase plate.) All bivalents show one chiasma.
(e) Meiosis—anaphase. (Side view.) Homologous chromosomes are now separating.

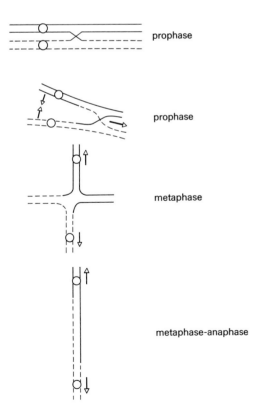

prophase

prophase

metaphase

metaphase-anaphase

Figure 21.3   Diagrammatic presentation of chiasma formation and separation of homologous chromosomes.

This binding together of homologous chromosomes is a necessary mechanical process to ensure that pairs of homologous chromosomes arrange themselves on the metaphase plate, and not single chromosomes. If the homologous chromosomes did not undergo this special physical

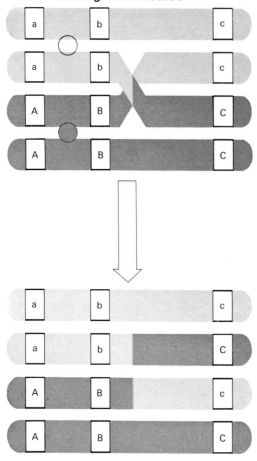

between the chromosomes are called chiasmata. Eventually the chromosomes have to separate from one another and Figures 21.3, 21.4 show how this occurs. As the chromosomes separate from one another the chiasmata move towards the end of the chromosome, and by the time the chromosomes have become attached to the metaphase plate the chiasmata have reached or nearly reached the ends of the chromosomes. We say that the chiasmata have terminalized.

The formation of chiasmata thus has a mechanical function in bringing homologous chromosomes to the metaphase plate in pairs. The process also has genetic effects. Each chromosome of a homologous pair that moves to the poles during anaphase is no longer identical to the corresponding chromosome in the rest of the body's cells, or to the chromosomes provided by the mother or father of which the latter are a replica. Because of the exchange of material between the chromosomes, the single chromosomes that move in anaphase contain a mixture of the genetic material originally supplied by the mother and father of the individual. Figure 21.5 illustrates the formation of new combinations of genes that results from the formation of a chiasma. Only six genes are indicated on the chromosomes—a, b, c, provided by one parent and A, B, C, by the other parent. After the formation of the chiasma there has been a recombination of these genes.

Figure 21.5   The formation of new combinations of genes resulting from chiasma formation.

union then they would arrange themselves on the metaphase plate as independent units, and when they started to move to the poles in anaphase they would do so quite randomly, resulting in gametes having an odd number of chromosomes. This kind of failure can result in serious disorders in the offspring (see page 250).

Figures 21.3, 21.4 illustrate the way in which the members of a pair of homologous chromosomes become physically united and how later they separate from one another. In 21.3 prophase the homologous chromosomes come together, each split into two chromatids. At one or more points of contact between the chromosomes, breakage occurs in the chromatids of the two chromosomes. These breaks quickly unite again but in such a way that the chromatid of one chromosome becomes united to the chromatid of the other chromosome. These physical bonds

Examples of patterns of inheritance

Having looked at the way that chromosomes behave during the formation of germ cells, we can now go on to see how this behaviour influences the inheritance of certain characteristics. We have seen that the members of a pair of homologous chromosomes are identical in their gross appearance under the microscope. They are also identical in the linear arrangement of factors—genes—which determine various aspects of body form and function. Thus at a particular point along the length of each member of a pair of homologous chromosomes, there is a gene that determines a particular feature, say eye colour. In other words there is a locus on each member of a particular pair of homologous chromosomes which determines eye colour. In this they are identical. However, the two loci may differ in that they determine a different kind of eye colour. At the locus on one chromosome there may be a gene which determines the development of blue eyes; at the same locus on the other chromosome of the pair there may be a gene which determines the development of brown eyes. In this example the effect of only one of these genes is expressed in the individual, i.e. the individual has brown eyes. The gene that determines brown eyes is said to be dominant to that for blue eyes; the gene that determines blue eyes is said to be recessive.

If, at a given locus, both chromosomes of a homologous pair carry identical genes, e.g. dominant genes determining brown eye colour, then the individual is said to be homozygous at this locus. If, however, one chromosome carries a recessive factor at the locus while the other chromosome carries a dominant factor, then the individual is said to be heterozygous at the locus.

Homologous chromosomes are thus very similar but they are not identical. In contrast the two chromatids that make up one chromosome are absolutely identical.

We have seen that in the case of eye colour the gene which determines brown colouration produces its effect whether it is present on one or both chromosomes of a homologous pair, i.e. it is a dominant gene. If one gene is dominant then its alternative form (allele) must be recessive. A recessive gene produces its effect only when it is present on both members of a pair of chromosomes. Some genes, however, are neither dominant nor recessive, and the appearance of an individual heterozygous for such a gene is

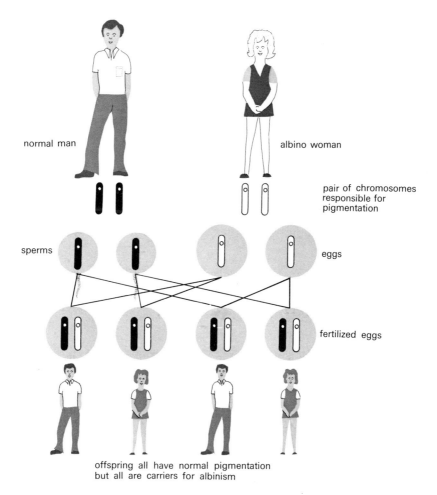

normal man

albino woman

pair of chromosomes responsible for pigmentation

sperms

eggs

fertilized eggs

offspring all have normal pigmentation but all are carriers for albinism

Figure 21.6   Mating of a normal man and an albino woman.
Only one pair of chromosomes is shown, that carrying the gene (or its mutant) responsible for skin pigmentation. Note that all the sperms of the man carry the chromosome responsible for normal pigmentation. Likewise all the eggs of the woman carry the same chromosome but with the mutant gene responsible for albinism. All fertilized eggs thus receive one of each of these two kinds of chromosomes. Because they all contain one chromosome carrying the normal dominant gene, all offspring will have normal pigmentation but will all be carriers for albinism.

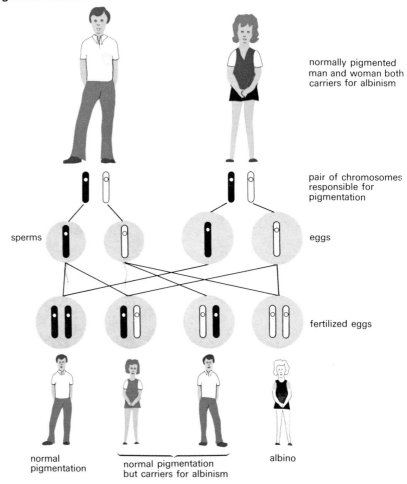

normally pigmented
man and woman both
carriers for albinism

pair of chromosomes
responsible for
pigmentation

sperms

eggs

fertilized eggs

normal
pigmentation

normal pigmentation
but carriers for albinism

albino

Figure 21.7   The mating of two normally pigmented individuals who are carriers for
the recessive gene which determines albinism. Their germ cells will be of two kinds, as
shown. There are four possible results of combinations of these germ cells. Although
only one in four offspring will be albinos, two of the others will be carriers for albinism.

intermediate in appearance between the homozygotes. So far we have mentioned characters
that are determined by the presence of a single
gene or gene pair; the inheritance of such a
character can be followed in a straightforward
way. However, there are many characters which
are the product of the interaction of many genes,
present on different chromosome pairs, and the
study of the inheritance of such characters is far
more complex.

Let us now consider a simple example of the
inheritance of a particular character to illustrate
the effect of the diploid state on both the
inheritance and expression of a mutation. Most
of us have seen albinos, individuals which show
a striking lack of pigment in the skin, hair and
eyes. This condition is due to a recessive mutation, which means that in order to develop this

condition an individual must carry the recessive
mutant gene on both members of an homologous
pair of chromosomes, i.e. he or she must be
homozygous for albinism. To produce an albino
the mutant gene must be present in the germ
cells of both parents; the gene may be present in
a homozygous state (i.e. the parent is an albino)
or in a heterozygous state (i.e. the parent has
normal pigmentation but carries the recessive
mutant gene on one of a pair of chromosomes).
Figures 21.6 and 21.7 show the transmission of
the gene determining albinism. Only one pair
of homologous chromosomes is shown, that
carrying the gene responsible for pigment
formation or its recessive mutant which is
unable to direct pigment production. Figure
21.6 shows the effects of the mating of a normal
man with a woman who is an albino (it does not

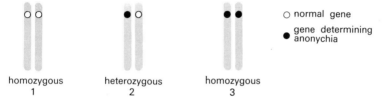

Figure 21.8   Possible combinations of genes determining normal and abnormal nail growth in a pair of homologous chromosomes.

in fact matter for our argument whether it is the man or woman who is the albino, for the outcome of the mating would be the same). Because albinism is a recessive condition, both of the albino woman's pair of chromosomes must carry the gene for albinism. In the reduction division during the formation of germ cells the chromosome number is halved, one of each pair of homologous chromosomes going to each daughter cell. All the eggs produced by the albino woman will carry the gene for albinism. All the sperms produced by the normal man will carry the gene which determines normal pigmentation. Thus *all* fertilized eggs will contain a gene that determines normal pigmentation, and none of the offspring will be albinos although *all* will 'carry' this recessive gene. For obvious reasons 'carriers' of recessive conditions are more common than individuals who express the

condition in their physical make-up, i.e. hetero-zygotes are commoner than homozygotes. In order to produce an albino it is necessary that an albino or a carrier of the gene should mate with another albino or carrier of the gene. The effect of the mating of two carriers of the gene, i.e. two heterozygotes, is shown in Figure 21.7. In the germ cells of both man and woman the normal and mutant gene will be present in equal proportions. The chances are that one in four of the offspring will be an albino, and although two out of four will appear normal they will be carriers of the mutant gene.

For purposes of comparison, Figures 21.8 and 21.9 show the transmission of a dominant gene. The inheritance of a dominant gene is characteristic. Whenever the gene is present its effects are shown in the individual, and the inheritance is readily shown by examining the

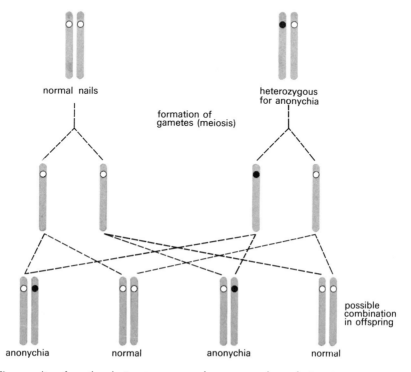

Figure 21.9   The results of mating between a normal person and one heterozygous for anonychia. Only the chromosomes determining nail growth are shown.

family tree. The example chosen is a mutant dominant gene that causes a rare condition called anonychia. In anonychia some or all of the nails of toes and fingers are absent or are present in a very rudimentary condition. There are three possible combinations of the normal and mutant gene on one pair of homologous chromosomes, and this is shown diagrammatically in Figure 21.8. Because the gene for anonychia is dominant then individuals 2 and 3 show the disorder of nail growth. The condition of anonychia is very rare and almost all individuals with the condition are heterozygous for the gene (2); this arises because of the remoteness of the chance of the marriage of two individuals who suffer from the disorder—the kind of union that is necessary to produce a homozygote. Figure 21.9 shows the result of the marriage of an individual heterozygous for the gene, with a normal mate.

The inheritance of sex

We have stressed the fact that each member of a pair of homologous chromosomes are identical in appearance. This is not true for a pair of chromosomes which are especially associated with sex. In the human male, this pair of chromosomes consists of a larger chromosome—

called the X chromosome—and a much smaller member—called the Y chromosome. In the female, the sex chromosomes consist of an identical pair of X chromosomes similar to the X chromosome of the male. The remaining chromosome pairs are called autosomes. The behaviour of the sex chromosomes during the meiotic division in the maturation of germ cells is shown in Figure 21.10. It is clear that the male produces two kinds of spermatozoa, one carrying X chromosomes and one carrying Y chromosomes. The female produces only one class of eggs, all containing an X chromosome. The sex of an individual is thus determined by the father, and at the moment of fertilization of the egg. If the egg is fertilized by a sperm bearing a Y chromosome then the sex of the individual will be male (XY) whereas a female (XX) results from the fertilization of the egg by a sperm bearing an X chromosome.

The Y chromosome is very important in the determination of the sex of an individual. In the absence of a Y chromosome the sexual development is female. In the presence of a Y chromosome the sexual development is male even if there is an abnormal number of X chromosomes (see also page 251). In addition to determining the pattern of sexual development, the sex

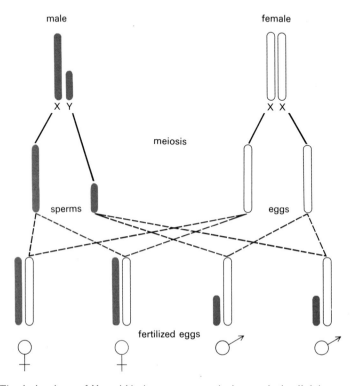

Figure 21.10   The behaviour of X and Y chromosomes during meiotic division.

chromosomes, particularly the X chromosomes, carry genes which affect body structures and functions which have no direct relationship to sexual development. These genes are rather special in that their inheritance is inevitably associated with that of sex. Whether or not an individual shows a particular condition may thus depend upon the sex of the individual. This phenomenon of 'sex-linked' inheritance is discussed more fully on page 257.

Genetics and medicine

In recent years the science of genetics, including that of human genetics, has made rapid progress. There is an increasing awareness of the importance of genetics to medicine, and a large number of genetically transmitted diseases are now recognized. It has been said that as many as one in ten of infants born in Britain have some genetically determined disorder; many of these are minor defects such as disorders of vision, but they may be major defects such as mongolism, severe mental retardation or some disorder of metabolism. In addition to diseases which are clearly transmitted by way of the genetic material, and there are at least a hundred of these, there are very many other disorders of health in which genetic factors play a part in their development. The importance of inherited diseases increases in developed countries where advances in standards of living and hygiene and the widespread use of various immunization procedures have demoted the old captains of death. More infants survive and more adults reach old age. We have seen that in such societies the so-called diseases of civilization become important—cancer, diseases of blood vessels and accidents. Increasing social and medical care also permit many who suffer from serious genetically determined diseases to survive and even to reproduce their kind.

Hereditary diseases are by no means always incurable. Curability often depends upon an understanding of the disturbance of complex physiological processes and patterns of development that result from the action of the particular inherited gene(s). Inherited diseases are becoming increasingly treatable. It *may* be possible to correct defects of physical development by surgery. Disorders of metabolism *may* be treatable by appropriate changes in diet or by the use of specific drugs. At the moment medicine cannot 'mend' the abnormal pattern of genes with which the individual starts his life, but progress in the various sciences is making it

possible more and more often to control the effects of the unfavourable genes. However, in the foreseeable future it seems likely that we may be able to attack some of these diseases at their root cause by means of 'genetic engineering'. Progress in this field is already afoot. In a Cologne hospital for children there are two sisters suffering from a very rare inherited disorder of metabolism called arginaemia. This disease is recognized by an abnormally high blood concentration of the amino acid arginine. The effect of this disorder in a child is profound; mental development is retarded and there may be epileptic fits and paralysis. It has been known for some time that laboratory workers in contact with a virus called the Shope papilloma virus sometimes develop low levels of the amino acid arginine in the blood. It was suggested that the virus might be able safely to introduce new genetic information into man to control excessive arginine levels. This information corresponds to the human gene normally responsible for regulating the manufacture of an enzyme called arginase which breaks down the corresponding amino acid arginine. The hypothesis has now been put to the test and the two sisters in Cologne have been inoculated with purified Shope papilloma virus, but the result of this desperate attempt to control the situation are not yet available. There can be no doubt that this is the forerunner of many attempts to artificially introduce genetic information into man to try to rectify genetic defects.

We will now look at examples of diseases that are clearly inherited, and then go on to look at other diseases the inheritance of which is not simple, mainly because various environmental factors are also involved in determining the development of the disease.

Diseases with simple inheritance

Diseases with obvious abnormalities of chromosomes

We have already discussed the significance of the reduction division in the formation of germ cells for maintaining the normal number of chromosomes of a species, and can now look at some examples of the effects of variations in chromosome number or structure in man. It has only recently become possible to make detailed examination of human chromosomes; indeed it was not until 1956 that the correct number of human chromosomes was established, i.e. twenty-three pairs including the sex chromosomes. In order to study human chromosomes,

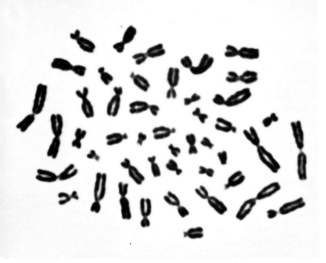

Figure 21.11　Photomicrograph of a cell growing in culture with growth arrested at metaphase. Each chromosome at this stage is made up of two chromatids joined at the centromere.

the first step is to obtain samples of living cells and culture these in the laboratory. These cells are usually white blood cells, skin cells or bone marrow cells. When the cells are multiplying in the artificial conditions of the laboratory, a

Figure 21.12　Preparation of a karyotype. A photograph of a cell at mitotic metaphase is being cut up, matching pairs of chromosomes being pasted on a sheet. (*By courtesy of the Wellcome Research Laboratories.*)

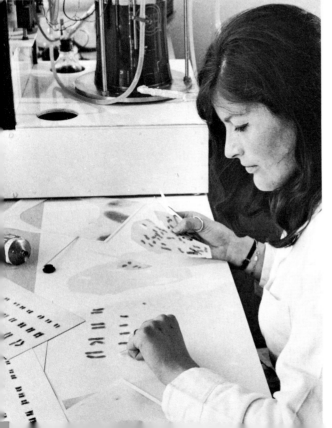

certain drug is added to the culture medium which has the effect of simplifying the study of the chromosomes of the cell. This drug, called colchicine, interferes with the formation of the spindle during cell division and has the effect of arresting cell division at the stage of metaphase, when the chromosomes are very conveniently distributed for observation. This action also increases the number of cells in the culture that show chromosomes, since *all* cells which entered mitotic division after the addition of the drug will be arrested at the stage of metaphase. The cells are now suspended in a weak salt solution; water enters the cells by osmosis and spreads out the chromosomes. The cells are then spread on slides, dried and then stained. Figure 21.11 is a photograph of one such cell. These photographs can be cut up and the individual chromosomes pasted on a sheet in matching pairs (Figure 21.12). Figure 21.13 is a picture of such a preparation showing matched pairs of chromosomes, each chromosome having divided into daughter chromatids which are still attached by the centromere. The two members of a pair of homologous chromosomes are matched by such features as length of the chromosome and position of the centromere. Such a preparation is called a karyotype and that shown in Figure 21.13 is that of a normal male, i.e. one pair consists of dissimilar chromosomes, the sex chromosomes (XY).

Non-disjunction of chromosomes

One cause of abnormal chromosome number in man is the result of an abnormality in the reduction division during the formation of germ cells. Figure 21.14 shows in a schematized form a normal and abnormal reduction division. On the left-hand side the pairs of homologous chromosomes (four in this example) first arrange themselves on the metaphase plate and then repel one another, so that during anaphase one member of a pair goes to one pole of the dividing cell and the other member goes to the opposite pole. Sometimes homologous chromosomes fail to separate in this way during anaphase and both go to the same pole of the dividing cell. This event is called non-disjunction of chromosomes and results in one daughter cell having two members of a homologous pair of chromosomes while the other daughter cell has neither. We will look now at what happens when non-disjunction occurs in relation to the sex chromosomes. If non-disjunction occurs during the development of eggs, it can lead to the formation of an egg containing two X chromosomes or to one

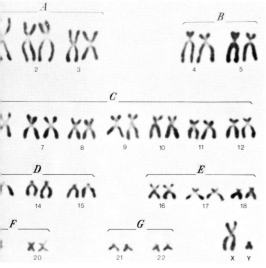

Figure 21.13 Karyotype of a normal male, XY.

containing no X chromosome. In the formation of sperms, non-disjunction can lead to sperms containing both X and Y chromosomes and to sperms containing neither of the sex chromosomes. When these abnormal gametes unite with normal gametes, a variety of abnormal chromosome complements results (Figure 21.15).

Individuals who show Klinefelter's syndrome (karyotype XXY) are usually outwardly normal

males except that the testes may be small and there may be some development of the breasts. The testes do not produce sperm and thus the individuals are infertile. Figure 21.16 shows a karyotype of a subject of Klinefelter's syndrome.

A karyotype with three or four X chromosomes is sometimes found when otherwise normal women are subjected to chromosome studies. The extra one or two X chromosomes do not usually interfere with normal development and fertility. There is, however, more chance of mental deficiency with extra X chromosomes, and this also applies to Klinefelter's syndrome. Because of the normal fertility of women with triple X, it is possible for the chromosome abnormality to be passed on to their offspring since their ova are presumably of two kinds, X and XX. An XX ovum when fertilized by a Y-carrying sperm will result in a male with Klinefelter's syndrome. If the ovum is fertilized by an X-carrying sperm, this will result in another triple-X female.

Individuals with a karyotype containing XO show the features which are called Turner's syndrome (Figure 21.17(a) and (b)). These individuals are outwardly female but the external genital organs remain small and the uterus is infantile. These deficiencies arise because the ovaries do not develop and this leads to a deficiency of female sex hormones. The failure of the uterus and other secondary sex organs to

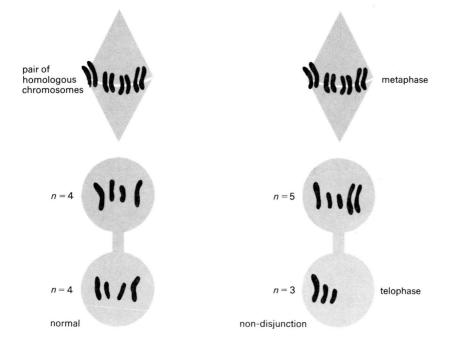

Figure 21.14 The process of non-disjunction of chromosomes.

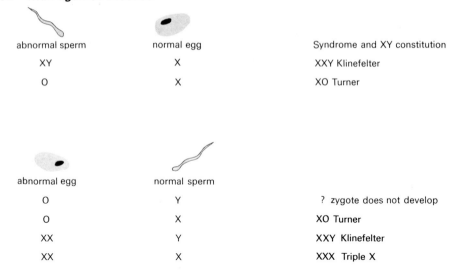

abnormal sperm	normal egg	Syndrome and XY constitution
XY	X	XXY Klinefelter
O	X	XO Turner

abnormal egg	normal sperm	
O	Y	? zygote does not develop
O	X	XO Turner
XX	Y	XXY Klinefelter
XX	X	XXX Triple X

Figure 21.15 The origin of sex chromosome anomalies. O refers to the absence of an X or Y chromosome.

develop normally can be rectified by giving sex hormones, although this does not, of course, restore fertility. There may also be abnormalities outside the reproductive tract, including 'webbing' of the neck, mental deficiency, dwarfism and an abnormality of the aorta.

Much more complex abnormalities of the sex chromosomes have recently been described. Some cases of Klinefelter's syndrome have been found to show XXXY or even XXXXY composition. Some males have a karyotype of XYY, and there have been several reports that males with this karyotype are more likely to have

violent and criminal natures. In 1965 one survey of 197 subnormal males with violent or criminal tendencies showed that seven had an XYY karyotype. XYY males are also unusually tall, and it has been estimated that a man more than 1.8 m in height has a one in two chance of having an XYY constitution. These findings, which suggest a genetic influence in criminal behaviour, raise important medico-legal issues, and in some murder trials a diminished responsibility has been claimed because of an XYY constitution.

From the above examples it is obvious that the body can tolerate gross changes in sex chromosome composition, far greater than could be tolerated for autosome number. The frequency of sex chromosome abnormalities is fairly high (see Table 23) but even more frequent is an abnormality of the autosomes which produces a condition called mongolism

Figure 21.16 Karyotype of an individual with Klinefelter's syndrome.

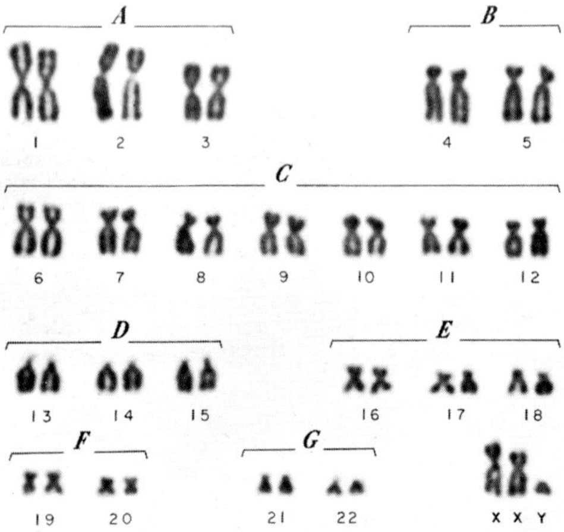

Table 23 Frequency of abnormal chromosome composition

Syndrome	Frequency
XXX	1/800 females
Turner's syndrome	1/2500 females
Klinefelter's syndrome	1/400 males
Down's syndrome	1/500 if the mother's age is 35–38 the incidence rises to 1/300 and this rises to 1/50 with increasing maternal age

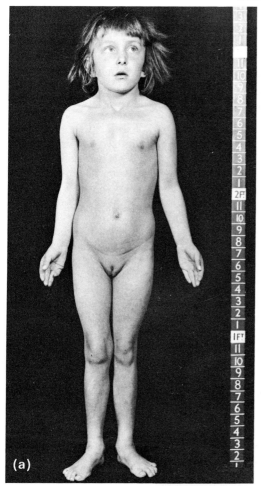

(a)

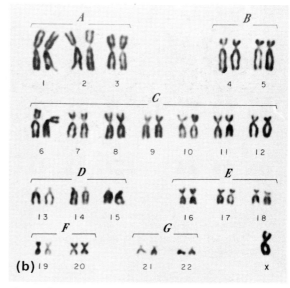

(b)

Figure 21.17   (a) (left) Turner's syndrome showing a webbed neck and deformity of the R. 5th finger. (The photograph was taken before treatment with hormones.) (b) (above) Karyotype of Turner's syndrome.

Figure 21.18 (below)   Mongolism or Down's syndrome. The top right-hand male is about eighteen years old, the bottom right-hand female is middle-aged. The discs on the foreheads of the babies are for identification in a survey.

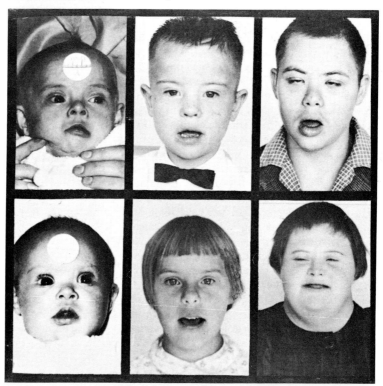

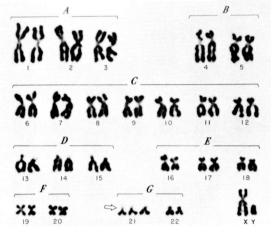

Figure 21.19 Karyotype of a mongol with trisomy of chromosome 21.

(Down's syndrome). The mongol shows severe mental retardation and abnormal physical development. Disordered growth of the skull produces a small skull which is flattened from front to back. The nose is short and flat and the mouth cavity is small, hence the protruding tongue (Figure 21.18). There may also be a squint, abnormal ears, cataracts, abnormal teeth etc. The heart may show defects in normal development, e.g. a persisting hole in the septum that normally completely divides the two ventricles. The commonest cause of mongolism is a non-disjunction affecting the autosomes producing three chromosomes of pair 21 instead of the normal 2, i.e. trisomy 21 (Figure 21.19). Additional autosomes produce more effects than do additional sex chromosomes—compare the defects of the mongol (trisomy 21) with those of individuals with an extra X chromosome (triple-X, Klinefelter's syndrome, XXY). Chromosome 21 is only a small chromosome, yet the presence of an additional 21 produces widespread defects in development. The cause of mongolism thus arises in the development of the germ cells, an abnormality in the reduction division which leads to an egg or sperm containing two members of chromosome 21. When this egg or sperm meets its partner containing one chromosome 21—the usual number for gametes —then trisomy 21 appears and the course of development is directed to produce a mongol. The karyotype of either mother or father of a mongol is usually perfectly normal and the chance of them having another mongol due to trisomy 21 is very small—only one or two per thousand, particularly if the mother is young. There is, however, another cause of mongolism

that is due to a different type of chromosome abnormality, a type that can be passed on from one generation to another by apparently normal 'carriers'. The chromosome abnormality is due to a translocation of chromosomes (see later) and these mongols are called translocation mongols. This type of inherited mongolism provides us with a good example of the use of chromosome studies in providing predictions to help parents of children born with genetic disorders to come to a decision about having further children. If chromosome studies of mother and father are normal and their mongol child shows trisomy 21, then the chances of these parents having a second mongol child are only one or two per thousand. If the mongolism results from translocation of chromosomes then the risks of having a second mongol are very much greater. With mongols born to mothers under the age of thirty, about four or five in a hundred are translocation mongols; there is an extra chromosome 21 but this is attached to another chromosome of the 13–15 group, producing a composite chromosome. Of these translocation mongols, half are due to causes operating during the formation of germ cells, i.e. trisomy 21 due to non-disjunction, with one of the extra chromosome 21 becoming fused to another chromosome (translocation). In this case the parents have a normal karyotype, and the chances of them having a second mongol are very small. However, in another 50 per cent of translocation mongols one of the parents is found to be a 'translocation carrier', and here the risks of having a second mongol are near to one in three.

Translocation

A whole range of abnormalities of human development can arise from breakage of chromosomes. A segment of a chromosome can be lost from the nucleus of a germ cell—a so-called deletion. The broken segment may become re-attached to its parent chromosome only after it has rotated through 360°, producing what is called an inversion. A broken segment may undergo non-disjunction so that one gamete has a segment of a chromosome duplicated. Breakage may involve more than one chromosome and members of two different homologous pairs may in fact exchange pieces of chromosomes; this is called translocation. Like non-disjunction, these major changes in the chromosomes are mutations, that is they produce a change in the genetic nature of the organism that results in a new variation. These major rearrangements of

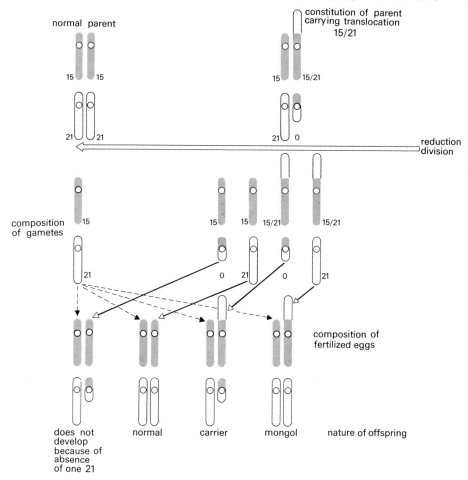

Figure 21.20 The inheritance of translocation mongolism.

the genetic information will understandably have profound effects on development when compared with the effect of mutation of a single gene. Often the change is incompatible with normal development and survival. Sometimes, however, this kind of chromosome rearrangement seems to have been important in evolution, and this is particularly true of inversions in which the total genetic information is unchanged, being merely redistributed among the chromosomes. Translocations also may be compatible with survival particularly if they are balanced translocations, i.e. with an extra segment on one chromosome being balanced by a corresponding deficiency in a chromosome of another pair. Figure 21.20 shows the cause of translocation mongolism, the exchange of chromosome pieces between chromosomes 15 and 21. The left-hand side of the figure shows the normal behaviour of the homologous pairs

of chromosomes 15 and 21 during the reduction division in the formation of gametes; all gametes contain one chromosome 15 and one chromosome 21. On the right-hand side of the figure is shown the effects of exchange of chromosome material between one chromosome 15 and one chromosome 21. When these chromosomes separate in the anaphase of the reduction division, four combinations are possible, as shown in the figure. When gametes carrying these combinations unite with normal gametes, the outcome varies. Some unions can result in normal offspring, some cannot develop, some produce a mongol and yet others can produce an apparently normal individual who is a 'carrier' for this type of mongolism. A translocation mongol has forty-six chromosomes, as does a normal person, but there is an extra chromosome 21 attached to chromosome 15. A 'carrier' of translocation mongolism has only forty-five chromosomes. The carrier has developed normally because most of the missing chromosome 21 has in fact been translocated onto chromosome 15. The only missing portion of this translocated chromosome is a small part close to the centromere (see Figure 21.20) and it is thought that this part of a chromosome carries little or no genetic information.

Summary

There exists a variety of chromosome abnormalities that can be detected by cytological methods. These mutations thus produce *visible* changes not only in various bodily features but also in the structure of the chromosomes. About one in a hundred of all live-born infants have some such chromosome abnormality. Probably even more embryos start off with chromosome abnormalities, but these are not compatible with normal development (particularly if there is a *loss* of chromosome material) and the embryo dies in utero.

Common effects of chromosome abnormalities are mental retardation and sterility. At the moment there is no treatment for such conditions; the only possible measure is *prevention* by giving appropriate advice to fertile individuals who carry chromosome abnormalities, e.g. carriers of translocation 15/21.

Diseases due to dominant, recessive, and sex-linked genes

These diseases are at present estimated to seriously affect about one in a hundred of all live-born individuals at some time in their lives. Most of the diseases are due to dominant genes, but some are due to recessive genes and a few are sex-linked. Most of the diseases due to dominant genes are sufficiently mild to be transmitted through several generations, but only about a third of them may be severe enough to prevent the affected individual from having children. By contrast, most of the serious recessive conditions prevent the affected individual from producing offspring.

Recessive conditions

We have already looked at the mechanism of inheritance of a recessive condition, that of albinism. This condition does not prevent reproduction, and one important feature of recessive conditions is that recessive genes can be passed on through many generations by means of apparently normal individuals who

are heterozygous for the condition. Only when two heterozygotes happen to marry one another is there a chance of the affected individual, the homozygote, appearing. We will refer back to this when we discuss the possible effects of the marriage of related individuals.

When an abnormal recessive gene is present in the homozygous condition, then the effect may be very serious and the individual may not survive long enough to marry and have children. Examples of such conditions are cystic fibrosis, infantile amaurotic idiocy and phenylketonuria. Cystic fibrosis (fibrocystic disease of the pancreas) is the most common of all diseases in this country which are due to recessive mutant genes that produce large effects. The disease affects about one child in 2000. The basic abnormality is that the mucus in the respiratory tract and digestive glands is abnormally sticky and the sweat glands produce a sweat which contains abnormally large amounts of salt. The main effects of this disease are caused by the sticky mucus. In the lungs the mucus tends to cause obstruction of the small air passages and this tends to lead to repeated chest infections. In the pancreas the ducts of the gland tend to become blocked so that there is a deficiency in the release of digestive enzymes; the digestion of fats and protein is thus incomplete and this affects the nutrition of the individual. In the past no cases of cystic fibrosis survived to adult life. Nowadays patients are being treated with pancreatic enzymes (obtained from animal glands) by mouth so as to improve the state of the digestion of fats and proteins. In addition, the introduction of a large range of antibiotics and other drugs that kill or damage bacteria means that the respiratory infections can be more effectively treated. Because of the frequency of this disease (1:2000), the prolonged nature of the treatment and the often frequent admissions to hospital for the management of respiratory infections, it imposes a fair-sized burden on medical facilities. The carrier rate in the population is about 1:20–1:25.

Phenylketonuria affects one child in 40 000 in this country and in Northern Europe. The basic defect is an inability of the body to convert the amino acid phenylalanine into another amino acid called tyrosine. This defect results in widespread changes in the body. About 80 per cent of affected persons are blue-eyed blondes who may have eczema. Very many have marked mental deficiency of a degree that produces what we call idiots or imbeciles. The remainder are usually mentally defective to a degree. The disease can be diagnosed by demonstrating the products of phenylalanine which appear in considerable amounts in the urine of affected individuals. The urine test is simple, and once this simple screening test was discovered it was found that one in a hundred of patients in hospitals for the severely mentally subnormal suffered from phenylketonuria. In Great Britain all infants are examined for this disease. The appropriate test reagents are impregnated on a strip of paper and a drop of urine or a wet nappy will turn the paper a characteristic colour if the urine contains abnormal amounts of the products of phenylalanine. Widespread testing is carried out because there is the possibility that if affected infants are reared from an early age on a diet free from phenylalanine, then relatively normal mental development may be possible. This practice is based upon the principle that the mental defect is not an essential part of the disease but results from poisoning by the by-products of phenylalanine. This is one of the rare instances in which one can prevent mental deficiency.

Diseases due to dominant genes

The inheritance of dominant genes is characteristic. Whenever the gene is present its effects are manifested in the individual and the inheritance is readily shown by examining the family tree. Many disorders have been shown to be carried by dominant genes; these include blindness (due to degeneration of the retina), porphyria, intestinal polyposis, dwarfism due to achondroplasia, hereditary spherocytosis (acholuric jaundice), Huntington's chorea and so on. We will look briefly at one example—familial polyposis of the large bowel. In this disease there are many small wart-like growths called polyps on the inner surface of the large bowel. These polyps appear in childhood, although they may cause no symptoms until the late teens or even later. The danger is that one or more of these polyps may transform into malignant tumours which spread and ultimately kill the patient. The risk is so great that once the condition is recognized the patient is advised to have all the affected bowel removed before cancer develops. The large bowel is removed and the end of the small intestine is made to open onto the surface of the abdominal wall (ileostomy), or the small bowel is joined onto the stump of the rectum if this is relatively unaffected by the disease. In spite of this apparently radical kind of treatment, patients are able to lead relatively normal lives. Children of individuals with the disease (who are almost always heterozygous for

the abnormal gene) have a one in two chance of developing the condition. The children can be told whether or not they carry the gene by examining the bowel for the presence of polyps (this examination is carried out by inserting an illuminated tube, a sigmoidoscope, up the rectum and into the colon). If they have no polyps then they do not carry the gene and their own children will be unaffected. If polyps are present then their own children will in turn have a one in two chance of developing polyposis and of needing surgical treatment. This disease is rather rare and one would expect this because it kills, certainly it used to kill prematurely, by causing cancer of the bowel.

Sex-linked conditions

In addition to determining the pattern of sexual development (i.e. to male or female), the sex chromosomes, just like the autosomes, carry various genes which affect body structures and functions having no direct relationship to sexual development. These genes are rather special in that their inheritance is inevitably associated with that of sex determination. Whether or not an individual shows a particular disease may thus depend upon the sex of the individual.

Sex-linked inheritance describes inheritance via the X chromosome. The genes responsible are carried only on the X chromosome and there are no corresponding loci on the Y chromosome. There are other possibilities, e.g. genes exclusive to the Y chromosome or genes represented on both X and Y chromosomes, but they are not of practical significance—at least in man. We can best illustrate the effect of inheritance of a character by way of the X chromosome by looking at a gene which determines an abnormal condition. If the male carries the abnormal gene then the condition will be apparent in the individual, i.e. it shows in the phenotype. There is no such thing as a recessive or dominant gene here, for all genes on the X chromosome which do not have normal genes on the Y chromosome will find expression. The situation is very different for the female who has a pair of homologous X chromosomes; in the female a sex-linked gene can be dominant, recessive or intermediate, as in autosomal genes.

One sex-linked recessive condition is an inherited deficiency of the enzyme glucose-6-phosphate dehydrogenase, which is necessary for the normal metabolism of red blood cells. As red cells age the enzyme content declines and the cells eventually are broken

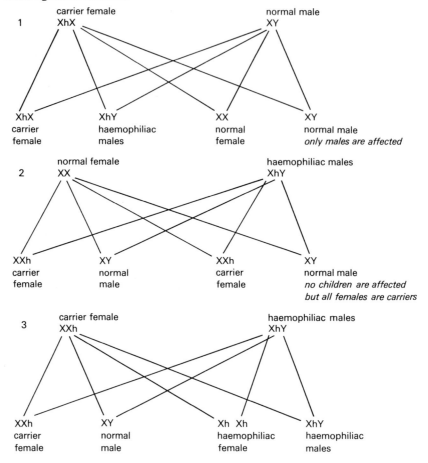

Figure 21.21 The mode of inheritance of haemophilia. Xh represents the X chromosome which carries the recessive abnormal gene determining haemophilia.

down. The inheritance of G–6–PD deficiency is sex-linked and may affect 10 per cent of negroes; it also occurs in Caucasians, and in these the deficiency may be more severe. It has been estimated that many millions of people are affected by the condition. The effect of G–6–PD deficiency is shown in a shorter survival of red blood cells in the circulation. Under normal conditions an individual with deficient enzyme may compensate for this shortened life of red blood cells by an increased rate of production of red blood cells from the bone marrow. But if oxidant drugs are given, e.g. sulphonamides for bacterial infections or antimalarial drugs, then large numbers of red blood cells are damaged and rapidly destroyed, producing an acute anaemia. These drugs are particularly dangerous in men carrying the factor (i.e. with no corresponding normal allele on the Y chromosome) and in women who are homozygous for the factor.

Most women who are heterozygous for the factor although they show some detectable deficiency of the enzyme in red blood cells, are not as prone to develop the anaemia.

Haemophilia is another example of a disease caused by a sex-linked recessive gene. It is a life-long bleeding disorder which affects males and is transmitted by apparently normal females. The bleeding is due to a complete or partial lack of an essential component of the blood-clotting mechanisms, a globulin in blood plasma appropriately named anti-haemophilic globulin. Haemophilia is a fairly uncommon disease; in its severe form it occurs in about one in every 7000 live male births, but if one includes more mildly affected patients the incidence rises to as many as one haemophiliac in every 3000–4000 live male births. With improvements in treatment it appears likely that the number of haemophiliacs in the community will steadily increase as they are enabled to live with their genetic deficiency. Figure 21.21 illustrates the inheritance of this condition. The recessive gene responsible for haemophilia is carried on the terminal part of the X chromosome. The human female has two X chromosomes but the human male has only one X chromosome which pairs with a shorter chromosome, the Y chromosome. In the male the terminal part of the X chromosome is unpaired, since the Y chromosome is shorter than the X. It is this unpaired region of the male X chromosome which carries the gene responsible for haemophilia. If a recessive gene is carried on this unpaired portion of the X chromosome in the male, then the condition will be expressed in the phenotype. In the female, however, since the X chromosome is paired along the whole of its length with another X chromosome, a recessive gene will always be paired with another gene; thus the female will only have the disease if she carries the abnormal gene on *both* X chromosomes (i.e. the homozygous recessive state). Females with haemophilia are extremely rare since to produce such a female, a female carrier (or female haemophiliac) would have to marry a male haemophiliac, and since the disease is uncommon such a combination is highly unlikely. However, females are important in transmitting the disease to their male offspring.

In about 30 per cent of men with haemophilia there is no previous history of haemophilia in the family. This might mean that there is a high mutation rate producing the disease or that the abnormal gene is in fact present in the family, but for various reasons, such as small families or few sons, the disease has not shown itself. Probably both factors operate. Haemophiliacs bleed seriously and persistently after injury because of failure of the clotting mechanism which normally operates to assist the halting of bleeding. Haemophiliacs may also bleed spontaneously, that is in the absence of obvious injury; this sort of bleeding characteristically occurs in joints and muscles, which is very painful and may lead to severe crippling if not treated early enough. Because of the life-long nature of the disease, with recurrent episodes of bleeding into joints and muscles or prolonged bleeding after even trivial injuries, with loss of time from school and work, the management of the disease has important social and economic implications as well as the more obvious medical ones. A variety of preparations are used to arrest bleeding in haemophiliacs, but all of them act because they contain anti-haemophilic globulin, the clotting factor deficient in these patients.

Diseases with a more complex inheritance

In the examples we have been discussing, the diseases are believed to be maintained in the population by means of recurring mutations. Hence it would be impossible to eradicate many of the diseases by the control of marriages or of the reproduction of affected individuals. Because of these spontaneous mutations, the diseases can crop up in families in which there has never been a previous case of the disease. This fact is of considerable importance to those concerned with public health because various factors in our environment are known to increase the rate of mutations, i.e. they are mutagenic. The control of these factors and the search for as yet undiscovered mutagenic agents is a vital responsibility of those concerned with our health. This activity will be discussed further in a later section.

In some inherited diseases there are other factors which operate to maintain the frequency of a particular gene at a high level from one generation to another. This is because the abnormal gene can paradoxically increase the fitness of the individual to withstand particular circumstances. Thus we have the unusual situation in which a gene damages and reduces fitness under some circumstances, and yet may have the reverse effect and increase fitness under other circumstances. The frequency of the gene in a population will depend on the balance of these forces. We call this a balanced polymorphic system.

One such condition which has been widely studied is sickle-cell anaemia. This disease is so-called because of the characteristic sickled shape of the red blood cells under certain conditions. These cells contain an abnormal form of haemoglobin, called haemoglobin-S. The disease results in a chronic anaemia which is punctuated by 'crises' in which the anaemia rapidly worsens due to a massive break-down of the abnormal cells in the circulating blood. The seriousness of the disease depends on whether an individual is heterozygous or homozygous for the gene. In the heterozygous condition, the gene results in nearly 50 per cent of the haemoglobin of the red cells being in the abnormal S-form. This fraction rises to much higher levels in the homozygous state, when the disease is often fatal. The gene responsible for this disease is very unevenly distributed in the world. In some areas it is *very* rare but in parts of Asia and Africa the frequency of homozygotes may be as high as 10 per cent. The reason for the accumulation of the gene in these areas is that the heterozygote for this trait benefits by having an increased resistance to malignant malaria. Such is the complexity of nature.

Factors governing the inheritance and distribution of other genes may be even more complex. There are many malformations of infants and diseases of later life, the inheritance of which may be complex and the expression of which is determined by the interaction of the genetic make-up with one or more factors in the environment. Many of the diseases in this class can be looked upon as the result of the action of certain environmental factors on an individual already susceptible to the disease by virtue of his genetic constitution. The genetic factor may be single recessive or dominant genes, or it may be the product of the action of many genes at a number of loci on the chromosomes. Conditions in which there is a genetic predisposition are many and varied, and include schizophrenia, manic-depressive psychoses, mental deficiency, pernicious anaemia, diabetes mellitus, some types of epilepsy, diseases of blood vessels, susceptibility to various infections, stillbirths, asthma and duodenal ulceration. The accurate assessment of the part played by genetic factors in these various conditions is exceedingly difficult. Studies of family trees and comparisons of health of identical twins are very important tools in trying to unweave the nexus of heredity and environment.

Mutations, mutagens and the effect of modern life on mutations

The mechanisms of heredity ensure that the offspring are similar to their parents. In the words of Dobzhansky heredity 'is a conservative force; evolutionary innovation demands that heredity be occasionally thwarted'. This thwarting occurs when a mutation takes place. We have seen a variety of examples of mutations in man, ranging from changes in the effects of single genes to relatively major changes in the number or composition of the chromosomes themselves. Major changes of the genetic material are often incompatible with normal development and survival. These major changes include duplication of chromosomes, losses of chromosomes or repatterning of chromosome segments by translocation. Most mutations, however, cause no change in the structure of the chromosomes that can be seen even with the most powerful of electron microscopes. The changes are in the individual genes, i.e. in the molecular structure of the minute sub-units of the hereditary material of the chromosomes.

All the mutations that we have considered in relation to human nature have been harmful. Indeed all mutations in all organisms are usually harmful. This state of affairs is inevitable if we consider for a moment the significance of the hereditary material. The complex array of genes in the nucleus of the fertilized egg carries the information that not only guides the development of this tiny cell into the complete organism but also enables it to survive and reproduce its kind in its particular environment, be it arctic tundra, arrid desert or the depths of the ocean. Any random change in the complex array of interacting genes is almost bound to result in an organism that is less fitted to survive in its own particular niche in the world. However, environments change and man himself has altered his own environment on a vast scale, and some genes that were unfavourable in the old circumstances may become favourable in the new; of course, the converse may be equally true. We have seen such an example in the case of the gene that determines the presence of an abnormal type of haemoglobin in the red cells (sickle-cell anaemia). In certain areas of the world this gene is relatively common because it confers some resistance to malignant malaria. In countries where malaria does not occur, only the damaging effect of the gene expresses itself and only rare individuals carry the gene. The decline in the frequency of this gene in non-malarious areas is due to loss of the gene by the death of individuals with sickle-cell anaemia (homozygotes) and to a somewhat increased mortality of the heterozygotes for this gene compared to normal individuals.

If natural selection carries out this role of 'weeding out' harmful genes, we may ask ourselves why it is that mankind suffers from so much hereditary ill health. The answer to this question can be given under three headings: the occurrence of harmful mutations, the less than perfect efficiency of the process of natural selection, and the effects of applying the advances of modern medical science in the treatment of individuals who suffer from hereditary illness.

The various genetically determined illnesses that occur in human populations do not all arise because of the inheritance of harmful genes from the parents; many occur in individuals who have no family history of such illness, and of these many are due to mutations that have occurred early in the development of the individual, possibly during the development of one of the germ cells from which he arose. This means that even when a genetically determined illness kills before the sufferer is able to reproduce, new cases of the disease may continually appear in the population because of recurring new mutations.

Even when a harmful gene does not kill the individual before he has a chance of producing offspring, natural selection may still operate to reduce this possibility. The individual may suffer from chronic ill health or may be otherwise less acceptable as a marriage partner, particularly if the disorder markedly alters the appearance of the individual. Achondroplastic dwarfs usually survive and enjoy fairly normal health, but they produce few children; this is due not only to the small pelvis of the female dwarf which makes for difficulty in childbirth, but also because many dwarfs remain unmarried. Thus some mutant genes are less efficiently passed on from one generation to another than is the corresponding normal gene. However, natural selection is much less efficient in removing harmful genes of a recessive character. Many individuals in a population may carry harmful recessive genes in a heterozygous condition (i.e. paired with a normal gene) without producing any effect on their general health or reproductive capacity. Natural selection can only operate when a gene manifests itself in the individual. These harmful recessive genes that are carried 'hidden' in the heterozygous state form what is called the 'concealed genetic load' of a population. This concealed load of recessive genes is immense compared with the visible genetic load that becomes revealed when two individuals heterozygous for the same recessive gene marry and produce children who are homozygous for the gene (but only one in four of their children will reveal the genetic defect). The recessive nature of many genetically determined diseases thus reduces the efficiency of the processes of natural selection in eradicating the gene from a population. The activities of man himself further hinder the process of natural selection by enabling affected individuals to survive and reproduce, individuals who would, in the absence of the benefits of modern medicine, die in their infancy or their youth.

Man not only hinders the forces of natural selection, he actually promotes the appearance of genetically determined diseases, either by contaminating his environment with substances that increase the rate of mutations or by means of social habits, such as the marriage of blood relations (consanguineous marriages), that encourage the revealing of the 'hidden genetic load'.

The effects of agents in the environment on mutation rate

Mutation takes place regularly in all species of organisms. Under 'natural conditions' individual genes mutate very rarely, perhaps once in 100 000–1 000 000 germ cells. However, since the number of genes in most organisms is very high the total number of mutations may be quite considerable. If we make a reasonable assumption that the 23 chromosomes in a human germ cell carry 10 000 genes, then one gamete in ten may carry a mutated gene. This then is the estimate of the 'natural' rate of mutation. During his evolution, particularly in that short period following the industrial revolution, man has so altered his environment that this 'natural' rate of mutation *can* be considerably increased. In the main this is due to the introduction of radio-active materials and chemicals that can stimulate mutations—the so-called mutagens.

Radiation

Much is known and much has been written about the effects of ionizing radiations in living organisms. Radiation is known to produce mutations in all organisms so far studied, and there is no reason at all for thinking that man might be an exception to this. For very obvious reasons it is difficult to estimate the effects of radiation in man, and it is easier to obtain information about bacteria or animals such as fruit flies that reproduce rapidly.

There are various natural sources of radiation that affect man and other organisms—cosmic rays, radiation from natural radio-active elements in the crust of the earth and in the air, and radiation from radio-isotopes that are normally present in the body. The dose of radiation to the soft tissues of the body from all natural sources of radiation averages about 0.1 rad per year (a rad is a unit of absorbed dose of radiation; one rad = 100 erg/G; a submultiple is the millirad, mrad = 10^{-3} rad) although the dose varies according to latitude, altitude and variations in the composition of soil and rocks. 0.1 rad/year is, then, an average dose of radiation from natural sources. Man's various activities in medicine (X-rays, radiotherapy etc.), occupations (radiographers, radiologists, workers in 'atomic-energy' institutions) and in war (nuclear explosions) can considerably increase this 'natural' dose of radiation for certain individuals. Table 24 shows the dose of natural radiation that reaches the gonads (ovaries or testes) compared with the dose received during various X-ray examinations.

Table 24

Examination	Gonad dose per examination (m rad)
X-ray hips	53–3600
X-ray femur	50–1650
X-ray pelvis	20–3580
X-ray kidneys (retrograde pyelography)	200–3800
Pelvimetry (measurement of pelvis)	76–2500
X-ray chest	0.01–450

(Annual dose from natural sources 100)
Data from 'Ionizing Radiation and Health' by Bo. Lindell and R. Lowry Dobson, *Public Health Papers 6*, World Health Organization. The wide variation in the measured values results from studies by different workers often using different techniques, exposing different numbers of films and in some cases shielding of the gonads of males with lead.

The average yearly dose from diagnostic X-ray examinations in technologically well developed countries is about the same as that from natural radiation, although for individuals the dose may be much higher and concentrated over a very much shorter period of time. When radiation is used to *treat* disease rather than to diagnose disease, larger doses of radiation may be used. This is particularly true when radiation is used to treat malignant tumours. Because of the serious nature of the illness for which the radiation is used, it is unlikely that long-term genetic effects will result. In many countries, however, some fairly harmless conditions such as acne, plantar warts and other skin problems may be treated by radiotherapy. Obviously this treatment should only be carried out with a full realization of the potential dangers and using special precautions to protect the gonads. Exposure to radiation in industries is subject to stringent regulations, but in some countries it is still permitted to use X-ray fluoroscopy in the fitting of shoes and this can involve considerable hazard both for the customer and the shop assistant.

Chemical mutagens

Much less is known about the genetic effects of chemicals that can stimulate the appearance of mutations. Two things, however, are certain: mankind is being exposed to an increasing variety of chemicals particularly in connection with medical treatment, food processing (preservatives, colouring and flavouring agents etc.) pesticides and so on; and a large number of chemical compounds can be shown to have genetic effects. Research in this field is still very fragmentary; many different types of organisms may be used in the studies—bacteria, moulds, fruit flies, mice, etc.—and different effects of drugs searched for (visible effects on chromosomes, abnormalities in development of the newborn, appearance of inherited single-gene mutations). It is very difficult to apply this information to man, for not all species respond in the same way to the same chemical.

The most powerful of all chemical mutagens which act on all test organisms belong to a group of compounds called the alkylating agents. These chemicals can produce effects in cells that are superficially similar to those caused by ionizing radiations—hence their name, radiomimetic drugs. The discovery of the radiomimetic action of these drugs arose out of wartime research on the chemical weapon called mustard gas which was first used in the 1914–18 war. Quite early in the investigations of the actions of alkylating agents it was found that, like radiation, the chemicals could stop cell division. Soldiers dying of mustard-gas poisoning showed virtual atrophy of the bone marrow and the presence of widespread ulceration of the small bowel; both of these tissues have a very rapid turnover of cells and it is these tissues that are affected first by any agent which interferes with cell division. The discovery in 1943 by Charlotte Auerbach that mustard gas could also produce true mutations was a finding of great importance.

Mustard gas is the parent compound of a whole range of alkylating agents. They are called alkylating agents because their prime action is to replace a hydrogen atom in a molecule with which they react by an alkyl group, $R.CH_2-$. All alkylating agents react by the formation of an intermediate compound bearing a positively charged carbonium ion, $-CH_2{}^+$. This positively charged carbonium ion can react with a variety of negatively charged centres in biological molecules; when a dose of alkylating agent is administered to an animal, most of the compound is 'mopped up' by biological molecules such as tissue proteins (including enzymes), phosphoric acid, and so on. The most important action of alkylating agents is, however, on the chemical substance of the genetic material itself, that substance called deoxyribonucleic acid (DNA). The DNA of a chromosome is a very long and complex molecule. It is a duplex

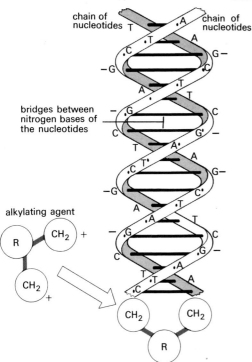

chain of nucleotides

chain of nucleotides

bridges between nitrogen bases of the nucleotides

alkylating agent

Figure 21.22 Mode of action of a molecule of an alkylating agent on the hereditary material (DNA) of the chromosome. The chemical can cross-link the two strands of DNA and thus disturb cell division.

structure consisting of a pair of intertwining strands. Prior to cell division these two strands separate, each going to a different daughter cell where each strand manufactures its partner to re-establish the 'double helix'. Some alkylating agents bear two reactive groups in their molecule, i.e. $CH_2^+ - R - CH_2^+$, and these bifunctional molecules can 'cross-link' two biological molecules. They can thus cross-link the two strands of the double helix of DNA and prevent the normal separation of the strands that precedes cell division. One can visualize (Figure 21.22) that it would take only one relatively small molecule of an alkylating agent to produce this effect in a very long molecule of DNA. Such is the sensitivity of the genetic material to alkylating agents. This sort of action can disturb cell division and cause breakage of chromosomes. Alkylating agents can also affect single genes, but we will not pursue the detailed biochemistry of this kind of effect.

In addition to alkylating agents, a large number of other chemicals have been found to produce visible changes in the chromosomes or invisible effects on single genes that can be detected only in the offspring of affected individuals. Many of these studies are carried out on micro-organisms, plants and fruit flies, and their relevance for human genetics is unknown. Certainly some substances do produce chromosome changes in man, substances such as LSD or methyl mercury, but again the significance of these effects is unknown. Recent work at the Karolinska Institute in Stockholm, for example, has shown that people who have eaten fish contaminated by methyl mercury (mercury levels ranging from 1–7 mg/kg fish, i.e. 1–7 parts per million) showed evidence of abnormally frequent chromosome breakages in cells. Methyl mercury is one of those persistent poisons that contaminate our environment. The mercury arises from industrial wastes that are discharged into waterways or into the sea. The inorganic mercury in the effluent is converted into organic mercury (methyl mercury) by the micro-organisms and minute plants and animals of fresh and sea water. As these minute organisms are eaten by larger animals the organic mercury is passed along the food chain, where it can become concentrated in the bodies of the larger fish that are eaten by man. The presence of methyl mercury (1–2 parts per million) in tinned tuna fish resulted in the condemning of vast stocks of this food in the U.S.A.

These examples serve to illustrate the great care that has to be taken before new chemicals are added to foodstuffs. The last example shows how our garbage may return to us in an unsuspected and dangerous guise. The tipping of industrial wastes (not merely radio-active wastes) into the vast oceans may *seem* to be a harmless practice, but in reality it may have potential far-reaching consequences for man's health in the future.

Consanguineous marriages and other patterns of behaviour

There are various aspects of human reproductive behaviour that can affect the number of children affected by genetic disease. Some habits (in particular marriage of blood relations) can increase the risk of bearing diseased children while others (e.g. efficient contraceptive techniques used in older women) can have the opposite effect.

The marriage of blood relatives increases the risk that characters that are determined by recessive genes or by polygenes will appear in the offspring. In terms that we have previously defined (page 261), consanguineous marriages tend to reveal the hidden genetic load of a population. Results of recent studies show that consanguineous marriages do not produce a greater number of miscarriages or stillbirths, but from birth onwards the death rate in children of such marriages is higher than that of a control group. There is also an increase in the number of children born with major congenital abnormalities. In one Japanese city it was found that in the offspring of first cousins there was a death rate of 116 per 1000 during the first eight years of life, compared to 55 per 1000 in controls. The number of major congenital abnormalities in children of first-cousin marriages was about double that of controls. Studies in America, where there is a lower total death rate, showed even greater differences. In one city the offspring of first-cousin marriages had a death rate of 81 per 1000 by the age of ten years compared with 24 per 1000 in controls.

In many communities first-cousin marriages are now uncommon (not more than 3 per 1000 marriages) and is still decreasing; but in some communities these marriages are still relatively common. One factor which probably affects the frequency of consanguineous marriages is the size of the family. A reduction in the size of families might result in a decrease in the frequency of consanguineous marriages; with fewer children in the various branches of a family tree and with increasing mobility of families, particularly in developed countries, there are fewer cousins, with fewer opportunities to meet and marry.

In developed countries there is an increasing tendency for women to produce their children while they are young, and then perhaps to return to work when they are in their thirties or forties. This pattern, which depends, of course, on efficient means of family planning, has various advantages for a community, not the least of which is that it can reduce the frequency of several inherited diseases which appear more frequently in the offspring of older mothers. Mongolism and disease due to Rhesus incompatibility of mother and foetus are well-known examples of this effect of maternal age. In mongolism the frequency of affected infants rises rather slowly until the mother reaches the age of thirty-five years (see page 252) but then it becomes very rapid as the mother gets near the end of her child-bearing period. The overall frequency of mongolism is about 1.5–2.5:1000, although there are geographical variations which *may* be due to differences in maternal age in different populations. In the age group 35–39 there is a 2–4 fold increase in the frequency of mongolism and this rises to a 5–10 fold increase

for the age group 40–44; after the age of forty-five there is a 10–20 fold increase in the frequency of mongolism.

Prevention and treatment of genetically determined disease

We have already mentioned many aspects of the control of these diseases and the future possibilities of nullifying the effects of some abnormal genes. The following is a list of the important preventative measures.

1. Control of exposure to mutagenic agents— X-rays and other ionizing radiations and chemicals.

2. Scientific study of the many substances used as drugs, food additives and preservatives to detect their ability to promote mutations, particularly in mammals. When suitable test procedures have been developed, legislation should follow to prescribe tests for mutagenic properties, particularly for newly introduced compounds.

3. Some radiomimetic chemicals are used in the treatment of various diseases but mainly for malignancies. These chemicals tend to be strongly mutagenic and this raises the question of whether patients under treatment should procreate. At the moment this is a small problem, at least in terms of the numbers involved.

4. Health education of the public about the known risks of consanguineous marriages and the effect of maternal age on genetic disease in the offspring. This education would be of little value in the absence of parallel developments of efficient and acceptable family planning services.

5. Genetic counselling. The implementation of many of the above measures awaits the development of government awareness and decisions, of scientific research and the establishment of appropriate health services. Genetic counselling is, however, a service that is available now for those individuals who need advice on the known risks of producing children that are affected by a particular genetic abnormality. These services will be discussed more fully in a later section (page 266).

6. Eugenics, which is the science of improving the human stock. Genetic counselling is one aspect of eugenics although the benefits of counselling are felt mainly by the particular

family. Eugenic measures are designed to improve the health of the population as a whole. At present the main aim of these measures is to reduce the total burden of genetic disease, and this aspect is called negative eugenics. Attempts to actually improve health—to improve such features as resistance to disease, intelligence or other attributes—are called positive eugenics.

Negative eugenic measures can never hope to eradicate completely the inherited burdens that handicap many individuals. Spontaneous mutations and the coming together of carriers of recessive genes will always bring about new cases of genetic disease. Even if every male haemophiliac were compulsorily sterilized, new cases of the disease would always appear, either because of spontaneous mutations in the germ cells of normal individuals or because a woman carrying the abnormal gene 'hidden' on one of her X chromosomes contributes the abnormal gene to one or more of her sons. The aims of negative eugenics are thus to try to *reduce* the frequency of hereditary diseases.

One obvious measure of negative eugenics is to discourage individuals from having children if they suffer from serious inherited diseases that carry a high risk of transmission to their offspring. This aim can sometimes be achieved by means of education and counselling. Some might argue that these individuals should be compulsorily sterilized or that pregnancies of such potentially dangerous unions should be compulsorily terminated. These decisions are vexed by moral and political issues and by a popular view of the inalienable right of every human being to reproduce his or her kind, whatever the consequences for the offspring or for the economic or medical burden to society as a whole. Compulsory measures have, however, been advocated, and sometimes used, for cases where genetic counselling and family planning advice (including *voluntary* sterilization) are likely to be ineffective. This is the eugenic problem of those individuals who suffer from severe degrees of mental retardation. There is clear evidence of a genetic influence in many mentally-subnormal individuals. These individuals moreover tend to have larger than average families and nowadays these children have an increased chance of survival because of improvements in medical and social care.

Positive eugenics does not really come within the scope of our present discussion but we will consider it briefly for the sake of completeness. Positive eugenics involves a planned programme to make the whole population (not just particular families) less prone to disease, more intelligent and so on. This sort of programme involves even more violation of the liberty of the individual than does negative eugenics. It might mean considerable restriction on the choice of a mate or even the use of artificial insemination of women using semen from a donor of optimum genetic constitution. Artificial insemination *is* carried out today, usually because a husband is sterile or because he is unable, for some reason, to impregnate his wife with semen. In the former case a donor's seminal fluid, and in the latter the husband's own seminal fluid is introduced into the neck of the womb of his wife. In the future it is possible that some forms of sterility in women may be treated by implanting into the womb of the barren woman an egg obtained from a normal woman. This procedure, like that of artificial insemination, could have important implications for the techniques of positive eugenics. However, in a world that is coping quite inadequately with the techniques of family planning to limit the astronomical growth of populations, these notions of 'positive eugenics' are mere pipe dreams. It is worth remembering, however, that in recent history positive eugenics of a sort was practised in Nazi Germany, involving not only the brutal elimination or sterilization of unwanted 'non-Aryan' (usually Jewish) stock, but also the pairing of chosen 'brood mothers' with approved males who showed the physical features of presumed excellence.

The treatment of inherited disease

Many of the diseases caused by genetic defects are virtually untreatable. It is, however, becoming increasingly true that a number of these diseases can be prevented or treated. We have looked at the treatment of that inherited metabolic disorder called phenylketonuria (page 256). Another inherited metabolic disorder, galactosaemia, can also be treated. If the diagnosis of galactosaemia is not made then early death is common, and even if the disease is not fatal there is a severe disability. Treatment consists in removing the sugar lactose from the diet; if this is done then physical and mental development are normal. Another example of a completely successful treatment of an inherited disease is the surgical correction of congenital pyloric stenosis. In this disease the pylorus, that part of the stomach that leads into the first part of the small intestine, is elongated and thickened. As it is difficult for food to pass through this thickened part of the stomach, the disorder shows itself by vomiting of feeds, beginning a few weeks after birth. This disease is inherited but in a rather complex manner. Before the advent of surgical correction of the defect, mortality was high, but in spite of this the disease maintained itself at a fairly high frequency, affecting as many as one in 150 in the population. The mortality of the disease is now very low following the introduction of a simple surgical procedure—Ramstedt's operation—in which the hypertrophied muscles of the pylorus are split, leaving the underlying mucous membrane intact.

Even if the genetically determined disorder cannot be completely corrected then considerable improvement in the condition is often possible. Congenital hare-lip and cleft palate and many orthopaedic disorders such as congenital dislocation of the hip or club foot can be considerably improved by means of appropriate treatment.

There is one special group of diseases in which there is an inherited susceptibility to certain drugs. The affected individual may be completely or relatively healthy until the particular drug is given, and then there may be disastrous consequences. General anaesthesia today commonly involves the use of a drug which relaxes muscles so that only small amounts of anaesthetic are needed, just sufficient to maintain unconsciousness. A commonly used muscle relaxant is one called 'scoline' (suxamethonium). This drug, like other muscle relaxants, paralyses all muscles, included the muscles used in breathing; this means that patients have to be artificially ventilated whilst they are under the influence of the drug. Most people metabolize and destroy this drug fairly rapidly, within ten minutes or so after receiving a relaxing dose, after which they begin to breathe using their own muscles. Some individuals, however, have a genetically determined abnormality of the enzyme in the body, called pseudocholinesterase, which destroys this relaxant drug. The action of the drug may be very prolonged in these individuals and sometimes normal breathing never returns and the patient dies. It is probable that the number of people who are sensitive to this drug is as high as 1:100.

We have already discussed the defect of enzymes in the red blood cells caused by a sex-linked recessive gene (page 257). Homozygotes for the gene may be extremely sensitive to some commonly used drugs, such as sulphonamides or antimalarials, and the use of these drugs results in a rapid destruction of many of the circulating red cells.

It is likely that the list of genetically determined sensitivities to drugs will grow rapidly and become a subject of great practical importance. Once these sensitivities are recognized then public health measures can be aimed at controlling their effects.

Genetic counselling

Genetic clinics

We can now go on to look at the main service available today for the prevention of genetically determined disease; this service is genetic counselling. From the preceding discussions it is obvious that the number of people who could benefit from genetic counselling is not enormous, but on the other hand the number is not negligible. Genetic counselling can not only prevent inherited disease, but it can also help the early diagnosis of these diseases; if parents who are likely to produce children who are at risk refuse to take contraceptive advice, then their offspring can be intelligently examined early in life with a view to determining the presence of inherited disease. Early diagnosis can be important because it enables treatment to be started early in life. In clinics that specialize in genetic counselling it has been found that the bulk of enquiries come from couples who have already had a child suffering from some disorder and who want some reassurance that there is little risk of another child being affected in a similar way, or who at least want to know the risks involved. The remaining 10 per cent or so of enquiries are from people with some abnormality in themselves or in their family history that they fear they will pass on to their children. This, then, is one aspect of genetic counselling, the advising of couples who come to the clinics for information about the risks of passing on particular disorders to their children. A second and potentially much more important aspect of genetic counselling is education of the public by way of health studies in schools, lectures to adults, and the spread of information by way of the mass media—newspapers and television. This reaching of large audiences is important in areas of the world where certain harmful genes are common in the population (e.g. sickle-cell disease or thalassaemia—see below) or where habits such as consanguineous marriages encourage the appearance of genetic ill health.

Our increasing recognition and understanding of genetic disease makes it more and more possible to give useful advice. One important advance is the ability to recognize carriers of harmful genes, that is those individuals who are outwardly healthy but who are able to transmit genetic disease to their offspring. In the study of mongolism we have seen how the advances in the study of human chromosomes has made it possible to distinguish between parents that are unlikely to have a second mongol child from those in which one partner carries an abnormal chromosome so that the chances of having a second mongol child are very high. Advances in biochemistry also allow us to make more accurate predictions. The commonest form of a disease called muscular dystrophy is due to a sex-linked recessive gene. In this disease the muscles gradually weaken and atrophy, and there is an increasing disability and deformity as the disease progresses. This progressive disease eventually results in death, often as a result of a chest infection in the weakened and inactive patient. Since the disease is determined by a sex-linked recessive gene (i.e. carried on the X chromosome) it is boys who are mainly affected (see the discussion of the inheritance of haemophilia, another disease due to a sex-linked recessive gene). Females who are heterozygous for the gene suffer no disability but they are capable of passing the disease on to their sons. When a family produces a boy suffering from muscular dystrophy, it is always a problem as to how to advise sisters who may carry the gene. In the past, sisters of boys with the disease could be told only that there was a one in two chance of them being a carrier and that the risk of any of their sons being affected was one in four. However, recent progress in biochemistry has shown that those who suffer from the disease have abnormally large amounts of a certain enzyme in the blood. This enzyme, creatine phosphokinase, arises from the degenerating muscles affected by the disease; even individuals who only 'carry' the gene (i.e. heterozygotes) show raised levels of creatine phosphokinase. It is now possible to tell most of the sisters of boys suffering from the disease whether or not they carry the abnormal gene. If they are found to carry the gene then the risk of producing a son affected by muscular dystrophy can be put precisely at a one in two chance.

It must be emphasized that a high-risk figure for affected offspring need not necessarily deter a couple from producing children, provided that treatment is available that will permit an affected child to lead a relatively normal life. A decision has to be taken with full regard for the background—medical, financial, social, psychological—of a particular family. The mentally stable woman without other children and per- haps with finances adequate to ensure domestic help may be able to cope well with the perhaps prolonged treatment of an affected child. If the woman has other children, affected or not, and is lacking psychological and/or financial stability then she may well be incapable of supporting the affected child through its treatment.

Genetic advice in populations with a high frequency of particular harmful genes

A few special clinics are quite unsuitable for countries where there is a high frequency of particular harmful genes. In tropical Africa there are some areas where the sickle-cell gene is carried by a quarter or more of the entire population; this size of problem requires planning at government level, although in this particular case genetic advice of any sort is rarely, if ever, available. Some governments, however, have responded to this kind of large-scale problem. In Italy there is network for the detection of the hereditary disease called thalassaemia and this consists of an institute in Rome and sixteen provincial centres which have facilities for the detection of the disease and for premarital counselling. Thalassaemia is an important inherited cause of anaemia due to a deficiency in the synthesis of the red pigment (haemoglobin) of the red blood cells. Individuals who receive the abnormal gene from both parents (i.e. are homozygous for the gene) either die before birth or suffer from a severe form of anaemia (Cooley's anaemia) and die, usually at an early age. Individuals who receive the gene from only one parent (i.e. are heterozygous for the gene) suffer from a mild anaemia called thalassaemia minor. There is no specific cure for thalassaemia although much can be done to treat the disease. Repeated blood transfusions may be needed for severe anaemia, and surgical removal of the spleen may help some cases; in areas where thalassaemia is common this sort of treatment could obviously impose a severe burden on medical resources. In Italy tests for the detection of carriers (i.e. those suffering from thalassaemia minor) are freely available and are applied especially to school children. The population is made aware by public propaganda of the dangers involved if carriers marry one another. If finances and services were available, the same measures could be applied to areas of the world where sickle-cell anaemia is common; this could lead to a dramatic fall in the number of cases even within a single generation.

Conclusions

The third Report of the World Health Organization Expert Committee on Human Genetics ('Genetic Counselling', World Health Organization, Technical Report Series, No. 416, 1969) made, among others, the following recommendations: 'Genetic counselling centres should be established in sufficient numbers in regions where infectious disease and nutritional disorders are being brought under control, and the relative importance of hereditary disorders is increasing, and in areas where genetic disorders have always constituted a serious public health problem.

In some parts of the world the high frequency of certain lethal or sub-lethal genes, such as those responsible for sickle-cell and thalassaemia, will require a special genetic counselling service for carriers, as well as suitable medical facilities for the care of afflicted individuals. Since genetic counselling centres and the specialized medical and laboratory services they require are an integral part of medical care, they should be covered by health and social insurance schemes.

It will not be possible to implement these recommendations unless trained personnel are available.'

22. Dental health and disease

Introduction

IN THE constitution of the World Health Organization, health is defined as 'a state of complete physical, mental and social well being and not merely the absence of disease or infirmity'. This applies to the whole human being and it includes all parts of the mouth. However, it is not possible to separate dental health from general health, for one can affect the other. Thus diseases of the teeth and gums can not only disfigure the appearance of an individual, so causing emotional and social problems, but they may also endanger general health. The converse is equally true, and general health, particularly the state of nutrition, can affect the teeth and their supporting tissues.

The aim of all care of the teeth and gums is not only to produce a mouth which is free of disease but also one that is positively healthy and beautiful. In the healthy mouth the teeth are regular and the 'bite' is normal, that is the upper and lower teeth fit together in the normal way. The teeth are creamy white without stains or calculus (tartar). There are no gaps in the rows of teeth. The gums are pink and firm and are closely applied to the necks of the teeth. The breath is sweet.

In this chapter we will look at ways in which the individual's own efforts, supported by expert dental care, can largely prevent two universal diseases, caries and periodontal disease. We will not consider abnormalities of the 'bite' that need expert dental treatment, except in so far as dental hygiene can prevent premature loss of teeth and remove one cause of abnormally placed and malfunctioning teeth.

The structure and development of teeth

The structure of a tooth and its supporting structures is shown in Figure 22.1. All teeth consist of two parts, the crown which projects above the gum and the tapering root (or roots) which fits into a cavity or socket, the alveolus, in the bone of the jaw. Where the crown and root meet is the neck of the tooth. Inside the tooth is a cavity, the pulp cavity, containing living soft tissues, blood vessels and nerves. The hard part of the tooth consists of three parts, dentine, enamel and cementum. Dentine (ivory) forms the bulk of the hard parts of the tooth. It is a hard, bloodless, yellowish material containing large amounts of minerals. It also contains a few nerve fibres and it is sensitive to touch, temperature changes and to the contact with sugary foods. In the crown of the tooth the dentine is surrounded by enamel. This hard white material, consisting almost entirely of rods of calcium salts, is the hardest substance in the body. It has no nerves or blood vessels. The cementum is a bone-like material that covers most of the tooth root.

The supporting elements of the tooth form the periodontium composed of the periodontal membrane, the bone of the tooth socket (alveolar bone) and the gums (gingiva). The tooth is suspended in its socket by the periodontal membrane. This membrane consists mainly of bundles of fibres (of collagen) that are embedded into the alveolar bone and the cementum. The

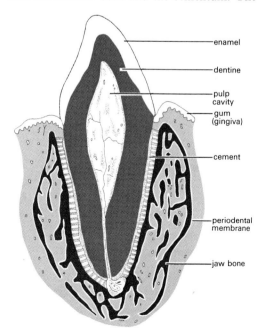

Figure 22.1 Structure of a mammalian tooth as seen in section.

gingiva (gum) is the pink tissue that surrounds the neck of the tooth. The normal gum is firm and stippled in texture, and it is attached to the tooth and bone by fibres of the periodontal membrane. There is a shallow crevice about 1 mm deep between the free margin of the gum and the tooth. In the healthy mouth the gum is closely fitted to the neck of the tooth. Extensions of the gum between the necks of the teeth form v-shaped wedges that are closely fitted to the surfaces of the teeth.

There is a great deal of normal variation in the age at which teeth appear (erupt) in the infant. At one rare extreme babies may be born with one or more teeth, and at the other extreme the first tooth may not appear until the child is thirteen or fourteen months old. Thus the age at which the teeth appear is no indication of the development of an infant. Table 25 is a list of the *average* age and order of the eruption of the teeth; wide variations from this average are not necessarily abnormal. These first teeth are called the milk or deciduous teeth, and they will gradually be replaced by the second or permanent teeth. The growth of the first teeth, with the stretching of the overlying gum followed by splitting of the gum to reveal the erupting teeth, is often accompanied by obvious pain, increased flow of saliva and irritability in the infant. In the past teething was blamed for many general disturbances of health—fevers, convulsions, diarrhoea and bronchitis. Indeed in the eighteenth and nineteenth centuries teething was registered as a cause of death of many infants. Nowadays no general disturbance of health is ever attributed to teething. To do so might result in a serious mis-diagnosis that might cost a life.

The twenty milk teeth of the infant are gradually replaced by the teeth of the permanent dentition. Extra teeth also appear so that the adult has 32 teeth consisting of 8 incisors, 4 canines, 8 premolars and 12 molars. At about the age of six years the child usually has some milk teeth and some permanent ones. Parents may not be aware of this state of affairs because the six-year-old's molars appear before there is any loosening of the milk teeth, and they erupt immediately next to the last deciduous molar. During the next six or so years the milk teeth are progressively lost and become replaced by the permanent teeth. Usually the front teeth are the first to be replaced, beginning with the lower ones. Indeed, sometimes the permanent incisors of the lower jaw erupt behind the milk incisors before these have been shed. The remaining teeth are replaced in an unpredictable order. Finally the third permanent molars (wisdom teeth) appear between the ages of seventeen and twenty-five, and sometimes these never erupt. The roots of the milk teeth are gradually eroded away inside the jaw until they have completely disappeared. The crown of the tooth then becomes loose and is easily pulled out by the child himself.

Dental caries (tooth decay)

Dental caries is a world-wide disease that affects almost 100 per cent of the population, particularly when they are young. The term caries describes the progressive degeneration and loss of the calcified tissues of the tooth—enamel, dentine and cementum. In a later section of this chapter we will be looking at another widespread, chronic, destructive disease—periodontal disease—that destroys the supporting tissues of the teeth. Both of these diseases may cause loss of teeth, disturbance of tooth function, infection, pain and disfigurement, with its accompanying emotional problems. There is one important common factor in the development of both of these diseases, and this is the formation on the tooth surface of a film of material called dental 'plaque'.

Dental 'plaque' and caries (Figure 22.2)

Dental plaque consists of a mixture of mucin, food debris, polysaccharides from food and bacteria, and enzymes; in this film the growth of bacteria flourishes. Bacteria in the plaque ferment sugar from the food and release acids close to the surface of the enamel of the teeth. The first stage in the development of caries is the loss of minerals from enamel by the action of this acid. Instead of being white and hard, the enamel is converted to a semi-translucent softer material that is gradually eroded away to expose

Table 25

Average age of eruption of first teeth

Teeth	Age at eruption (months)
Lower central incisors	7.5
Upper central incisors	9.5
Upper lateral incisors	11.5
Lower lateral incisors	13
Upper first molar	15.5
Lower first molar	16
Upper canines	19
Lower canines	19
Lower second molars	26
Upper second molars	27

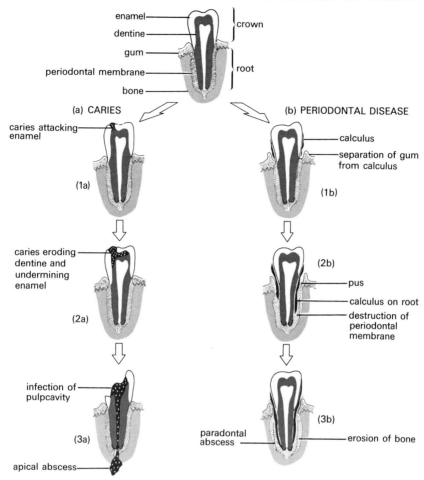

Figure 22.2   The progression in dental diseases (a) caries and (b) periodontal disease.

the inner tissues of the tooth, first of all the dentine. The dentine is broken down to a rubbery brown material, teeming with bacteria and giving off an offensive smell. The destruction of the softer dentine can be rapid, so undermining the harder enamel which now tends to collapse on biting. Once the barrier of enamel has been breached, the process of decay progresses relentlessly unless dental treatment is carried out. The progressive destruction of the dentine eventually exposes the pulp of the tooth to invasion by bacteria. The pulp becomes infected and this causes sharp severe pain that is aggravated by hot or cold fluids or by the presence of sugar in the mouth. When tissues are infected, inflammation follows. Inflamed tissues swell and there is little room for swelling in the pulp cavity. The pressure within the cavity rises and this contributes to the pain. The

rise in pressure also slows down the flow of blood in the pulp, and the living tissues of the pulp gradually die, that is the pulp becomes gangrenous. The death of the tissues of the pulp—which include nerves—usually results in the disappearance of pain, and this encourages a false sense of security. The destructive process, however, has not finished. Infection may now spread to the root of the tooth and result in the development of an abscess around the tooth. Although the tooth is now dead and without sensation, the infected and inflamed jaw bone becomes painful and any movement of the dead tooth in the socket causes severe pain. A general disturbance of health appears; the patient becomes feverish, sweats and feels miserable. Eventually pus may force its way into the soft tissues of the mouth and it may drain into the mouth cavity through the mucous membrane.

Factors influencing the development of caries

Age

No age is immune to caries but the disease is *mainly* one of childhood and adolescence. The periods of greatest carious activity are five to eight years (in the milk teeth) and twelve to eighteen years (in the permanent teeth).

Diet

It is not possible to rid the mouth of the bacteria that start the decay process. The bacteria can, however, be deprived of fermentable sugars and they can be prevented from accumulating in the high concentrations in which they occur in the dental plaque applied to the enamel. These aims can be achieved by attention to the diet and to oral hygiene.

Sugars are particularly important in the development of caries. Sweet things stick to the teeth for a long time after being taken into the mouth, and they provide a rich source of fermentable material for the bacteria in dental plaque. Sugars are, of course, gradually washed away from the tooth surface by the action of saliva, and the acids produced by bacterial action can be neutralized by alkali in the saliva. However, saliva is not produced continuously at a high rate. Between meals the rate of secretion of saliva falls so that sweet sticky foods eaten at this time are much less likely to be cleansed away by saliva. Compared to our ancestors we consume enormous quantities of sugar, as much in one month as they consumed in years. Thus for dental health it is best to reduce the intake of sweet foods, particularly between meals. Roughage in the form of firm vegetables and fruit helps to clean plaque from the surfaces of teeth, and it is helpful to finish a meal with this sort of food. One recent cause of rapidly developing caries —so called rampant caries—has appeared in infants who are given dummy-feeders containing undiluted fruit syrups which results in a sugar-coating of the teeth for hours at a time.

In this section we are *presuming* that the diet contains adequate supplies of vitamins, minerals and protein; these are as essential for the normal development of teeth as they are for the normal development of the entire organism. Nutrition is most important in the pregnant woman, the infant and the young child, when most of the teeth are undergoing formation and calcification. Once the teeth have erupted into the mouth cavity, nutritional factors become less important. When enamel and dentine are fully formed they are acellular and without blood, and are no longer very susceptible to the effects of deficiencies in the diet, although the growth and health of the gums, bone and other periodontal structures continues to be influenced by the diet throughout life.

Oral hygiene

Cleaning the teeth is a familiar phrase, but what may be involved in the process varies widely from one person to another. Many children reach adult life without ever having been shown how to clean the teeth and gums thoroughly. Indeed many young children up to the age of six or so are unable to clean their teeth adequately, even when supervized, and the parent may have to carry out this task. Adequate cleaning takes several minutes and involves systematic progression over the various surfaces of the teeth. In the process of cleaning the front and back surfaces of the teeth, the brush should be first placed on the gum and then swept onto the tooth surface. This action stimulates the gums and removes food debris from the gum margin and plaque from the tooth surface. Thus the brush moves downwards on the upper teeth and upwards on the lower teeth. Brushing from side to side is a poor substitute for it fails to stimulate the gums, it misses the space between the teeth and it wears the teeth out at the necks. Moreover it tends to push food debris under the gum margin. Sixteen surfaces should be cleaned:

1. front of upper front teeth,
2. front of upper right cheek teeth,
3. front of upper left cheek teeth,
4. back of upper front teeth,
5. back of upper left cheek teeth,
6. back of upper right cheek teeth,
7. biting surfaces of right cheek teeth,
8. biting surface of left cheek teeth,

and the same in the lower jaw. At each position the brush should be swept over the tooth surface at least three times. The brush head will not cover all the teeth in each one of the sixteen sections, certainly not in adults. This means that thorough cleaning will involve a minimum of fifty-four brush movements, and twice that number in adults. It is impossible to carry out these manoeuvres in less than a minute. In adolescents and adults, further cleaning is usually needed because of the effects of perio-dontal disease (see page 275). The shrinkage of the gum away from the teeth, particularly that part of the gum that projects in a point between the necks of the teeth, produces gaps between

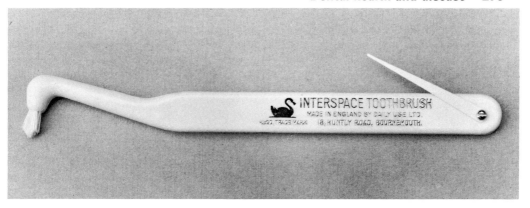

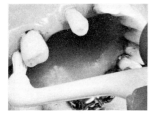

distal surfaces of
molars,

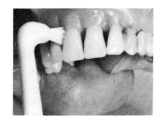

interdental spaces,

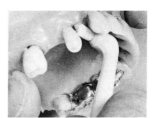

the mesial and distal
surfaces of insulated
teeth,

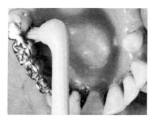

fixed bridgework,

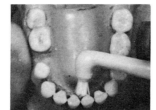

the lingual surfaces of
the lower front teeth,

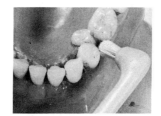

crowded teeth,

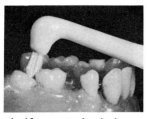

half-erupted wisdom
teeth,

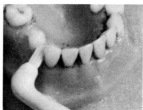

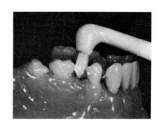

and narrow gaps.

Figure 22.3　The inter-space brush and its uses. (*Photographs supplied by Dr F. Engel.*)

the necks of the teeth. These gaps have also to be cleaned, by means of special inter-space brushes, medicated wooden sticks or dental floss (Figure 22.3). This cleaning process should be carried out after every meal.

Many types of toothbrush are available on the market, made of nylon or bristle with flat or shaped heads, and soft, hard or medium textures. It does not seem to matter whether brushes are made of nylon or bristle but the texture of the brush has some bearing on the cleaning properties. Hard-textured brushes are certainly best for removing dental plaque although they may damage the gums if they are not properly used, that is with pressure on the brush varied according to whether the head is on the gum or the tooth surface. Medium-textured brushes would seem to be the best compromise. It is important to note that a toothbrush will no longer clean efficiently after about three months of use, and sometimes long before this time.

Dental caries and fluoride

Fluorine is a very common element in nature. It is the seventeenth most abundant element in the earth's crust. Because it is a very reactive substance, it is never found as the free element. Invariably it is combined with other substances to form fluorides such as fluorspar (calcium fluoride, CaF_2), apatite (mixed calcium phosphate and fluoride, $3Ca_3(PO_4)_2.CaF_2$) and cryolite (Na_3AlF_6). These compounds are not very soluble, but they yield some fluoride to the water that percolates through soils and rocks containing them. The natural content of fluorides in water and foodstuffs varies widely in different parts of the world depending upon the chemical nature of the soil and rocks. Surface waters usually contain less than one part per million of fluoride, although underground waters usually contain higher levels if they have seeped through rocks containing compounds of fluorine.

When drinking water contains one part per million of fluoride, the amount of fluoride consumed per day is about 1 mg. Foods supply less fluoride than water unless much sea fish is eaten. The body can, to a degree, regulate its fluoride content, and excess fluoride is excreted, mainly in the urine. The fluoride of the body is concentrated mainly in the bones and teeth, where it becomes incorporated into the crystals of apatite that forms the hard inorganic component of these tissues. Teeth containing fluoride are much less likely to develop caries, and the more fluoride present, the more resistant the teeth become. Of course, other factors influence the susceptibility to caries, particularly the nature of the diet and the standard of oral hygiene. Drinking waters containing less than one part per million result in merely a postponing of caries for a period varying from five to ten years. Slightly higher levels result in a marked reduction of caries that may continue into adult life. Many countries of the world have started schemes for the addition of fluoride to drinking water to bring the concentration of fluoride up to one part per million. Some districts in Great Britain have now had fluoridated water for fourteen years. A report has been published on the effects of the first eleven years of fluoridation (*Reports on Public Health and Medical Subjects*, No. 122, Her Majesty's Stationery Office). This report shows that five-year-old children living in areas with a naturally high fluoride content have nearly two-thirds less dental caries than those in low fluoride areas. American studies confirm these results and show that fluoridation halves the incidence of caries at ages five to twelve years. This effect is reflected in the cost of dental care, the cost being halved. After twenty-five years of fluoridation the benefits extend into adult life.

In Britain there has been considerable opposition to the artificial fluoridation of water supplies, mainly from a small group of individuals, members of the National Pure Water Association (Offices at Thorpe End, Almondbury, Huddersfield). This group continues to oppose fluoridation of water in spite of the fact that health authorities in many parts of the world have confirmed the benefits of fluoridation and the absence of any risks at the recommended levels. Even in regions where the natural levels of fluoride in water are eight times that of the recommended level of one part per million, there has been no evidence of any harmful effects on general health. The vigorous activities of this small group may well prevent the fluoridation of the water supplies of large areas of Great Britain. The National Pure Water Association issues, from time to time, various pamphlets and articles to further their cause. Their most recent publication is a booklet, '11 Years of Fluoridation; Ineffectual and Unsafe; Errors and Omissions in Government Report'. Only someone with a good knowledge of the wide literature on fluoride, health and disease would be able to counter many of the claims in this booklet. The Department of Health and Social Security has prepared a series of notes giving point-by-point answers to the arguments in the Association's booklet. The World Health Organization supports fluoridation; the 1969 World Health Assembly passed a resolution recommending fluoridation as a desirable measure after a careful scrutiny of the evidence from many countries. This evidence is presented in a World Health Organization monograph, 'Fluorides and Human Health', *Monograph Series no. 59*.

Toxic effects of fluoride

The facts about the effect of small amounts of fluoride on dental health are clear. It is also true that excessive amounts of fluoride can be dangerous. A fatal dose of fluoride is in the region of 2.5–5 grammes, and usually results from the accidental swallowing of insecticides containing fluoride salts. In order to obtain this dose of fluoride from fluoridated municipal water, one would have to drink 2500 litres of water, and this without excreting any! However, sub-lethal doses of fluoride when taken over a long period of time can have damaging effects, producing a condition called fluorosis. In fluorosis the bones become abnormally dense and may be thickened. There may also develop abnormal calcifications of the soft tissues that are attached to bone, in ligaments, tendons or muscle. Mottling of the tooth enamel (dental fluorosis) also occurs. This consists in a mild mottling of the teeth—small paper-white opaque patches in the enamel. In severe cases there may be deep-brown or black stained pits in the enamel that give the teeth a corroded appearance. Fluorosis has *never* been demonstrated when the daily intake of fluoride is less than 2 mg. Even with an intake of twice this quantity, fluorosis of the enamel is seldom seen. In areas of the world where the fluoride content of water is high and where dental fluorosis is frequently seen, a natural intake of fluoride of over 8 mg per day is common. Advanced and crippling effects of skeletal fluorosis occur only in individuals who have been exposed daily for up to twenty years to an intake of 20–80 mg of fluoride a day. It is important to emphasize that none of the chronic effects of excess fluoride intake have ever been seen with a municipal water supply fluoridated with one part per million of fluoride. Many natural waters all over the world contain fluorides well in excess of this level without any damaging effects on the population.

The way in which fluoride protects the teeth from caries is not definitely settled, but it seems that two actions of fluoride may be involved. First, fluoride reduces the solubility of dental enamel in acid. Second, fluoride inhibits the action of bacterial enzymes that are responsible for the production of the acid. One can show the first effect outside the body by washing a tooth with a solution of fluoride and then treating the tooth with acid. This tooth will lose less of its minerals in the acid than will an untreated tooth. As for bacterial activity, it is well known that fluorides can inhibit some enzymes, and it has been shown that when pure cultures of bacteria from dental plaque are grown in a medium containing fluorides, they produce less acid from sugars than do control bacteria grown in a medium which is free of fluorides.

Periodontal disease

Periodontal disease is one of the most widespread diseases of mankind, and no area of the world is free of it. It is not a spectacular disease. It does not affect the very young, nor does it usually cause pain or death, but it makes life miserable for many middle-aged and old people and causes unnecessary loss of teeth. This disease of the supporting tissues of the teeth deprives many people of all their teeth long before old age. Most people, even in developed countries, regard this state of affairs as inevitable. This attitude is shared, if not in mind then in practice, by many health educationalists and dentists.

However, the disease is not inevitable, and research into methods of prevention and treatment shows that provided the public is educated in these matters and provided that education is followed by the seeking of early dental care, then this widespread disease with its serious effects on the teeth could be considerably reduced.

Let us first look at the structures in the mouth that are affected by the disease. The term periodontium describes all the elements that support a tooth, the cementum, periodontal membrane, the bone of the jaw and the gums (gingiva). These structures have already been described (page 269). Here we can look briefly at some aspects of the biology of the periodontium that are relevant to their normal function and to the disease process. First, let us look at the periodontal membrane itself. An important function of this membrane is the transfer of the forces of chewing from the teeth to the jaws. The orientation of the individual fibres in the periodontal membrane depends on the direction of the force that is applied to a tooth. Increased chewing activity can to some extent increase the strength of the membrane, but over and above a critical force the membrane becomes damaged, and indeed the tooth may now adjust its position to one where conditions are more favourable. When the membrane is damaged by disease, the supporting function is disturbed and the tooth becomes loose.

The shallow crevice between the gum (gingiva) and the tooth is very important in relation to periodontal disease, for it is here that the first stages of the disease usually start. In the perfectly healthy mouth, the epithelium of the inner part of the gum should be very closely attached to the surface of the tooth. As we will see later, this state of affairs alters considerably when periodontal disease attacks the mouth. Fortunately the epithelium of the gum has very great capabilities in defence and in healing.

Dental plaque and periodontal disease

Malnutrition can produce disease of the periodontium, particularly when the diet is deficient in protein and vitamins, especially vitamin C. Swollen bleeding gums are a typical feature of scurvy, caused by a deficient intake of vitamin C. Certain hormonal states (e.g. pregnancy) and drugs can also produce disorders of the periodontium. These causes of periodontal disease are, numerically at least, of little importance in the development of the widespread degeneration of the periodontium that damages the teeth of most people, provided they live long enough. The most important single factor is the failure of hygiene of the mouth to remove food and bacterial growth from the surface of the teeth. Teeth that are not regularly and efficiently cleaned develop the thin white film called dental plaque. We have already seen that this contains various materials, but most important it contains large numbers of living bacteria. In the deeper layers of the film the bacteria may die, and calcium salts are deposited from the saliva to form a hard calculus (tartar) that becomes firmly attached to the tooth. The plaque is a living film which can grow in thickness and can also extend below the gum. Although these bacteria are non-pathogenic in the usual sense of the word, they are present in the highest possible concentration and in constant close contact with the soft tissues of the gum. The presence of these bacteria and their toxins invariably leads to degeneration of the epithelium lining the gum crevice and to inflammation of the gum. White blood cells (mainly polymorphonuclear leukocytes) migrate from the tissues to attack the bacteria in the crevice of the gum. The rate of growth of the plaque depends on the rate of multiplication of the bacteria and the success of the resistance of the host, but if the upward growth of the plaque is not stopped then it may reach the tip of the tooth root well within a normal life span, destroying the supporting periodontal membrane as it does so and loosening the tooth. Calculus may also develop in the plaque under the gum and this further aggravates the disease process, causing shrinkage of the gum away from the tooth—the cause of 'growing long in the tooth'. In addition, the presence of plaque and calculus causes progressive absorption of the bone that surrounds the root of the tooth; the tooth socket thus enlarges and contributes to the loosening of the tooth (Figure 22.2).

This is the course of periodontal disease. A variety of factors encourage the development of the disease, and some of these factors can be remedied. The kind of food eaten is important in relation to dental hygiene. Raw and fibrous foods help to prevent the accumulation of plaque and calculus by their scouring effect during chewing movements. Soft foods have little cleansing action and indeed may be swallowed without any mastication. Overcrowding of teeth also interferes with natural or artificial cleansing and increases the stagnation of food debris on and between the teeth. Mouth-breathing may also be important because it dries the food debris on the tooth surface; in the normal mouth the food debris, bacteria and the products of bacteria are subjected to the diluting and cleansing action of saliva, but mouth breathing interferes with this function. The design of fillings and appliances can also encourage the development of periodontal disease. Thus poorly designed fillings can lead to such narrow spaces between the necks of teeth that they are uncleanable. Removable appliances (false dentures or appliances to alter the position of the teeth) also favour stagnation and interfere with the diluting and cleansing action of saliva, particularly when they are not removed at night and are infrequently removed for cleaning.

The effects of periodontal disease

In the mouth affected by periodontal disease the gums become reddened and may be thickened. The gum tends to bleed, particularly after the use of a toothbrush or after probing by the dental surgeon, and pus may be squeezed out between the teeth and gum margin (pyorrhoea). As the disease extends, the gum is no longer firmly applied to the surface of the teeth; the gum 'recedes' and becomes 'pocketed' and the teeth appear to grow in length. As the supporting structures are gradually destroyed the tooth loosens. This progress of the disease is illustrated diagrammatically in Figure 22.2.

Distribution of periodontal disease

We have already noted that periodontal disease is one of the most widespread diseases of mankind, and it rivals dental caries as a major dental disease. No country is free of the disease. Wherever the disease has been studied, it has been found that severe and destructive disease increases progressively with age. The disease may start as early as puberty, and many individuals show extensive destruction of the periodontal tissues before the age of twenty years. The importance of the disease can be appreciated from surveys carried out by the American Dental Association which indicate that in men over the age of thirty-five and women over the age of forty, periodontal disease is responsible for between two and three times as many extractions of teeth as dental caries.

Prevention and treatment of periodontal disease

Since the destruction of the supporting tissues of the teeth is irreversible, prevention is obviously an important aspect of control. Provided that there has been a normal development of the periodontium (assisted by an adequate balanced diet for the pregnant woman and infant) the formation of dental plaque and calculus are the most common direct causes of periodontal disease. All measures aimed at preventing the formation of these deposits should be undertaken. Some of these measures can be carried out by the individual. These measures include the introduction of raw and fibrous foods into the diet to help clean the teeth and gingiva during mastication; these should be introduced into the diet as early an age as possible. However, thorough cleaning of the teeth and gums is the most important factor, performed after every meal, or at least twice a day. Tooth brushing can, if properly carried out, remove plaque from the teeth, gum margins and crevices. If plaque is removed then calculus cannot develop, but the use of the toothbrush cannot usually remove plaque from between the teeth. In children the projection of the gum between the teeth—the interdental papilla—is usually firmly adapted to the teeth and special cleaning between the teeth is not usually needed, but in older children and adults where there is evidence of some inflammation of the gum, some form of interdental cleaning is indicated. When the interdental papilla has contracted away from the teeth then interdental cleaning is probably the most important part of teeth hygiene. Special interspace brushes are available but in most cases other aids in the form of interdental sticks, elastic bands or dental floss (a medicated thread) are indispensible.

This personal care of dental hygiene must, however, be supplemented by the attentions of the dentist. Ideally every person from an early age should have regular examinations of the teeth and gums, preferably twice a year, to see if any disease is present, for treatment, and to check if the individual's methods of cleaning the teeth and gums is being effective. The dentist will remove any hard deposits of calculus on the surface of the teeth both above and below the margin of the gum, together with the dental

plaque. The dentist can also treat any dental condition that is encouraging the development of periodontal disease. For the management of established periodontal disease, thorough scaling and polishing of the teeth and the maintenance of perfect oral hygiene by the patient are the fundamentals of treatment.

Dental health education

A programme for dental health is, or should be, part of any general health education. It is important to realize that many factors will determine the success or failure of dental health education. First and foremost, dental health services must be readily available and they should not be too costly to the individual. To a degree these requirements are met in Great Britain, where many groups receive free dental treatment under the National Health Service. Free treatment is available to children under sixteen, expectant mothers or mothers who have borne a child in the last twelve months, and to young people between sixteen and twenty-one years who are in full-time attendance at schools or colleges. For others a nominal charge is made for a course of dental treatment, not exceeding £1.50 (except where dentures or other appliances are needed). A grant to meet the cost of dental treatment or dentures is paid by the Department of Health and Social Security to anyone receiving a supplementary pension or allowance.

Even were dental services freely available with no cost to the individual, it is unlikely that this alone would produce a radical improvement in the state of dental health. People have to understand and desire the benefits of new dental health behaviour. They have to want to protect their teeth. Some value their teeth little and regard the degenerative diseases of teeth and gums as a natural and inevitable course of events. Modern dentures are so comfortable, efficient and acceptable to one's relatives and friends that there may be little incentive to carry out dental hygiene several times a day, and to attend regularly for treatment that may be uncomfortable if not actually painful.

In the past, education seems in general to have failed to alter the *laissez faire* attitude to dental diseases. Information about dental health is given to many teachers and children, but this alone is not an effective method of obtaining the appropriate change in behaviour. The problem is by no means unique to dental health education; accidents, cancer of the lung, chronic bronchitis and venereal diseases continue to increase in frequency in spite of widespread publicity about methods of prevention. Health education has not only to provide information but it has to encourage the development of attitudes that will lead to appropriate changes in behaviour. This is a complex educational problem in which one has to take into account the many forces that affect the behaviour of individuals. These forces vary from one social or economic class to another. It is, for example, well known that people from lower educational, occupational and income groups care for their teeth less than do those of higher status. The provision of free dental services does not necessarily change this state of affairs. One has to choose educational techniques appropriate to the kind of individual. The arousing of fear is one educational weapon. People need some emotional arousal before they will take action. It is necessary to remove the fear of dental treatment itself (modern dentistry can be remarkably painless) and replace it by fear of painful and offensive degenerative diseases of the teeth and gums. There is no doubt that established disfigurement of the teeth and gums can lead to emotional and social problems.

It should not be impossible to persuade the beauty-conscious youth of today's affluent societies that progressive dental diseases lead to loss of teeth and a deterioration in personal appearances. When teeth are extracted there is a gradual absorption of the bony tissues of the jaw that supported the teeth. This can lead to a considerable change in the contour of the face that is by no means beautiful; and artificial dentures, although they may be comfortable and efficient, are not things of beauty unless they are made by a dental technician with an artistic flair. Artificial teeth made so that they have a natural and attractive appearance that match the face of the wearer are an expensive luxury for the few.

Much research remains to be done on methods of obtaining changes in health behaviour. One important influence is certain. Parents everywhere have an important effect on the behaviour of their children in all areas of health. If parents were adequately educated when they attended a dentist for treatment, then this *could* have marked effects on the dental health of their children. Unfortunately some dentists still think in terms of treatment and repair rather than in terms of education and prevention, and this attitude is encouraged by the way that dental practice is organized and financed.

23. Diseases of civilization
I Blood vessels

Introduction

IN THE following three chapters we will be looking at new kinds of epidemic diseases which appear in industrialized countries such as North America and Europe. These diseases are cancer, diseases of arteries (especially of the coronary arteries), and accidents. In terms of the total number of deaths in the world, these diseases are not of supreme importance. Sixty or so million people die every year, and of these deaths less than ten million are caused by diseases of the blood vessels and by cancer, that is about the same number of people who succumb from tuberculosis and malaria. The modern 'captains of death' only take the helm in countries where economic wealth leads to improvements in nutrition, preventative medicine (e.g. immunizations and other public health measures) and in the treatment of infectious diseases. Individuals in these countries, protected as they are from the major communicable diseases, have a life expectancy of sixty-five to seventy-five years. In *any* society, diseases of blood vessels and cancer are commoner in the older age groups. In societies where many people live beyond the age of fifty, it is inevitable that these two diseases should become important killers; in fact they account for about two-thirds of all deaths in both sexes. Industrialization not only allows people to live longer and die of heart diseases or cancer but it brings with it new killers in the form of accidents; these accidents are not only the sort caused by drowning or falls that may occur in any society, but they include accidents that are the result of the sophisticated electrical gadgets, heating systems etc. that abound in our homes, of the machinery of industry and of the lethal weapons in the form of cars, lorries and buses that hurtle along our ever-busier streets and highways.

Death from diseases of blood vessels, cancer and accidents do, of course, occur in the so-called developing countries of the world—the name for undeveloped countries where poverty, malnutrition and overcrowding are matched by inadequate personal and public health services. Life expectancy is naturally less than in developed countries and many individuals die from a combination of malnutrition and infectious disease in infancy and early childhood. Indeed, nearly half the total deaths in the world occur in this young susceptible group in Latin America, Africa and Asia.

Having put the modern 'captains of death' in perspective, we can now go on to look at the nature of these diseases. These three big killers have one thing in common, the fact that the development of preventative measures is still in its infancy, particularly in relation to disease of blood vessels. We will however, whenever possible, look at ways in which these 'captains' can be demoted.

Arteriosclerosis

Just a glance at Table 26 should be adequate to stress the importance of diseases of blood vessels as a cause of death in Great Britain, and a very similar pattern can be seen in data from other developed countries. Figure 23.1 shows the distribution of the three major 'captains of death' according to age, and it is obvious that diseases of blood vessels affects mainly the middle-aged and elderly. This term 'diseases of blood vessels' covers a wide range of disorders and these are listed in Table 27. The table also illustrates the importance of particular arterial diseases, especially arteriosclerosis, and the increasing control of one particular kind of heart disease caused by rheumatic fever (page 73). We will now look mainly at the chronic progressive degenerative disease of arteries that we call arteriosclerosis, at its possible causes, its effects, and the prospects for prevention.

The term arteriosclerosis covers what we loosely call degenerative disease of arteries. There are, in fact, several kinds of this disease, but by far the most important variety is one that is called atheroma or atherosclerosis. The importance of atheroma is that without any doubt it is the commonest disease of arteries that leads to thrombosis of the arteries, that is the development of a blood clot in the lumen of the vessel. Obstruction of an artery by means of a blood clot results in destruction or at least severe damage to the tissues which this artery supplies with blood. If the artery supplies a

Table 26 Ten major causes of death (percentage values of all causes), 1965, England and Wales

Causes of death	Percentage value of all causes
1. Arteriosclerotic heart disease (including coronary disease)	21
2. Cancer	19.5
3. Vascular disease affecting the central nervous system	14
4. Diseases of the respiratory system	12
5. Accidents (including suicide)	4.5
6. Diseases of the digestive system	2.5
7. Diseases of the uro-genital system	
8. Congenital malformations	1
9. Diabetes mellitus	
10. Tuberculosis	0.5

Table 27 Death from various diseases of the heart and blood vessels in 1954 and 1964, England and Wales

Causes of death	1954	1964
Rheumatic fever	299	61
Chronic rheumatic heart disease (the aftermath of an attack of rheumatic fever)	8596	6171
Arteriosclerotic and degenerative disease of the heart		
1. arteriosclerosis of coronary arteries	67 844	106 290
2. other causes of degenerative heart disease	60 162	34 419
Hypertensive disease (raised blood pressure)	20 573	13 195
Disease of arteries	12 043	14 989
Generalized arteriosclerosis	10 035	10 911

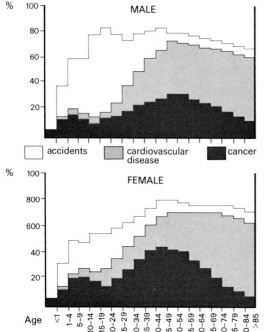

Figure 23.1 Mortality from cancer, cardiovascular diseases, and accidents (percentage of total mortality per age group) in males and females, 1962–63.

vital organ such as part of the heart or brain, then local destruction of the tissue which is normally nourished by the artery can, and often does, lead to death. Atheroma typically affects the larger arteries such as the aorta and its main branches, but it also affects some medium-sized arteries such as those that supply the heart (coronary arteries) or brain (cerebral arteries); this is of course very unfortunate in view of the vital nature of the organs supplied by these medium-sized arteries, and accounts for the lethal effects of atheroma.

The disease is present to some degree in almost all adult members of a community, indeed the early signs of the disorder are said to appear at birth. Many authorities in this field of medicine feel that there has been no serious

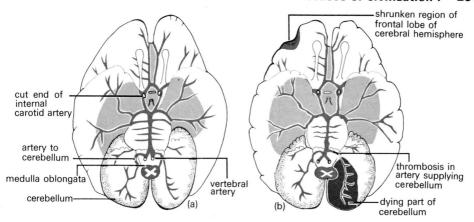

Figure 23.2 (a) Normal blood vessels in the brain and (b) the effects of arteriosclerosis on the brain.
The brain is drawn from the under-surface showing the main blood supply from the internal carotid arteries and vertebral arteries. On the right-hand side are shown some of the possible effects of arteriosclerosis. The arteries are irregular in outline due to scarring. The right frontal lobe of the cerebral hemisphere has a depression, the result of removal of dead tissue following an old thrombosis of an artery supplying this region. There is a recent thrombosis in an artery on the left side supplying the cerebellum. The part of the cerebellum affected dies and various symptoms appear due to disordered cerebellar function.

increase in the amount of atherosclerosis in the community, but what has happened is an increase in the complications that the disease gives rise to, i.e. to obstruction of affected blood vessels by clots. In Jamaican and other poor native communities, extensive atherosclerosis is still found at post-mortem examinations but this condition does not commonly give rise to obstruction of blood vessels by clots, i.e. disorders such as heart attacks (coronary thrombosis) or 'strokes' (cerebral thrombosis and haemorrhage). What appears to have happened in developed areas of the world is that various factors in the environment of man have made it more likely that blood clots will develop in vessels damaged by atherosclerosis. We thus have to look at two processes, first, the development of atherosclerosis itself, and second, factors which encourage the development of clots in the damaged vessels that lead to those disastrous consequences of heart attacks or strokes.

The appearance of atheroma (Figure 23.3)

Atheroma produces several visible changes in the structure of an artery. When one cuts open a healthy aorta the inner surface is pale, smooth and glistening. Atheroma may show itself as yellow fatty streaks lying under the thin, semi-transparent layer of cells that line the aorta (the endothelium). These fatty streaks also occur in smaller arteries where, far from blocking the vessel, they may weaken the wall, allowing it to stretch. A second kind of change in the wall of arteries is an accumulation of fatty cells surrounded by dense fibrous tissue. When one looks at the inside of an aorta affected in this way, the lining is seen to be studded by irregular, raised white patches. The white colour is given by the bloodless fibrous tissue that surrounds the fatty material. Later in the evolution of the disease, the smooth epithelial lining of the aorta becomes ulcerated over the patches of atheroma, so that the blood comes into direct contact with the fat and fibrous tissue in the patch of atheroma. This exposure of the patch has two effects. First, calcium salts from the blood become deposited in the fat and fibrous tissue to produce hard calcified patches in the wall of the blood vessel. A second effect is to promote clotting of blood over the patch. The clotting of blood is an extremely complex event involving many different factors, but one important reason why blood remains fluid in vessels is the presence of the smooth lining to the vessel wall. If fresh blood is collected into glass tubes that are lined with a smooth layer of wax, the blood clots form more slowly than when collected in an uncoated tube; so it is with blood vessels. Wherever the lining of blood vessels is rough then clots are likely to develop. This happens because blood

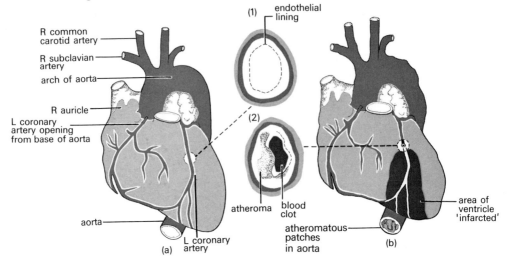

Figure 23.3   (a) Normal blood vessels in the heart and (b) the effects of arteriosclerosis on the heart.
The heart is drawn from the front and shows the left and right coronary arteries. A low-power section of the normal left coronary artery is shown in (1). In the right-hand sketch there is a thrombosis in the left coronary artery resulting in infarction (death due to deficient blood supply) of part of the ventricular wall. (2) shows a section of the affected left coronary artery indicating obstruction of the lumen of the artery by atheroma and blood clot.

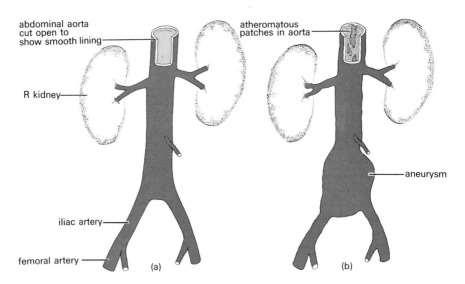

Figure 23.4   (a) Shows a normal abdominal aorta and some of its main branches. (b) Shows atheroma of the aorta and an aneurysm of the aorta and origins of the iliac arteries.

platelets (an important source of the chemical substance that 'triggers off' the clotting process) tend to stick and accumulate on the rough surface.

The development of atheroma

The commonly accepted explanation for the development of atheroma is called the 'encrustation' theory, which was put forward as long ago as 1842 by a man called Rokitansky. According to this theory, the patches of atheroma develop from patches of blood clot (fibrin) which have encrusted the inner lining of the blood vessel. It is thought that these patches of fibrin become covered over by the epithelial cells of the inner lining of the blood vessels (the endothelium), i.e. they are taken into the wall of the blood vessel. Here the patches of fibrin degenerate and fat is deposited in the area; this is followed by a fibrous reaction around the patch.

Factors in the diet may be important in this progression. Some people feel that a fatty diet (particularly if it contains fats from animals) leads to the production of the yellow streaks of fat in the wall of the vessel. Fat may produce its effect in another way, by increasing the tendency of the blood to coagulate and so deposit patches of fibrin on the walls of the vessels—the presumed first step in the development of atherosclerosis.

The effects of atheroma

The possible effects of atheroma are illustrated in Figures 23.3 and 23.4. Obviously the size of vessel affected and the organ which the vessel supplies with blood are important factors which determine the effects of atheroma. One effect is the gradual obstruction of the lumen of the vessel by a patch of atheroma; this is most likely to occur in the medium-sized vessels supplying the heart or brain. Obstruction may, however, develop very suddenly in these vessels if a clot develops on a surface of an exposed patch of atheroma or if a haemorrhage occurs in a wall of a blood vessel which has been progressively weakened by atheroma. In large vessels the weakening of the wall by atheroma may lead to progressive stretching of the vessel and the formation of an aneurysm—a local dilatation of the artery. These aneurysms may rupture or they may be the seat of clotting, due to the abnormal eddy currents set up in the cavity which encourage platelets to stick to the wall and trigger off a local clotting process. Clotting of blood in an aneurysm may be harmless, but it may have disastrous effects if large pieces of clot break off and are carried away in the blood stream to reach smaller blood vessels. Aneurysms can also produce effects by pressing on surrounding structures; a large pulsating aneurysm may thus press on and damage nerves, other blood vessels, the oesophagus, and indeed the relentlessly pulsating mass may even gradually erode away bony structures. A rarer consequence of atheroma in a large vessel is the formation of clots over the eroded patches in the wall of the blood vessel and the separation of pieces of clot that may reach the brain or other important structures. We call the freely circulating piece of blood clot an embolus.

Of these various effects of atherosclerosis—obstruction of a vessel by atheroma or by superimposed thrombosis, aneurysm formation and embolus—obstruction of the coronary arteries is by far the commonest complication. In 1954 over 67 000 people died of disease of the coronary arteries, and in 1964 this figure rose to over 106 000. In a fifteen year period the disease has increased four-fold, and this increase is not explained by a more accurate diagnosis. The particular complication of atherosclerosis thus deserves some more detailed attention here.

Coronary artery disease

The classical picture of coronary artery disease is seen in the case of the middle-aged man with coronary atherosclerosis who develops a thrombosis overlying a patch of diseased vessel. The least serious effect of this clot will be the appearance of pain in the chest coming on during exercise or emotional excitement. Any muscle of the body will give rise to pain if it is exercised without an adequate blood supply. When atherosclerosis blocks a major artery in the leg, severe muscle pain will occur during exercise. This pain is called intermittent claudication. When the heart is involved in a similar process, we call it anginal pain or simply angina. With more complete obstruction to the blood supply of part of the heart, severe pain occurs even at rest, and the area of muscle supplied by the blocked vessel may die; this is a 'heart attack' or myocardial infarction (an infarction describes death of tissue caused by obstruction to blood supply).

Myocardial infarction is a serious illness and of all patients with a first heart attack about 40 per cent will die in this attack; in fact 20 per cent of all patients will die within one hour. These early deaths are usually due to electrical changes in the damaged heart muscle that lead to a disordered ineffective type of contraction of the ventricles, called ventricular fibrillation. Major efforts are being made to try to prevent these potentially avoidable deaths by means of special 'coronary-care' ambulances and coronary units in hospitals which can detect the warning signs of abnormal heart rhythms that often precede ventricular fibrillation. Certain drugs can be used to abolish these abnormal heart rhythms, and even ventricular fibrillation or complete 'standstill' of the heart can be treated by passing a direct-current shock across the chest wall.

Of those who do not die because of abnormal heart rhythms, many others will die from some other effect of myocardial infarction. Sometimes so much of the heart muscle has been destroyed that the heart can no longer work efficiently as a pump, and progressive 'heart failure' develops. Sometimes clots of blood develop in the heart chamber overlying the dead or dying patch of muscle, and if these float off into the blood stream they may block vessels to vital organs such as brain or kidneys.

These, then, are the gloomy prospects of myocardial infarction. Centres all over the world are trying both to improve the treatment of heart attacks and to discover the factors that convert a symptomless atherosclerosis into a potential killer. We can now look at the factors which are thought to influence the development of coronary atherosclerosis and its complications.

Age

From the studies of the coronary arteries of individuals killed in accidents, it seems that coronary atherosclerosis increases with age. Indeed, some people regard coronary artery disease as an inevitable consequence of growing old, like going bald or grey.

Sex

There is, however, a sex difference in the frequency of coronary artery disease, at least in the young. Women before the menopause (i.e. before about forty-five years) rarely suffer from heart disease. It has been suggested that this is due to a protective effect of the female sex hormones. After the menopause there is an abrupt increase in blood fats (cholesterol and triglycerides) and also a rapid increase in the number of women affected by coronary artery disease. If the ovaries of a woman have to be removed before the age of thirty-five years, the risk of prematurely suffering from coronary artery disease is so great that the woman is usually treated with sex hormones (oestrogens).

Diet

Many believe that the kind of diet we eat is a very important factor in determining the development of coronary artery disease. Atheroma in arteries contains fats, and in some animals fed on a high fat diet the diseased parts of the arteries are very rich in fats. Moreover, patients with symptoms of coronary artery disease often have abnormal amounts of lipids (fats) in their blood. Some individuals have an inherited disorder shown by abnormally high blood levels of the lipid called cholesterol (hypercholesterolaemia); sufferers from this disorder have an increased risk of developing coronary artery disease and may develop symptoms while still in their teens.

This kind of evidence has led some physicians to believe that the fat content of the diet is important in determining the development of coronary artery disease. There are many kinds of fat in the diet, and the so-called 'saturated fats' have come to be regarded as the most dangerous. A saturated fat is one in which the fatty acid chain of carbon atoms has no free valency bonds remaining, for they all have hydrogen atoms attached to them. These fats are usually of animal origin (butter and lard) and are firm, not soft or liquid. Unsaturated vegetable fats are artificially saturated (by 'hydrogenation') during the manufacture of margarine. A high intake of saturated fats can lead to a rise in the amount of cholesterol in the blood. It is difficult to know at what level the blood cholesterol becomes important in determining the development of coronary artery disease. In patients with *very* high levels (more than 350 mg/100 cm^3) there is a quite exceptionally high risk of developing symptoms of coronary artery disease, even when these patients are young women. However, there are a large number of cases of heart disease due to atheroma where the blood cholesterol levels have been well down in the normal range. In these cases other factors must be operating to produce symptoms of the disease. It is thought that cholesterol in the blood produces its effect by increasing the 'stickiness' of blood platelets; this makes them more likely to settle down on the wall of blood vessels and trigger off a local clotting process which ultimately leads to the characteristic picture of atherosclerosis and its complications.

In spite of the fact that individuals with high blood cholesterol levels are more prone to develop coronary disease, there is no evidence available that changes in the diet aimed at reducing the blood cholesterol levels in patients already suffering from the disease can in any way alter the outcome. There have been several studies in which groups of patients with coronary disease have eaten special diets—some for as long as five years—reducing the cholesterol intake (i.e. no butter, no margarine, lard, fat meat, cheese, egg yolk etc.) and increasing the intake of unsaturated fats, but the mortality of these treated groups was not statistically significant from control groups who did not diet. There are, however, various drugs which can artificially lower blood cholesterol levels. One drug called cholestyramine traps cholesterol in the bowel and prevents its absorption into the blood. Another drug is clofibrate which lowers blood cholesterol by suppressing the actual synthesis of the substance in the body. Several trials are being carried out to see if these drugs will help patients with coronary disease to live longer and also to see if healthy people can avoid developing heart disease.

Heredity

Heredity is one important factor in the development of coronary artery disease. Its influence is seen most clearly in patients with familial hypercholesterolaemia. Even without this inherited abnormality of blood, cholesterol hereditary factors are important. If a man has one parent who died suddenly of coronary disease then he is twice as likely to suffer a myocardial infarction himself compared with a man without a family history of the disease. If both parents suffered from premature coronary disease then the risk of a man suffering a myocardial infarction is increased by a factor of about five. Thus a bad family history should alert the physician when he is confronted by an apparently healthy man. This familial tendency may be due to the inheritance of diseases such as diabetes mellitus or hypertension that promote the development of coronary atheroma, or to the inheritance of a certain pattern of coronary arteries that results in eddy currents of blood about the mouths of branches of the arteries leading to the premature formation of atheromatous patches.

Smoking (see also page 298)

There is no doubt that heavy cigarette smokers are much more likely to develop general atherosclerosis and in particular coronary artery disease than are non-smokers, pipe-smokers and those who have stopped smoking. It has been estimated that people under the age of forty-four who smoke more than twenty-five cigarettes a day are nearly fifteen times more likely to die of heart disease than are non-smokers. The risk is lower with fewer cigarettes smoked and with increasing age, but the risk is still apparent. However, like so many of the factors that are involved in the development of atherosclerosis and the conversion of this disease of blood vessels into the killer disease coronary thrombosis, not all the patients dying from coronary disease are heavy smokers.

Social and economic class

It used to be thought that the kind of person most likely to suffer from coronary artery disease was the professional man or the successful business man. Recent surveys of hospital records show, however, that no social class is protected and that the disease is mainly one of the skilled artisan.

Psychological factors

There have been many studies of the relationship between personality, psychological and emotional stress and coronary artery disease. It is, however, very difficult to measure such things as 'stress', and many of these studies have not been very meaningful. In spite of the problems of quantifying stress, there is a general agreement that psychological and emotional stress is often an important factor in triggering off an attack of angina pectoris and sometimes even a myocardial infarction. Many Darby and Joan deaths may be caused in this way.

Physical exercise

Some studies have shown that the more a person is physically active at work, the less chance there is of suffering from the effects of coronary artery disease (e.g. bus conductors are less likely to have myocardial infarction than are bus drivers). However, these views are not shared by everyone; indeed every physician has seen cases where *excessive* physical exercise in someone with diseased coronary arteries can actually precipitate a myocardial infarction. A classic example of this effect of severe exertion is seen in the middle-aged man who tries to push his car out of a snow drift.

The effect of other diseases

The presence of certain other diseases can considerably increase the risk of a person developing a coronary thrombosis. Diseases such as diabetes mellitus and hypertension (raised blood pressure) are cases in point. The American Society of Actuaries (1959) found that men under fifty with a blood pressure of about 170/100 were twice as likely to die from coronary artery disease as men with normal blood pressure.

Discussion

The triumphs of modern medicine in industrial

societies make it difficult to realize that we are unable to prevent (and often unable to treat effectively) the major killing disease of these societies. It is true that it may be possible to prolong life for a few years for someone who has had a myocardial infarction, but these successes have minimal effects on the rapidly increasing death rate from coronary artery disease. These deaths, often in young or middle-aged men, have profound effects on family life and on the economics of our community, and we are in urgent need of preventative measures to stem the flood.

We are in obvious need of much more information about the various factors that may interact to convert a fairly harmless non-thrombosing kind of arteriosclerosis into a killing thrombosing arteriosclerosis. The results of long-term trials in large numbers of individuals of the effects of reducing blood cholesterol levels (by diet or drugs) are eagerly awaited. But are we making full use of the information that is already available? The answer to this question is an unequivocable 'no'. We know the effects of cigarette smoking, the lack of physical exercise and of obesity, but information alone is not enough. 'At risk' patients should be specifically warned of the risks that their way of life brings, and doctors should and are showing examples by giving up cigarette smoking. Governments are very slow to react to this kind of information, for they fear a loss of their popularity and revenues, and in spite of murmurs of 'infringement of human liberties' they would have been quick to act if tobacco had been a foodstuff. In that case it would have been banned years ago and on *far* stronger evidence than that which led to the banning of cyclamates and tinned tuna (in the U.S.A.). It is estimated that if only half of all adolescents, young adults and middle-aged men became non-smokers and physically active, then the total mortality in men could be reduced by a factor of 10 per cent within a relatively short period of time. This would save annually about 1000 per million male members of the population.

The day will surely come when it will be as routine to advise a young man about coronary prevention as it is to immunize children against infectious diseases or take detailed care of a pregnant woman throughout her pregnancy.

24. Diseases of civilization II Cancer (malignant tumours)

Introduction

IN DEVELOPED countries of the world diseases of blood vessels, cancer and accidents are dominant causes of death from childhood to old age (Figure 23.1); in industrialized countries diseases of blood vessels and cancer account for two-thirds of total mortality in both sexes, and their importance is increasing, particularly in men.

What do we mean by the terms tumour, malignant tumour and cancer? We use the term tumour to describe a mass of abnormally arranged cells that can appear in virtually any tissue of the body. The most typical property of a tumour is in the behaviour of its cells. The cells of a tumour no longer obey the 'laws' that normally govern the growth and multiplication of cells of the tissue in which the tumour appears. The cells of a tumour continue to multiply in the absence of any need for repair or enlargement of the tissue or organ. In the adult, normal tissues do not grow. They maintain a steady number of cells. In some tissues such as the liver this steady state is achieved without much cell division because the cells of the organ do not die. In other normal tissues, such as the bone marrow or skin, cells are continually being lost from the tissue; they are shed from the surface layers in the case of the skin or lost into the blood stream in the case of the bone marrow. These tissues achieve their steady state by means of a division of cells at a rate which is just enough to maintain the number of cells. Normal cells show to varying degrees a property called 'contact inhibition' which means that when cells are in close contact with one another they do not divide. We do not understand the nature of this mechanism, but certainly tumour cells lose this property to a variable extent, so that they continue to divide under the most close-packed conditions. Tumour cells may differ from normal cells in other ways—in their appearance, biochemistry and in the number or shape of the chromosomes in the nucleus. Tumour cells do not usually grow and multiply at a faster rate than normal cells, indeed they do not need to divide rapidly in order to produce a large mass of tumour tissue. Each cell division

of a tumour cell doubles the number of cells, one cell becoming successively 2, 4, 8, 16, 32, 64 and so on; only forty successive divisions are needed to convert one cell into 1 000 000 000 000 cells weighing about a kilogramme!

Benign and malignant tumours

Tumours are divided into two main groups, benign ('innocent') and malignant ('cancer'). This distinction is of the utmost practical significance. Benign tumours are usually slow-growing masses of cells that gradually compress the normal tissues that surround them, but they show no tendency to invade the surrounding healthy tissues. These compact, well-defined masses of cells can develop in any body tissue— breast, brain, lung etc. If they are unsightly or are causing trouble by pressing on surrounding tissues, they can be removed with every prospect that they will not return or affect the health of the individual.

Malignant tumours differ considerably in their behaviour from benign tumours, and they have quite a different significance for the health and life of the person carrying them. Cells from the malignant tumour invade surrounding healthy tissues, and often they penetrate lymph channels and blood vessels. Once malignant cells penetrate into these fluid circulations, they can be distributed widely in the body. Many of these circulating malignant cells die during their journey around the body, but some settle down and 'colonize' various tissues and organs. In these tissues the cells multiply and produce new masses of malignant tissue. This process of spreading of a malignant tumour is called metastasis, and distant colonies are called metastases. Once metastasis has occurred then eradication of the tumour becomes very difficult, and often impossible, to achieve. The symptoms of cancer vary enormously according to the place where the cancer first appears and upon the kind of organs that become colonized by metastases. Sometimes the malignant tumour may spread in this way so rapidly that the first evidence of the presence of the tumour may be those that are caused by metastases, particularly if the metastases appear in a visible structure, such as the skin, or affect such a vital organ as the brain.

We are here going to be concerned with the causes and prevention of cancers rather than with the complexities of signs and symptoms of various cancers. However, it must be emphasized that cancers vary considerably in the symptoms they cause, the ease with which they can be diagnosed and in the chances of successful treatment. Thus cancer of the skin differs as much from cancer of the lung as does chicken pox from smallpox. Cancer of the skin is visible to the eye, is usually diagnosed early and it can be readily and successfully treated. Cancer of the lung is more insidious in the way that it shows itself, and by the time symptoms or changes in the X-ray appearances of the chest have developed the condition is often beyond any hope of successful treatment.

The terminology of malignant tumours is complex, unnecessarily so for our present purposes, and we will use the term 'cancer' for all malignant tumours, although strictly speaking this name is usually reserved for certain kinds of malignant tumours that arise in the epithelial tissues of the body.

Causes of cancer

The known causes of cancer are many and varied. When we do know the cause of a particular kind of cancer the information comes from such studies as the effect of certain occupations, habits such as smoking and the influence of deficiencies in the diet and inheritance. There is an increasing interest in the geographical distribution of cancers, and it is hoped that these studies will throw new light on the factors that make certain types of cancer commoner in certain parts of the world or in certain communities. The causes of cancer are also being studied in animals. The effects of all manner of factors—chemicals of various sorts, radiation, hormones and viruses that *may* cause cancers in man—are studied in experimental animals. It is hoped that this kind of research will ultimately reveal the way in which cells become converted into those of a malignant tumour and how this change can be prevented or treated. However, there is already a great deal of information available about particular causes of cancer, and much of this information has still to be put to use to prevent cancer.

Known causes of cancer

Many factors in the environment that can trigger off malignant changes in a cell have already been identified. These factors are called 'carcinogenic agents' or 'carcinogens'.

Chemical carcinogens

The first chemicals which were recognized as causes of certain cancers in some individuals are those present in soot, coal tar and mineral oils. As long ago as 1775 Sir Percival Potts described the first occupational cancer, cancer of the scrotum in chimney sweeps. Later on, when coal tar was being made by the distillation of coal, cancer of the skin became fairly common in workers who were exposed to the tar. Mineral oils were also found to be carcinogenic. When 'shale oil' was used as a lubricant in the Lancashire cotton-spinning mills, cancer of the skin of the abdominal wall and scrotum began to appear in those workers whose clothes became splashed with the oil. In the late nineteenth century, bladder cancer began to appear in workers engaged in the production of synthetic dyestuffs. Later it was found that particular aromatic amines such as benzidine, aniline and α-naphthylamine were the culprits. The list of known chemical carcinogens has progressively lengthened and include the following:

1. Coal distillation and fractionation products, e.g. tar, pitch, creosote, anthracene oil, tar oils and soot, which contain aromatic polycyclic hydrocarbons, produce cancer of the skin and lung.
2. Distillation and fractionation products of shale oil, soft coal, petroleum and hydrogenated coal oils, including tar, asphalt cutting oils and crude waxes, which contain aromatic polycyclic hydrocarbons and other carcinogenic substances, produce cancer of the skin and lung.
3. Aromatic amino-, nitro- and azo-compounds (e.g. α-naphthylamine, 4-aminodiphenyl, some of their analogues, benzidine and 3,3′-dichlorobenzidine) produce cancers of the bladder; some products of chromium- and nickel-ore produce cancers of the lung and nasal sinuses.
4. Inorganic arsenicals produce cancer of the skin.
5. Asbestos produces cancer of the lung.

The polycyclic aromatic hydrocarbons have received the most attention as chemical carcinogens, for these substances are produced in a variety of ways that ensure their presence in our environment. Not only are they responsible for certain occupational cancers (e.g. in the tar industry and in the manufacture of petroleum) but they are present in the atmosphere of any urban society, as well as in tobacco smoke, in solvents used for many processes and in the smoking and preparation of food.

Physical factors

Ionizing radiations

The relationship between ionizing radiations and cancer is well known. Many of the pioneer workers with X-rays died of cancer, and detailed evidence has been collected from Nagasaki and Hiroshima which links the development of leukaemia with the exposure to radiation from atomic bombs. Some radio-active elements are concentrated in the bones and lead to the appearance of bone cancer. An outbreak of this type of cancer appeared in girls who were employed in a factory painting the dials of watches with a luminous paint containing radium and thorium. As the girls painted they sucked the tips of their brushes to bring the bristles to a point. In this way they swallowed small amounts of the radio-active materials over long periods, and many of them succumbed to bone tumours which developed one to five years after exposure to the carcinogen.

Ultra-violet light

Excessive exposure to sunlight is known to produce cancer of the skin of the exposed parts. The risk is greatest with those who have white skin that does not tan easily. Cancer of the exposed parts of the skin is thus commoner in white people in Australia and South Africa than in white people in temperate climates such as our own.

Smoking, dietary habits, food additives, personal hygiene etc.

There is clear evidence of a connection between tobacco smoking and cancer of the lung. There is a clear relationship between the number of cigarettes smoked and the likelihood of developing lung cancer, and moreover, when smoking is discontinued the liability to lung cancer decreases in proportion to the number of years in which the habit has been discontinued. Tobacco tars are known to contain carcinogenic hydrocarbons, and in experimental animals these tars cause cancer when they are painted onto the skin. By the stopping of smoking, hundreds of thousands of lives could be saved each year; this is such an important subject that a separate chapter is devoted to it.

In certain parts of the world the habit of chewing betel nuts or nass (a mixture of tobacco, lime, ash and butter) is very common. In these areas cancer of the mouth and pharynx is a comparatively common form of cancer.

It is easy to imagine that factors in the diet or drinking water might be responsible for cancers of the stomach or intestines. So far no single factor in the diet has been identified as a cause of gastro-intestinal cancer. On the other hand, certain deficiencies in the diet seem to play a part in the development of some cancers. In women who suffer from a special form of iron-deficiency anaemia, cancer of the pharynx is common, and cancer of the thyroid gland is commoner in areas of the world where there is a deficiency of iodine in the water. Dietary deficiencies, particularly of the B-vitamins and protein, may well be important in determining the development of cancer of the liver.

The possible dangers of food additives (colourings, flavours, stabilizers etc.) and food contaminants (e.g. pesticides) has caused concern in recent years. Over the course of the years a number of substances used as food additives or pesticides have been withdrawn because they were shown to cause cancers in experimental animals. Obviously extreme caution must be exercised before any new substance is added to food; the number of new additives proposed for use throughout the world is so large that there are not adequate facilities for testing their effects in animals. Moreover, the absence of a carcinogenic action of a substance in a particular experimental animal does not necessarily mean that the substance is safe for man. The same problem arises with the use of substances in cosmetics and household products such as cleaning agents.

Carcinoma of the neck of the womb (cervix) in women and carcinoma of the penis in the man have been related to sexual habits, absence of circumcision in the male and the lack of attention to personal hygiene (i.e. washing of the genitalia). Cancer of the penis is often attributed to retention of the secretion called smegma, behind the prepuce of the penis. Cancer of the penis is virtually unknown in circumcised Jews (in whom circumcision is carried out a week after birth) and is rare in Moslems (in whom circumcision is carried out between the ages of four and fourteen years). Circumcision would appear to give complete protection against development of cancer of the penis; if circumcision is not carried out then scrupulous attention to personal hygiene is of great importance.

The latent period in the action of carcinogens

An important feature in the action of all these various carcinogens is that there is a 'silent' or 'latent' period between exposure to the carcinogen and the appearance of the cancer. This period varies from one carcinogen to another. Chimney sweeps took twenty years to develop scrotal cancer from contact with soot, while many people whose whole bodies were exposed to radiation (e.g. from nuclear 'fall-out') developed leukaemia ('cancer of the bone marrow') in about five years. This latent period creates problems for the identification of the role of various carcinogens, for it gives ample time for a patient to forget about exposure to a particular agent. Moreover, a person may change employment several times and be exposed to different kinds of carcinogen before eventually succumbing to the effects of one of them.

Hereditary predisposition to cancer

For most of the commoner types of cancer there is little or no evidence of any inherited tendency to develop the disease. There are, however, a number of rare types of cancer in which there is a strong genetic influence. One example of this kind of cancer is intestinal polyposis caused by the inheritance of a particular dominant gene (see page 257).

Diseases of metabolism and cancers

There are various disorders of the body's metabolism that can increase the risk of developing some kinds of cancer. Thus over 90 per cent of all cases of primary cancer of the liver (i.e. cancers originating in the liver, *not* metastases in the liver) occur in individuals whose liver is damaged by malnutrition or alcoholism.

Hormones and cancer

Over the years there has been considerable controversy over the possible part played by hormones (particularly the female sex hormones called oestrogens) in the development of certain kinds of cancer, e.g. of the breast or uterus (womb). In recent years concern has been expressed over the use of sex hormones in contraceptive pills, cosmetic creams etc. Certainly some cancers in experimental animals can be provoked by the administration of hormones, but only after massive doses of hormones, given over a long period of time, and then only in certain susceptible strains of animals. In human disease hormones appear to be only rarely involved in the production of cancers. There is one rare tumour of the ovary that produces massive amounts of oestrogen, and this may sometimes be followed by the appearance of cancer of the tissue that lines the cavity of the uterus.

Although hormones are rarely a cause of human cancer, they may stimulate the growth of existing cancers. Just as the normal healthy breasts, uterus or prostate gland are dependent on sex hormones for their growth, so may it be with cancers developing in these tissues; one can make use of this 'hormone-dependence' of certain cancers in treatment. Cancer of the prostate gland was the first human cancer to be treated by means of hormone treatment. Many cancers of the prostate are just as dependent on male sex hormone (testosterone) for their growth as the normal gland. If the source of male sex hormone (the testes) is removed by castration then there is often a dramatic change in the cancer and its metastases; these shrink in size and symptoms disappear. Nowadays it is not usually necessary to castrate a man to deprive his body of male sex hormone. The testes can only function normally and produce testosterone (and sperms) in the presence of a growth factor in blood that comes from the pituitary gland, that small gland lying under the brain. This growth factor is a mixture of two hormones (gonadotrophic hormones). The output of gonadotrophins from the pituitary gland is regulated by various factors, an important one being the amount of sex hormones in the blood. When the amount of sex hormones in the blood falls the pituitary gland produces more gonadotrophins to stimulate the testes, and vice versa. Oestrogens are the most potent of all hormones in suppressing the output of gonadotrophins from the pituitary. Small doses of oestrogen are thus as efficient as castration in preventing the production of testosterone by the testes; this sort of treatment is appropriately called 'chemical sterilization'.

In recent times other types of cancer, e.g. of breast or uterus, have been fairly treated by hormones of one sort or another. Unfortunately cancers that often start off by being hormone-dependent, and thus are responsive to this kind of treatment, may change their character as the disease progresses so that their growth becomes independent of the presence of hormones.

Viruses and cancer

There is great interest being shown in viruses that have been shown to cause cancers in animals. These are the oncogenic viruses. Intensive research is now exploring the possibility that certain human cancers may be caused by virus infections. This problem is discussed more fully on page 32.

Precancerous states

There are some changes in certain tissues, particularly epithelial surfaces, which are not in themselves malignant but which often lead to the development of cancer. The recognition of these changes is important, because if they are diagnosed and treated early enough it is possible to prevent the development of cancer. These precancerous states include 'papillomas' (wart-like growths) of the bladder and larynx, polyps in the colon (see page 257) and changes in the epithelium covering the neck of the womb (cervix). The neck of the womb can readily be inspected and smears of cells painlessly removed for examination under the microscope (Figure 24.1). Cancer of the cervix appears to develop over a period of many years. First of all there is the presence of abnormal epithelial cells that can be readily seen in the 'cervical-smear'. The main change in the cells is in the appearance of the nuclei which become enlarged and show variation in size and shape. The nuclei also take up more stain than the nuclei of normal cells. If these cells are found in a 'cervical-smear' then a more detailed examination is carried out, and a cone-shaped piece of epithelium is removed for microscopic examination. In the absence of cancer cells in the tissue, the patients are examined at regular intervals so that if cancer develops it can be treated in its early stages, when the chances of completely successful treatment are very high. The role of 'screening' tests for the diagnosis of early cancer is discussed more fully on page 293. This kind of cytological study can be used to diagnose other forms of cancer; sputum, stomach contents and urine can all be easily obtained and examined for the presence of cancer cells.

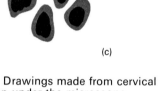

(a)

(b)

(c)

Figure 24.1 Drawings made from cervical smears as seen under the microscope.
(a) From a healthy cervix. These cells are similar to those obtained from inside the cheek. The dead sloughed cells have a regular pale staining nucleus.
(b) Cells of a suspicious smear. The nuclei are irregular in size and more darkly stained than in (a). A patient with this type of smear would be examined at regular intervals, for a life-time if necessary. Many will later show normal smears. About a third of patients with this type of smear will later develop definite 'positive' smears and will need some form of treatment.
(c) Cells of a positive smear. This patient would need a 'biopsy', i.e. a removal of a piece of epithelium from the cervix. If this showed cancerous cells invading the tissues underlying the epithelium then treatment would be needed—radiotherapy and/or surgery. Note the deeply stained nucleus with marked variation in size and shape. The ratio of nuclear/cytoplasmic volume is markedly reduced compared with cells of (a) and (b).

Summary

We have seen a variety of factors that may trigger off the development of some kinds of cancer. Unfortunately very many cancers develop without any apparent cause. Where causes *are* known then this can lead to the most successful approach to the control of cancer, that is its prevention. The avoidance of known chemical and physical carcinogens would dramatically reduce the number of certain kinds of cancer (e.g. lung cancer), while an improvement in the nutrition of the undernourished millions of the world would help to control primary cancer of the liver. This aspect of the control of cancer is so important that we will consider it in detail in the next section. Finally, a second method of cancer prevention is the detection and treatment of conditions that are known to lead to cancer; thus the routine use of periodic examinations of the cervix by means of 'smears' could make cancer of the cervix a preventable disease—a disease which kills about 3000 women each year in Britain. The treatment of this and other forms of precancerous states forms a cornerstone of cancer prevention.

Cancer control

The control of cancer can be considered under the following headings:

1. Prevention, including (*a*) the elimination of, or protection against, any factors known, or believed to be, carcinogenic— this aim may be achieved by the education of the public in cancer prevention, industrial hygiene and legislation against a proved carcinogen—and (*b*) the diagnosis and treatment of precancerous lesions.
2. Diagnosis, in which mass screening of either the general population (e.g. mass radiography) or the screening of special groups who are 'at risk' (e.g. in certain industries) have an important role to play.
3. The treatment and after-care of the cancer patient.

The prevention of cancer

We have already mentioned many of the chemicals, physical factors and habits that are likely to lead to the development of cancer. The general public and workers in industries in which there are special risks, should be made aware of the dangers of exposure to carcinogens, and if voluntary control of a carcinogen cannot be achieved then legislation may be imperative. In the past, cancer educational campaigns have laid stress on trying to correct wrong ideas about cancer and on encouraging individuals to pay attention to certain symptoms or signs that might indicate the presence of a cancer, so leading to early diagnosis with its increased chances of successful treatment. Table 28 shows the differences in the five-year survival rate for cancers in different parts of the body when they are treated at early and late stages of development. In the World Health Organization Report on the Prevention of Cancer (*World Health Organization Technical Report Series*, no. 276, 1964) is the comment that 'with increasing knowledge of aetiological factors and of

precancerous conditions, it is time for cancer education to swing to positive preventative measures. The Committee feels that cancer education should aim at encouraging the use of the word 'cancer' so that discussion can be free from secrecy and emotional embarassment. The fact that cancer is by no means an incurable disease should be re-iterated. The warnings that cancer education might create cancerophobia have proved a myth'. Since the publication of the report there has been progress in achieving this swing to positive preventative measures. The mass media of communication are increasingly discussing these problems, and few people in developed countries of the world can fail to have heard of the risks of smoking and air pollution or the value of 'well-woman' clinics. However information alone is not enough; as many general practitioners will no doubt testify, cancerophobia and anxiety states are a real risk when education is not fully supported by legislation or by adequate facilities for mass screening for cancer. To an impartial observer it must surely seem folly to harrass a population about the risks of a particular carcinogen, and yet at the same time permit the free sale and advertizing of the carcinogen, particularly when the carcinogen (tobacco) is a drug of addiction.

Industries would appear to care more for their workers than do governments for the general population. This attitude of industries may not be entirely philanthropic, for there is always a risk that a worker who develops a cancer attributed to the action of some industrial carcinogen may try to claim heavy compensation. Workers require, and often receive, a clear explanation of the risks to which they are exposed, and of the reasons for the various protective measures that have to be carried out in the particular industry; these measures may include the mechanical handling of articles, removal of fumes, 'monitoring' of chemical or radiation contamination, protective clothing,

Table 28 Survival rates for cancers when treated at early and late stages of development

Position of cancer	Percentage of survivors 5 years after treatment	
	Early stage	*Late stage*
Bladder	50	15
Breast	75	10
Cervix of uterus	70	10
Larynx	75	5
Mouth	60	5

dust control, washing facilities, periodic medical tests etc.

There are few examples of legislation introduced to deal with the use of an industrial carcinogen, although the manufacture of some carcinogens, e.g. of α-naphthylamine in the dye industry, has been stopped on a voluntary basis. There are, nevertheless, a number of highly carcinogenic industrial products which are still being manufactured and used commercially, and expert committees have recommended that every effort should be made to persuade or compel industries to stop producing these chemicals and find less dangerous substitutes for them.

In some countries, including Britain, legislation ensures the compulsory notification of cases of occupational cancer. Even with this legislation, it is difficult to obtain a true estimate of the number of occupational cancers because of the long latent period of many of the cancers. During the latent period workers may change their occupation, move to different parts of the country or even emigrate.

The diagnosis and treatment of precancerous lesions

We have already mentioned various conditions which are precancerous. If these conditions are recognized and treated, then it may well be possible to prevent cancer. There are many possible symptoms and signs that are due to precancerous conditions in various parts of the body—in the skin, mouth, pharynx, oesophagus, stomach, colon, female reproductive organs, and breast. Health education can increase the population's awareness of symptoms and increase their willingness to consult a doctor for what might seem to be trivial matters; however, many general practitioners will probably respond to this sort of statement by an affirmation of the fact that they are already overburdened by trivia. Obviously a well-staffed health service is needed for this aspect of cancer prevention.

The detection and diagnosis of cancer

It is impossible and probably inadvisable to teach laymen the symptoms of the commoner cancers. What can be done is to concentrate on symptoms or signs that in all cases should lead to a consultation with a doctor. These symptoms and signs include the following:

1. a lump in the breast or discharge from the nipple;
2. chest pain, persistent cough, blood in sputum, breathlessness, loss of weight;
3. indigestion, loss of appetite;
4. changes in bowel habits or the presence of blood or mucus in the faeces;
5. irregular or heavy menstrual periods, vaginal discharge, vaginal bleeding after intercourse;
6. blood in the urine, discomfort or difficulties in passing urine;
7. chronic ulcers or lumps in the skin or in the mouth, tongue and throat, enlarged lymph glands in the neck, arm-pits or groins, hoarseness of the voice.

For any one of these symptoms or signs there may be a variety of causes. Every woman with a lump in the breast does not have cancer, and certainly few women who present themselves with a story of vaginal discharge will prove to have cancer of the cervix. These symptoms should, however, be taken seriously and efforts made to exclude cancer as a cause of the symptoms.

We are not going to consider the kinds of investigations which are used to detect cancer in an individual patient who attends his doctor with particular symptoms. Instead we will look at methods of screening for cancer in populations. There are a variety of types of mass screening in operation in different parts of the world. A complete screening operation involves inspection of the entire skin surface and all accessible body cavities (mouth, throat and rectum), a chest X-ray and urine examination; in females the breasts are examined, cervical smears are taken and a pelvic examination made, while in males the prostate gland is felt via the rectum. If there are any suspicious symptoms or abnormal findings in the above tests, then other investigations may be added such as X-rays of the stomach or bowel, examination of the sputum for cancer cells, X-ray of the breasts (mammography) etc. A full examination of this kind is obviously a costly affair and is usually applied to restricted, usually wealthy, groups of individuals. It has been found that fairly simple examinations, with more special examinations included only if there are suspicions of serious underlying disease, can detect a considerable proportion of accessible cancers. These screening surveys have proved their worth in countries such as Hungary and the U.S.S.R.

We come now to surveys of more limited aims. Mass radiography, originally instituted for the detection of pulmonary tuberculosis, has detected an impressive number of lung cancers in some surveys. In Japan, screening for gastric cancer—a very common disease in that country —is carried out on a large scale in some areas by means of mobile X-ray units. Improvements in the techniques of examining sputum for malignant cells are proving of value is detecting *early* malignant changes in the lungs (X-ray changes are often a *late* feature of lung cancers) and the technique has been found useful in the chromate industry.

Special clinics for the detection of certain cancers of women (breast and cervix) have been set up in some areas of Great Britain (and in North America and Scandinavia). In Britain the number of women dying each year from these diseases is some 10 000 from breast cancer and a further 3000 with cervical cancer. The successes of treatment of cancer of the breast and cervix (by surgery, radiotherapy and drugs) has shown no improvement in recent years, and it seems important to direct efforts towards early diagnosis or prevention of the diseases. Cancer of the cervix must now be regarded as a preventable disease. Breast cancer can be detected by simple palpation of the breasts (and individuals can be readily taught the technique) or by temperature scanning of the breasts with an infra-red detector. For the latter examination patients are undressed to the waist and sit for ten minutes in an air-conditioned room at 19 °C. The scan takes about five minutes and produces an instant record. Further information can be recorded by taking an infra-red photograph of the breasts. These examinations detect areas of the breast with an abnormal flow of blood which is reflected in the temperature of the area. Breasts can also be examined by means of X-rays (mammography), but in areas where there are not enough staff or equipment the examination is reserved for women with an obvious lump, or a woman with large breasts in whom it is easy to miss small abnormalities. An annual examination of the breasts is recommended, particularly for certain 'high-risk' groups (i.e. women over thirty-five years, those with a history of breast disease or a family history of breast cancer, and single or married women who do not have children). In a recent report of a screening programme ('Is screening for cancer worthwhile? Results from a well-woman clinic for cancer detection', J. B. Davey et al., *British Medical Journal*, 3, 1970, 637–718), 1768 women were screened for breast and cervical cancer in the year of May 1968 to April 1969. The screening consisted in a brief questionnaire, examination of the abdomen and pelvis by a gynaecologist, cervical and vaginal smears, and examination of the breasts by a second medical officer.

The breast examination included temperature scanning with an infra-red detector. Breast cancer was detected in fifteen patients (8.5 per 1000); none of these patients were aware of any abnormality, although a lump could be felt by the doctor. Early carcinoma (i.e. non-invasive) of the cervix was found in a further eight patients (4.5 per 1000).

If most pre-cancers and symptomless invasive cancer of the cervix can be discovered and treated, then the death rate from cancer of the cervix should inevitably fall. So far, no surveys have been able to show that there has been a drop in mortality rate, although in Canada it has been reported that there has been a decrease of 54 per cent in the number of cases of invasive cancer of the cervix, in a population in which half of its female members were regularly screened for carcinoma of the cervix over a period of eight years.

Unfortunately the spread of the facilities for cervical screening is limited by expense, particularly that of training and maintaining the number of pathology technicians that are needed for examination of the smears. It is hoped that a machine for the automatic preliminary screening of smears will be available in the next few years. The machine will be able to work about ten times as fast as the technician—and for twenty-four hours a day. The aim of the machine is to pick out the one in twenty or so slides that show signs of abnormality, and these will then be examined in the usual way by the technicians.

The examination of urine for the presence of malignant cells is an important way of controlling cancer of the bladder, and should be a routine in groups who are at special risk, such as workers in some dye industries. The available techniques of cytological examination of the stomach contents are too time-consuming to be of general use in the detection of cancer of the stomach. There is urgent need for some method of mass screening for this common and dangerous cancer.

The treatment and after-care of the cancer patient

The treatment of cancer should follow diagnosis as early as possible. At the present time surgery and radiotherapy are the mainstay of treatment. For a few types of cancer, certain drugs and hormones are also used (see hormone-dependent cancers, page 290). We cannot here discuss the details of treatment of the various kinds of cancer, but two points need emphasis. First the outlook for completely successful treatment, as opposed to temporary arrest of the disease, varies widely from one kind of cancer to another. For some kinds of cancer, particularly in the early stage of the disease, the prospects of complete cure are very high. Second, many people are in fact cured of cancer; it has been estimated that about 30 000 people are cured of cancer each year in Britain alone.

The after-care of the cancer patient who has received treatment is very important. Sometimes prolonged after-treatment, often with radiation, is necessary, and periodic medical check-ups are used to check the development of complications or the occurrence of relapses of the disease. Rehabilitation, particularly the care of mental health, is a vital, and sometimes neglected, aspect of after-care.

25. Diseases of civilization
III The smoking disease

Introduction

THE second report of the Medical Committee of the Royal College of Physicians of London, *Smoking and Health Now* (Pitman, London, 1971) has recently been published. It is a document of the utmost importance, and should be in the possession of anyone who is either concerned with the education of children or who is in a position to demand or initiate legislation against the sale or use of tobacco. In the words of the report, 'cigarette smoking is now as important a cause of death as were the great epidemic diseases such as typhoid, cholera, and tuberculosis that effected previous generations in this country'. The greatest achievement of modern medicine has been the control of infectious diseases by the use of vaccines and antibiotics. New epidemics of heart disease, lung cancer, bronchitis and emphysema, now take a vast toll of human life. No vaccines or antibiotics will prevent deaths from these diseases. The remedy is far simpler. The avoidance of tobacco smoking, in particular cigarettes.

The known facts about the effects of tobacco smoking

The effects of cigarette smoking as a cause of disabling illness and shortening of life are well known, and have been verified by many studies in a score of countries. These effects are fully described in the above report, and they are summarized below.

Shortening of life

Cigarette smokers have shorter lives than non-smokers; the shortening of life is in proportion to the number of cigarettes smoked. For non-smokers the chances of dying before the age of sixty-five are about one in five; for heavy cigarette smokers the chances of dying before the age of sixty-five are double the figure, i.e. two in five. The earlier in life that smoking begins, the greater is the risk. A study of the life expectancy of American men showed that whereas a non-smoker at the age of forty has an average life expectancy of 34.5 years, for those who smoke 1–9 cigarettes/day, 10–19 cigarettes/day and 20–39 cigarettes/day the life expectancies are, respectively, 30.2 years, 29.3 years and 28.7 years, i.e. a man of forty who smokes heavily loses, on average, about six years of his life.

Smoking and cancer of the lungs

In the last fifty years, cancer of the lung has changed from being an uncommon to a major cause of death, particularly in men, and this trend is international. The change has occurred during a period when the deaths from other forms of cancer have shown little change, or in some cases have even declined. In the U.S.A. deaths from lung cancer have steadily risen from below five per 100 000 of the male population in 1930, to forty per 100 000 in 1965. In this same period, the number of cases dying of cancer of the stomach fell from about thirty to ten per 100 000 of the male population. A similar trend has occurred in England. Figure 25.1 shows the changes in the death rate from cancer of the lung in British men, between the ages of forty-five and sixty-four, compared with the death rate from other forms of cancer.

In 1968 about 27 000 men and 5500 women died from lung cancer. It has been estimated that if there is no change in the numbers or kinds of cigarette smoked then by the 1980s some 35 000–40 000 men will die each year from this disease. By this time the number of female deaths from lung cancer will have reached 10 000–15 000 per year.

Women do seem to be less liable to cancer of the lung than men, even when they smoke the same number of cigarettes, but as in men, the risk for women increases with the number of cigarettes smoked. Women's smoking habits have, however, differed from those of men. In the past British women have tended to begin the habit later in life and inhale less. In America women do not, like men, smoke cigarettes to the end where the 'tar' is concentrated during smoking, and more of them smoke filter-tipped cigarettes and those with a low nicotine and 'tar' content.

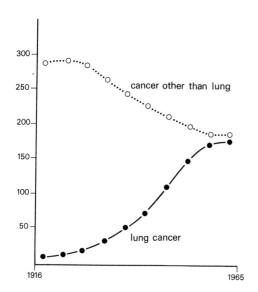

Figure 25.1 Death rates from lung cancer and other forms of cancer from 1916–65. Figures are per 100 000 men between the ages of 45–64.

Table 29 Death rates per 100 000 from bronchitis in some European countries (1952)

Country	Death rates per 100 000
England, Scotland and Wales	207.2
Portugal	43.1
Germany	22.5
Netherlands	20.9
France	9.1
Denmark	6.9

Great Britain occupy an unenviable position as far as these diseases are concerned, for she heads the list of countries when these are arranged in order of mortality rates from bronchitis—see Table 29.

During the early stages of bronchitis there are recurring attacks of cough and phlegm, usually following common colds, sometimes occurring every year. The phlegm may be clear and small in amounts, but at times, particularly after a cold, it is profuse and yellow or green due to the presence of pus. As the disease progresses there is a narrowing of the air passages which causes difficulty in breathing. At first this breathlessness may be temporary, and may be capable of being relieved by drugs that act on the muscle in the wall of the airways or by anti-biotics that clear up chest infections. Later the patient may enter a phase of constant breath-lessness; such patients cannot walk except about the house and may be unable to sleep unless they are propped up in a chair. Emphysema makes this condition worse. Emphysema describes a change in the structure of the lungs in which the walls of the tiny air spaces (alveoli) are broken down to produce larger air spaces. A lung in which this change has occurred has less surface area of respiratory membrane for the exchange of oxygen and carbon dioxide with the atmo-sphere. When this happens more air has to be moved in and out of the chest to produce the same degree of exchange of gases. When the demands for gas exchange increases, as in exercise, then difficulties arise and the patient becomes very distressed. The blood vessels of the lungs may be so damaged by these pro-gressive changes in lung structure that the right chamber of the heart becomes stressed by having to pump blood through the damaged lungs. Eventually heart failure is added to the picture of chronic bronchitis and emphysema.

Other factors in the production of lung cancer

Over the course of years, controversy has raged over the role played by air pollution (fog and fumes) in the appearance of epidemics of lung cancer. Although lung cancer is commoner in urban than in rural areas, this difference can no longer be regarded as being simply due to differences in the amount of air pollution. Moreover, although the air pollution in our cities has steadily fallen in recent years, the death rates from lung cancer have persistently risen.

Certainly some forms of air pollution found in certain industries increases the risk of develop-ing cancer (e.g. asbestos dust, chromates, nickel, products of coal distillation, see also page 288), but the number of people affected in this way is too small to have much effect upon the total number of deaths from this disease.

Smoking, chronic bronchitis and emphysema

Chronic bronchitis and emphysema are common ailments which kill over 30 000 men and women each year in the United Kingdom. Deaths from these diseases is usually preceded by years of progressive disability at the end of which the individual may be unable to take a few steps without distressing breathlessness and cough.

Cigarette smoking

The importance of cigarette smoking in the

development of each of these stages of chronic bronchitis is becoming clear. The presence of cough, phlegm and recurring chest infections are all associated with cigarette smoking. The more a person smokes, the more likely is he or she to develop these changes. Indeed smokers so commonly have a cough with phlegm that they come to regard this state of affairs as normal. Individuals with normal bronchi and lungs do not, however, suffer from cough. When cigarette smokers stop smoking they cough less and become less liable to develop chest infections. When the disease has progressed far and lung damage and emphysema have appeared, giving up smoking cannot improve the breathlessness although it may still reduce the cough and the production of phlegm.

There is little doubt that smoking greatly increases the risk of illness, disability and death from chronic bronchitis and emphysema. On the other hand it is obvious that cigarette smoking is only one cause of this disease. There must be other factors which make the British so susceptible to this disease which killed so many people long before the smoking habit was popular. The Report on Air Pollution by the Royal College of Physicians concluded that life-long exposure to air heavily polluted by coal smoke contributes to the special liability of British cigarette smokers to develop severe bronchitis. There must obviously be other as yet unidentified factors which make this so typically a British disease, for bronchitis is commoner in country areas of Great Britain than it is even in urban areas of Scandinavia, Finland and the U.S.A. The important point, however, is that these disabling and killing diseases are, to an important degree, preventable. Control of air pollution and the giving up of the smoking habit would save very many lives, and working hours, lost by these diseases.

Smoking and diseases of the heart and blood vessels

We have already discussed the factors that seem to be involved in the development of coronary artery disease in Chapter 23. We can here re-iterate that coronary artery disease is a common cause of death in developed countries (it killed 31 000 people in the United Kingdom alone in 1968) and that smoking is one of the factors in causing the development of this disease.

The risk of dying of coronary artery disease for smokers of cigarettes is two to three times greater than that of non-smokers. This risk is not

as great as that of developing lung cancer (in the U.K. for men who smoke over thirty cigarettes a day the risk of dying of lung cancer is over thirty times that of non-smokers). However, since coronary artery disease is so common, the total number of premature deaths which are associated with the smoking of cigarettes is very large.

In addition to its effects on diseases of the coronary arteries, the smoking habit also affects other arteries of the body. Generalized atherosclerosis with its effects such as intermittent claudication and strokes are commoner in cigarette smokers than in non-smokers.

Smoking and other conditions

Smoking may affect health in a variety of other ways. Smokers are more liable to cancers of the mouth, pharynx, larynx, the oesophagus, and bladder; they are more likely to die from peptic ulcers and tuberculosis of the lungs than are non-smokers. Many fires are due to the smoking habit; in the U.S.A. studies have shown that 16–18 per cent of deaths in fires had resulted from fires caused by smokers. Pregnant women can affect their unborn children in a variety of ways by smoking; these mothers are more liable to have a miscarriage, to have a stillborn baby, or one that dies soon after birth. A recent publication in 'Nature' indicates that in women who smoke during their pregnancy, the number of their children affected by congenital heart disease (i.e. abnormal development of the heart and great vessels) is 7.3 per 1000, i.e. 50 per cent higher than among children born to non-smokers. There is the obvious possibility that it may be associated with other abnormalities of development in children.

Why do people start to smoke and why do they continue with the habit?

Most smokers start their experiments with tobacco in childhood or adolescence. A variety of factors may combine to bring about these early experiments, factors such as curiosity, bravado, and a need to create the appearance of being grown-up, particularly if parents and other relatives smoke. These first experiments usually create unpleasant sensations of nausea and giddiness, and it seems obvious that fairly potent social or psychological pressures must be encouraging the individual to persist with these unpleasant experiences before ultimately he finds some physical pleasure from the habit.

Sooner or later the individual develops tolerance to the effects of nicotine on the body, and dependence often develops (see page 330). Recent studies have shown that a teenager need smoke only twice to have a 70 per cent chance of smoking for the next forty years, provided that he lives so long. Smokers go on smoking because they find the habit satisfying and they soon begin to feel a sense of deprivation or because of craving when they are without a cigarette. Most people smoke to obtain nicotine and they do not find nicotine-free cigarettes satisfy.

Physical dependence on nicotine accounts for the fact that smokers persist with the habit even when they are fully aware of the risks they run and even when they wish to give up smoking; indeed they may have made at least one unsuccessful attempt to give up the habit. This behaviour is typical of a dependence disorder. Smoking is clearly associated with other dependence disorders; the bulk of alcoholics (92 per cent) and heroin addicts (99 per cent) are smokers, compared with 58 per cent of the general population who smoke. Very few smokers (about 2 per cent) do so only occasionally; the vast majority eventually become addicted and thus regular, dependent smokers. Drug-dependent individuals need help to overcome the habit, and they are not receiving enough of this help either from health authorities (because of limited finance and staff) or from governments (because of ignorance or apathy, or more probably a concern of members for their political lives and for the vast revenues from tobacco sales).

Types of smokers

Smokers have been classified in a variety of ways according to the number of cigarettes smoked, whether they inhale smoke or not, and whether they smoke regularly or intermittently. Another type of classification describes the kind of enjoyment derived from the habit. Psychosocial smoking describes the habit where the rewards are all psycho-social, indeed there may be very little intake of nicotine. This type of smoking occurs mainly in adolescence and almost invariably it progresses to a type of smoking which produces sensory rewards, such as the pleasure of mouth contact (indulgent smoking) calming effects (tranquillizing smoking), stimulating effects to reduce fatigue during monotonous tasks, such as long-distance driving, or to increase alertness for creative

tasks (stimulation smoking). In these types of smokers the frequency of smoking varies according to the physical or mental situation. In addictive smoking, smoking frequencies vary little with mood or activities and a persistent high intake is necessary to achieve a constantly high level of nicotine in the blood. After an interval of about half an hour of non-smoking, the individual becomes ravenous and feels a craving for a cigarette.

Stopping smoking

About 18 per cent of smokers eventually become ex-smokers. In the younger age groups, the ex-smoker status is a rather unstable one and the individual may readily revert to the habit. However, with advancing age there is a progressive increase in the number of ex-smokers; at the age of seventy it has been estimated that some one in three of those who were regular smokers have given up the habit.

The reasons for giving up smoking are various. Most smokers need to have some personal experience of the effects of smoking such as cough, breathlessness, sore throat, indigestion, repeated colds, before they decide, or are persuaded, to give up the habit. These personal experiences seem to be far more potent persuaders than statistical evidence of the real risks to health and life. Expense is another factor in giving up smoking, although this affects mainly adolescents or those on restricted income. Other, although at the moment minor, factors include the need to show example to others (e.g. in doctors, nurses, teachers, parents) or the influence of social pressure (of parents, relatives, colleagues etc.). Many of those who try to give up smoking fail in their attempt or, if successful, return to the habit after months or even years. An important reason for this failure is the 'withdrawal effects' (see also page 330) which include intense craving, irritability, anxiety and difficulties in sleeping and concentrating. Various measurable physical changes may occur during this period, such as sweating, fall in blood pressure and pulse rate, and changes in the stomach and intestines. That these psychological and physical changes are due to deprivation of nicotine is shown by the fact that they can be relieved by an injection of nicotine.

During this withdrawal period, smokers can be helped by the support of their doctor. Unfortunately there is no effective drug or psychological treatment (and this includes hypnotism) that can be shown to have any advantage over moral support and encouragement during the withdrawal period. The withdrawal process is in fact a learning period, when the individual has to achieve a way of living without smoking. The aim should be to stop smoking as quickly as possible; 'cutting down' is only a means to an end, for it cannot remain indefinitely. *Only* when smoking has stopped can the withdrawal symptoms gradually disappear and the feeling of a need to smoke under particular circumstances disappear, circumstances that include the after-meal period, telephone conversations, social outings or times of personal stress.

For those who cannot give up smoking unaided, further support is available from specialized clinics. Reports of success in these clinics have varied widely from 30–60 per cent. Even a 30 per cent success rate is a considerable achievement, for these clinics deal with individuals who have been unable to give up smoking unaided. Research is needed to find ways of improving these success rates. Some of the failures are due to social pressures; the individual returns to a family or place of work where smoking still continues. A gain in weight may also undermine the decision to give up smoking. This is unfortunate, for the risks of smoking are far greater than those of obesity; furthermore, obesity is easier to manage than cigarette-dependence. Every effort should be made to understand the reasons why an individual smokes and the kind of situation that re-inforces and maintains his smoking.

The prevention of diseases due to smoking

In theory, the prevention of these diseases is simple—the prohibition of tobacco. If tobacco had been a food, a pesticide or a drug, it would have been banned years ago. The situation is, however, complicated by political and financial issues and by the vast extent of nicotine-dependence. The most recent report of the Royal College of Physicians came to a conclusion which some may regard as over-cautious. The report concludes that 'it is, of course, impracticable to prohibit a habit to which so many people are devoted, for this could lead to large-scale evasion with consequences that could be as grave as with those of the prohibition of alcoholic drinks in the U.S.A. While maintaining individual freedom of choice, every effort must be devoted to persuading smokers of cigarettes to take the only sure means of reducing the risks they run, which is to give up smoking. At the same time the tobacco manufacturers must be encouraged in their efforts to develop products that will not be so injurious as modern cigarettes, so that the dangers to those who cannot or do not wish to discontinue the habit may be diminished.' This conclusion, in a report that begins by an assertion that the deaths and illnesses caused by cigarette smoking have now reached epidemic proportions and 'present the most challenging of all opportunities for preventative medicine in this country', sounds less than adequate.

There is as yet no safe cigarette (although some may be safer than others) and no way of identifying those individuals who are at special risk from smoking. This means that every effort must be made to discourage people from starting or continuing the habit. In spite of the brief outburst of publicity via the mass media which followed the publication of the major reports linking smoking with various diseases, there seems to have been a general lack of appreciation of the *exact* risks of smoking. People *must* have the information so that they know the level of risk and can compare it with the risks associated with other activities such as are experienced by drivers or pedestrians on roads, by housewives in the home, or by housewives on a contraceptive pill. Unfortunately it would appear to be difficult for even responsible information media to maintain an impartial and unemotional attitude when it comes to estimating risks. A recent report of the dangers (to an infinitely small number of women) of contraceptive pills containing more than 50 microgrammes of oestrogen led within hours to the withdrawal of these tablets from the market and to a spate of television programmes and news flashes on the subject. These responses resulted in much concern and the abandoning by many women of a safe and extremely effective method of contraception. This state of affairs arose in spite of the fact that authoritative estimates of the dangers of contraceptive pills have been put at a similar level to that of smoking one-third of a cigarette once a day for three weeks out of four. Another way of comparing this risk of the contraceptive pill is to equate it with the risks of death in men from playing football and cricket. When we come to lung cancer, it appears that few people realize that this disease kills over four times as many people as do road accidents.

Realistic and persistently applied information about the risks of cigarette smoking should help both to prevent individuals from starting the smoking habit and to persuade some smokers to give up the habit. It is important to make clear that by giving up smoking, people can lose the increased risks of the various smoker's diseases gradually over a period of ten or more years (see Figure 25.2). For those who continue to smoke unwillingly and against their better judgement, special help must be made available. A few clinics were set up after the first report of the Royal College of Physicians on Smoking and Health, but most of these have been now discontinued. At the time of writing, six months after the first impact of the second Report on the Royal College of Physicians, little progress seems to have been made in this field.

For individuals who do not wish to give up smoking or who are unable to do so, the risks can be reduced by changes in their smoking habit which include the following:

1. smoking pipes or cigars (moderate smokers have a risk of the smoker's illness only slightly greater than that of non-smokers);
2. smoking fewer cigarettes, inhaling less, leaving a longer stump and taking the cigarette out of the mouth between puffs;
3. smoking a brand of cigarettes with a lower tar and nicotine content (the Consumers' Association proposes to publish information about the tar and nicotine content of major brands of cigarettes on sale in the U.K.).

The latest report of the Royal College of Physicians makes a variety of other recommendations which includes suggestions about the removal of cigarette vending machines, prohibition of gift-coupon schemes, more restrictions on smoking in public transport, places of entertainment etc. and the reduction of insurance premiums for non-smokers.

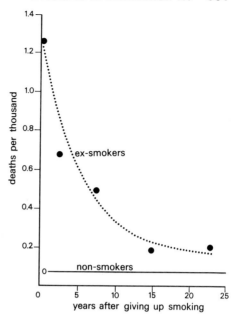

Figure 25.2 Death rates from lung cancer at various intervals after giving up smoking, compared to the death rate from lung cancer in non-smokers. (*Data from a study by British doctors.*)

Whenever there exist a variety of remedies for a particular disease, doctors usually comment that this means that probably none of the remedies is very effective. This would appear to be the case for the remedies for the smoker's disease. The real remedy is perhaps in the hands of politicians, but if this is so, they will probably hold on to it for some time to come.

26. Diseases of civilization IV Accidents

Introduction

WE HAVE already seen that as the tide of infectious diseases recedes in developed parts of the world, new threats to life and health become important, threats that include cancer, coronary thrombosis and mental illness. One of these new 'epidemics' is the menace of accidents. Death by accident is becoming important not just because death from other causes has decreased; accidental death and injury rates are *increasing* in many countries as individuals fail to adapt to changing patterns of life and as the complex and potentially dangerous products of modern technology invade every niche of our lives—on roads, in the air, in our factories, homes, schools,

Figure 26.1 Each year in Europe, between one-ninth and one-quarter of all workers have a disabling accident. In the U.S. out of a total of 91 000 accidental deaths from all causes, almost 14 000 are due to industrial accidents. This photograph was taken in the Siemens-Schuckert factory in Vienna where the works safety engineer and workers staged a series of accidents that should not happen. (*WHO photo by Kopetzky.*)

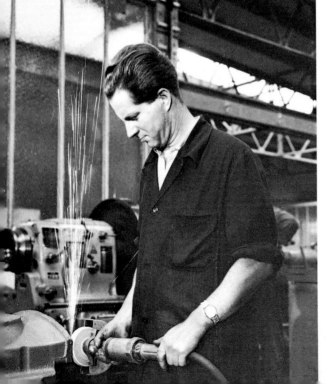

laboratories and places of entertainment (Figures 26.1, 26.2).

Among the definitions of the term accident in the concise Oxford Dictionary are included 'event without apparent cause, unexpected, chance, fortune.' It is unfortunate that such a word as accident should be used to describe an increasingly important cause of death and injury. The word implies that these deaths and injuries are unavoidable and that individuals are involved by chance happenings. Nothing could be further from the truth. Just as some individuals, because of their age, occupation and habits, are susceptible to particular infections and other diseases, so it is with accidents (Figures 26.3, 26.4). Even when a group of similar individuals is exposed to the same risks, some will be more likely to be damaged or killed by accidents. This state of affairs is not necessarily due to the operation of chance or 'fate'; some individuals, because of their psychological make up, lack of information, training or intelligent foresight, are what we call 'accident-prone' (Figure 26.5). Accidents *can* be prevented, and our attitude about the role of 'chance' and 'fortune' in accidents must be replaced by an awareness of the importance of ignorance and carelessness as contributory factors in accidents. The term 'death by accident' might well be replaced by 'death due to negligence'.

The size of the problem

It is important for us to have a measure of the threat from any particular cause of death and illness, in order to examine its importance for a society and to arouse some interest and research in the provision of medical care and preventative measures. As in the case of so many diseases, we are rather uncertain about the real hazard to life, health and the social economy presented by accidents. Many accidents, particularly those that occur in the home or those that do not result in death or serious injury, are not reported, and indeed many countries do not publish detailed analyses of accidents. Because of these problems, the World Health Organization requested member countries to publish statistical material on

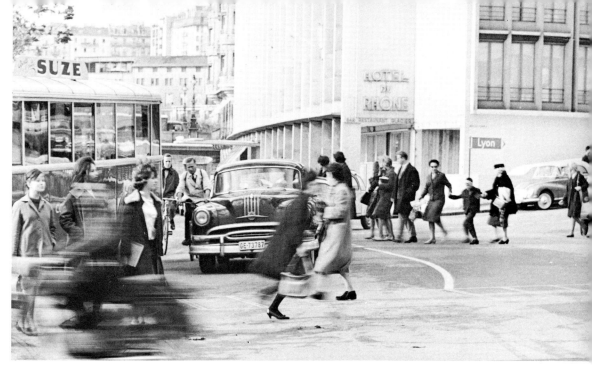

Figure 26.2 This picture was taken in a city in Europe and shows a strange ballet of pedestrians and vehicles at a street crossing. Both kinds of road users are seen to be at fault. The town has some 200 000 inhabitants and in 1960 road accidents killed 54 people, including 25 pedestrians. (*WHO photo by Jean Mohr.*)

deaths caused by accidents. Table 30 shows the reports of some of the countries that provided the information to the World Health Organization, and a glance at this table will confirm that accidents are indeed an important cause of death.

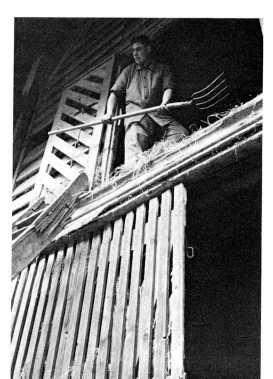

Figure 26.3 Country people are exposed to many accidents. The farmer's home is also his workplace and combines the dangers of both. The photograph shows a loft, pitchfork, and doubtful ladder. (*WHO photo by Eric Schwab.*)

Figure 26.4 Children are at risk from accidents. Photograph shows a child exploring the environment around his home; he approaches an open gate which leads to further dangers. (*WHO photo.*)

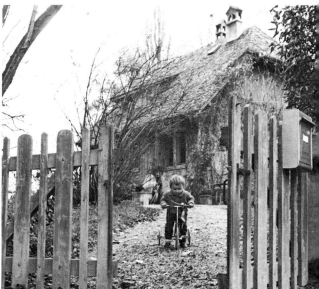

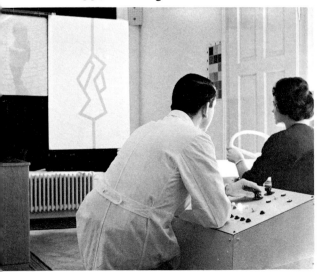

Figure 26.5 Research workers have been trying to discover the personality of the principal actor in road tragedies, i.e. the driver. The co-ordination of the driver's reactions is investigated by means of an apparatus which simulates driving conditions, Pictures on the screen enable distraction to be studied. (*WHO photo by Eric Schwab.*)

Accidents in the home

In this chapter we are going to look mainly at accidents in the home. Domestic accidents form a large proportion of deaths from all accidents (see Table 30); in the Netherlands, for example, deaths in women from accidents in the home account for 87 per cent of all non-transport accidents. These accidents, however, do not attract the same public interest as the drama of aircraft or train disasters or the concentrated outbreak of accidents to children that occur on Guy Fawkes night in Great Britain. We are constantly reminded on television and radio of the number of deaths and non-fatal accidents that occur on our roads, particularly during holiday periods. Furthermore, the accidents that occur outside the home are subject to many control measures and to common and general laws that enable the injured or relatives of the dead to be compensated if the injury is caused by the negligence of another. Penalties for the negligence of employers who expose their workers to risks, or for drivers of cars who drive dangerously or under the influence of drugs or alcohol stimulate the taking of pre-cautions. However, the home is a potentially dangerous place where the occupants are rela-tively unprotected by the law. Few publicity or educational campaigns have been directed at the home in an attempt to reduce the toll of death and injury.

Definition of accident

We all feel we know what an accident is; how-ever, it is difficult to define the term precisely. In 1957 the World Health Organization defined an accident as 'unpremeditated event resulting in a recognizable injury' and later they elabor-ated the definition to 'an event, independent of the will of man, caused by a quickly acting extraneous force, and manifesting itself by an injury to body or mind'. However, one can readily find exceptions to these definitions. Thus some accidents are far from rapid in their action, e.g. some drugs, or the effect of exposure to cold in the elderly. Many accidents are far from independent of the will of man, as seen in

Table 30 Deaths due to all accidents, to non-transport accidents and to domestic accidents in several countries in 1960

Country	All accidents	Non-transport accidents	Domestic accidents
Canada	9403	5074	2235
Netherlands	4212	1989	1294
Norway	1569	1000	594
United Kingdom	20 660	12 264	7769
U.S.A.	93 806	49 628	24 068

Data from special World Health Organization inquiry (World Health Organization, 1963). See also figure 23.1, page 280.

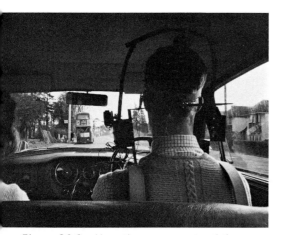

Figure 26.6 Here the movements of the driver as related to movements of the vehicles are being studied on recording instruments. (*WHO photo by Philip Boucas.*)

many accidents to children which arise from their unsupervized explorations of the home environment. The definition of the term 'domestic' is equally difficult, particularly if one compares different cultures, for what is the 'home' for a nomadic tribe, for a community living on barges or for communities living on houses suspended over the sea on stilts?

Domestic accidents as a cause of death or injury

Table 30 indicates that domestic accidents are a formidable cause of death in developed countries. In most western countries, accidents are the leading cause of death among persons under forty-five years of age. We know that accidents in the home loom large in these

accidental deaths, indeed in some age groups (e.g. one to four years) they are the most important cause of accidental death.

The magnitude of the effect of accidents can be expressed in ways other than the crude death rates per annum. Table 31 shows the relative importance of deaths due to domestic accidents and tuberculosis in 1960. Tuberculosis is a disease which has receded under the impact of economic development and the force of public health services in the west. A glance at the table is enough to indicate that domestic accidents are a more important cause of mortality than is tuberculosis in many developed countries. This situation is somewhat of a paradox, for while domestic accidents are a source of interest to few educationalists and doctors, tuberculosis still commands considerable attention with mass radiography, B.C.G. vaccination, routine examination of pregnant women and so on. Table 32 shows another way of expressing the effect of accidental deaths, not in terms of numbers of deaths but in terms of loss of working years caused by death (calculated on the maximum expectation of life). At a time when the American population was worrying about cancer, obesity and coronary heart disease, their country was losing more working years from accidental deaths than from any other killer.

The effect of changing patterns of living

Even quite small changes in the pattern of community life can present unexpected dangers to life and health in the home. These changes are most rapid in the developing countries of the world where an individual can move from a tribal existence into a sophisticated technological culture within a short period of time.

Table 31 The importance of domestic accidents and tuberculosis as a cause of death in various countries in 1960

Country	Domestic accidents	Deaths from all forms of tuberculosis
Canada	2235	823
Hungary	927	3097
Ireland	140	468
Netherlands	1294	325
United Kingdom	7769	4058
U.S.A.	24 068	10 670

Data from 'Domestic Accidents' by E. Maurice Backett, *Public Health Papers*, No. 26. World Health Organization.

Table 32 The effect of accidents and various diseases in America (1945) expressed as the number of thousands of working years lost by death

Cause	Working years lost (thousands)
Accidents	1980
Heart disease	1892
Cancer	1155
Tuberculosis	1144
Cerebrovascular disease	465

(Data modified from 'Domestic Accidents' by E. Maurice Backett, World Health Organization)

Even smaller changes in the pattern of life of a village, such as the digging of deeper wells, drainage trenches and the like, present new dangers which are poorly recognized even by adults.

Even in developed countries, new hazards are continually appearing, by-products of affluence and a still advancing technology. The widespread use of plastic bags for wrapping all manner of goods resulted in many deaths in children (and some in adults). Many of the bags are large enough to go over a child's head and then the thin airtight pliant film of plastic can readily block the mouth and nose and cause death by suffocation. Nowadays, plastic bags often carry a warning of the dangers to children. The home is rapidly becoming a complex workshop containing sophisticated and potentially lethal equipment including electric grinders, blenders, cutters, tin openers, toothbrushes, television, radio, hedge-cutters, drills etc. Many of these operate at very high voltages. New forms of heaters, new fuels, and water supplied at high temperatures create further dangers. Attempts to introduce these advances into old buildings with primitive electric wiring systems, inadequate ventilation and the like can be potentially disastrous.

Domestic accidents in the developing countries

In trying to assess the importance of domestic accidents as a cause of death and injury, we have looked mainly at the developed countries of the world. Much less information is available from the developing countries of the world, but the indications are that here also accidents, including domestic accidents, are an important cause of death. Technological evolution is likely to increase this burden as new hazards are presented to unsophisticated individuals.

The effects of non-fatal accidents

The recorded numbers of deaths caused by accidents represent the 'visible tip of the iceberg' of the accident problem. We are not sure of the size of the invisible submerged part of the iceberg, for many minor accidents are not reported and do not appear in any statistics. However, minor or near-accidents are none the less important in any study of the causes of accidents or in the development of methods designed to prevent them.

We are here looking at what is called the 'morbidity' of non-fatal accidents—that is their effects on health, employment, schooling, loss of work, cost of medical care and so on. We know that in these terms the effect of non-fatal domestic accidents is considerable. The Royal Society for the Prevention of Accidents in the United Kingdom estimated that two million domestic accidents occur in Great Britain each year that require in- or out-patient treatment in hospital. This is an annual rate of one in twenty-six of the population and does not include those who were treated by a general practitioner. The cost to the Health Service must obviously be very considerable. The effects on the economy of the country in terms of days of work lost is no less impressive—see Table 32.

Table 33 The number of fatal domestic accidents in young children and the elderly expressed as a percentage of total fatal domestic accidents (1960)

Age group	Sex	Percentage of total fatal domestic accidents
0–4	Male	15
0–4	Female	6
65 plus	Male	54
65 plus	Female	77

Individuals at risk

We have seen enough data to indicate the importance of domestic accidents as a cause of death and morbidity—loss of health, schooling, loss of working hours etc. We can now go on to look at the types of individuals that are at special risk and the ways in which the home environment can bring disaster to the individual. Obviously those people who are most in the home are most likely to be injured or killed in domestic accidents. However, not all those who are habitually in and around the home are at equal risk; very young children (particularly males) and the elderly (particularly females) are especially prone to accidents (see Table 33). These special groups apart, it is also clear that other groups of the population suffer severely from domestic accidents; about 20 per cent of all domestic accidents were in young and middle aged adults (1964). The effect of these deaths in young and middle-aged individuals obviously has not only serious consequences for the economy but also drastic personal effects on their families.

Factors in addition to age alter the suscept-ibility of particular groups of individuals to domestic accidents. Poverty and a poor standard of living tend to result in poorer people having more serious accidents and, moreover, they probably take longer to recover from the effects of the accidents. Poverty results in poorer housing conditions which include steep danger-ous stairways in old tenement properties, im-provized cooking and heating equipment, anti-quated electric wiring systems and so on; it also results in overcrowding and often in the inadequate supervision of young children.

The nature of domestic accidents

If we look at the nature of domestic accidents we can see where are the main dangers in the home. Table 34 shows the proportion of fatal domestic accidents due to various causes in several countries. The table shows a similar pattern for the various countries, with falls, poisoning and fires being important causes of fatal domestic accidents in all countries (there are also some special dangers for each country such as firearms in the U.S.A. and drowning in Japan). We will now go on to look at these various causes of fatal domestic accidents and the ways in which accidents might be prevented, paying particular attention to falls, fires and poisoning.

Falls

Table 34 illustrates clearly that falls are a very important cause of fatal domestic accidents. The elderly woman is particularly at risk; in 1962 of over 3200 domestic accident deaths due to falls in England and Wales, 89 per cent were in persons above sixty-five years, two-thirds of whom were females. Many of these falls in elderly women occur from falls at the same level, i.e. while walking, standing or sitting. One does not have to fall from a high window or ladder for the accident to result in death. Of course, in younger people falls from heights are more

Table 34 Causes of fatal domestic accidents in several countries in 1963
(figures are percentage of total)

Country	Poisoning (and gassing)		Falls		Machinery		Fires etc.		Hot substances etc.		Firearms		Drowning		Others	
	M	F	M	F	M	F	M	F	M	F	M	F	M	F	M	F
England and Wales	25.1	19.1	45.2	61.9	0.1	0.1	8.1	10.1	1.3	0.9	0.7	0.1	1.6	0.8	17.9	7.0
U.S.A.	8.5	5.7	35.4	51.3	0.5	0.1	25.9	26.6	1.3	1.3	7.3	1.9	2.3	1.7	18.9	11.4
Canada	10.9	6.4	29.7	49.2	1.3	0.3	22.8	20.9	1.2	1.8	4.1	0.9	1.9	1.3	28.2	19.3
Japan	15.8	14.7	18.5	22.1	0.4	0.1	16.3	21.1	4.1	4.7	0.2	0.1	11.0	11.4	33.7	25.8

Source: World Health Organization (1956).

Note. One important cause of domestic accidents not clarified above is suffocation (with food or mechanical). This cause varies from 7 per cent (England and Wales) to 21 per cent (in Japan).

important. In addition to the elderly woman, there are two other groups at special risk from falls. These are the young male toddler busy exploring his home environment and the middle-aged male engaged in carrying out house repairs.

The prevention of falls involves many changes in our attitudes and in the construction and furnishing of our homes. The use of really safe stepladders, modern windows that turn inwards for cleaning so that it is not necessary to sit on the window ledge, and stairways that are not too steep and are well lit and equipped with a firm handrail, would all help to reduce the number of fatal falls. Highly polished floors are often regarded as necessary for hygiene and elegance, and this applies not only to our homes but also to our public buildings—including hospitals. Non-slip polishes are an obvious answer to the problem, but these are not as efficient as one could hope for. Certainly, carpets that are placed on smooth or slippery surfaces should have a non-slip back.

The elderly who are most likely to suffer a fatal fall are ill equipped to cope with potentially dangerous environment of the home; failing vision, arthritic joints, loose-fitting slippers and walking sticks with shiny tips all increase the likelihood of falls. Bones become increasingly brittle with advancing age, and fracture of the neck of the femur is a common enough result of a fall, even from a standing or sitting position. Although this fracture itself does not usually have an immediately fatal outcome the surgery or prolonged bed rest that must follow carries high risks for the elderly. For the protection of children much more positive measures must be taken, such as gates at the top and bottom of stairs, efficient fencing around holes, ditches and the like which may be in the surroundings of the home.

Burns and scalds

Burns and scalds are a very important cause of domestic accidental death. In Japan burns and scalds are the most important cause of accidents (see Table 34) and in the U.S.A. a similar state of affairs exists; in 1960 fires and burns were the principal cause of accidental deaths in the home in all age groups except the very young up to one year old and the elderly (sixty-five plus). In England and Wales there are about 9000 fatal domestic burns a year, and these affect mainly the very old and the young. Burns in the elderly are particularly dangerous, and even fairly small areas of burns can cause death.

The most common cause of fatal domestic burns is the firing of clothes, which accounts for over 50 per cent of cases. Falling into the fire and widespread fires in a building each account for about 10 per cent of cases. Open domestic fires are the chief danger in the home, and this accounts for the increased number of burning accidents in the cold season. In countries where central heating systems are commoner than open fires, burns due to the firing of clothes are rare.

Many people do not realize that fires in the home can kill by asphyxiation with poisonous fumes long before the actual fire reaches the body. An important way of preventing deaths from fires is the education of individuals to evacuate a burning building as quickly as possible (page 313), even if the fire does not seem to be extensive. This aspect of the prevention of fatal accidents is discussed more fully in the section on Accident Prevention.

Poisoning (including gassing)

In most developed countries of the world, poisoning is second or third in importance as a cause of fatal domestic accidents. Moreover this killer is increasing in importance. Scotland seems to lead the world, with poisoning (and gassing) accounting for over 30 per cent of fatal domestic accidents. In England and Wales the figure is over 22 per cent, and for the U.S.A. it is 16 per cent.

In England and Wales the dangers from poisoning and gassing is lowest in the age groups five to fourteen years and it then increases with age. In the older age group, poisoning by domestic gas accounts for a large fraction (70 per cent plus) of all poisoning and gassing deaths. In the youngest age groups (up to four years) the greatest risk is from poisoning—from medicines and household material (bleaches, cleaning fluids, caustics etc.).

The introduction of natural (North Sea) gas into Britain should change the importance of gassing as a cause of accidental death. Natural gas consists of methane with a minor proportion of other gases. A recent report on this gas (Ministry of Technology, 1970 *Report of the Enquiry into the Safety of Natural Gas as a Fuel*, London, H.M.S.O.) concludes that it is non-toxic. Leakage of this gas from pipes and appliances should not therefore cause poisoning. Of course, if an individual walks into an atmosphere consisting almost entirely of methane—as sometimes happens in coal mines—then asphyxiation and deaths would very rapidly follow, but this condition is not likely to occur in houses or other premises from the leakage of natural gas.

The use of natural gas does not increase the risk of fire or explosion provided that appliances are correctly designed, installed, maintained and operated. It is important to note that natural gas needs more oxygen (about seven per cent more) to produce the same amount of heat as does town gas. When natural gas is used, it is thus even more important to have an adequate supply of air for combustion and to have a properly functioning flue. Indeed, in any room where heating is provided by the combustion of some material—gas, coke, coal, oil etc.—there must always be enough ventilation to ensure adequate combustion of the fuel, to remove potentially dangerous gases, carbon monoxide particularly (that insidious killer that asphyxiates by progressively combining with the pigment of red blood cells so as to prevent them from carrying oxygen from the lungs to the body tissues), but also irritant gases such as sulphur dioxide, and to maintain the supply of oxygen in the atmosphere at normal levels.

Suffocation

Accidental death due to suffocation usually occurs in the form of choking over food in either the very young or in the very old who are already weakened by some other disease. This is not an important cause of death. In 1962 there were 558 deaths from 'suffocation' at home in England and Wales, and 341 of them were due to choking over food. We have already mentioned the dangers of plastic bags. Another risk is the habit of leaving infants alone with a feeding bottle in the mouth; the risks of inhalation of liquid food to the air passages with a fatal outcome is considerable.

Electrocution

This is a form of death that occurs only in developed countries where homes are supplied with high voltage currents. The number of deaths from this cause has steadily increased in Great Britain as the consumption of electricity has increased. In the period 1901–1904 there was an average of about eleven deaths a year from electrocution, and this rose to about 137 deaths a year in the period 1960–64. Many of these deaths occurred in the home. There are many people who feel that 240 volts a.c.—the general voltage in Europe—is unnecessarily high and dangerous, and many appliances can be adapted to work efficiently at far lower voltages. In the

home small children and 'do-it-yourself' males are the chief victims of fatal electrical accidents; in 1962, of the forty-nine domestic electrocutions thirty-one were in males.

Accidental hypothermia

Hypothermia is said to occur when the temperature of the body falls below 35 °C. When this occurs, urgent treatment is necessary to save the life of the person. In the home, accidental hypothermia most commonly affects the very young infant (especially the premature) and the elderly. The power to generate heat and the ability to conserve heat are very much reduced in an immature infant. These babies move little and lose heat over their comparatively large surface area; they thus quickly take on the temperature of their surroundings, becoming hot or cold according to the air temperature. Over-heating is fairly easy to recognize because the baby becomes restless and flushed, but a slow downward drift in body temperature is much more insidious and the baby may be thought to be just sleeping when in fact it may be in an hypothermic coma. This danger is a well recognized one, and mothers usually receive enough guidance from the doctor, midwife or health visitor on the dangers of a cold room. However, it is often not realized how steadily warm a bedroom must be to maintain a normal temperature in an immature baby; it must be about 29 °C, and in many homes this sort of temperature may be difficult to achieve.

Similar dangers for the elderly are now well recognized. It is estimated that about 9000 old people are admitted to hospital with hypothermia in England and Scotland each year (about half of which are over sixty-five years old). This figure does not include those treated at home or those who are found dead at home. The mortality of this condition is high; depending upon the severity and duration of the hypothermia it ranges between 30 and 80 per cent. Many cases of hypothermia are in old people who fall and then remain for several hours on a cold bedroom floor before being found, or in those elderly people who are socially isolated and who are likely to suffer a long period of exposure to cold before they are discovered. Many old people cannot provide adequate heating, either because of poverty or because of illness or physical disability. In addition many illnesses (strokes, heart attacks and the like) which may affect an old person living alone are likely to be complicated by hypothermia if the illness occurs in the winter months.

The prevention and early detection of accidental hypothermia is a challenge to the health and social services. Death from this cause can be prevented if individuals have enough money to buy fuel and heating appliances, and if old folk at risk are advised of the dangers of cold and are provided with some regular human contact. Hypothermia has probably often passed unrecognized because the normal clinical thermometer does not register below 35 °C. A thermometer reading down to 24 °C should be carried by general practitioners, home nurses and the like.

The prevention and control of domestic accidents

General

Domestic accidents can and should be attacked at all levels of organization in a society. These levels of attack are enumerated below.

1. *Legislation*, e.g. the Fireguards Act of Great Britain which requires that new fires are properly guarded; this law cannot, however, ensure that fireguards are correctly used, and only if a child under twelve (or under seven in

Figure 26.7 Internal combustion, electricity, atomic energy and their endless applications can be used without excessive danger only if the safety laboratories keep abreast of developments. New gadgets need to be tested. In Britain, over 3000 standards have been established by the British Standards Institution for a wide variety of goods. Here the electrical insulation of the connections in a washing machine are being investigated. (*WHO photo by Patrick Ward.*)

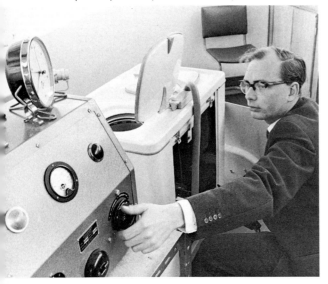

the case of Scotland and Northern Ireland) is injured by burns from an inadequately guarded fire can the person in charge be prosecuted. In Great Britain the safety and quality of much of our home equipment—cooking and washing machinery, fires, electrical appliances etc.—is ensured by standards set up by the British Standards Institute (which has its own advisory committee on personal safety) (Figure 26.7). Only appliances that achieve required standards are allowed to be sold with the Mark of Approval attached; that the quality of these appliances does in fact match the standards is ensured by laws such as the Consumer Protection Act of 1961. The law also operates indirectly by way of public health legislation aimed at making the environment safe; thus some responsibility for accident prevention is placed on public health authorities. However, these duties of public health authorities are not fully carried out, for these authorities have traditionally been heavily concerned with the prevention of communicable diseases, and moreover there are obvious difficulties for their personnel to freely enter and inspect the home environment.

2. *Voluntary bodies.* A number of voluntary bodies such as the British Royal Society for the Prevention of Accidents and the Fire Protection Association are very actively concerned in the prevention of accidents. These bodies urge legislation, collect information and statistics and design health education and propaganda services. In addition to the work of these voluntary bodies, consumer protection associations are playing an increasing part in educating for safety as well as in coercing manufacturers to comply with safety standards. In many countries, including Great Britain, there are Government-sponsored consumer councils with important advisory functions.

3. *Action at the level of the family and the individual.* When we come to the particular family and the individuals in it there are two aspects of control; first, the general design, lighting etc. of the home and the safety of particular features (electrical fittings, fires, poisons—cupboards and the like) and second, the education of individuals to avoid accidents. The alteration of the behaviour of individuals so as to avoid accidents is the most difficult of all aspects of accident prevention. We know very little of how to improve 'risk-taking' behaviour or the reasons why, in groups of apparently similar individuals, some are more 'accident-prone' than others. Certainly no amount of training will be of much avail if any of the senses

of sight, hearing, or touch are defective. Every effort should be made to ensure that the elderly, who are so at risk from accidents, should have defects of sight corrected by spectacles or cataract operations, or defects in hearing corrected by suitable hearing aids, or surgery if this is indicated. Unfortunately, defects in smell, which are usually impossible to correct, are common enough in the elderly and must contribute to deaths from gassing and fires. After ensuring that the individual's senses are as corrected as far as possible (note that only about one in five of elderly people in Great Britain who would benefit from removal of cataract(s) make use of the services provided free under the National Health Service), the next aim is the training in the proper use of the senses in the detection of 'danger signals' in the home. In planning any training programme it is very important to distinguish between children, adults and the elderly. Through their past experience, adults are often able to *anticipate* a dangerous situation or an accident. An adult may well anticipate the potential dangers of, say, a polished or wet floor, of an unsupported ladder propped against a wall, or of using a mirror fitted above an open fire. Young children do not have this ability to predict situations—it has to be learned, and a completely safe environment would not provide an adequate learning situation for a young child. Obviously children must be protected from serious hurt, but to some extent they must be allowed to explore and learn for themselves what is dangerous and what is not, of course under the watchful eye of an adult. This supervized exploration should be increasingly combined with training in the recognition of danger (Figure 26.8). There are many lessons, however, that cannot be learnt from trial and error—for example, tasting of poisons, probing of power points, and falls downstairs.

In schools, the training that has begun at home should be extended by formal lessons in accident prevention and by 'in situation' experiences in model kitchens and workshops and roads (Figure 26.9). This kind of education can be 'fed back' into the home if children carry out project studies in their own homes. If all children took home the check list given at the end of this chapter, and with the help of a parent went through the various items, a very apt learning situation would be created in which child, parent and school might well benefit. Where the infant, the handicapped and the elderly are concerned, training is important not only for the individual but also for the person(s) in charge of the individual.

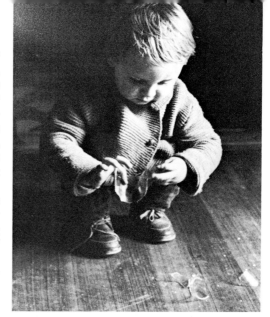

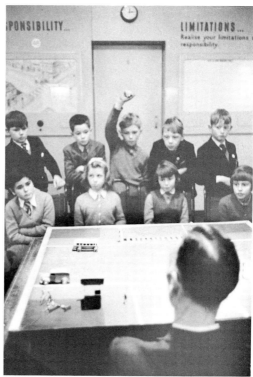

Figure 26.8 (top)　Michael among the hazards of life at home. (*WHO photo by Jean Mohr.*)

Figure 26.9 (bottom)　Accident prevention specialists consider it just as dangerous to frighten children with real dangers as with imaginary ones. Instead children should be encouraged to build a simple self-defence system into their everyday behaviour. Safety education is recommended as a part of general education everywhere. Around a magnetic table with moving models, these school children learn to cross a street. (*WHO photo by Philip Boucas.*)

We can now go on to look in some detail at the prevention of accidents, classified according to cause.

Fires, suffocation, burns and scalds

Legislation

Attempts to protect individuals against accidental burning in the home by legislation have not been too successful. In order to punish the law must have information, and this information is not readily available without the right to inspect homes. The Heating Appliances (Fireguards) Act, 1952, of Great Britain, requires that all new fires purchased after that date be fitted with guards. The Children and Young Persons Act of 1948 makes it an offence to leave a child under twelve years of age in a room with an inadequately guarded fire. However, this law has only very rarely been enforced, in spite of the fact that infringements of this law must reach astronomical figures.

Prevention of fires

1. *Materials of houses.* It is important to be aware of flash-prone ceilings and wall panels of compressed paper board, untreated fibreboard etc. or materials prefinished with highly inflammable lacquers. Certain acoustic and plastic tiles are extremely inflammable. Whenever possible, non-flammable or flame-retarding furnishing fabrics should be used. It is now illegal to sell children's nightdresses of highly flammable material.

2. *Smoking* (cigarettes, etc.) is an important cause of domestic fires—about 3000 a year. Smoking when one is liable to go to sleep is always extremely hazardous. There are on the market cheap ashtrays that exclude air and that cannot be spilt.

3. *Electrical heaters and electricity wires* are an important cause of domestic fires. Even the electrical heater—particularly the bar heater—with a fitted guard, does not always protect clothing from getting between the meshes of the guard and igniting. Space heaters of the blow type, in which the electrical elements are completely enclosed, are far safer, particularly for children and the elderly.

The over-heating of domestic circuits is a great fire hazard, particularly in old houses where the circuits become progressively unable to cope with the load of new appliances that are added to the home. The most important danger sign is when fuses keep blowing. It is important to note that fuses in an electrical circuit are very important in the prevention of fires. The purpose of the fuse is that the soft wire should melt and cut off the supply of electricity when the wire becomes overloaded and threatens to heat up and start a fire. Some people make the error of inserting fuses of larger diameter, even to the extent of putting a hairpin across the points. The only certain thing that these measures do is to remove the protection afforded by the fuse and increase the risk of a fire started from over-heated wires.

Every child should be taught the significance of the insulation around electric wires. Worn electric cords carry not only a risk from electrocution but also the risk of fire from sparks between two wires. In many homes there are electric extension cords running under carpets, tacked down with staples, or passing over pipes or rough edges. Wherever electric cords are exposed to friction in any form there is a risk of baring of the wires, and this may result in the sparking that leads to fires.

4. *Matches, petrol etc.* About one in twelve of all extensive house fires in Europe are caused by children playing with matches. The moral is obvious. In these fires easily ignited fuel oils are often involved. When highly volatile liquids such as petrol, hair sprays etc. are exposed to air, the vapours formed can explode if they come into contact with the smallest spark or fire—and these sources of heat need not be in the same room as the inflammable vapour. These liquids are increasingly used in homes, in dry-cleaning tasks, as paint cleaners and strippers, and in various hobbies. If highly inflammable liquids have to be stored in or around the house, they should be kept in closed containers that are not within the reach of children, and never in glass bottles that can shatter and rapidly produce a highly explosive vapour. When they are to be put to use, they should be in a well ventilated area where vapours cannot accumulate and where there is no risk of contact with sparks or flame. Whenever possible it is best to try to find a non-inflammable alternative for a particular cleaner or solvent.

5. *Burns from boiling water and fat.* These burns can in large measure be prevented by using utensils that are so designed that they tip and spill only with difficulty. These specially designed utensils include flat rough handles on pans, pans with a low centre of gravity, kettles that will not spill or even pour unless a spring-

loaded trigger is pulled, and frying pans deep enough to prevent fat from flying from the pan when wet food is added. To safeguard children, all flames and hot plates should be at least three feet above the ground, and no hot pans should be left on stoves with their handles within the reach of children.

Minimizing the risk of fire

We have looked briefly at some of the ways in which fires can be prevented. We now have to consider how the risks of an established fire can be minimized. In the first place there is a need for people to be aware of the risk of smoke, which in many cases asphyxiates people before the fire ever reaches them. Smoke is a mixture of various poisonous gases; the actual nature of the mixture depends upon the kind of material burning. Potent killers in gases from burning materials include carbon monoxide, hydrogen sulphide, ammonia and hydrocyanic acid. The colour and density of smoke is no indication at all of its danger. The important point to grasp is that wherever there is smoke, there is potential death from asphyxiation; this means that the evacuation of a burning building is very urgent.

Second is the importance of the existence and knowledge of safe escape-routes. All individuals in a house should be aware of safe escape-routes in case of fire. The greatest problem is, of course, from upper floors; however, inexpensive and well designed home fire-escape ladders are available, both of portable and permanent kinds. The Fire Protection Association (see bibliography) recommends various kinds.

Third, all who are old enough or are able enough should know how to telephone for help, clearly giving the family name, number and name of the street and nature of the fire, waiting after giving this information to see if the person answering the phone has understood or has any questions.

Fourth, early warning systems increase the chance of survival and of limiting the fire. These systems are common enough in industry, and many home owners are now installing automatic fire detection and alarm equipment. Of course, their greatest value is at night when the alarm can awaken one from sleep. Details of recommended systems are included in the Fire Protection Association's 'Fire Protection Equipment for the Home'. It is important to note that an automatic fire alarm system is triggered off by a heat detector and it does not react to smoke and fumes.

Family fire drills are an extremely sensible precaution to ensure that all members of a family know what they have to do in the case of fire, although it would seem that few parents ever take this precaution. Family fire drills and a 'Fire Quiz' for children are admirably discussed in *Stay Alive* by Jean Carper and Elizabeth Gundry, Macgibbon and Kee, 1967.

Obviously very small fires may be readily extinguished in the home and prevent extensive damage to the property or loss of life. If, however, there is the slightest doubt of one's ability to extinguish a fire, it is far safer to evacuate the premises and call the fire brigade. Although water may be effective in extinguishing many small fires, it is not very effective for inflammable liquids such as oil or petrol, and of course it is positively dangerous if the fire starts in an electrical appliance or a wire while it is still connected to the electrical supply. Two types of home fire extinguishers are available, one an asbestos blanket and the other some type of container containing an extinguishing material such as carbon tetrachloride, baking powder or a carbon dioxide generator. The asbestos blanket excludes oxygen from the burning material by covering it with a non-flammable layer. These are effective and safe to use for small fires. In the case of the various containers, their safety and effectiveness varies considerably depending upon the size of the container and the nature of its contents. Extinguishers are easy to come by from hardware shops or from door-to-door salesmen. Many are 'aerosol types' releasing carbon tetrachloride or baking powder, and are reasonably priced. Unfortunately most of them contain far too little material—probably not enough to extinguish a burning chip pan. Others may be positively dangerous, either because of the risks of aerosols themselves or because the contents are poisonous, e.g. carbon tetrachloride. It is thus important to choose an extinguisher that one knows to contain enough material to put out a small fire. Details of fire extinguishers made to British Standard specifications can be obtained from the Fire Protection Association.

Poisoning

Every year about five hundred people die of poisoning; many of these are children and many more than this number are made ill by poisons and need treatment in hospital.

The number of poisonous substances on the consumer market (medicines, detergents, dyes, paints, insecticides, disinfectants, cosmetics etc.) is enormous. In the U.S.A. it has been estimated that there are 250 000 toxic or potentially toxic proprietary products on the market, excluding drugs prescribed by doctors. No parent, indeed no doctor, can keep abreast of this mounting number of potentially dangerous material that may litter our cleaning cupboards, medicine chests, handy-man kits, garages and greenhouses. The problem is so acute that special 'poisonous-reference' centres have been set up in various parts of the country to advise about potential poisons or the treatment of accidental or deliberate poisoning. Of course, some poisons are far more toxic than others, and some materials, such as hydrocyanic acid or salts of the acid which may be used by amateur entomologists or in other hobbies, are so poisonous that the most extreme caution is needed in their use. It does help to know the degree of risk involved in using various materials, but this must not lead one to suppose that a bottle of some cleaner, polish, hair dye etc. which has no warning label is necessarily safe. The safest line of action is to regard anything that is not intended to be eaten as a food as a potential poison, and to regard any medicine as poisonous (see list).

There are special hazards when tablets containing dangerous drugs resemble sweets, or when bottles that normally contain soft drinks are used to store detergents, caustics, petrol etc. All poisons should be kept in special containers. When there are young children in a household, this precaution is vital. All drugs should be kept in a medicine chest with a lock. When there are children in a household it is best not to use a cupboard under the sink for household cleaners and detergents—these should be kept on a high shelf. Poisons are also found around the house in the form of insecticides, weed killer, rodenticides etc. in greenhouses or garages, and in the form of poisonous plants in the garden. No part of any plant in a garden can be regarded as safe to eat unless it is specially grown to be eaten. Many common garden plants are poisonous, such as bulbs of hyacinths, narcissus, daffodil, larkspur, monkshood, autumn crocus, lily of the valley, iris, lupin and foxglove. Ornamental shrubs and trees are often poisonous, e.g. daphne berries, wisteria seed pods, laburnum seeds, broom seeds, yew berries and foliage, all parts of laurels, rhododendrons, azaleas, yew, twigs and foliage of wild and cultivated cherries, holly and privet berries and oak foliage and acorns.

Doctors and nurses automatically check the label of any medicine to be given to a patient; this check includes the name of the drug, its strength, dose and often its date of manufacture and batch number. Accidents that result from a failure to carry out such simple precautions may have profound effects not only on the patient but also on the doctor's future career. Many people do not realize how easily errors can arise when choosing a bottle from a collection in a medicine cupboard, where bottles of similar shape may contain materials that differ very much in their safety. At one time bottles containing substances for external use—iodine, linaments etc. were both coloured and ridged; in the light their deep purple or green colour was an efficient warning signal and in the dark their ridged surface carried the same message. Nowadays linaments containing the highly poisonous oil of wintergreen may be distinguished only by a red label or some warning message on the bottle.

Below is a list of some ways in which child poisonings may be prevented.

1. Keep all medicines (tablets and bottles) in a locked cupboard. Take particular care of drugs that are regularly used, e.g. aspirin, iron tablets and sleeping tablets that accidentally may be left on dressing tables or bedside tables.

2. Before giving a dose of medicine *always* read the label beforehand. Never be tempted to rely on a sense of touch or smell in choosing the right bottle in the dark.

3. Do not use jam jars, soft drink bottles etc. for storing potential poisons.

4. Do not tell children that a medicine is a sweet. Encourage a cautious attitude to cleaning materials, insecticides, weed killers etc.

List of common household poisonous substances
> Adhesives
> Agricultural chemicals (many)
> Anti-freeze
> Antiseptics (some)
> Bleaching fluid
> Brake-fluid
> Cleaning fluids particularly caustic soda, corrosives etc.
> Cosmetics (hair dyes, permanent wave solutions, nail-polish remover, perfumes etc.)
> Disinfectants (most)
> Drain cleaners (many)
> Fire extinguishers
> Indelible inks and dyes
> Insecticides and fungicides
> Paraffin

Paints (N.B. also painted surfaces
and painted toys if paint contains
lead)
Rodenticides
Weed killers

Gassing

Death from gassing may result from the toxic effect of the unburnt gas itself—e.g. bottled propane or butane or coal gas—or from carbon monoxide poisoning from inefficiently burnt gas or coal or other solid fuels.

Heating by means of coal gas is very common, and apart from fires there are several dangers. First, fittings often leak small amounts of gas which remain undetected, particularly by the elderly in whom the sense of smell may be impaired. Second, taps are sometimes not easily turned completely on or off so that at times not all the burners light, a fact which may not be noticed. Automatic taps that close with a bayonet action and are spring loaded for safety—i.e. they are not easily turned on accidentally—are a great improvement. There is evidence that in many rooms where gas is used for heating or cooking, there are potentially dangerous concentrations of carbon monoxide. Regular inspection and maintenance of appliances and the provision of adequate ventilation could prevent many accidents.

Suffocation

Suffocation is a cause of accidental death mainly in children and the elderly. Inhaling vomit is the usual cause of these accidents. The importance of not leaving infants alone with a feeding bottle in the mouth has already been mentioned. In older children round sweets of about 2–3 cm in diameter are often the cause of choking which may be fatal. Small children should not be given this kind of hard sweet, nor should they be given small nuts, e.g. peanuts or raw peas, since these can be readily inhaled, particularly if a child runs and stumbles with them in the mouth. These small food particles readily pass into one or other of the main bronchi and cause the collapse of a lung or a lung abscess.

Electrocution

In considering accidental electrocution it is important to stress two things. First, the effect of an electric shock depends on the amount of current which flows through the body and not necessarily upon the voltage of the electrical supply. Second the body behaves as a salty solution of electrolytes enclosed in a leathery container; the greatest density of current flow through the body is a long straight line joining two points, one the electrical contact and second the point of exit (earthing) of the current. In order that current can flow through the body these two points are vital. Obviously one cannot be electrocuted without a point of contact with electric current, but it is equally true that one cannot be electrocuted if the current cannot flow out of the body, i.e. if there is no 'earth'. Thus one might touch a 'live' appliance such as a faulty cooker or television set without suffering from an electric shock provided that one is standing on wood or carpet; but touch this appliance whilst at the same time touching a water pipe or radiator, so that the circuit is complete and current flows through the body to earth, and one may be fatally electrocuted.

Normal dry skin has a fairly high resistance to the inward flow of current into the body. If the skin is wet or sweating then the resistance falls dramatically and greatly increases the chance of suffering from a fatal shock if a 'live' object is touched. In fact nearly all shocks at home are precipitated by water because this is such a good conductor of electricity. Thus shocks commonly occur in the bathroom or kitchen. Classically the bathroom electric heater is a source of current that electrocutes a person in the bath—sometimes by the electric radiator actually falling into the bath. Nowadays even more electrical appliances may be used in the bathroom, such as the electric toothbrush or shaver. It is very important that the floors of bathrooms should be of a non-conducting material, that any appliances which 'must' be used in this room are regularly serviced, and that the electricity supply should be controlled by external switches or by pulling a cord.

All electrical equipment should be regularly serviced by a *qualified* person. When buying electrical goods it is best to choose only those tested and found free of shock and fire hazard; these goods bear the BEAB (British Electrical Approvals Board) label. *All* electrical appliances should be earthed.

People die from electric shock because of asphyxia, respiratory arrest or ventricular fibrillation. Often a person is held on to the source of an electric current by the contraction of muscles which are stimulated by the current. If the current passes through the chest the muscles of the chest wall contract and breathing movements become impossible so that asphyxia results. Even after the flow of current has stopped breathing may fail to return to normal, and this may be due to the flow of current through the brain-stem which controls breathing. An important cause of death from electrocution is due to ventricular fibrillation, a condition in which the ventricular muscle of the heart fails to contract and relax in the normal rhythmic manner; in ventricular fibrillation the muscle of the heart contracts irregularly and ineffectively, and the flow of blood from the heart stops. This is the commonest mode of death in electrocution, and rapid treatment to restore the circulation is necessary if the patient is to survive. In the home this treatment must take the form of external cardiac massage and mouth-to-mouth artificial respiration. In this country external cardiac massage has gained wide acceptance and has been adopted by the voluntary first-aid organizations. This treatment does not, however, guarantee recovery—probably less than 20 per cent will recover using treatment with external cardiac massage, even from trained persons—and in some cases the vigorous compression of the chest wall may itself cause serious damage. It is probably easier to prevent ventri-

cular fibrillation than to treat it. One method of prevention is rapidly to disconnect the current from the appliance by means of what is called a low-voltage earth leakage circuit breaker. The principle of this device is shown in Figure 26.10. In (a), under normal conditions the current flows through the appliance between live and neutral. The current thus flows through the two primary coils in the circuit, producing equal and opposite magnetic fluxes in the core of the circuit breaker. In (b), someone has accidentally touched the live side of the circuit so that part of the current flows to earth through his body. Since some current is now flowing through the body of the person touching the appliance, the current in the primary coils 1 and 2 are now unequal. The magnetic fluxes induced are also unequal and current will be induced in the secondary coil 3. This induced current in secondary coil 3 is made to operate the relay R which immediately disconnects the current. This kind of safety device for electrical appliances is used in some countries and is being tried experimentally in Great Britain.

A brief check list of measures for the prevention and control of domestic accidents*

The following list, which is presented in the form of single questions, is intended to be illustrative and elementary rather than exhaustive and technical. It illustrates some precautions that might be considered in a highly developed country, and is intended to provoke discussion among those likely to be involved in home visiting and domestic accident prevention.

Social policy

1. Are all possible uses being made of existing safety legislation?
2. Are there any new laws (or regulations) directed at maintaining standards of construction and equipment?
3. Are all the voluntary agencies mobilized (including key persons in the community and 'pressure groups' such as accident prevention societies)?
4. Are newspapers, radio and posters exploited?
5. Are consumer protection associations supported?
6. Do engineers, architects, electricians, sanitarians, etc., know their obligations?

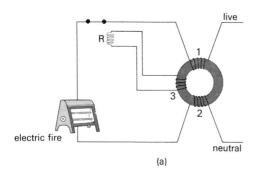

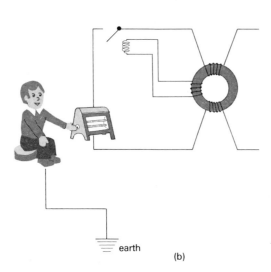

Figure 26.10 Principle of low-voltage earth leakage circuit breaker.

*Reproduced from 'Domestic Accidents', *Public Health Papers* No. 26. World Health Organization, Geneva, by kind permission of Professor E. Maurice Backett, the author, and the World Health Organization.

The individual and risk taking: recognition of danger

1. Are the special senses (eyes, hearing, balance) functioning as well as possible? (Provision of hearing aids, operations for cataract, etc.)
2. Are both parents and children being instructed in how to recognize common dangers?
3. Have health personnel (nurses, health visitors, physicians and sanitary workers) been mobilized to play their part?
4. Are the specially vulnerable groups well known?
5. Has the schoolteacher been asked to help? (The experimental home, trial and error games, etc.)
6. Have the elderly been instructed about and shown the common dangers?
7. Are those in charge of vulnerable persons fully trained?

The agent and the environment
(examples only)

Surroundings of the house

1. Are all wells, ditches, drains and pits properly covered or otherwise guarded?
2. Are there in the neighbourhood any old wells etc. covered with wood that may now be rotten?
3. Are overhead electricity supply lines accessible to children?
4. Have small children been supplied with buoyant clothing?
5. Is clothing likely to impede escape from water?
6. Is the property adequately fenced?

The kitchen

1. Are all electrical insulations up to standard?
2. Are any electric points accessible to young children?
3. Are any electric contacts possible between the source of current, the individual and the water supply?
4. Are all electrical gadgets earthed?
5. Are all electric points fitted with a separate fuse?
6. Is there adequate lighting?
7. Are all high-speed cutting devices foolproof?
8. Is domestic water delivered at over 60 °C?
9. Are open flames (cooking stoves, etc.) less than three feet from the ground?

10. Are all cooking utensils broad at the base?
11. Do all cooking utensils have low centres of gravity?
12. Do all cooking utensils have rough, short or detachable handles?
13. Do ovens have double doors and an inside light?
14. If coal gas is used, is there adequate ventilation?
15. Has the pipe system been checked for leaks?
16. Have old persons been tested to see if they can smell coal gas?
17. If kerosene (paraffin) is used, how is it stored?
18. Is food kept separate from household cleansers, etc.?
19. Can electric kettles easily be pulled over by their cable or knocked over by hand?
20. Is the floor particularly slippery when wet?
21. How are heights reached?
22. Are matches near a heat source or within access of children?
23. Are only safety matches used?
24. Where are oils and waxes stored?
25. Do can openers leave raw-metal edges?
26. Do powered washers and driers switch off automatically when opened?

The bathroom

1. Are all sources of electric current outside the room or suitably earthed and covered?
2. Can any electric point be reached while in contact with water?
3. Is the floor slippery when wet?
4. Are there handrails to the bath, etc.?
5. Is there a bell, or could a call be heard?
6. Is the water delivered at over 60 °C?
7. Is the bath too high for easy access by some occupants of the house (e.g. children and old people)?
8. How is the bathroom heated? Are electric heaters used?
9. If the water heating is by coal gas, are ventilation and safety devices functioning?

The stairs

1. Are the stairs too steep?
2. Are they well lit?
3. Are they regular and straight and of uniform height?
4. Are there loose coverings?
5. Are there firm handrails on both sides?
6. Are there smaller or larger steps at bottom or top?
7. Is there a loose carpet at the bottom of the stair-case?

8. Is there a switching system of lights so that the stairs can always be negotiated in the light?
9. Are there any loose boards or steps?
10. Is the stair-carpet pinned securely to the floor at the top and bottom of the stair-case?
11. Do any doors open on to the stairs?

The living-room

1. Is the electricity supply fool-proof?
2. Is the floor polished?
3. Are the floor coverings easily moved?
4. Are they backed by rubber?
5. Are the edges of the floor coverings fixed securely?
6. Is there an open fire?
7. Are heaters and fire adequately guarded?
8. Is the fire well enclosed?
9. Is the fire well ventilated?
10. If utility gas is used, is the pipe system intact and are the taps functioning correctly?
11. Is the system efficiently ventilated in case gas escapes?

The bedroom

1. Electrical installations and floor coverings—same questions as above.
2. If the occupant is an elderly person, is the bed too high for easy access?
3. How is the room heated? (If by utility gas, same questions as above.)
4. Where are drugs stored? Are they out of reach? Are they labelled?
5. If the occupant is an elderly person, how near is the bedroom to the toilet?
6. Is lighting adequate?
7. Are ashtrays safe?

The toilet

1. Are floor coverings adequate and non-slip?
2. Are handrails installed (particularly if there are elderly persons in the household)?
3. Is the toilet shared with other households and does it have to be reached by going up or down stairs?

The workroom or workshop

1. Are power tools (particularly drills, saws and wire brushes) adequately protected?
2. Are power tools adequately earthed?
3. Does lighting reach normal industrial standards?

The garage

1. Is ventilation adequate?
2. Can the car be reversed into the garage?
3. If the garage is also used as a car workshop, can the car engine be run easily when the garage doors are closed?
4. Is the floor level?
5. Are inspection lamps, battery chargers etc. earthed?
6. Is petrol stored?

General points to be checked

1. The clothing of small children (nightdresses particularly) should not be inflammable.
2. The shoes and slippers of elderly people must fit well and have rubber or plastic soles and heels.
3. Portable heaters—electric or oil—should be space heaters with enclosed elements.
4. Upstairs windows should not be accessible to small children, and it should be possible to clean them from within the room.
5. Access to roof spaces should be by fixed ladder. The space itself should have a floor.
6. Safety rings should be set into high walls, chimneys, etc., for outside working.
7. Colour codes on all wiring must conform to standards.
8. Wiring and fusing standards must be high.
9. Fire exits must be available, as well as some means of extinguishing fires.
10. The integrity of gas systems must be checked regularly.
11. Air conditioning systems (particularly if using gas) must be checked regularly.
12. Walking sticks, plastic bags, medicine cupboard locks, domestic equipment (washing machines, vacuum cleaners, etc.), television and radios, and step-ladders should all be checked regularly.
13. The structural features of balconies should be sound.
14. Unused medicines should be safely destroyed.
15. Garden tools, particularly power tools (e.g. hedge-trimmers), should be inspected.
16. Volatile domestic solvents, paints and caustic alkalis should be safely stored.
17. All floors should be checked for irregular or loose boards etc.
18. All ashtrays should be of the bowl type—preferably totally enclosed.
19. Large sheets of plate glass should be clearly visible.

Minimizing the effect of domestic accidents

Communications

1. Are there telephones or other methods of communication available—particularly to old people?
2. Do those most at risk (or those in charge) know how to use them?

The family

1. Are all members of the family mobile?
2. Can they escape from or deal with common dangers?
3. Can they swim?
4. Do they understand first-aid and resuscitation?

Medical aspects

1. Are medical care facilities and, in particular, first-aid services available?
2. Are emergency transport (ambulance, car) services available?
3. Are special casualty services (e.g. burns units and poison units) available?
4. Are rehabilitation services available?

Economic aspects

1. Does insurance for all members of the family cover all accident risks, medical care and compensation for unemployment due to injury?
2. Does legislation allow for compensation or other redress?

27. Venereal disease

Introduction

VENEREAL disease is a world-wide problem. In many countries there has been a persistent rise in some venereal diseases, which have now reached epidemic proportions. Britain is no exception to this problem, as shown by the number of patients attending Venereal Disease Clinics; in 1964 there were about 153 000 people attending these clinics and by 1969 this figure had risen to over 230 000. In the following pages we will be looking briefly at the nature of common and important venereal diseases, and we will pay special attention to measures aimed at controlling these diseases.

Definition of venereal disease

The term venereal describes an infection which is spread from one person to another by and during sexual intercourse or contact. The sexual contact may be between individuals of the opposite sex (i.e. heterosexual) or between individuals of the same sex (homosexual). There are, however, some definite exceptions to this rule. Some infants are infected with syphilis from the mother while they are still in the womb. Blood which contains the infective organisms can also transmit the disease; syphilis has been reported on rare occasions as being caused by transfusions of blood or by tattooing. Fortunately individuals suffering from syphilis are routinely barred from acting as blood donors in Great Britain. Babies may also suffer gonococcal infection of the eye by contamination with the infected vaginal secretions during the process of birth. Transmission of the diseases other than by sexual contact or by the above mentioned special situations, is rather rare. It is highly unlikely that simple contact with an infected person can cause a venereal disease.

About a dozen diseases are capable of being transmitted during sexual intercourse. Of these diseases only three—gonorrhoea, syphilis and chancroid—are defined *in law* as venereal. However we will make no distinction between *legal* venereal diseases and sexually transmitted diseases. Of these twelve or so diseases gonor-rhoea and syphilis form the bulk of the problem, and most of this chapter will be concerned with these two diseases. Other diseases such as chancroid (soft sore), lymphogranuloma venereum and granuloma inguinale are very uncommon in Great Britain (except in immigrants) and are more often seen in tropical and subtropical parts of the world. We will, however, be looking at two 'newer' venereal diseases—diseases which have fairly recently been recognized as commonly transmitted during sexual intercourse. The first of these two diseases is non-specific urethritis. The term non-specific means that no particular cause has been found for this malady—no bacterium, virus or other micro-organism has been isolated from cases of this disease. The second is a disease called trichomoniasis—an infection caused by a minute protozoan parasite called *Trichomonas vaginalis*. There is increasing evidence that this is *often* transmitted during sexual intercourse.

There are yet other diseases which, although not regularly transmitted during sexual intercourse, may occasionally be so transmitted. These diseases are usually those of the skin—scabies, lice, genital warts etc.

Gonorrhoea and syphilis

Gonorrhoea and syphilis have been known for centuries, although they were recognized as two distinct diseases as late as 1793. The diseases have, through the centuries, waxed and waned. A virulent epidemic of what we know to be syphilis raged in Europe from the end of the fifteenth century to the middle of the sixteenth century. The disease is thought, by some, to have been introduced into Europe in the fifteenth century by the return of Columbus' men suffering from 'Indian measles'. Tens of thousands died in the hundred years or so of this European epidemic.

Syphilis

Syphilis is caused by a micro-organism called *Treponema pallidum* (Figure 2.4). This organism

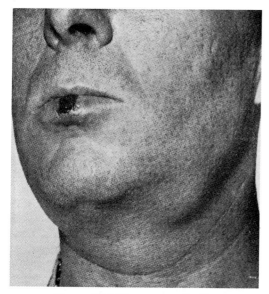

Figure 27.1 Chancre on the lip.

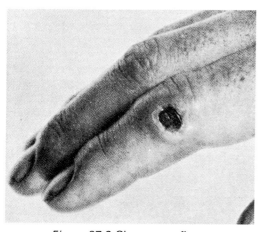

Figure 27.2 Chancre on finger.

is a spirochaete, an elongated, flexible creature twisted spirally along its long axis. This is a purely human parasite; it dies very quickly when allowed to dry, and it has proved quite impossible to culture the organism in the laboratory.

Syphilis is a disease of a very chronic nature, with widespread damage of tissues occurring over the years. From the beginning of the disease the organism is widespread in the body tissues, and many different organs may become involved —e.g. skin, aorta, spinal cord and brain, bone etc.—producing conditions which may mimic many other diseases in the fields of medicine and surgery.

This disease is nearly always acquired by direct contact, usually venereal. Indirect transmission of the disease by clothing, drinking

utensils etc. is extremely rare for the reason mentioned above—the very brief life of the organism outside the human body. Syphilitic women transmit the disease to their unborn children because the spirochaetes can pass across the placenta from mother to foetus, resulting in foetal death or the birth of an infant whose various body tissues are damaged in ways which produce the 'stigmata' of congenital syphilis—see below. With the exception of congenital syphilis, the disease is marked by three stages—primary, secondary and tertiary.

The primary phase of syphilis follows the introduction of the spirochaete through a small abrasion in the skin or mucous membrane, usually as a result of sex contact. The spirochaetes begin to multiply in the tissues and rapidly spread throughout the body, even before the first signs of infection appear at the place where the spirochaetes entered the body. This incubation period, before the first signs of the disease appears, may vary widely from ten to ninety days but is usually two to four weeks. The first sign of the disease is one, sometimes several, sores called chancres. A chancre is a rounded, regular, usually painless ulcer. Most chancres appear on the genitalia; in the female these may pass unnoticed if they appear in the internal parts such as the cervix (neck of the womb) or on the wall of the vagina. Chancres can, however, be found on any part of the body surface—e.g. lip, tongue, tonsils, eyelid, nipple, finger (Figures 27.1, 27.2). In the absence of treatment, the chancre slowly heals in three to eight weeks, leaving a thin scar.

The secondary stage of the disease usually begins six to eight weeks after the beginning of the primary stage, although occasionally the delay may be as long as a year or more. This secondary stage has many possible features which include slight fever, skin rashes, a sore and ulcerated throat, general enlargement of the lymph glands of the body and often disorders of bone, eye and other organs. The skin rashes vary greatly in their character and can mimic many other skin diseases (Figures 27.3, 27.4, 27.5). During the secondary stage of the disease, which usually lasts about two years, the patient may be highly infectious, particularly from the moist lesions of the mouth and skin. It is, however, important to note that both the primary and secondary stages of this disease may be very inconspicuous or brief, and they may not be noticed by the patient.

After the second year of the disease, syphilis enters the tertiary stage when the patient is usually non-infectious. There may be no

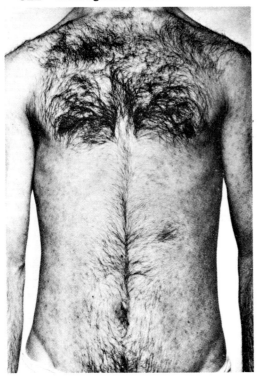

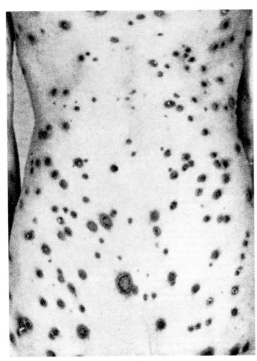

symptoms due to the disease for many years and indeed the patient may die from some quite other condition. During this stage of the disease many tissues of the body may become damaged by the infection. It has been estimated that about 70 000 people in the world die each year from the late effects of syphilis, although this is probably a marked underestimate of deaths due to this disease. It is thought that if syphilis is untreated, one in thirteen people will develop syphilitic heart disease (with aneurysms of the aorta (Figure 27.6)—see page 283 for description of an aneurysm), one in twenty-five will become crippled or incapacitated, one in forty-four will develop syphilitic insanity and one in two hundred will become blind. This situation, in a world where syphilis is a common disease in undeveloped nations, is serious; the maximum frequency of syphilis in Africa during the period 1950–60 was in Basutoland, where over 1000 in every 100 000 of the adult population over sixteen suffered from early syphilis.

Syphilis is obviously a serious disease for the individual, and it is by no means an uncommon disease. In the United States, the National Health Survey produced evidence that 4.4 per cent of white males, 3.6 per cent of white females, 22.9 per cent negro males and 3.6 per cent negro females had positive blood tests for the disease. Maximum rates of syphilis for various regions of the world during the period 1950–60 have been estimated as 1232 per 100 000

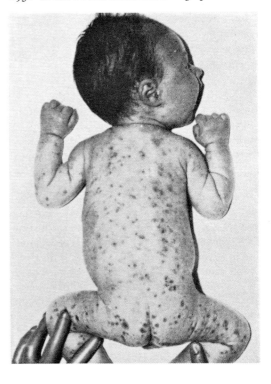

Figure 27.3 (top)   A rash of secondary syphilis

Figure 27.4 (bottom)   A rash of secondary syphilis.

Figure 27.5 (right)   Congenital syphilis with generalized rash.

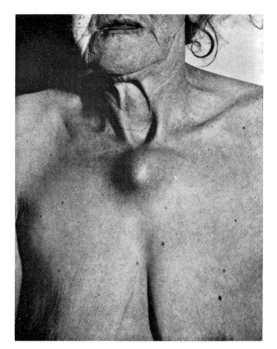

Figure 27.6 Syphylitic aneurysm of the aorta. The pulsations of the aneurysm are eroding away the upper part of the sternum.

in Basutoland (Africa), 340 per 100 000 in Columbia (America), 3687 per 100 000 in the Sudan (Eastern Mediterranean) and 53.6 per 100 000 in Yugoslavia (Europe). In some parts of the world, including Great Britain, syphilis is slowly decreasing in frequency. In 1964 there were 3775 cases of syphilis seen in Venereal Disease Clinics in England and Wales; this figure fell to 3413 in 1969. Part of the success in this 'control' of syphilis is due to the fact that precise diagnostic tests are available, using blood samples, even when there is no evidence of infection. It is thus possible to screen large groups of the population for evidence of this disease—groups such as pregnant women, blood donors and couples seeking medical examinations before marriage. The situation is the reverse of that seen in gonorrhoea, where the only proof of infection is to isolate the bacterium— the gonococcus—from the patient. In many women gonorrhoea produces no symptoms and they do not seek diagnosis or treatment; even if they do seek treatment, diagnosis may not be easily made. This difference in the ease of diagnosis between syphilis and gonorrhoea is one of the reasons for the rapidly accelerating growth of gonorrhoea in many countries.

Treatment of syphilis

Penicillin is the drug of choice for the treatment of syphilis in all of its stages, although there are alternative antibiotics or drugs for those individuals who are 'sensitive' to penicillin. In the treatment of early syphilis ten to twenty daily injections of penicillin cures more than 95 per cent of cases. Some patients are, of course, uncooperative and will not return for treatment after one or more injections, and so some venereologists use a single large dose of a long-acting penicillin which is also very effective. Obviously the patients are also instructed to avoid sexual intercourse till tests show that they have been cleared of the disease.

The treatment of early syphilis is thus simple and straightforward. Treatment of late syphilis, in which the heart or other organs have become damaged, is more complicated; in-patient treatment in hospital is usually necessary, and surgery may be needed for strengthening a damaged aorta or for damaged joints. Congenital syphilis is easily prevented by the administration of penicillin to the syphilitic woman who is pregnant.

Gonorrhoea

Gonorrhoea is a venereal disease of increasing importance, and it now reaches epidemic proportions in many countries. Like all venereal diseases it was common during and after the Second World War, and in 1946 the number of cases of gonorrhoea diagnosed in clinics in England and Wales was 47 343. Following this there was a rapid post-war decline in its importance, so that by 1954 the number of cases was 17 536 per year. Since 1954 the number of cases has risen almost every year. The Annual Reports of the Chief Medical Officer of the Ministry of Health gives figures for England and Wales of 36 665 in 1964, 41 829 in 1967 and 51 260 in 1969. These figures underestimate the true incidence of the disease, for they do not include cases treated by general practitioners or specialists in private practice, or cases treated by Medical Officers in the armed forces. In the U.S.A., reported cases of gonorrhoea rose from 216 476 in 1957 to 375 606 in 1967. In the world population it has been estimated that the number of new cases of gonorrhoea exceeds 60 million each year. In a later section of this chapter we will discuss the probable causes for this new epidemic.

The organism responsible for gonorrhoea, the gonococcus, is a strict parasite of man and is

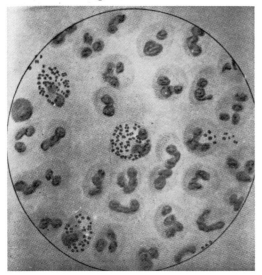

Figure 27.7 Photomicrograph of a Gram-stained slide showing typical Gram-negative diplococci within pus cells (white blood cells).

never found free in nature. The disease can only be diagnosed by finding these organisms in secretions from the genital tract (Figure 27.7) or in cultures of the secretions in the laboratory. It is a difficult organism to culture in the laboratory, and media enriched by blood, serum or other materials is necessary. After culture of the organisms in the laboratory, a firm diagnosis also depends on certain biochemical reactions carried out by the organism.

In adults the disease nearly always results from sexual intercourse with an infected person. In children infection can occur in other ways such as sharing a bed with infected parents, and the newborn may be infected during the process of birth. In the past epidemics of the disease have occurred in children's hospitals because of some failure in nursing care, such as inadequate disinfection of thermometers, bed pans etc.

The incubation period of the disease is short, usually about five days, although it may vary from two to ten days. The symptoms of the disease vary considerably between the sexes. In the male there is a burning feeling in the penis with discomfort on passing urine. Later there is a yellow discharge. These local symptoms may also be accompanied by fever, headache and a feeling of being generally unwell. The symptoms in the male may be more severe because the gonococcus infects accessory structures of the male reproductive system such as the prostate gland or the epididymis, and swelling and abscesses may occur in these infected areas. If the disease is untreated, various tissues may

become severely damaged, perhaps the most disabling of which is a local constriction of the urethra which makes for difficulty in passing urine. Disorders of joints and eyes may also occur.

In the female there may be no symptoms of gonorrhoea of the genital tract. Up to 50 per cent of cases of acute and uncomplicated cases of gonorrhoea in women fall into this category, and many of these women are detected only because their male partner has developed symptoms. The commonest sites of the infection in women are the urethra and the cervix (neck of the womb). The infection can spread from the cervix to the body of the womb and then to the Fallopian tubes, which may become filled with pus. This extension of the infection may have immediate or late serious consequences. Infection of the Fallopian tubes can cause a general pelvic peritonitis—with fever and abdominal pain. The late effects of Fallopian tube infection can include obstruction of these tubes so that they can no longer transport the eggs from the ovaries into the body of the uterus, i.e. the woman becomes sterile.

We have already seen that symptoms may be absent, or not enough to attract the patient's attention, in about half the cases of acute and uncomplicated gonorrhoea in the female. When symptoms do occur, they consist mainly of a scalding or burning pain on passing urine. There is a discharge from the opening of the urethra but women do not usually notice this because of the presence of normal secretions. Infection of the cervix usually passes without any symptoms, but sometimes there is a feeling of low backache or abdominal discomfort. In severe infections of the neck of the womb there may be a profuse yellow secretion which is enough to cause the women to complain of vaginal discharge. Some of the complications of acute gonorrhoea—infection of the Fallopian tubes, pelvic peritonitis or abscess—have already been mentioned. There also may be complications in the external genitalia, usually of one or more of the glands that open into the region of the external genitals.

In untreated cases a state of chronic gonorrhoea may develop which may be extremely difficult to diagnose because the gonococcus tends to disappear from the secretions of the genital tract. Sometimes the only evidence of the nature of this condition is that the woman has recently infected a male partner. If the gonococcus has reached the cavity of the pelvis it may cause much chronic ill health, with recurring attacks of lower abdominal pain and a low-grade fever, or painful, heavy or irregular periods. If both Fallopian tubes have been involved in the infection, sterility is likely.

The treatment of gonorrhoea

The introduction of various drugs e.g. sulphonamides and various antibiotics, has revolutionized the treatment of gonorrhoea. We have seen that the early dramatic successes with sulphonamides was short lived due to the development of sulphonamide resistance by the gonococcus (page 99). Nowadays sulphonamides are successful in some 15–30 per cent of cases, although the recent use of sulphonamide-trimethoprim mixtures produces far better results (see also page 215).

The introduction of penicillin caused the virtual abandoning of sulphonamides for the treatment of gonorrhoea. The gonococcus was found to be one of the most susceptible of bacteria to the action of penicillin, and small doses completely cured most cases. Nowadays, the gonococcus is less sensitive to penicillin, and larger doses of the drug are needed to clear the infection. There are other antibiotics which are also active against the gonococcus, drugs such as streptomycin, tetracyclines and erythromycin. The advantages of some of these drugs is that they are not very active against *Treponema pallidum*, so that they do not suppress the diagnostic signs of syphilis—for some patients may contract both diseases simultaneously. Thus the treatment of gonorrhoea without complications is straightforward. A more difficult problem is the treatment of the effects of chronic infections such as strictures (localized narrowing) of the urethra in the male or chronic pelvic infection in women. During the course of treatment patients should avoid sexual contacts until they have been pronounced free of infection.

Non-specific urethritis in males

This condition is a common disease of males which may sometimes closely mimic an acute attack of gonorrhoea. There is little doubt that the disease is spread by intercourse, but no organism has been isolated from patients. Like gonorrhoea the disease has increased in numbers, and in 1969 it was diagnosed in over 41 000 males in Venereal Disease Clinics in England and Wales.

After an incubation period which is thought to be eight to fourteen days (sometimes longer) the disease appears with symptoms of inflammation of the urethra. Often there is only a burning discomfort on passing urine but the symptoms may be more severe, with a discharge that makes the disease indistinguishable from gonorrhoea. The disease can only be diagnosed by exclusion, i.e. from the absence of any pathogenic bacteria in the urine or in the urethral discharge. The disease will gradually disappear over the course of weeks even without treatment, although nowadays a drug (e.g. streptomycin, sulphonamides, tetracyclines) is usually given to shorten the period of discomfort and reduce the risk of infection of others.

In the female the disease may be present without any symptoms, and may be diagnosed only on the knowledge of infection in a male partner.

Trichomonal infections

Figure 27.8 is a drawing of a minute motile protozoan that may infect the uro-genital tract of men and women. When infected secretions are examined freshly under the microscope, typical jerky movements of the creatures can be seen.

Infection by this organism is fairly common, although its true incidence is difficult to estimate. Studies of various groups of women—e.g. those attending birth control clinics, gynaecological or venereal disease clinics, and women prisoners—

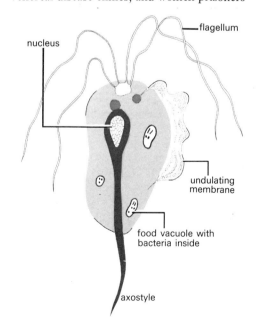

Figure 27.8 H.P. sketch of the flagellated protozoan parasite *Trichomonas vaginalis.*

have found numbers ranging from 0–70 per cent of women examined. The highest figure, 70 per cent, was in a group of over 200 women prisoners, most of whom had been drug addicts or prostitutes. It is reasonable to suppose that the male partners of infected women may also be infected, although the isolation of the organism from men without symptoms may be difficult. Various studies of male partners of infected women have found that in 19–70 per cent of the men it was possible to isolate trichomonads. The importance of these findings is that whenever a woman is treated for a trichomonal infection, her male partner should receive treatment simultaneously.

Infection in women

This infection can occur at any age, but it usually occurs during the years of sexual activity. The minute protozoa are nearly always transmitted during sexual intercourse; however, occasionally infection may occur from borrowed clothing, towels, splashes from water closets or from secretions recently deposited on a lavatory seat. When the disease is first diagnosed it may have been present for a long period, so that there may in fact be no history of recent sexual activity.

In most women the infection is of the vagina. Although the infection may produce no symptoms, most individuals complain of a vaginal discharge, usually thin, yellowish and offensive. This discharge may cause inflammation of the vulva and soreness between the thighs. In some cases the urethra is also infected and there may be discomfort on passing urine. The disease is diagnosed by seeing the organisms under the microscope in a fresh sample of secretions and by culturing the organisms in the laboratory.

The treatment of this condition has been greatly improved by the introduction of a drug called metronitazole ('Flagyl') which is taken by mouth in the form of tablets. A seven-day course of this safe drug clears over 80 per cent of cases without any local treatment to the urogenital organs. Of course, both sexual partners are treated simultaneously, even if it proves impossible to isolate the organism from one of them.

The control of veneral diseases

Syphilis

We have seen that in Great Britain at least, cases of syphilis have decreased somewhat in recent years (from 3755 cases in 1964 to 3413 in 1969) in spite of an increase in the total population. There are various reasons for this state of affairs, which contrasts strongly with the virtual epidemic character of gonorrhoea. Syphilis can be readily diagnosed from blood tests (for the presence of antibodies and other changes in blood proteins) even when there is no real evidence of the infection such as sores or skin rashes. A blood test for syphilis is a routine feature of the examination of pregnant women, and treatment of infected individuals has thus virtually abolished congenital syphilis.

The main reservoir of syphilis appears to be in prostitutes of either sex, and very many of these are in London. The practice of prostitution has declined in recent years. A survey in 1969 showed that only about one in ten of known contacts of men with gonorrhoea were prostitutes. Nowadays the kind of men that have need of prostitutes include older men, the sexually perverted and foreign visitors. The rest of the sexually promiscuous community now have no need of prostitutes. These features, the easy diagnosis of syphilis and the declining contact of the new generation with the known reservoir of syphilis (prostitutes), could account for the control of the disease in Britain.

Gonorrhoea

A variety of factors would seem to have combined to increase the spread of gonorrhoea.

Social factors. Patterns of sexual activity

An absence of sexual activity is a sure guarantee of the freedom from venereal disease, although few would suggest this as a remedy for the situation. A stable sexual relationship with one person, either inside or outside marriage, is also a good guarantee of freedom from these diseases. A stable sexual relationship is more likely to occur in the group over twenty-five years of age. Gonorrhoea is becoming increasingly a disease of the younger age groups; the clear increase in the number of pregnancies and abortions in unmarried young women reflects the increasing sexual activity, if not promiscuity, of young people. In some groups there is now considerably less restraint on premarital sexual activity, restraint that was formally imposed by family and public opinion and by the authority of the Church. Indiscriminate and brief sexual relationships in which one partner may not even know the other's name or address creates considerable difficulties for the tracing of infected individuals, a technique that has had much success in the control of venereal diseases (see below). Nowadays many individuals no longer fear these diseases; they do not feel any stigma attached to their condition, they are treated kindly and sympathetically at venereal disease clinics and they feel assured of a simple straightforward cure for any infection that might result from a casual sexual relationship.

Homosexuals may sometimes be very promiscuous. This pattern of behaviour is in part due to social, if not legal, pressures which prevent the establishment of a stable sexual relationship between two homosexuals. In the homosexual societies that have established themselves in major cities all over the world, the homosexual is likely to contract both syphilis and gonorrhoea simultaneously during his activities.

Travellers and immigrants

The increased mobility of people is one important factor in the spread of venereal disease. Promiscuity tends to appear in travellers all over the world, even when the separation from the regular sex partner is only for a short period. Commercial travellers have been subjected to many 'music hall' jokes on this subject, but they are by no means the only group at risk.

Immigration of single men from Asia and the Caribbean is one factor in the spread of venereal disease in Britain. The more recent organization of immigrants as family units will probably reduce this problem.

Ignorance

In spite of recent popularization of health subjects by television and magazines and by the emergence of a more liberal attitude to the discussion of venereal disease in the general public, many surveys have shown widespread ignorance about venereal disease in young people. There is obviously a need for more education on this subject, which includes information about the risks of promiscuity, about the early symptoms of the disease, where to go for treatment, and the assurance that the individual will be treated sympathetically and in confidence.

Medical factors

There are various medical factors which contribute to the failure of control of venereal diseases, not the least of which is a deficiency of money and manpower to control what is,

numerically at least, one of the most important communicable diseases. The diagnosis and treatment of these diseases is not always as straightforward and simple as may be thought from the accounts in the preceding pages. The lack of symptoms of gonorrhoea in many females and in some male homosexuals is certainly a problem, and there is a great need for a screening method for this disease which can be carried out without examining the genital organs. The increasing resistance of some strains of gonococci to penicillin is also a problem, one that is worst in the war areas of the Far East. In addition to the need for better diagnostic tests for gonorrhoea, there is an urgent need for the development of vaccines which could prevent these diseases. Unfortunately there is no experimental animal that can be reliably infected with the gonococcus. In view of the fact that many natural infections with the living organism fail to produce any immunity, the chances of immunizing with dead gonococci seems remote.

Methods of control

Health education

Since not all sexually active men and women, young or old, married or unmarried, will be faithful to one partner, it is important that sex education should begin before puberty. Children should be fully aware of the risks of promiscuity, risks that include unwanted pregnancies, venereal disease and difficulties in personal relationships. Insofar as venereal diseases are concerned they should at least know the early signs of gonorrhoea and syphilis, and where they can obtain information, advice and treatment, i.e. at 'special clinics' attached to most hospitals, where their confidences will be respected.

Treatment of contacts

When venereal disease has been diagnosed in an individual, it is important to try and trace the sexual contacts of the patient so that these contacts can be offered the opportunity of medical examination and tests for venereal disease. In some cases the original patient searches out the contact and hands on a 'contact slip' which carries a warning that the person may be suffering from venereal disease and gives details of where they may seek advice. This method is certainly not 100 per cent successful and brings in at best only a quarter of the infecting or infected contacts; with very promiscuous individuals or in infections picked up on travels or holidays, the patient may not know the name or address of the person who infected him.

More recent advances in contact tracing have involved the cooperation of local health authorities who have seconded social workers to find contacts or to trace patients who have failed to complete a course of treatment. Using this method it is possible to trace contacts living in other areas of the country, and through the Department of Health and Social Security international contact tracing is possible. In the U.S.A. this approach has been carried even further; here the 'cluster technique' is used in which not only sex contacts but also friends of the patient, who may be promiscuous, are offered treatment.

The prevention of veneral disease by drugs, vaccines and contraceptives

There is no satisfactory method of preventing venereal disease. No vaccine is yet available for either syphilis or gonorrhoea. In the Far East the World Health Organization is studying the use of 'antibiotic foams' for vaginal use by promiscuous women. However, the prevention of disease by means of drugs has never been popular with most doctors, for it carries risks of the evolution of drug-resistant strains of microorganisms, and it can lead to the patient becoming allergic to the drug so that the drug can never again be used in the patient, even for a life-endangering infection. The only device which offers *some* protection is' the use of a condom by the male partner.

28. Drug abuse and drug addiction

Introduction

Definition of the term drug

FOR the purposes of this chapter the term *drug* will be used for any chemical substance, either natural or synthetic, which can alter the psychological state of an individual (changes in mood, consciousness, behaviour etc.) and which may be abused to the detriment of the individual and of society. These drugs are classified as follows:

1. tobacco—this is such an important subject as to be the subject of a separate chapter,
2. alcohol,
3. morphine-type drugs (opiates), e.g. morphine, opium, heroin and synthetic substances with a morphine-like effect such as pethidine and methadone,
4. barbiturate-type drugs, e.g. pentobarbital, secobarbital, meprobamate, glutethimide and chlordiazepoxide,
5. stimulants such as cocaine and amphetamines (amphetamine, dexamphetamine, metamphetamine, phenmetrazine, diethylproprion),
6. hallucinogens, e.g. LSD, mescaline, psilocybin.

Drugs in the history of man and in different cultures today

Throughout the recorded history of man each society has had drugs capable of producing profound effects on mood and behaviour. In each society there have always been some people who have failed to follow the general pattern of using the drug, in that they have taken more of the drug, or have taken it for different reasons or in different situations from the majority of users. In this sense, the phenomenon of the misuse of drugs is as old as man himself. The notion that a particular drug is being abused varies during the history of a culture and between cultures. Even in one particular culture the attitudes to the drug vary, the drug being acceptable in one situation but its use frowned upon or severely punished in another situation. In our society chronic intoxication with alcohol is generally regarded as an abuse of alcohol, and yet extreme degrees of intoxication are acceptable in certain situations, e.g. rugby-club sprees or 'stag' parties. Similarly society regards the use of barbiturates as a sedative before sleep as perfectly acceptable, but to use the drug in a different social setting would be regarded as abuse.

Different cultures tend to have different drugs that are regarded as acceptable or reprehensible, and the same drug may be used for very different reasons in different cultures. In western culture the use of cocaine for any reason other than its restricted medical applications (as a local anaesthetic or vasoconstrictor) is regarded with disfavour, and is indeed a punishable offence in law. In fact this stimulant drug is not often abused in our culture; amphetamines, which are cheap and relatively freely available, take the place of cocaine. This state of affairs contrasts strongly with that found in some areas of South America. In the Andes the chewing of coca leaves (the source of cocaine) is practised by about 90 per cent of the adult male population. Similar cultural differences are found with morphine-type drugs. In western cultures the use of morphine, heroin and the like, is regarded as serious drug abuse, and yet in many eastern countries opium is an accepted part of the culture as an aid to relaxation and meditation.

Compulsive abuse of drugs and drug dependence (addiction)

In 1964 a World Health Organization Scientific Group on the Evaluation of Dependence-Producing Drugs defined drug dependence as 'a state arising from the repeated administration of a drug on a periodic or continuous basis'. This term drug dependence is used to describe all types of drug abuse, and the term itself carries no notion of the degree of health risk to the individual. The report goes on to state that 'individuals may become dependent upon a wide variety of chemical substances', and these chemicals include drugs that stimulate or depress the nervous system. 'They are capable of creating a state of mind in certain individuals which is termed psychic dependence. This is a psychic

Table 35 The effects of various drugs

Drug	Psychological dependence shown by craving and compulsive use	Pronounced psychic effects on administration of the drug	Tolerance	Physical dependence
Alcohol	+	+	+	+
Tobacco	+	−	+	+
Morphine and similar drugs	+	−	+	+
Cocaine	+	+		
LSD	+	+		
Amphetamines	+	+		
Marijuana	+	+		
Barbiturates	+	+	+	+

drive which requires periodic or chronic administration of the drug for pleasure or to avoid discomfort. . . . Some drugs also induce physical dependence, an adaptive state characterized by intense physical disturbances when administration of the drug is suspended.' In simple terms, people take drugs repeatedly either because of an intense need for the state of mind that the drug produces (psychological dependence), or because their bodies have become so 'used' to the presence of the drugs (addiction) that they become ill when the drugs are not available (the withdrawal or abstinence syndrome). The kind of disorders that appear when a drug–dependent person is deprived of his drug vary according to the nature of the drug, but range from the relatively mild restlessness and irritability of the tobacco smoker to the catastrophic bodily and mental changes that occur in individuals who are physically dependent upon heroin, morphine or barbiturates.

Drugs are not equally likely to produce this problem of physical dependence (see Table 35). Some drugs, such as heroin, if taken over a period of time regularly produce physical dependence, whereas other drugs such as barbiturates and alcohol only occasionally do so; however, since the consumption of alcohol and barbiturates is enormous compared to heroin, physical dependence upon these drugs is a common problem. The use of amphetamines and marijuana is very rarely associated with the development of physical dependence, while the use of cocaine and LSD is completely free from this risk. In spite of the dramatic sufferings that are experienced by the physically dependent addict when he is deprived of his particular brand of poison, physical dependence is easier to treat than psychological dependence. Long

after an individual has been weaned from physical dependence on a drug, some personal or social problem may drive him back to seek the mental release that comes from using the drug.

Drug tolerance

Physical dependence on drugs is closely linked with a feature called tolerance. Tolerance develops when a drug produces decreasing effects on an individual, so that larger and larger doses may have to be taken to produce an effect similar to that produced by the original dose. Tolerance is a pronounced feature of the use of morphine-like drugs, barbiturates and alcohol.

Why people become compulsive users of drugs

An individual's initial contact with a drug is determined by many kinds of factors such as curiosity, the presence of mental illness, chance contacts and the accessibility of a particular drug, which in turn will be determined by the society and sub-stratum of society in which the individual lives or moves. What is even more difficult to understand is why some people will have no wish to repeat a drug-taking experience while others will become compelled to use the drug time and time again. When a drug such as alcohol produces pleasurable effects, we can perhaps sympathize with the one user in 500 who eventually becomes an alcoholic; we can understand that the effects of alcohol are being used to relieve psychological and social pressures. In the case of heroin our understanding and compassion are stretched. Few normal people who are not in severe pain experience any pleasant feelings after taking the drug, indeed the experience may be most unpleasant with nausea and vomiting. Even many confirmed addicts to these drugs describe their initial experiences with the drugs as being unpleasant. It would seem that any pleasant effects of such drugs have to be learned. Most workers in this field have concluded that anyone who can persist with the very unpleasant initial effects to uncover relaxing or pleasurable effects must have some psychological disorder that was present before using the drug.

Once a person has become physically dependent upon drugs such as alcohol, morphine or barbiturates, then the reason for continued use is all too clear. Individuals continue to take these drugs in order to avoid the devastatingly unpleasant effects that appear on withdrawal of the drug. The whole of an individual's existence comes to be devoted to the seeking and taking of drugs, to the detriment of normal social activities, work and personal hygiene. Even if this physical dependence is treated, psychological dependence may drive the individual back to the use of a drug whenever life presents its problems.

It appears that individuals with very different psychological problems may use the same drug and obtain different effects from it. This is not to say that a particular kind of drug is not more effective in producing a particular psychological effect—be it the relief of anxiety or depression, or the obtaining of a positive 'thrill'—than is another drug. Alcohol and barbiturates, by reducing the activity of 'inhibiting' parts of the mind, tend to aggravate mental conflicts, and addicts to these drugs tend to 'work out' their problems in aggressive acts. In contrast drugs such as morphine and heroin seem to suppress the sources of anxiety, making the addict adapt passively to his problems. These differences in the action of drugs explain why some addicts to heroin or morphine will refuse to accept the 'relief' given by alcohol although this would be a more socially acceptable way of solving their problems.

In recent years there has been an increasing awareness that it is the nature of the drug user rather than the nature of the drug which is of paramount importance in addiction. Many addicts have personality problems long before their first contact with drugs, and some addicts are in the early stages of serious mental illness such as schizophrenia. There are many individuals with similar problems who have made their adjustments to life without the aid of drugs,

i.e. there are more potential addicts than there are addicts. The reason for this state of affairs is unknown.

Alcohol

Alcohol has the distinction of being the only drug producing marked psychological effects which is sociably acceptable in many countries, particularly in the West. Alcohol plays an enormous role in our social and economic life and, although only one in 500 partakers will become an acute alcoholic, the harm produced by this drug is more devastating to the individual and to society than any other single drug. It has been estimated that there are about one hundred thousand acute alcoholics in England and Wales, and that the upkeep of these individuals (and their families) who are in prison or who cannot work, cost the nation in the region of £6 million a year. Less acute alcoholics are more numerous and probably cost, in terms of absenteeism etc., another £35 million a year. Alcohol is a vital contributing factor in 1200 deaths and 50 000 injuries on the roads each year. Many crimes are committed under the influence of alcohol. In 1968 there were 2719 receptions of men and 206 receptions of women in to prisons for drunken offences. Of an average day, the police and courts deal with more than 200 public drunkenness offences.

There are a number of special problems that are seen in the chronic alcoholic that are related to the ability of alcohol to supply the body with calories but without at the same time supplying the necessary vitamins and essential amino acids. Widespread disorders of the body's metabolism follow this chronic deficiency of vitamins and amino acids, and degeneration of peripheral nerves, disorders of vision, cirrhosis of liver and mental changes can result.

Tolerance and physical dependence

Most alcoholics start off as ordinary social drinkers, although there are a few who relate their addiction to their very first contact with the drug. The chronic intake of alcohol produces tolerance so that higher blood levels of alcohol are needed to produce the same mental effects; eventually the person becomes physically dependent upon the drug. Why so few people who drink socially become alcoholics is not known with any certainty. Certainly there is a positive correlation between alcoholism and states of anxiety occurring before the age of eighteen years, caused by the death of a parent, separation or divorce. Intact homes can also fail to give children the affection and support they need, and generate the chronic anxiety and feelings of inferiority that are common to alcoholics.

Alcoholics have been divided into various classes according to their psychological make-up. Some alcoholics appear to be so normal, apart from their alcoholism, that one cannot hang a psychiatric label on them. The outlook for these individuals is very good and many of them can be rehabilitated. Not so for the many 'neurotic' alcoholics burdened with anxiety states, depression, phobias and the like, or the alcoholics with some underlying mental disease such as schizophrenia or a psychopathic personality—insincere, unreliable individuals who are incapable of feeling guilt or shame for anything that they do. These individuals, crippled by personality disorders and mental illness, are much more difficult to treat, and they may need prolonged psychotherapy and support by institutions such as Alcoholics Anonymous.

An alcoholic may not appear to be drunk in the accepted sense of the word, and his or her true problem may not become apparent unless alcohol is withdrawn. Then all the symptoms of chronic alcoholism appear; the pulse increases in rate, trembling and sweating occur and there may be a fit. Insomnia is a problem and hallucinations, both auditory and visual, may occur. After prolonged and heavy use of alcohol, withdrawal produces the full picture of what is known as delirium tremens. A few hours after the last drink then weakness, anxiety, perspiration and trembling appear. There may be cramps and vomiting. The subject now begins to 'see things', at first only when the eyes are closed but later even when they are open. These visual hallucinations may be terrifying. At this stage, on about the third day of withdrawal, fever and extreme exhaustion develops and sometimes generalized fits. These withdrawal symptoms are, however, self-limiting, and if the patient does not die of heart failure or extreme exhaustion he recovers in five to seven days without treatment.

The treatment of alcoholism

As in the case of the treatment of all drug addictions, the management of alcoholism falls into two phases, withdrawal of the drug and re-habilitation of the patient. There is certainly no 'cure' for alcoholism. If a cure existed then a 'cured' alcoholic would be able to drink in moderation, but such a treatment is unknown; the recovered alcoholic is always one drink away from alcoholism.

There are a variety of treatments available that include physical procedures and psychological techniques (individual and group psychotherapy, hypnosis etc.). The first stage is the withdrawal of alcohol, which can be immediate or gradual. During this phase large doses of vitamins are needed to make good the long period of malnutrition, and tranquillizing and sedative drugs are used to allow the patient to relax and sleep. Following this 'detoxication' the patient may be subjected to deterrent therapy to disrupt the drinking pattern or make the intake of alcohol a very disagreeable experience. Vomiting is an important part of these methods, and the patient is given drugs to make him vomit whenever he takes alcohol. Following these forms of deterrent therapy, psychotherapy, usually in groups, perhaps aided by hypnosis, can re-inforce the individuals intention to avoid the use of alcohol. Unfortunately there is a lack of doctors who are genuinely and actively interested in this problem, and lack of resources, so that voluntary organizations such as the National Council on Alcoholism and Alcoholics Anonymous play a large part in the rehabilitation of alcoholics.

Morphine-type drugs

Before the 1939–45 war, addiction to 'opiates' was something of a medical curiosity. The vast majority of these addicts were patients who had received one of the opiates—morphine, heroin etc.—for a painful condition and had become so-called 'therapeutic addicts'. In addition, there were some doctors and nurses who were addicted to the drugs. Today this type of addiction is no longer a curiosity; although the number of *known* heroin users is statistically negligible (estimates are between 400 and 2000 in this country) the problem threatens to be of increasing importance. Therapeutic addicts on the whole still use morphine but the non-therapeutic addicts, which now form the bulk of this population, take heroin.

By about 1960 addiction to heroin had begun to increase, with new addicts being recruited mainly from adolescents, both working class and middle class. This pattern of change from morphine to heroin followed a similar change in the U.S.A. Indeed the patterns may be directly linked, for the introduction of Canada's new penal Drug Code in 1958 led to the flight of about seventy addicts to Great Britain, although by the mid-sixties most of these had either died or had returned—voluntarily or deported—to Canada. The arrival of these addicts coincided with the shift óf interest of teenagers from the violent world of groups of gangs to the gentler world of contemplation and inner experience. The scene was set for a greatly increased interest in and use of drugs that modify mood.

The medical use of heroin is in the management of severe pain, and it is a drug that is often chosen for use in 'terminal illnesses'. Weight by weight it is certainly more potent than morphine, and this is of economic importance for the 'pusher' of drugs, i.e. he can sell more doses. A myth has grown up that heroin has a special mood-lifting effect. Most normal individuals cannot however distinguish between the effects of morphine or heroin. Indeed, most normal people feel no hint of pleasure before the vomiting that the first dose of heroin or morphine brings about. The main function of heroin, or any of the other opiates, for the addict is the releasing effect from anxiety; this effect of heroin appears to be 'learned' by the addict, the risk of the drug is with the kind of person who uses it.

Heroin alone, even in doses as high as ten to fifteen grains a day (a therapeutic dose of heroin for severe pain is about one-quarter of a grain) probably is not intrinsically damaging. However, like alcohol, opiates act as addictive agents first of all by depressing primary drives of pain, hunger, thirst and sex. Irregular and incomplete meals, insanitary living and insanitary injection of drugs into veins, all take their toll on health. The kind of disorders that result from this way of life include jaundice (by the transmission of the virus of serum hepatitis from borrowed syringes), malnutrition, venereal diseases, infections of the skin, veins and blood stream from contaminated syringes, coma from accidental overdose, pulmonary tuberculosis and pneumonia.

Tolerance. Physical dependence

The user of heroin usually finds that he has to progressively step up the dose of the drug to produce the same effect. Drug tolerance has developed. Continued use of the drug inevitably leads to physical dependence. When this happens the user finds that four hours after the last dose of heroin, he becomes anxious and develops a craving for the drug. He knows that if he does not soon receive another dose of heroin he will become acutely ill. His whole life now revolves around seeking sources of the drug, for heroin is now needed not only to relieve anxiety but to maintain his physical well-being.

The picture of withdrawal

'Withdrawal sickness' from heroin or the other opiates is a shattering experience for the addict. In the case of heroin symptoms appear early, about four hours after the last dose. The individual becomes restless and anxious, and craves for the drug. After eight hours the individual yawns, sweats and both eyes and nose discharge fluid. These symptoms progress in intensity, and at about twelve hours there is dilatation of the pupils, gooseflesh, trembling, hot and cold flushes, aching muscles and bones and a complete loss of appetite. At about eighteen to twenty-four hours the patient is now unable to sleep, utterly restless and wretched. Fever develops, both pulse and breathing rates increase and a feeling of nausea appears. These features increase in intensity and to them are added vomiting, abdominal pain and diarrhoea. Neither eating nor drinking, and losing large amounts of fluid in sweat, vomit and diarrhoea, the addict rapidly becomes emaciated. This utter misery can be terminated at any stage by means of an intravenous injection of heroin (or other appropriate opiate according to the form of the addiction). However, if the drug is not repeated after about six hours then the same cycle of events inevitably recurs. In the absence of this sort of treatment the symptoms of withdrawal gradually subside by the sixth or seventh day, although the patient is left in a very weak and nervous condition.

The heroin (or opiate) addict as an individual

Most studies of heroin addicts have shown that heroin addiction is most likely to occur in individuals with grossly abnormal personalities, abnormalities that were present long before the start of drug taking. These disorders show themselves in persistent antisocial or asocial acts and attitudes, immaturity, hypersensitivity, passivity and an inability to develop stable personal relationships. American studies have also shown the importance of social-economic deprivation and family backgrounds of disturbed personal relations in the addicts in America.

The use of other drugs such as marijuana or amphetamines may or may not predispose an individual to the use of opiates. Certainly there is evidence that association with addicts exposes *susceptible* individuals to the use of drugs. Experimentation with drugs, even in a casual way, can be disastrous if it occurs at a time when the person is in low spirits or in another way psychologically vulnerable, e.g. after a quarrel with a lover or spouse, or after a bereavement.

Some uncommon addicts may pursue their way of life for many years, sometimes for twenty years or more, without undue mental or physical harm. These individuals use the drug regularly to relieve anxiety and to prevent withdrawal symptoms from appearing. At the other extreme there are adolescents who are dead after a few months. No one really knows the number of addicts who die because of their addiction, indeed we do not know the number of addicts at risk. Certainly many do die because of their addiction (accidental overdose, infections etc.) or because of the mental state which led them into addiction (suicide, murder, accidents etc.). In New York about 350 deaths a year occur among 35 000 addicts.

Treatment of heroin (and opiate) addiction

As in the case of alcoholism, treatment of heroin addiction consists of withdrawal of the drug followed by rehabilitation. The drug is not usually completely withdrawn, rather it is gradually tailed off and replaced by another opiate taken by mouth. This opiate is usually one called methadone. Methadone is itself a drug of addiction, and physical dependence to it develops. Methadone, however, produces milder withdrawal symptoms; it also has a longer duration of action than heroin. Heroin tends to be taken at three to four hour intervals whereas methadone can be given once daily on an out-patient basis. If enough of methadone is given then the patient loses the desire to take heroin; furthermore, when methadone is given orally under supervision at an out-patient clinic there is no surplus of the drug to be sold on the 'black-market'. Under the influence of methadone many addicts have been socially rehabilitated and been able to resume some productive work. Methadone can and often is abused; addicts sometimes take it erratically and in combination with other drugs by the intravenous route. This is not what was intended by the workers who developed the methadone-maintenance system. In Britain at least (not in the

U.S.A.), some addicts have been maintained on controlled doses of heroin itself. This is, however, a controversial issue, and involves the risk of addicts selling any surplus and so spreading addiction to other individuals. The liberal prescription of heroin and other drugs will soon be a thing of the past, and only certain doctors will be allowed to prescribe heroin for addicts.

The after-care of the treated heroin addict may be a prolonged affair and will be the responsibility of the new Treatment Centres. Following the withdrawal of heroin, the patient may have a variety of problems which need management by physical rehabilitation, psychotherapy, occupational therapy, industrial training, counselling and advice in various places such as out-patient clinics or a half-way house. There are various self-help groups in the U.S.A., and similar ones may well develop in Britain. In America there is, for example, Narcotics Anonymous modelled on Alcoholics Anonymous, and Synanon, a voluntary organization which sponsors groups of addicts living in communities which support themselves; in these communities there is no drug taking.

Barbiturates

The consumption of barbiturates in western societies is enormous. In 1968 the number of prescriptions for them in the United Kingdom under the National Health Service was reported to be 24 700 000 (this does not include their use in private practice or in hospitals). Barbiturates are thus 'acceptable' drugs to both doctors and patients alike. The danger of accidental or deliberate overdosage with these drugs is not realized by many people; self-poisoning with barbiturates is one of the commonest causes of urgent admission to hospital—there are about 8000 cases of barbiturate poisoning each year. What very many people do not appear to realize is that barbiturates are the most commonly used drugs of addiction with by far the most addicts.

The actual numbers of people who use these drugs compulsively is not known, but they certainly exceed the number using opiates. Illegal traffic in these drugs is common, and many opiate users frequently make use of barbiturates to boost the effects of 'weak' heroin; these individuals become physically dependent upon both drugs. Alcoholics may also use barbiturates to remove the trembling of alcohol withdrawal.

There are many different types of barbiturate and barbiturate-like drugs available. The way in which these drugs are used varies, and ranges from infrequent 'sprees' of severe intoxication, lasting a few days, to the daily use of large amounts of the drug; when the drugs are used daily and in large amounts then considerable time and ingenuity is needed to ensure a constant supply. The original contact with the drug may, for example, have been via a doctor's prescription for barbiturates to relieve insomnia. Gradually the dose may be increased at night and then the individual adds a few tablets for sedation in the morning. Eventually the whole life of the addict revolves around the procuring and taking of barbiturates, with all the associated physical and social decline that typifies other forms of addiction.

Addiction to barbiturates differs from that to opiates in several important respects. Barbiturates tend to be taken until the individual is intoxicated; his object is personal oblivion. Both the acute and chronic effects of mild intoxication with barbiturates resemble those of alcoholic intoxication. The intoxicated person is sluggish and thinks, speaks, understands slowly. He may be highly emotional, irritable, quarrelsome or morose. There may be crying or laughing without any provocation, and personal habits become untidy. The mind may become dominated by ideas of persecution or suicide. In chronic barbiturate intoxication there may be changes such as double vision, squint, difficulty in accommodation, dizziness, disordered walking, abnormal reflexes, skin rashes and kidney damage.

Tolerance, physical dependence, and withdrawal symptoms

Chronic intoxication with barbiturates results in both tolerance to the effects of the drug and physical dependence. Although individuals may become tolerant to some effects of barbiturates, the lethal dose is not much greater in addicts than it is in normal individuals. This means that accidental poisoning and death may occur at any time, as may deliberate suicide.

When the addict has become physically dependent on barbiturates, then withdrawal of the drug produces catastrophic changes even more severe than those seen after the withdrawal of heroin. Over the first twelve to sixteen hours after withdrawal, as barbiturate disappears from the blood the patient may seem to improve, becoming more alert and better behaved. Soon, however, he becomes increasingly restless, anxious, trembling and weak. Abdominal cramps, nausea and vomiting may now appear.

The patient may be so weak that he cannot get out of bed, and even if he is able to stand he is likely to faint. Convulsions may occur, the patient becoming rigid and falling down with thrashing limbs and with the involuntary passing of urine and faeces; seizures may occur in rapid succession. If the patient survives these stages of withdrawal then mental disorders—psychoses—appear. Anxiety increases, sleep may become impossible and there are visual hallucinations—usually in the nature of persecutions. The patient may be so disorientated that he may not know where he is or what time it is. During this delirium, which occurs between the fourth to seventh day of withdrawal, agitation and a rise in temperature may lead to exhaustion and heart failure. The withdrawal symptoms, even if untreated, usually begin to clear by the eighth day, although hallucinations may persist for some months. During the early stages of withdrawal the symptoms can be stopped by doses of barbiturates, but once delirium develops barbiturates may be of no help.

Although public opinion still has a tolerant and accepting attitude to barbiturates and their users (most people regard barbiturates as standard equipment of a medicine chest) the medical profession is becoming increasingly aware of the dangers of these drugs and the need for control (e.g. *British Medical Journal*, Vol. I, 1971, No. 5742, 'Cutting down on barbiturates'). The voluntary ban or restriction on the prescribing of amphetamines will surely be followed by similar voluntary control of barbiturates. After all the bulk of prescribing for these drugs is for relatively harmless conditions e.g. insomnia, for which there are a range of simple remedies. Alternative sleeping drugs are available, and though some are undoubtedly safer as far as gross overdosage is concerned, it is still too early to say whether they are free from the risks of psychological and physical dependence.

Amphetamines

There are now more than fifty preparations of amphetamine substances on the market. These are issued either alone or in combination with other drugs, notably barbiturates. The well known ones include amphetamine itself, dexamphetamine (Dexedrine), methyl amphetamine ('Methedrine'), phenmetrazine ('Preludin'), diethylproprion ('Apisate', 'Tenuate'), 'Drinamyl' and 'Anxine' (mixtures of amphetamine and barbiturate).

Amphetamines produce widespread effects on the body. Most of the effects are similar to those that are produced when we experience fear or excitement, i.e. a rise in blood pressure and pulse rate, dilatation of the pupils, relaxation of the smooth muscle of the bowel, bladder, bronchioles, and the secretion of a thick saliva. In the nervous system, amphetamines increase mental alertness and produce a sense of well-being as well as decreasing sensations of hunger and fatigue. These actions on the nervous system were the reasons for the use of amphetamines during the war. Millions of tablets of amphetamines were issued to both German and Allied troops to support them during periods of physical and mental exhaustion.

In medical practice amphetamines have, over the years, been used for many different conditions, e.g. in the treatment of epilepsy (to counteract the drowsiness of other drugs which may be used), barbiturate poisoning, drug addiction, including alcoholism (to offset sleepiness and lethargy), psychopathic states, behaviour disorders in children, enuresis (bedwetting), obesity and depression. The commonest use of amphetamines has probably been for the treatment of obesity, where the drug is used in an attempt to reduce appetite. Amphetamines have thus been widely used drugs, and in 1959 some $5\frac{1}{2}$ million National Health prescriptions were for amphetamines and phenmetrazine (Preludin). Even after several years of widespread concern about the liberal prescriptions for these drugs, the figure was over 3 million prescriptions in 1969, and this in England alone.

Amphetamines are irreplaceable only in one condition, a *very* rare disease called narcolepsy, in which there is a compulsive desire to sleep. In 1968 a working party of the British Medical Association considered that amphetamine compounds appear to have no place in the modern treatment of depression. Their widespread use in the treatment of obesity is also regarded as being unsound and unsafe. In October 1968, as a result of Home Office pressure, there was a nation-wide voluntary ban on the prescription of Methedrine (a liquid preparation that can be injected) except by hospitals. Later, when it was discovered that powdered amphetamine sulphate could be dissolved in water and injected, the ban was extended to this preparation. A voluntary ban on the prescription of *all* amphetamines was advocated at the B.M.A.'s Annual Representative Meeting in 1970. This was put forward by an Ipswich doctor, a city in which, for the past year and a half, general practitioners and all hospitals have been refusing to prescribe amphetamines except on rare occasions, and then only at several days notice, because no stocks of the drug are held by pharmacists. This voluntary ban, pioneered at Ipswich, has now spread to other parts of Britain. One major British drug company has stopped production of amphetamine compounds and has recalled stocks from chemists and wholesalers so that they can be destroyed.

In amphetamine compounds we have a drug that is virtually useless in medical practice but which has been so widely prescribed as to cause serious abuse of the drug. Doctors alone cannot be held responsible for this state of affairs in a society in which patients demand pills as a right, for every trivial ailment. When people take amphetamines in doses which are in excess of those prescribed by doctors, they do so because they wish to experience the psychological effects of the drug, the elevation of mood and reduction of inhibitions. The side-effects of large doses include marked euphoria, restlessness, rapid speech, anxiety, disordered walk, dry mouth, raised pulse rate and irregular heart action and rise in temperature, perhaps leading to profound collapse. One severe side-effect is amphetamine psychosis; the patient in this state has vivid hallucinations and ideas of persecution which may readily lead to a mis-diagnosis of schizophrenia. So common are ideas of persecution by the police that Swedish workers have called it police paranoia. The psychosis lasts a few days until the drug has been excreted from the body.

The war experiences in Japan, where large numbers of children were giving themselves intravenous injections of methyl amphetamine, drew attention to the dangers of dependence on the drug. Most of the cases that developed amphetamine psychosis were dependent upon the drug. This dependence is mainly a psychological one, although some studies have indicated that a form of physical dependence may also occur. By measuring the pattern of electrical activity from the brains of amphetamine users, it has been shown that the normal electrical behaviour of the brain may be disturbed for days or weeks after withdrawal of the drug.

The kind of people who tend to abuse amphetamines are adolescents out for a 'kick' or middle-aged women with problems of obesity or depression. These women initially obtain their supplies legitimately from their doctors. Amphetamines are cheap and readily available to young people. Although only a small proportion of the adolescents experimenting with amphetamines or amphetamine-barbiturate mixtures will become drug-dependent, in view of the widespread use of the drugs the total number of drug-dependent young people is likely to be formidable. The effects on personal and social life of this drug dependence may be profound, with involvement in illegal acts to obtain supplies, abnormal behaviour or law-breaking under the influence of drugs, suicidal attempts in the phase of withdrawal depression, and the disruption of work and family life.

The treatment of individuals who take large amounts of amphetamines, and who are clearly dependent on the drug, usually needs admission to hospital for withdrawal treatment, followed by psychiatric rehabilitation.

Cocaine

The abuse of cocaine, once a serious problem, is now rare in western countries. Cocaine has limited uses in medicine and then only in hospital practice, so that the drug is not easily available to the potential addict. The main effect of cocaine is elevation of mood, and this often reaches intense excitement. There is marked decrease in hunger and an indifference to pain. As in the case of amphetamines, one does not need to suffer from a disordered personality to experience these effects of the drug on mood. The action of the drug is relatively brief, but if the dose is large enough a psychosis may develop, similar to that of amphetamine psychosis. Unfortunately the persons suffering from a cocaine psychosis may act out his delusions and become aggressive to his alleged persecutors.

Tolerance or physical dependence are not features of the effects of this drug, certainly not when the drug is used by people with normal personalities.

Marijuana (cannabis)

Cannabis, a drug which is obtained from the flowering tops of Indian hemp plants, is a very ancient drug, and has been widely used in Africa and Asia. Usually the hemp plant is cut, dried and incorporated into cigarettes, but the drug can also be drunk or eaten. Many confusing names are used for this drug; 'grass' and 'pot' are common slang terms and a marijuana cigarette is a 'stick', a 'reefer' or a 'weed'. Like many other drugs, cannabis is used for different reasons in different cultures. In India the Brahman uses the drug to help in his meditation and prayers, whereas in the West a typical pot smoker of the city uses it, like alcohol, to ease his social contact and increase his enjoyment of the external world.

When marijuana is smoked, the effects occur within a few minutes and these effects are short lived. After swallowing the drug the action is more delayed, by up to one hour, and the effects may persist for several hours. The physical effects of the drug are usually slight. The pulse rate usually increases somewhat and the blood pressure rises slightly. Reddening of the eyes may occur and urine may be passed more frequently. An increase in appetite often occurs, and occasionally there may be nausea and vomiting or diarrhoea. The fatal dose of the drug is probably many times larger than that which is ever likely to be taken under ordinary circumstances.

The psychological effects of marijuana, which are the reasons for taking the drug, are impossible to describe succinctly. These effects vary according to the personality of the user, the dose, the way the drug is administered, the circumstances in which the drug is used, and on the individual's previous experience of the drug and his skill as a smoker. The individual who is experienced in marijuana smoking can usually regulate the dose so as to get the effect he wants without intoxicating himself. He is seeking a mood of pleasant euphoria, a dreamy state of altered consciousness in which ideas seem uncontrollable and freely flowing and in which things long forgotten may be remembered. Perception of time may be altered and minutes may seem to be hours. For those who have had no previous experience of the drug these feelings may cause unpleasant anxiety. When larger doses are used acute intoxication may occur. The individual experiences marked changes in mood, usually a change to a feeling of extreme well-being and excitement. If this state occurs the individual may become increasingly restless, talkative, with outbursts of uncontrollable laughter for little apparent reason. Sometimes the effect of a large dose produces the opposite effect, with a withdrawn, dreamy or depressed state being predominant.

There has been considerable debate as to whether marijuana can produce a psychotic state or not. The accuracy of the diagnosis of marijuana psychosis has often been doubted; in North America and Britain drug users often take several drugs simultaneously so that it is often difficult to know whether a psychosis is due to marijuana or to some other drug such as amphetamines or LSD. However, many workers in this field now feel that a psychosis can develop from the use of marijuana alone. This psychosis may closely resemble acute schizophrenia, with a disturbance of consciousness, hallucinations and feelings of 'dual personality'.

Physical dependence

Informed medical opinion is moving towards the view that there is no convincing evidence that there are long-term harmful effects from the use of marijuana. This is not to say that if marijuana were freely available, cheap, and with no social prohibitions, that no one would become psychologically dependent upon it to the detriment of their social and physical well-being. There is at the moment no evidence of 'tolerance' to this drug or of physical dependence.

The dangers of the use of marijuana, apart from obvious conflict with the law, is that an intoxicated individual may commit suicide or, in a state of utter euphoria, walk under a bus or out of a window. These accidents do, however, seem to be rare. Possibly a greater risk is that familiarity with this drug and of people who use it may lead to experimentation with other drugs that lead to physical dependence and physical and social deterioration. In this country at the moment, there is little doubt that most users of marijuana never progress to heroin. A more serious immediate danger is that the use of marijuana introduces the individual to a deviant 'sub-culture' which not only experiments with drugs but which may also be sexually promiscuous, unambitious and 'work-shy'.

Hallucinogenic drugs

According to the Poisons Regulations (Hallucinogenic drugs) 1964, made under the Poisons Act of 1962, Hallucinogenic drugs means one of the following:

> Dimethyl tryptamine
> Lysergic acid diethylamide
> Mescaline
> Psilocybin
> Psilocin

In the West the abuse of hallucinogens is restricted to lysergic acid diethylamide (LSD); this most potent and readily available hallucinogen is the only drug considered in this section.

Hallucinogens have been used to alter consciousness or mood in connection with religious practices of American Mexican Indians for many centuries. Indians use the peyote cactus as their source of the hallucinogen called mescaline. Other plants also provide natural sources of hallucinogens. The action of the first synthetic hallucinogen was discovered in 1943 by Hoffman. In the course of laboratory studies with LSD, Hoffman had a very unusual experience. He was 'seized by a peculiar sensation of vertigo and restlessness. Objects, as well as the shape of my associates in the laboratory, appeared to undergo optical changes. I was unable to concentrate on my work. In a dream-like state I left for home where an irresistible urge to lie down overcame me. I drew the curtains and immediately fell into a peculiar state similar to drunkenness, characterized by an exaggerated imagination. With my eyes closed, fantastic pictures of extraordinary plasticity and intense colour seemed to surge towards me. After two hours this state gradually wore off'. Hoffman had not deliberately swallowed LSD but he suspected that this drug with which he was working had been the cause of this experience. He now decided to test this idea, and took what he thought would be a safe dose— a quarter of a milligramme—by mouth. We now know that this is indeed a large dose of this most powerful of all mind-affecting substances; it can produce detectable effects in doses as small as 20 microgrammes. A quarter of a milligramme understandably produced spectacular effects on Hoffman.

By about 1950, LSD was being used by psychiatrists in treating a wide variety of psychiatric problems. Some psychiatrists themselves have taken the drug to try to feel something of what it is like to be a schizophrenic. The use of the drug continues today in a few centres, but it is no longer regarded as a 'new wonder drug' capable of helping to cure all manner of mental ills. In the phrase of one psychiatrist, LSD 'does no more than break down the mind's established defences to let the conscious see the unconscious'. This vision of the unconscious with its labyrinth of fears and guilts may be too much for an individual to handle alone, and the consumption of this drug in solitude is fraught with dangers, particularly for the unstable people who are attracted to its use. Some individuals have committed suicide under its influence or have become psychotic.

It was in the U.S.A. that LSD was first used outside medical control. The drug was received with great enthusiasm by groups of individuals seeking liberation from the fetters of mass living and the mass media. These groups were, and are, often led by psychologists or formed of students or middle-class intellectuals. It has been estimated that in 1966 about four million Americans took LSD. It was only a question of time before

LSD became an instrument of British sub-cultures, and it has been linked particularly with the 'Hippie' movement. Despite the Poisons Regulations of 1967 it is very likely that the use of LSD in Britain is increasing, particularly in groups where drug addiction is common or in communities such as University students or Colleges of Further Education, and especially Art Colleges.

The dose of the drug is so small that it is often taken as a drop of liquid on a sugar lump or soaked onto a fragment of blotting paper. The action of LSD occurs within thirty minutes of swallowing it and the effects reach a peak in about an hour or two, and then subside over the next hours, although there may be some after-effects which persist for many hours or days. The predominant effects of the drug are mental rather than physical, and they have already been described in Hoffman's first description. The visual and emotional changes and the emotionally charged fantasies may cause considerable alarm, especially if the drug has been secretly administered to an individual. These after-effects are particularly dangerous if, after return to relative normality, the effects of the drug rapidly return when the person is at work, driving a car or in some other responsible situation requiring full attention. Some people have had psychotic reactions after LSD and there are some reports of these being permanent in some cases. Feelings of persecution (paranoia) are the commonest psychotic reactions.

The long-term dangers of LSD

Addiction to the hallucinogenic drugs is one of misuse rather than physical addiction, for people do not become physically dependent on these drugs. Misuse involves taking the drug without medical supervision during the period of action of the drugs. A few individuals become so fascinated by the effects that they use the drug repeatedly. Many of these regular users claim that it has beneficial effects on their personality—including freedom from pressure and over-ambition. Not all these regular users are unstable personalities, and in fact those individuals who do not wish to repeat the experience of LSD are those who fear loss of control during the release of unconscious fears and guilts.

A potential long-term hazard of LSD has recently been described. LSD is capable of producing chromosomal damage in cells growing in tissue culture. In two young men, heavy users of LSD, was found the 'philadelphia' marker, an abnormal chromosome which appears in cases of myeloid leukaemia ('cancer' of the bone marrow). In experimental animals LSD has been found to cause abortions or abnormalities in the offspring. There is obviously the distinct possibility that LSD may be the cause of abnormalities in babies of mothers who have taken the drug, or that LSD may be a cause of cancer.

In spite of the laws regulating the use of LSD, the disapproval of many members of society including responsible medical opinion, and the possible damaging effects of the drug (psychosis, suicide, cancer and abnormalities in children) it is likely that more and more people will experiment with the use of this drug. It is obvious that the user of this and other drugs should be actively discouraged. If, in spite of this discouragement, individuals will persist with the use of LSD, they should be clearly aware of the possible risks involved, and in particular the risks of taking the drug alone or in company in which no members are free of its influence. If an LSD experience gets out of hand then medical assistance should be sought, for there are drugs which can counteract the effects of LSD.

How to identify a drug addict

The identification of drug addiction in an individual is becoming an increasingly important facility, particularly for hospital and family doctors, parents and teachers. Addicts may present their problem to society in a variety of ways, and sometimes the nature of their disorder may go unrecognized for many years, particularly if they have a fairly normal mental and physical constitution and have access to a regular supply of the drug(s) to which they are addicted. Conditions such as coma (due to an overdose) or a psychosis, are obvious ways in which their problems may manifest themselves, although even here mis-diagnosis of the condition, e.g. as the case of schizophrenia, are understandably common. The following list includes changes in behaviour or appearance that may be noticed in the heroin addict. Many of these features are also common to other forms of drug addiction.

1. Changes in social and personal habits:
   (a) loss of interest in physical appearance, e.g. failure to shave, wash or change clothes;
   (b) giving up organized social activities e.g. dances, sports etc.;

(c) poor work record, repeatedly changing jobs, giving up work entirely;

(d) spending long periods in the bedroom,

(e) unexpected absences from home— obtaining supplies of drugs from doctors, clinics, fellow addicts, hanging around chemists and toilets;

(f) frequent use of the telephone—contacting the drug users' sub-culture, checking on supplies of drugs, arranging meetings, parties etc.;

(g) poor appetite.

2. Evidence of the use of syringes and the habit of boiling up tablets of heroin in water in a spoon for injection:

(a) blood stains on the clothes,

(b) teaspoons and fully burnt matches lying around.

3. Physical effects of the drug or of the way of injecting the drug.

(a) an attack of jaundice (due to the virus of serum hepatitis, transmitted in a trace of blood in a borrowed syringe);

(b) inflamed veins, scarred veins, abscesses;

(c) loss of weight, infections such as tuberculosis.

4. Diseases resulting from the way of life of the drug addict, e.g. venereal diseases.

Various adolescent problems and mental illness (depression, schizophrenia) may produce some but *not* all symptoms of drug addictions. Disappointments in love affairs may lead to a poor appetite, irritability and perhaps some loss of interest in social activities. Early schizophrenia may produce many of the symptoms common to drug addicts, but schizophrenics do not make new friends or receive and make many telephone calls, nor do they show physical evidence of the use of drugs. These various possibilities must obviously be kept in mind before seriously considering that an adolescent with a problem is using drugs.

29. The growth and control of human populations

Introduction

THE volume of publications on the growth of human populations, food problems, and the need to limit population growth by controlling fertility, increases almost as steadily as the world population itself. Ever since Malthus's 'Essay on Population' (1801) these problems have received attention by all manner of individuals, including politicians, geographers, agronomists, economists, social scientists and experts in public health. Malthus warned us that, since populations increase geometrically whereas agricultural production does not, populations would grow to the limit of available resources and maintain the world in poverty. He gave the estimate that the human population might double itself every twenty years, provided that there were no checks by war, famine, epidemic disasters or self-restraint. His message went unheeded; progress in the techniques of agriculture and the development of the New World in North America seemed to improve the prospects of the human race. These developments were, however, only a temporary palliative.

possible because of an increase in the rate of food production. The rate of food production has not, however, matched the growth of population, so that half the individuals of the world now live in a state of semi-starvation (Figures 29.2, 29.3).

In spite of international concern, which dates from the Conference at Hot Springs called by President Roosevelt in 1943 (from which sprang the Food and Agriculture Organization—FAO —of the United Nations), the situation continues to deteriorate. The population of India, for example, will grow more in the next ten years (an additional 165 million) than it did in the first fifty years of the twentieth century (123 million). To put these figures into more comprehensible terms we can say that the population of India grows by about 50 000 per day, or more than the population of Australia each year. The problem is a world-wide one and the United Kingdom, for example, increases her population by about 1000 per day. This may seem of little consequence compared to India's contribution. It is, however, a vast challenge, for each individual person in the U.K. consumes at least forty times as much of the world's economic resources as each individual person in India. A

The population explosion

In 1801, at the time that Malthus published his essay, the world contained 1000 million people. It had taken some 200 000 years of human history to achieve this number, but it took only a further 100 years to double this figure to 2000 million, and only a further thirty years to treble this figure to 3000 million. The world population now grows at a rate of some 70 million a year. This is the population explosion (Figure 29.1).

The reason for this sudden rate of increase in population growth is well known. The explosion has happened mainly because of the control of infectious diseases by means of vaccines, antibiotics and a host of public health measures (see Chapters 6–10). In some parts of the world the birth rate, traditionally high, has remained high, so producing a progressive widening in the margin between births and deaths. Of course this increase in population has only been made

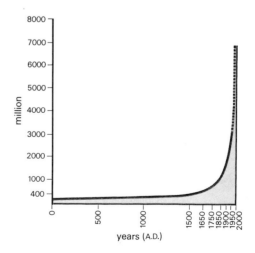

Figure 29.1 The population explosion. Solid line—estimated population of the world from A.D. 1 to A.D. 1960. Interrupted line— projection of population to A.D. 2000.

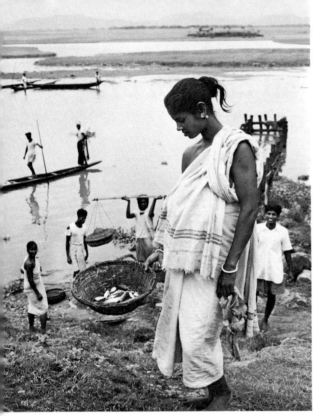

further problem is that each additional person in the U.K. will contaminate the environment on a vast scale compared with the additional person in India.

The future prospects

The population explosion is here, and little has been done to try to halt the explosive force of geometric progression. India led the world in 1951 as the first nation to declare a Government commitment to family planning; since this time it is estimated that over 3 million intra-uterine devices (IUDs—see page 348) have been inserted and up to $6\frac{1}{2}$ million sterilizations have been performed. It is estimated that this deliberate national policy of family planning has averted about 9 million births. Malcolm Potts, in his Tenth Darwin Lecture in Human Biology, put this figure into perspective when he said that 'the net consequence of the Indian family planning programme is that the country will reach in December the situation it would have reached in May if no family planning had ever taken place'. The outlook is truly pessimistic, for the problem in India is in fact a world-wide one.

It seems unlikely that, with the present resources that are diverted to family planning, the population explosion can be halted. Improvements in agricultural production have given only a temporary pause in the race against starvation, and although there is considerable room for agricultural expansion and economic growth, it is clear that in certain areas of the world the growth of population is quite out of hand. The explosion will continue until famines, disease and war exert a braking force on population growth, although to have significant global effect these forces would have to annihilate many millions of people.

In the meantime increasing numbers of people will live in overcrowded miserable conditions, on the verge of starvation. The social consequences of this state of affairs are, of course, profound. In Latin America, for example, where the population has doubled since 1930, 'unconscious infanticide', i.e. death of children due to lack of concern and control, is a major problem. In Santiago, Chile, sixty of every 1000 first born children die in their first year; for the third and fourth born this death rate increases to 100 in every 1000 children. The main cause of this staggering mortality in the pre-school child appears to be due to the lack of the mother's concern. Out of every 100 deaths in Latin America, 44 are of children under five

Figure 29.2 (above)   More than half the world's population are victims of hunger or malnutrition in one form or another. One continent where grave food and nutrition problems persist is Asia. Here, the diet is often deficient in animal products such as fish, eggs, and milk. In this region the consumption of such animal products is less than one-third of what it is in the U.S. and Europe. The photograph shows an Indian fisherman's wife examining the meagre day's catch.
(*WHO photo by Sharma.*)

Figure 29.3 (below)   A victim of Kwashiorkor—the African name for a disease of young children whose food contains little or no protein. The victims are unforgettable; the piercing eyes, bloated belly, and match stick legs. (*FAO photo.*)

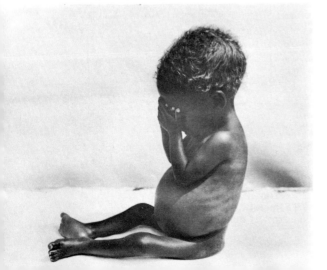

years old. In the overcrowded towns and cities of South America, the rate of *criminal* abortion is very high (16–20 per cent of women) and one reason for this state of affairs is the serious housing problem. When governments and religious bodies fail to face the realities of the population explosion and take effective action, these are the sorts of solutions by which individuals try to solve their problems. Unconscious or conscious infanticide, criminal abortion, poverty, starvation, epidemic disease, social disintegration and war would seem to be the inevitable consequences of overpopulation.

The solution to these problems does not lie in family planning alone, indeed some authorities feel that it is already too late to solve the crisis by this method. The remainder of this chapter will, however, be devoted to the technique of controlling human fertility. It is beyond the scope of our discussion to deal with the resources of agriculture, international co-operation, or the reasons why nations continue to divert vast resources in maintaining either an armed peace or in the pursuance of the policies of war.

Family planning

In its widest sense, family planning includes not only the limitation of the family to an optimum size by contraception but also the assistance of those couples who have difficulties in starting a family. Whether we like it or not doctors are not entirely the servants of the politicians and population experts; in spite of the population explosion many doctors continue to devote a great deal of time and resources to the promotion of fertility in that not inconsiderable number of couples who, for one reason or the other, are infertile. We will, however, restrict our discussion of family planning to its negative aspects, the restriction of human fertility, i.e. contraception.

The methods of contraception

These can be classified as follows:

1. mechanical or chemical methods,
2. oral contraception—'the pill',
3. intra-uterine contraception—IUDs,
4. abortion,
5. fertility control by periodic abstinence, the rhythm method,
6. sterilization.

Recent advances in contraceptive techniques have provided a wide range of materials and methods; however, the perfect contraceptive that is suitable for use in *all* individuals has yet to be found. Indeed, 'couples in 1970 must use a range of second-rate methods of birth control . . .' and 'women in developed countries, as well as those in developing countries, must now pay the penalty of the previous apathy and antagonism to scientific family planning' (Malcolm Potts, 'Against Nature', *Biologist* Vol. 17 No. 4).

Mechanical and chemical methods

Mechanical methods are amongst the oldest contraceptive techniques although some of them, notably the condom, are probably the most widely used contraceptives in the world.

Mechanical methods in the male

The mechanical technique used in the male is called the condom or sheath. The basis of this technique is that the penis is covered by an impermeable sheath which prevents semen from reaching the vagina. The earliest condoms were made from the intestines of animals. These were replaced by ones made of rubber or latex and more recently of plastic. Condoms are made in a variety of materials and thicknesses and sizes; some are disposable whilst others are washable and re-usable; some have a 'teat' at the end in which semen is collected, while others have a plain rounded end; some are packed dry and powdered while others carry a thin layer of lubricant.

In use the condom must be applied to the erect penis before intercourse. Some condoms have a natural rim incorporated into the base to help it to keep in position during intercourse. For maximum protection it is best to use it with a spermicidal cream. The use of the condom confers an additional benefit in that it also offers a degree of protection against the transmission of venereal diseases.

This method of contraception can fail for a variety of reasons, the commonest of which is tearing of the sheath. Obviously the production of condoms needs a high level of quality control. Other causes of failure are due to the way in which the condom is used. The condom may, for example, be applied too late in love-play. The failure rate of this method of contraception is quoted as about three pregnancies per 100 woman-years.

Side-effects of this method of contraception are extremely rare. In a few instances a man or wife may be sensitive to the rubber material of the condom or to the powder used to dust it. Some individuals may dislike this method of contraception, e.g. because it interferes with 'sensation'. Given a high quality product used with a chemical spermicide, this is one of the most effective and widely used methods of contraception. A population council survey in the U.S.A. showed that about 27 per cent of couples using contraception were using the condom. This method is being increasingly used in developing countries of the world.

Mechanical methods in the female

Mechanical methods in the female are devices which act as a barrier preventing the access of semen to the neck of the womb. They come in many shapes and sizes. Because of variations in the shape and size of the internal female genital organs (particularly affected by childbirth) and because of the presence of various disorders, these mechanical devices have in the first instance to be chosen and fitted by a doctor or nurse. The woman is then instructed in the way they are to be used. The various types that are in general use are described below.

Diaphragm (*Dutch cap*)

The diaphragm is a thin rubber dome attached to a metal, circular, rubber-covered rim. The rim is flexible and the whole diaphragm can be compressed and inserted into the vagina. Before insertion the cap is smeared with a spermicide and then placed into the upper reaches (vault) of the vagina (Figure 29.4). It is held in position partly by the tension in the spring and partly by vaginal muscle tone. Diaphragms come in various sizes, ranging from 45–100 mm in diameter, and it is important to have the correct size fitted. When there is difficulty in inserting

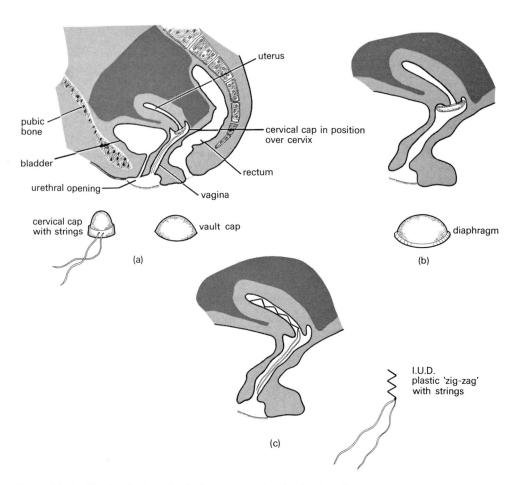

Figure 29.4 Mechanical method of contraception in the female.
(a) Cervical cap and vault cap, (b) diaphragm, (c) I.U.D.

the diaphragm, a curved and notched 'stick' can be used to insert the appliance. In some women, e.g. in those who have had severe tears during childbirth, the diaphragm does not stay in position well enough and an alternative has to be chosen.

Cervical cap (Dumas, see figure 29.4)

This cap of rubber, plastic or metal, fits closely around the cervix (neck of the womb). In order to use this cap the individual must be able to reach her cervix with her fingers. The cervix must be healthy to use this cap. Like the Dutch cap, the initial fitting must be carried out by a doctor or nurse.

Vault cap

This cap is larger than the cervical cap. The cap sticks to the roof of the vagina by suction, and covers the cervix. Again the patient must be able to reach the cervix with her fingers, and the correct size of cap has to be fitted.

Fittings of caps

In all cases, the type of cap chosen for a particular individual is fitted by a doctor after an examination of the pelvic organs and after a view of the cervix has been obtained and a cervical smear taken for cytology (if this is possible). The patient is then taught how to insert the cap, using it with a spermicidal cream or jelly. When the woman is familiar with the technique of inserting the cap, she returns to the doctor with the cap in place so that he can check if it is in its correct position. The woman inserts the cap before intercourse and leaves it in place for six to eight hours afterwards. The position of the cap must always be checked. The woman returns at intervals for the cap to be checked for wear and size.

Provided that the cap is used in the correct way and consistently, it offers a good degree of contraceptive protection. Figures of failure rates quoted vary from two to fifteen pregnancies per 100 woman-years. Side-effects are rare and are usually due to reactions to the material of the cap or of the spermicide used.

Chemical spermicides

A variety of chemical spermicides are available. These act by immobilizing sperm on contact with the chemical, or by producing an impenetrable foam around the neck of the womb.

The spermicides come in the form of pessaries, tablets, jellies, creams and aerosol foam. Some of them come with a special syringe-type applicator carrying a long nozzle. These products are tested for efficiency and safety by the United Kingdom Family Planning Association and by the International Planned Parenthood Federation, who keep a supply of tested spermicides. Used alone as a contraceptive, they have a failure rate as high as twenty-five pregnancies per 100 woman-years. Although they have the advantages of cheapness, simplicity of use and the lack of need of a pelvic examination, they are best used in conjunction with a condom or one of the female mechanical methods of contraception.

Oral contraception

The ability of certain sex hormones to prevent the liberation of eggs from the ovary has been known since the 1930s. No one seriously considered using sex hormones as contraceptives until the classical studies of Rock, Garcia and Pincus were published in 1957. These workers were attempting to treat a group of infertile women in whom there was no obvious cause for their infertility. Their aim was to try to stimulate the growth of the uterus by means of sex hormones (oestrogen and progesterone), a state of affairs that occurs during natural pregnancy. In most of these women ovulation (i.e. the release of eggs from the ovaries) was prevented by this treatment. Incidentally—at least to our story—14 per cent of these women became pregnant some months after stopping hormone treatment. Following on from these studies the first trials of oral contraceptives (hormones), i.e. the pill, took place in 1965 in Puerto Rico. The results of these trials were so successful that within a few years oral contraceptive pills were in regular use in many countries of the world. Today there are at least 1.25 million in Britain (out of the 10.5 million women aged between fifteen and forty-four) who are taking an oral contraceptive.

Components of the pill

The chemicals that are used in contraceptive pills (we will, hereafter, abbreviate this to 'the pill') are synthetic hormones, oestrogens, progestagens (i.e. having an action similar to the natural hormone called progesterone) and related compounds. In the normal woman these hormones are produced mainly by the ovary, and they are responsible for the development and maintenance of the structures of the sex organs (breasts, vagina, uterus etc.) and for the rhythmical changes that occur in the lining of the womb that lead to menstruation. Some pills contain a mixture of oestrogen and progestagen. These are the combined tablets that are taken from the fifth to the twenty-fifth day of the menstrual cycle (day five being that following the end of the menstrual period which normally lasts four days). After completing the three-week course of tablets, a menstrual period starts in a day or two and then the new course of the tablets is commenced after completion of the menstrual period. In another method called the 'sequential system', oestrogen tablets are taken from the fifth day, either for fifteen days or for eleven days, and then a tablet containing a mixture of oestrogen and progestagen is taken for the last five or ten days of the cycle. Other types of tablet and systems have also been used, such as low-dose *continuous* progesterone (taken daily for as long as contraception is required), or 'morning after' oestrogen, taken in fairly high doses for four to six days after intercourse. These systems are not, however, in general use, and the 'morning after' type of pill is still experimental.

How do these hormones prevent pregnancy?

During a normal pregnancy the ovaries of a woman do not release eggs. This dormancy in egg production is due to the lack of the necessary growth factors that reach the ovaries from the pituitary gland. These ovarian growth factors (gonadotrophins) are not produced by the pituitary gland during pregnancy. The pituitary gland (or more accurately that part of the brain that controls the pituitary gland—the hypothalamus) is very sensitive to the amount of sex hormones that are present in the circulating blood. When the 'level' of circulating sex hormones fall (as occurs for example after the menopause), the pituitary steps up its output of gonadotrophins, as though it were 'attempting' to restore the activity of the ovaries of the elderly woman. The reverse happens when the blood 'level' of sex hormones rises; the pituitary responds by cutting out its release of gonadotrophins. This state of affairs occurs in pregnancy; the placenta produces large amounts of both oestrogen and progesterone and these hormones ensure that the supply of gonadotrophins to the ovaries is cut off. Egg production by the ovaries thus ceases during pregnancy.

This situation that occurs during a normal

pregnancy is mimicked by the pill, and both oestrogen and progestagens can inhibit ovulation by this method, provided that the dose is high enough. It seems clear, however, that the pill can prevent conception in other ways. The lining of the womb—the endometrium—is also altered by the pill, particularly when the hormones are given sequentially—(see above). The endometrium may become thin and obviously ill-equipped to receive and nurture a fertilized egg. Another effect of the pill may be seen in the character of the mucus which is present in the cervix (neck of the womb). The character of this secretion fluctuates throughout a normal menstrual cycle. Immediately after menstruation there is little mucus, but under the influence of the increasing amounts of oestrogen in the blood stream which is being released from the

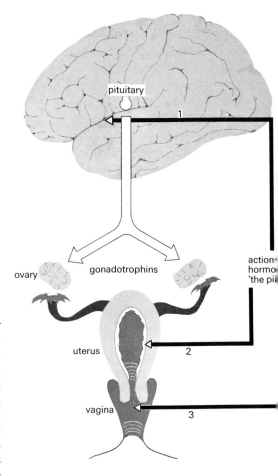

Figure 29.5 Sites of action of the hormones in the contraceptive pill.
(a) Cut-out of production of gonadotrophins by the pituitary gland, (b) endometrium,
(c) character of mucus produced by the neck of the womb.

ovaries the mucus becomes copious and clear. At a point midway in the menstrual cycle—the point of release of an egg (or eggs) from an ovary—these changes reach their climax. This type of mucus is ideal for the penetration by sperms on their way to the uterine cavity. After ovulation, however, the kinds of hormone released by the ovary change. The remnants of the structure (follicle) which released the egg are transformed into a short-lived gland, the corpus luteum, which produces the hormone called progesterone. Under the influence of progesterone the fluid in the canal of the neck of the womb becomes cellular and tough—the cervical 'plug'—which is 'hostile' to the penetration by sperm. This natural change can be produced by taking large enough amounts of progesterone by mouth, and even smaller doses of the progesterone can prevent the effects of naturally produced oestrogen on the cervical mucus. These various effects of oral contraceptives are shown in Figure 29.5.

The effectiveness of oral contraceptives

If tablets are taken according to directions, this method of contraception is virtually 100 per cent effective in preventing pregnancy.

Side-effects of contraceptive pills

Various possible side-effects of the pill have been described. Minor side-effects, such as nausea and breast tenderness or fullness, are usually only a temporary nuisance and tend to occur in the first few cycles of taking the drug, eventually settling without treatment. Headache may also occur and true migraine may be aggravated. Depression is another effect that has been described in some cases. A few normal women have a rise in blood pressure while taking the pill, and if the woman already suffers from high blood pressure (hypertension) it may be made worse by the pill. This is one reason why women on the pill should have regular medical supervision.

Changes in the menstrual cycle, e.g. irregular bleeding or disappearance of menstrual periods (amenorrhoea), occasionally occur. These side-effects need medical advice and possibly a change to another type of pill. A gain in weight is a fairly common side-effect.

Real risks to health

There is no evidence to indicate that oral contraceptives are a 'cause' of cancer of the breast or cervix. The only real risk to health and life is deep vein thrombosis and cerebral thrombosis. In these conditions a clot of blood develops in a blood vessel. The vein affected by thrombosis is usually one in the leg or in the pelvis. The risk of venous thrombosis is that a piece of clot will detach itself and pass up with the main stream of blood in the veins to the heart. The clot may pass through the heart into the pulmonary arteries which supply the lungs with blood. If a large clot passes into a pulmonary artery it may completely block the artery or one of its branches. This condition is called pulmonary embolus. It is a potential killer if the clot is a large one. In the case of cerebral thrombosis the clot develops in an artery, and the consequences depend on the size of the artery and upon the part of the brain which the artery supplies with blood.

These untoward effects of the pill have been much publicized and have caused much concern (see also page 300). The evaluation of risks is a complex affair, but the mortality associated with the use of oral contraceptives (or indeed the IUD) are certainly no greater than the risks of pregnancy itself. In a previous section (page 300) we have compared the risk to that of males playing football or cricket, or of the risks of smoking one-third cigarette once a day for three weeks out of four. (See Tables 36 and 37.)

Supervision of individuals on oral contraceptives

For obvious reasons the decision to start oral contraception has to be taken jointly by a woman and her doctor after discussion of the benefits and possible risks of the technique. For the vast majority of women the benefits of oral contraception outweigh any possible disadvantages. This initial contact with the doctor should include the taking of a full medical history and a physical examination that includes

Table 36 Death rates per million (England and Wales, 1957–61) in men and women aged 20–24 years, from certain causes

Cause	Males	Females
All causes	1126	514
Road accidents	434	59
Drowning	32	3
Suicide	67	33
Murder	8	5
Oral contraceptives	–	13

Table 37 Death rates from cerebral thrombosis and pulmonary embolism in users and non-users of oral contraceptives, compared with the risks from some other causes (figures for 1966, England and Wales)

Death rates	*Women aged 20–34 years*	*Women aged 35–44 years*
Annual death rates per 100 000	60.1	170.5
Death rates per 100 000 healthy non-pregnant women from pulmonary or cerebral thrombo-embolism:		
users of oral contraceptives	1.5	3.9
non-users	0.2	0.5
Death rate per 100 000 pregnancies	22.8	57.6
Death rate from cancer per 100 000 women	13.7	70.1

the recording of blood pressure, examination of the breasts and pelvic organs and a cervical smear. There are certain reasons why a woman should not take the pill. These reasons include cancer of the breast (the growth of which *might* be stimulated by the hormones) and severe hypertension.

When a decision has been made to start on the pill, the woman usually sees her doctor some time during the second or third cycle of the treatment so that it is possible to check that all is well and that the woman is taking the pill as prescribed, and also to ensure that both she and her husband are happy with this method. After this check then a six-monthly examination is all that is necessary, unless, of course, the woman experiences side-effects from the use of these drugs.

Intra-uterine contraception

Contraceptive devices that are inserted into the body of the uterus have been in use for many years. They were first made of metal or silkworm gut and were used for the purposes of contraception in Germany in the 1920s. Because of a variety of complications—excessive bleeding, infections, expulsion of the device, pregnancies, abortions, perforation of the uterus—they fell into disfavour in western countries although they still continued to be used in certain countries such as Japan and Israel.

Interest in intra-uterine contraception revived in 1959 with the publication of two independent reports on the long-term safe and reliable use of two types of intra-uterine rings, one made of silkworm gut, the other made of metal or moulded plastic. A variety of devices are now in use. In Great Britain the commonest kind is called Lippes' Loop. This is a plastic

zig-zag which is introduced into the uterus through the neck of the womb by way of a plastic cylinder. There are two threads attached to the tail of this plastic device and these protrude through the cervix so that one can readily check the position of the device or remove it by pulling on the cords.

Mode of action

It is by no means clear how these devices prevent conception. Various suggestions have been put forward—blocking passage of sperm to the Fallopian tubes, prevention of ovulation, prevention of a fertilized egg from entering the uterine cavity, causing chronic inflammation of the lining of the womb—only to be subsequently rejected. We can only say that the presence of the device makes the environment of the uterus 'hostile' either to fertilization of the egg or the implantation of fertilized egg into the lining of the uterus.

Insertion

These devices are usually inserted as an outpatient procedure, and usually without an anaesthetic. Before insertion the woman is told that the IUD, like most other methods of contraception, is not 100 per cent successful, and that with any method a few women have complications. She should also know how to obtain advice in the event of a complication occurring as an emergency.

Complications

1. Pregnancy. The occurrence of pregnancy with the Lippes' Loop has been recorded as

0–6 per cent in the first year of use; with all devices the pregnancy rate tends to increase with further years. If a pregnancy occurs when a loop is in place perhaps about one-third will miscarry (abort) spontaneously.

2. Expulsion. The Loop can be and often is expelled from the body of the uterus, usually at the time of menstruation, when the muscular activity of the uterus is greatest. For one type of device, Lippes' Loop expulsion occurs in 5–32 per cent of women in the first year.

3. Bleeding and pain. These effects sometimes make it necessary to remove the loop.

4. Increased vaginal discharge.

5. Serious side-effects. Serious side-effects that result in death are fortunately rare. Mortality has been estimated at about 2 per 100 000, i.e. a figure which is comparable to the risks of the pill. These serious side-effects include perforation of the uterus, infection and ectopic pregnancy i.e. pregnancy outside the body of the uterus, usually in the Fallopian tubes.

Choice of the IUD as a method of contraception

There are a variety of medical or gynaecological reasons which make it unwise to use the IUD as a method of contraception. The presence of these conditions can be ruled out at the clinic for inserting the device. In general only the woman who can appreciate the importance of symptoms which may develop and the need for regular follow-ups at a clinic should be fitted with an IUD. Some workers feel that the use of IUDs in a primitive society may be unwise.

Fertility control by periodic abstinence— the rhythm method

Fertility and the menstrual cycle

The human female is not fertile throughout the duration of the menstrual cycle. Fertility is restricted to about four days during the cycle at the time when an egg is liberated from the ovary. In order to discover which is the fertile period, it is necessary to know both the time of ovulation and the period of survival and fertility of both egg and sperm.

The menstrual cycle

During a woman's active reproductive era, menstruation ('periods') occurs at intervals of approximately twenty-eight days; the length of a cycle is counted from the first day of one period to the first day of the next. Each woman tends to have her own rhythm (cycle length) and any cycle length between three and five weeks may be accepted as normal. Individual women, however, tend to vary in the length of the cycle. These variations are greater in adolescence and in the few years before the menopause. Every woman who says that she has a perfectly regular cycle can usually be shown to have occasional cycles which vary by as much as two days less or more than their usual cycle provided that accurate records are kept. A convenient way of describing the menstrual cycle of an individual woman is in terms of a fraction, e.g. 4/28, where the numerator refers to the duration of the flow and the denominator to the length of the cycle from the beginning of one period to the beginning of the next.

Ovulation and the menstrual cycle

For various reasons, not the least of which is contraception, it is important to know if a woman is ovulating during her menstrual cycle and at what part of the cycle ovulation is occurring. There are various ways in which doctors can determine the presence and timing of ovulation, but here we will restrict ourselves to the use of observations which the woman herself is capable of making. Up to 70 per cent of women have some symptoms at the time of ovulation which they can be trained to recognize. Many women experience some lower abdominal pain for twelve to twenty-four hours just before or after ovulation, and this pain may be linked with the actual rupture of a follicle in the ovary releasing an egg and a small amount of blood to the cavity of the pelvis. Some women also experience a slight loss of blood or mucus tinged with blood at the time of ovulation. It may occur together with ovulation pain, but the two can occur independently. A more reliable method of dating ovulation in most women is, however, a daily charting of body temperature.

Figure 29.6 shows a temperature chart during the menstrual cycle of a normal woman who ovulates during the cycle. In the beginning of the cycle the body temperature is low but after ovulation the temperature begins to rise. This rise in temperature is due to the effect of the

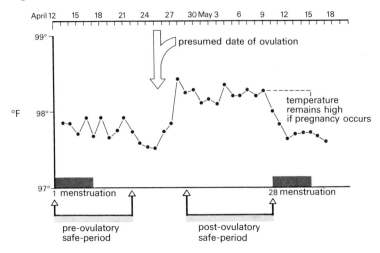

Figure 29.6 Temperature records during a menstrual cycle showing the 'safe' periods.

hormone progesterone liberated from the corpus luteum, which develops from the remnants of the erupted follicle after the release of the egg. The exact relationship between ovulation and the rise in temperature is not known; what does seem to be certain is that as soon as the temperature has been elevated for forty-eight hours, the ovum is no longer capable of being fertilized. This is known from studies of artificial insemination (i.e. when sperm from the husband or a donor is artificially introduced into the woman's vagina); conception does not occur if artificial insemination is performed more than two days after the rise in temperature. Normal women occasionally have cycles in which they do not ovulate, but these cycles are more common in the early and late years of menstruation. In these cycles—called anovulatory cycles—there is no rise in temperature. A further variation on the normal bi-phasic temperature chart occurs if a woman becomes pregnant. In such a woman the temperature chart shows the normal rise in temperature on ovulation, but this continues (Figure 29.6) because of the continuing production of progesterone by the corpus luteum, and later by the placenta.

The safe period

Obviously there are two parts of the menstrual cycle in which conception is unlikely to occur. One of these parts is before ovulation, the other begins two days after ovulation (see Figure 29.6). This second 'safe period' is the easiest to recognize because of the rise in body temper-

ature that occurs around the period of ovulation. We have already seen that after the temperature has been raised for forty-eight hours the egg is no longer capable of being fertilized. For women who can produce reliable daily temperature records, restriction of intercourse to this infertile period, beginning after forty-eight hours of rise in temperature, has proved an effective method of contraception; impressive figures of failure rates as low as 0.8–1.4 pregnancies per 100 woman/years of use have been given from some surveys.

Extension of the safe period to the pre-ovulatory period

Although it is easy enough to recognize when ovulation has already occurred by means of temperature charting, it is much more difficult to *predict* ovulation and so to use the days before ovulation as a 'safe period'. Usually a 'calendar method' is used to predict ovulation, using information from previous menstrual cycles. In order to use this calendar calculation the menstrual cycle *must* be regular. However, even when cycles *are* regular this does not necessarily mean that the timing of ovulation is necessarily regular. Because of these reasons the use of the part of the cycle before ovulation as a 'safe period' carries higher risks of pregnancy. In calculating the infertile period before ovulation, it is necessary to estimate the *earliest* day of ovulation from previous temperature records; the day of ovulation is regarded as four days before the earliest recorded day on which there is a rise in temperature (see Figure 29.6). To this must be added three days, to take into account the fact that the sperms deposited in the genital tract can survive and fertilize an egg released several days later. Thus, looking at the temperature chart in Figure 29.6 the rise in temperature occurred on 29 May. Ovulation is presumed to have occurred on 25 May. Taking into account the period of survival of sperm, the safe period before ovulation would be 12–22 May, i.e. the first ten days of the menstrual cycle.

Summary

We can conclude that there are two infertile parts of the menstrual cycle, one occurring before ovulation the other following an interval after ovulation. The post-ovulatory infertile period is easier to recognize because of the rise in body temperature which follows ovulation. The pre-ovulatory infertile period is more difficult to assess and has to be calculated from information about previous cycles. The risk of pregnancy is inversely proportional to the length of the 'safe period' which is used. The risk is least for those using the post-ovulatory infertile periods. The risks associated with this method of contraception are not those of the method, but those of the risks of failure, i.e. the risks of pregnancy itself (see Table 37).

Sterilization

Medical attitudes to sterilization have changed considerably in recent years, particularly since the implementation of the Abortion Act. Although oral contraception can offer a virtual 100 per cent success rate, there are some women in whom these drugs are inadvisable. If these women are likely to run serious risks to life and health should they become pregnant, or if they are likely to produce children with defects or inherited disease, then sterilization of the woman, or her husband, is usually seriously considered (in Great Britain at least). Simple and safe methods of sterilization are available for both women and men, even under the influence of a local anaesthetic.

Legal aspects

In Britain the legal position of sterilization is rather obscure, for there has never been a case which has been tested by the Courts. There seems little doubt, however, that the Courts would regard sterilization as legal, even if only for a convenient method of birth control, provided that it is carried out only after both partners have had the nature and effects of the operation explained to them.

Methods of sterilization

Female

In the female sterilization is usually achieved by either tying, cutting or burning the Fallopian tubes. This operation can be done very conveniently a few days after the birth of the last child, when the uterus is still an abdominal organ and the tubes are easy to reach. Recent advances in sterilization have produced a simple and safe technique that disturbs the patient very little and needs only a short stay in hospital. In this technique the 'cold light telescope' is introduced into the abdominal cavity through a small opening. Under this direct vision it is possible to divide each Fallopian tube by a heating electric current (diathermy).

Male sterilization

Male sterilization, as a contraceptive technique, is a recent development. In 1960 the Medical Defence Societies in Britain were advised that male sterilization was not unlawful. Soon afterwards the Simon Population Trust launched a successful campaign to make doctors and the public more aware of the technique. In April 1971, the Secretary of State for Health and Social Security announced that vasectomy (male sterilization) could be carried out under the National Health Service if the health of the husband or wife was in danger. Thousands of these operations have already been performed, and the demand for the operation exceeds the services available. The operation is regarded as a 'simple, safe, aesthetic, efficient and cheap method of achieving permanent family limitation' (Pauline Jackson et al. 'A Male Sterilization Clinic', *British Medical Journal*, Vol. 4, No. 5730, 1970). In India male sterilization has been carried out on a large scale to promote the aims of population control.

In Britain the couples are usually interviewed to determine whether or not this kind of contraception is in the best interests of the family. The merits of both female and male sterilization are discussed, and if the operation on the male is decided upon then both husband and wife are given information about the operation and its effects—that the operation has to be regarded as irreversible (although in some cases it is possible to repair the damage and restore fertility) and that sexual activity remains unchanged. The operation takes only fifteen to twenty minutes and is carried out under the effect of a local anaesthetic. The principle of the operation is to divide the tubes (vasa deferentia) which conducts sperms from the testes to the base of the bladder. After the operation some other form of contraception is needed until stored sperms disappear from the semen—and this has to be checked by microscopic examination of this fluid. Semen continues to be produced after the operation, for the bulk of this fluid comes from the prostate and other excessory glands, although it does not contain sperms.

The place of sterilization

In view of the fact that 70 000 or so *therapeutic* abortions are carried out in England and Wales each year, it is obvious that many people do not use the existing and efficient methods of contraception. The reasons for this kind of personal irresponsibility are many. What is clear is that, until the ideal contraceptive is available and is used, sterilization will continue to have a significant place in family planning. For some women in whom the risks of pregnancy are great, sterilization can offer much.

Abortion

Abortion is the deliberate termination of a pregnancy before the twenty-eighth week. Although for two-thirds of the world's population abortion is either prohibited entirely or is allowed for only narrowly defined medical reasons, abortion is still a widespread and secret way of controlling fertility. In Britain and Scandinavian countries (2 per cent of the world's population) the laws regarding abortion are more liberal. In Britain abortion to protect the health of the mother has been legal since 1938. In 1968 the new Abortion Act came into force, but only after a long and bitter legislative struggle. According to this new British act, abortion is permitted after two doctors have certified that the continuance of the pregnancy would involve risk to the life or physical and mental health of the woman, even if the risk is very slight. This law also permits abortion if the birth of the child would endanger the physical or mental health of the woman's existing family or if the child would be born defective. These are indeed liberal indications for abortion. In view of the difficulties of weighing up the medical and social facts in any individual case, it is little wonder that the interpretations of the new Act vary from one

doctor to another. Among the medical reasons given for carrying out legal abortions in Britain, psychiatric problems predominate. A number of abortions are now carried out for non-medical reasons, such as youth and immaturity of the pregnant woman, large existing families, problem husbands ('away from home', drug addicts, violence, etc.) and financial and housing problems.

In Japan, China and most countries of Eastern Europe (one-third of the world's population), abortion is permitted either at the request of the pregnant woman or on broad social indications. In some countries the number of abortions have increased so much that it might be thought that abortion had displaced contraception as a method of birth control. In Hungary in 1967 there were 187 500 legal abortions compared to 148 900 live births. The fall in the birth rate resulting from the liberal abortion laws has caused some countries (e.g. Rumania and Bulgaria) to re-introduce some restriction on abortion. This vast increase in the number of legal abortions has only been made possible by a considerable improvement in the safety of the operation. In Japan and Eastern Europe the mortality of legal abortions has fallen to 1–4/100 000; the reasons for this low mortality is that these countries prohibit abortion after the third month of pregnancy, except for medical reasons. In countries such as Sweden and Denmark, which permit legal abortion at later stages in pregnancy, the death rate has been considerably higher, and in Sweden it was 39 per 100 000 in the period 1960–66. In Britain the total number of abortions carried out during the first eight months of the operation of the new Act was 23 641. In the last quarter of 1968 there were 9163 legal abortions with 12 deaths. In the first quarter of 1969 there were 10 513 legal abortions with 5 deaths. The new British Abortion Act appears to have had considerable impact overseas. Canada, South Australia and Singapore have since liberalized their abortion laws, and so have many states of America; the law in New York is even more liberal than it is in Britain.

Legal abortion usually involves a day in hospital, a general anaesthetic and the emptying of the contents of the womb. The womb is emptied, particularly in the early months of pregnancy, by stretching the neck of the womb, viewed via the vagina, and then scraping or sucking out its contents. Another method, used particularly if the operation is carried out after the third month of pregnancy, is to open the abdominal wall and cut into the body of the womb and then scrape out its contents. The risks and complications of these procedures include those of the anaesthetic itself, haemorrhage and infection. Various other methods of emptying the womb are in use, and much interest is being shown in the use of a new group of drugs that can stimulate the womb into powerful contractions so that it empties itself without the need for surgery. There seems little doubt that simpler and safer methods of producing abortion will come into general use during the next few years.

The pros and cons of abortion

Abortion as a way of controlling fertility, is unpopular to many people, not least to some gynaecologists who have to routinely carry out these destructive operations. There seems little doubt that if abortion were to become free on demand then it might replace contraception as a method of controlling family size. To many this would be a retrograde step. Certainly it would be a costly method of fertility control, both in terms of resources and human life. For a fuller discussion of the pros and cons of abortion, including moral and ethical arguments, the reader is referred to the bibliography.

Illegal abortion

So far we have not mentioned criminal (or illegal) abortion. Many criminal abortionists rely on damaging or destroying the embryo by mechanical means and then waiting for the uterus to become active and expel its contents. The risks of criminal abortion depend upon the skill of the operator and the circumstances under which the operation is done. The risks are similar to those of legal abortion, such as haemorrhage, infection (which may be followed by sterility), perforation of the uterus, air or fluid emboli (see page 283) and effects on the mind of the woman (e.g. depression). The risks are, however, greater than those of legal abortion and they have been estimated to be in the region of 1–1000 in a developed country. Illegal abortion becomes less frequent when a country is liberal in its indications for legal, therapeutic abortion; illegal abortions do not, however, disappear entirely.

The promotion of family planning

In January 1965 President L. B. Johnson in his State of the Union address said 'five dollars invested in birth control is worth a hundred dollars invested in economic growth'. In the year following this address the Declaration of Population was signed by twelve world leaders, and in 1968 further signatories were added. This Declaration on Population marked an important step in man's evolution—the recognition that the survival of the human race depends, among other things, on the ability to control his own fertility. The political, religious and educational problems in encouraging family planning are very complex. In many segments of societies there is traditional resistance to the ideas of population control. The medical profession itself has been criticized for its conservative influence. It is unfortunate that many modern methods of population control (the pill, IUDs, abortion) need medical supervision. Many doctors, already overburdened by their traditional role of saving life, are unsympathetic to family planning, and understandably so when this involves the routine destruction of living embryos. It would be preferable if the control of family planning were to be in the hands of a specialist branch of the medical profession, in which only those devoted to the ideas of family planning, and unfettered by religious or ethical scruples, were members. This would leave those devoted to the saving of existing lives to pursue their true vocations.

It is impossible to discuss barriers to the promotion of family planning without mention of the influence of the Roman Catholic Church. The attitudes of this Church have been a serious obstacle to the control of population growth, particularly in South America, France and South Ireland. Pope Paul's encyclical, Humanae Vitae, clearly stated that *without exception* the primary and legitimate purpose of marriage is for the purpose of procreation. This encyclical was not delivered *ex cathedra*, i.e. it is not regarded as being 'infallible', so that for each Roman Catholic the ultimate authority on contraception is his or her own conscience. The Roman Catholic Church does not, however, seem to disapprove of the rhythm method of contraception. This method does not involve the deliberate use of a barrier between egg and sperm—merely the 'wasting' of sperm at the time when the chances of conception are known to be remote. Such are the niceties of philosophical arguments.

Ignorance and fear are still potent forces that prevent the promotion of family planning, even in developed countries of the world. It is important that women have knowledge not only of the various methods of contraception but also of the risks of failure and the possible side-effects of the methods. If possible side-effects are not explained in advance, the appearance of these effects—e.g. weight gain with oral contraceptives or bleeding and discomfort with the IUD—then this can lead to the woman discontinuing with the method with the obvious risk of an unwanted pregnancy. Moreover, the fears and disappointments that these experiences produce can lead to a spread of misinformation among the woman's friends and thus bring a particular method into disrepute. The effect of this kind of misinformation or misrepresentation can be profound if mass media (television, newspapers etc.) are involved (see discussion on the side-effects of the pill, page 300). Ignorance and prejudice about contraception can all too easily be re-inforced by fear, e.g. will the use of a particular contraceptive make my wife unfaithful, effect my desire and potency, cause future sterility, effect the health of any child that may result from a failure of the method, cause cancer, cause thrombosis, encourage promiscuity among the unmarried and so on. Great care must be exercised in the use of 'fear' as a method of promoting family planning (or any other aspect of health education)—fears of the effects of repeated pregnancies on the health of the mother, and in causing poverty and malnutrition. When people are frightened they use one of man's most primitive methods of dealing with a difficult situation; they reject the information, denying that it is true or casting it away from the conscious mind into the depth of the unconscious. Those who fail to solve their fears in this way may become anxious or depressed. It is difficult indeed to know how people will respond to propaganda based on fear, to take the appropriate positive

action, i.e. to use contraceptives, stop smoking, to take out life insurance policies, or buy fire extinguishers for their homes.

Of increasing importance in many countries is the vexed question of the teaching of family planning to adolescents. Whilst a general study of the growth of human population and agricultural needs engenders no opposition, the teaching of contraception *per se*, particularly if it attracts too much public attention, is fraught with risks for teachers, doctors and publishers. In spite of the sexual activities of adolescents, which are all too clearly revealed by the increasing number of unwanted pregnancies, venereal diseases and abortions, society tends to frown upon the teaching of the aims and methods of family planning to this age group. On the other hand it is clear that increased knowledge alone is not enough to promote the aims of family planning. One of the main barriers to the wider acceptance of contraception in the world has been a lack of *motivation* at all levels of societies.

The force of geometric progression of the world's population needs stronger restraints than are available at the moment. More acceptable, efficient and safer methods of contraception are urgently needed. The resources diverted to population control need to be greatly increased. Moreover it would be a great advantage if these resources were employed by specialists, not only in the techniques of family planning but also in the arts of persuasion, leaving the bulk of doctors and educators to pursue their traditional roles in society.

30. Mental health

Introduction

THE bulk of this book has been concerned with physical diseases of many kinds and the way in which vaccines, antibiotics, public health measures, health education and the like can be used to reduce the total of physical suffering and to promote health. In this last chapter we turn to mental and spiritual aspects of health. The amount of space that is devoted to this topic in no way reflects the importance of mental and behavioural disturbances as agents that can cripple the individual and the society in which he lives. In many developed nations it is estimated that nearly 50 per cent of all hospital beds are occupied by the mentally ill, and that as many as ten per 1000 of the population are suffering from severe mental disorders. Rapid social and cultural changes in developing countries also bring with them their toll of mental disorders. In these countries, ill-equipped as they are to cope with even the basic requirements of adequate food, clean water and efficient sanitation, these disorders will inevitably continue to devastate the lives of individuals and drain the human resources of nations.

The treatment of mental disorders and the promotion of mental health forms 'the other half', the 'dark side' of medicine. After centuries of ignorance, prejudice and empirical treatment (i.e. treatment based on results rather than understanding, Figure 30.1) and the segregation of the mentally ill in institutions, this dark side of medicine is slowly rotating to come under the impact of concern, compassion, scientific scrutiny and rational treatment. One of the outstanding developments of mental health services is the trend away from 'custodial care' of individuals in institutions, and towards active treatment with the aim of returning the individual as soon as possible to the community, where he receives the support and encouragement to live as normal a life as possible. We are still ignorant of the causes of many mental disorders and indeed of the way in which various treatments produce their effects, but there is a growing realization that the frequency of some mental disorders depends upon social structure and forces, and the way that other people and institutions in society respond to these mental disorders.

A look at the 'spectrum' of mental illness

The term mental and behavioural illness covers a vast range of disorders which, compared to physical illness, can differ from one another in terms of effects or chances of cure as much as the common cold differs from cancer of the lung. In this section we can do no more than review briefly and in patches the range of mental and behavioural disorders; wherever possible we will indicate possible methods of the prevention of these disorders.

Figure 30.1 Photograph showing a 'dance of possession' employed by African medicine men to 'treat' certain forms of mental illness. The accelerating rhythm of the dances and the music induces a hypnotic state, terminating in unconsciousness. (*WHO photo.*)

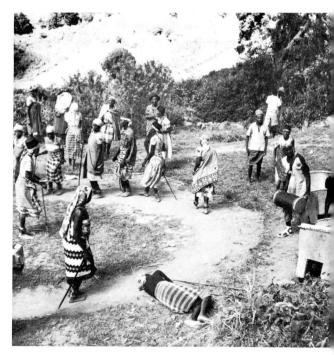

Constitutional disorders

In this group of illnesses are mental disorders in which constitutional, i.e. inherited factors, are important. We can regard these disorders as extreme variations of the normal personality.

Individuals with sub-normal intelligence

These individuals are called mental defectives and exist as all grades from idiots who are so defective as to be completely unable to guard themselves against common physical dangers, to feeble-minded persons who need *some* care and control for their protection or for the protection of others. The borderline between the mental defective and the normal individual is, of course, vague, and the transition between the two continuous. The definition of the term mental defective (oligophrenia) is thus disputed, but many take a point of I.Q. 70 to distinguish the mental defective from the individuals at the lower range of 'normal' intelligence. The number of individuals who have an I.Q. below 70 is somewhere between 1 and 3 per cent of the population. Individuals with an I.Q. between 50 and 70 are the high-grade mental defectives—the 'feeble-minded' or 'morons'—whereas those with an I.Q. of less than 50 are the imbeciles, and at the lowest part of this range are the idiots.

The causes of mental deficiency are varied. The severest cases of mental deficiency—the imbeciles or idiots—often result from forces operating during and after birth—e.g. brain damage during birth, injury or brain disease in infancy and deficiencies of thyroid hormone (cretinism). These individuals tend to occur in otherwise normal families, i.e. there is no constitutional (genetic) factor operating. In considering any individual imbecile or idiot this can, however, never be assumed, for in this group there are in fact many forms of mental deficiency which are subject to simple Mendelian forms of inheritance. Many of these genetically determined causes of mental deficiency are transmitted as recessive genes on the autosomes (see Chapter 21). In view of the nature of recessive genes and the small family size in developed countries, it often happens that a mentally defective individual is the only person affected by the disorder in the whole family. In this group there are also various autosomal and sex chromosome abnormalities (see Chapter 20). Another possible cause of this degree of mental deficiency is survival after brain damage caused by Rhesus incompatibility between mother and infant.

When we come to the less severe forms of mental deficiency we find that inherited factors are much more important, and factors operating after birth are uncommon causes of this condition. The mode of inheritance of the gene(s) which determines this grade of mental deficiency is by no means simple, and probably these conditions are due to the inheritance of several genetic factors. An added complication in the study of these individuals is that feeble-minded mothers create an unfavourable environment for the mental development of their offspring; thus in addition to the effects of inherited genes there may be added an inhibiting environmental factor.

Treatment and prevention of mental deficiency

The possibilities for treating the mental defective are very limited. There are a few individuals in which the cause of mental deficiency can be corrected provided an early diagnosis is made. One such example is phenylketonuria, an inherited disorder (see page 265). Another treatable cause of mental deficiency is cretinism caused by a deficiency of thyroid hormones. These hormones are vital for normal physical and mental development, and if the condition is not diagnosed early and treated with the hormones then the individual becomes a cretin, a mental defective who fails to attain normal adult stature or sexual maturity (Figure 30.2). These special individuals apart, there is little that can be done to improve the level of intelligence of the mental defective. What can be done is to ensure special training facilities to enable the defective to make full use of whatever potentialities he or she may have. Special schools and institutions can achieve much in stimulating the performance of the less severely mentally handicapped.

From the discussion of the known causes of mental deficiency, it is obvious that the main way of controlling this problem lies in *prevention*, e.g. improved obstetrical care to reduce the risks of brain damage during birth and to prevent disease resulting from Rhesus incompatibility, and efficient contraception in those families likely to produce more defectives. Unfortunately the high-grade defectives (who are common enough and make up to 2 per cent of the general population) are the least capable of controlling their propagation.

Constitutional disorders of personality and instinct (homosexuality)

By 'personality' we mean distinctive personal

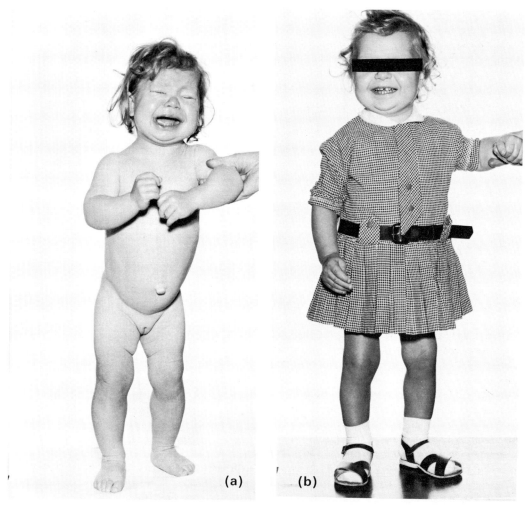

Figure 30.2 The little girl in photograph (a) is a cretin. The effects of six months treatment with the hormone thyroxine is seen on the right in (b).

characteristics of one individual, the person as he is known to his friends. In spite of the difficulties of defining the normal personality, there is general agreement that there may be many unusual and abnormal individuals. Although these individuals may not be classified in generally recognized mental disorders, their recognition has great social and psychiatric importance. They may, for example, be more likely to develop certain mental illnesses (e.g. schizophrenia, hysteria, depression or anxiety). There may also be difficulties in social relationships and their activities may bring them into conflict with the law.

An attempt to untwine the nexus of influences that guide the development of the personalities, normal and abnormal, would be doomed from the outset, certainly in a book of this size. We will restrict ourselves to some brief observations of two types of personality defects—the psychopath and the homosexual.

Psychopathic personalities

The main feature of psychopathic personalities lies in their anti-social or asocial behaviour. The psychopath acts without regard for consequences in the fulfilling of his immediate desires. In fulfilling these desires—which may change repeatedly—the psychopath frequently gets into social and legal difficulties, although these difficulties do not prevent him or her from repeating the experience, i.e. he fails to learn from experience. These activities often lead to a drift into a criminal way of life. Of course, not all criminals are psychopaths, but an appreciable number are, particularly of the group of 'persistent' offenders—bigamists, prostitutes, seducers, confidence men etc. Criminal activities are more likely to occur in a group of psychopaths who are aggressively anti-social. In them is a complete absence of shame or guilt for their actions.

The factors that mould an individual into this kind of personality are complex and incompletely understood. As in the case of so many personality and behaviour disorders, attempts have been made to explain the origins in the nature of the upbringing. These attempts are by no means always successful, and many psychopaths seem to emerge from backgrounds which could in no way be regarded as a cause of their abnormal development. There may indeed be a variety of causes of psychopathy, even in one individual—constitutional (inherited), physical and psychological causes. Certainly there appears to be a strong constitutional element in many psychopaths (see page 252 for a discussion of the effect of chromosome composition on criminal behaviour), and a family history of the same disorder is a common experience. Psychopaths seem to attract one another as marriage partners, and this situation sets in train a sequence of events that leads to the appearance of psychopathy in their children. Not only do these children run the risk of inheriting factors that may lead to this kind of personality disorder, but they are nurtured in an unsettled environment in which there are no stable models on which to match their own developing personalities.

Homosexuality

Homosexuality is a disorder of 'instinct' which can, and often does, cause great personal problems for the individual, particularly if he or she lives in a society which does not tolerate, or even actively punishes, overt homosexual behaviour. These conflicts with family or society as a whole may, in turn, bring their toll of mental illness—anxiety and depression, which may lead to suicide.

The origins of this disorder of instinct have been hotly disputed for years, and ideas have changed as science and medicine have progressed. With the discovery of the vital role of sex hormones in determining the kind and intensity of sexual behaviour in animals, it was inevitable that these findings should have been applied to human sexual behaviour. Some early workers, for example, thought that they might be able to transform a male homosexual into a normal heterosexual individual by treatment with a male sex hormone (testosterone). This

kind of treatment, however, has no influence on the *direction* of the sexual impulse (i.e. towards males or females); it does, in fact, intensify sexual activity in its original direction. The emergence of psychoanalytical studies and the results of the observations made by anthropologists on primitive peoples (e.g. Margaret Mead) brought new attitudes to homosexuals. Now the causes were seen to lie in the early formative years, in the child's relationships within the family. Thus if a young boy developed in a family with a dominant mother and a pathetic inadequate father, then the boy might refuse to model himself on the male representative within the family and turn to the female; this kind of family situation came to be regarded as the seed bed of homosexuality.

We still have no clear understanding of the nature of the forces that direct an individual's developing sexual impulses into unusual channels. Like the situation in mental deficiency, it is likely that a variety of factors are involved, both constitutional and environmental. With homosexuals we are dealing with a large group of individuals, and although estimates vary it is certainly a numerically more important group than the mentally defectives. Recent important clues about the mechanisms of sexual differentiation in animals may be significant for our understanding of the causes of sexual deviation in man. In lower animals it is known that a tiny area of the brain (the hypothalamus), which overlies the pituitary gland, is critically important for various aspects of sexuality, for it regulates not only the timing of the onset of physical sexual maturation but also sexual behaviour. In the rat and other mammals the hypothalamus in the newly born animals is apparently sexually indeterminate, and is capable of differentiating into either male or female type irrespective of the kind of gonads (i.e. ovaries or testes) that the animal possesses, provided that it is given the appropriate conditions. If the ovaries or testes are removed from newly born animals the hypothalamus continues to differentiate into the female type, capable of initiating sexual rhythm and behaviour of the female, provided that ovarian tissue is grafted into the animal at a later date. The main factor which determines the direction of differentiation of the hypothalamus is the presence or absence of male sex hormone. If male sex hormone is administered early in post-natal life, then the hypothalamus differentiates into the male type, irrespective of whether or not the animal is genetically female and possesses ovaries. Thus if a newly born female rat is treated with male sex hormones, the hypothalamus differentiates into the male type. If a male rat is castrated at birth or shortly afterwards, the hypothalamus differentiates into the female type in the absence of male hormone.

The implications of these findings for our understanding of human sexual abnormalities are by no means clear, but it seems possible that abnormal behaviour such as homosexuality may, in some cases, be due to some relatively minor defect in the nature or amount of circulating hormones at a critical stage in the development of the individual. Homosexuality arising in this way would certainly have a deep constitutional origin and would probably be extremely resistant to any type of treatment. Homosexuality is certainly an extremely difficult and often impossible condition to treat; indeed most homosexuals are resistant to attempts to change their nature. Apart from those few individuals who feel a desperate need to try to alter the direction of their sexual impulses, it is far kinder and more successful to try to help them adapt to their defect and the problems to which it gives rise, i.e. make them happy homosexuals.

Mental disease caused by physical factors acting after birth

We now turn to mental disorders in which environmental factors, acting after birth, are of importance. 'Mind' and body interact with one another in complex ways, the one invariably affecting the other to some degree. This reciprocal relationship gives rise to two classes of disease. One class is a series of mental disorders in which physical factors are a prime or at least contributing factor in determining the disease. These mental diseases are listed below. A second class of disorders of physical conditions in which causative or aggravating factors are in the realm of the mind or emotion are the psychosomatic illnesses, and are a subject of a later section of this chapter. The following is a list of physical conditions which may give rise to mental disorders:

1. Debilitating physical illnesses may give rise to a vague type of mental illness given the name of 'organic neurasthenia', which is typified by features such as fatigue, irritability, headaches and anxiety.
2. Nutritional deficiencies, particularly deficiencies of vitamins. One type of mental illness of this type is given the name of Korsakow's psychosis, in which defects of memory and appreciation of relationships in

time are prominent features. This particular mental illness occurs most commonly as a complication of chronic alcoholism, but other causes of vitamin deficiency as well as poisoning by some metals (e.g. lead) can produce the same picture. Most cases improve markedly with doses of vitamins, particularly those of the B group, given in high enough doses over a long enough period.
3. Drug addiction (see Chapter 28).
4. Head injury and epilepsy.
5. Syphilis. A proportion of untreated cases of syphilis (possibly about 5 per cent) develop the condition known as dementia paralytica (general paralysis of the insane). In this condition there is progressive deterioration of the personality, both in intelligence and character. Usually the disease develops gradually in many people and the possible early symptoms include deterioration in the memory, changes in eating, drinking and sexual habits, and irritability. As the disease progresses the individual becomes more and more indolent and apathetic. This disease is preventable, by adequate treatment of early syphilis. Even in the late stages some improvement usually occurs following treatment with penicillin or some other appropriate antibiotic.
6. Senile dementia. The normal processes of ageing usually result in changes in the outlook and behaviour of the individual; to some degree both emotions and memory become blunted. When these changes involve a progressive disorganization of the whole personality, with severe disturbances of memory, we call the condition a senile psychosis or dementia. To some degree these changes can be linked with degenerative changes in the brain and its blood supply. These individuals are common enough in mental hospitals. The condition may progress rapidly, sometimes after a bereavement or a physical illness, the individual becoming physically feeble, unable to follow a conversation, with mood swinging from senseless hilarity to irritability and suspicion with periods of feelings of persecution. Personal habits and hygiene progressively deteriorate. The outlook for these patients is poor and little can be done to halt the progressive deterioration.

Schizophrenia

The term schizophrenia covers a range of psychotic illnesses characterized by a disintegration of the personality (but not necessarily of the intellect) in the absence of any known form of brain damage. In most cases the disintegration is progressive, unless it is halted by treatment. Cases of schizophrenia make up a large group of patients in mental hospitals— about half the beds in mental hospitals, or one in five of all hospital beds.

There are many ways in which this disease can show itself, indeed on some occasions the disease may be diagnosed by exclusion. If we are presented with an individual whose mental disorders cannot be explained by the presence of any physical illness or other form of mental or personality disorder then the question inevitably arises whether or not we are dealing with a schizophrenic. The basic disorder in a schizophrenic is one of his idea of 'self'. To a greater or lesser degree he loses contact with reality and he withdraws into a world of fantasy. Disorder of thought processes, particularly abstract thoughts, may be so marked that the individual may believe that his thoughts are being 'stolen from my head'. Hallucinations and delusions are indeed common symptoms. The causes of schizophrenia are hotly disputed and a number of hypotheses have been put forward. In a proportion of schizophrenics there are biochemical abnormalities, and an abnormal chemical appears in the urine of a proportion of cases of acute forms of the disease. It is by no means clear whether these changes are causes or effects of the disease. There are almost certainly hereditary factors at work; when one of a pair of twins develops the disease then the other member is more likely to develop the disease if he or she is an identical twin (monozygotic) than if he or she is non-identical (dizygotic).

Furthermore, the relatives of a schizophrenic are more likely to develop the disease than is the rest of the population. Of course these observations do not *necessarily* indicate that genetic factors are operating; some schools of thought argue that the family influence is very important in determining the development of the disease. The influence of a schizophrenic mother in this respect has received a notorious reputation. Professor Munro in a recent article on the subject 'Current Views on Schizophrenia', *The Practitioner*, Vol. 205, Sept. 1970, concluded 'in general it is probably true to say that schizophrenia cannot occur in most cases unless a genetic predisposition is present. Even if the predisposition is present, however, it is possible that a favourable upbringing may prevent its expression'.

Schizophrenia is increasingly a treatable condition, especially if it is diagnosed early; early treatment can prevent most cases from progressing into a permanent and incapable invalidism. Various drugs are available that can *halt* the illness in most cases. For some severe cases this treatment is started in hospital, but every attempt is made to return the patient to his home environment (unless this is thought to be harmful to his condition). The amount of outpatient supervision that is needed varies from one individual to another; if support is adequate it seems that many of the recurring break-downs that need hospital treatment can be prevented.

In view of the genetic factors which seem to be involved in this disease, many doctors discourage schizophrenics from having children, even if they have had only a single attack of the disease. In the case of brothers and sisters of the schizophrenics, advice about parenthood can only be given by a closely collaborating team of family doctors, a psychiatrist and a genetic counsellor, who can weigh up the environmental and genetic factors in the individual case.

Manic-depressive psychoses

These illnesses, like the schizophrenias, are difficult to define in clear terms. Mild cases of this psychosis may be readily missed or misdiagnosed. In its classical form this psychosis shows itself by the appearance at different times in the same individual of swings of mood, sometimes of depression and sometimes of excitement (mania). Often there is a period of normality between these swings of abnormal mood, and indeed there may be a fairly regular rhythm in these periods of normality and mood change. Commonly an individual may show only one type of mood change.

The disease may occur at any time in life, but most commonly it occurs in the thirties and attacks may be brought on by a range of factors— by infections, by menstruation, childbirth, the menopause, operations etc. The symptoms of depression are simple and easily overlooked; failure to recognize depression in mental illness is a common mistake, both by relatives of the patient and by his doctor. There are two aspects of depression, physical changes and mental symptoms. The physical changes include a lowering of energy and activity, and the individual becomes easily fatigued. Characteristically there is a reduction of sexual activity and a disturbance of sleep pattern which consists of frequent and early waking. Usually there is also a loss of appetite and a loss of weight. The mental symptoms run parallel to these physical changes, with a loss of interest and confidence so that the individual feels unable to cope with normal social activities; indeed he may become withdrawn and anxious to avoid the company of others. This withdrawal into the self may lead to exaggerated feelings of unworthiness and guilt. An important feature of depressive illness is that every depressed person, whatever the cause of the depression, is a potential suicide risk.

The manic phases of this illness may develop gradually, but if it follows a depressive phase the onset can be very sudden. In this phase the personality becomes expansive and self-assertive. The individual may become very talkative and unusually familiar with strangers. Physical activity increases; he or she may get up early in the morning and bustle about the house, carrying out as many chores before breakfast as would normally fill a whole day. Social life runs at a hectic and chaotic pace, with unnecessary telephone calls, telegrams, rapid changes in plans, striking up acquaintances with complete strangers met in buses, bars etc. With life running at such a pace the individual becomes intolerant of any frustration or obstacle in achieving his ends. Quarrels and brawls are likely. The tempo of this existence increases as the individual progresses into frank mania, with shouting, dancing, incoherent rapid speech, uncontrollable hilarity, violence and lack of sexual restraint, with exhibitionism and even open masturbation in public. Like the depressive phase of the illness, the manic phase eventually tends to resolve spontaneously.

In this disease a clear genetic influence is at work. In view of the difficulties in exactly defining and diagnosing the illness, there is a considerable variation in estimates of the risk that an individual will succumb to the illness when a near relative has been diagnosed as a manic-depressive. When one member in a family is affected, the chances are about one in ten that brothers or sisters will be similarly affected, and this risk becomes greater if one of the parents is a manic-depressive. These uncertainties create a problem when it comes to genetic counselling; each case has to be judged on its own merits, taking into account a full family history and the severity of the disorder. Many manic-depressives have unusual talent, and they may well feel that their gifts or unusual experiences more than compensate them for the burden of mental illness.

Anxiety and depression

Anxiety and depression are common enough

symptoms in many different kinds of mental illnesses. Frequently, however, they are present as dominant features that characterize a mental illness. These two states are by no means mutually exclusive and, for example, anxiety is often a prominent feature of a depressive illness. Depressive illnesses and anxiety states form the bulk of mental illness seen in a general community, and much of the time of a general practitioner is taken up in dealing with them.

The anxiety state

In the anxiety state there is always a mixture of both psychological and physical elements, although one may dominate the other. The physical features of the anxiety state are similar to those experienced in fear—palpitations, sweating, a rise in pulse rate and blood pressure, giddiness, trembling, diarrhoea and an increased output of urine. Other physical features may occur after prolonged anxiety—headaches, nausea, loss of appetite and other digestive disturbances and difficulties in sexual life. The psychological counterpart may include a feeling of apprehension, depression of spirits, insomnia and changes in memory and the ability to concentrate. The whole world, including the patient, may seem to have changed and become unreal or unfamiliar. Sometimes the anxiety may be focused on special situations—fears of certain kinds of travel or being in crowds, or of certain objects or of disease, particularly of cancer.

These various symptoms may fluctuate. Sometimes they may disappear for a period but they may suddenly increase in intensity to reach a state of panic. All the while the patient may well realize that these physical and mental reactions to life are quite disproportionate and unnecessary. They have, however, arisen without any conscious effort on the part of the patient, and they persist after prolonged and rational discussion.

The causes of these abnormal forms of anxiety are complex and undoubtedly vary from one individual to another. There seems to be some constitutional element in some cases which causes the individual to develop anxiety under *any* stress. Physical factors may also play their role, influences such as occur in long continued physical stress, head injuries, puberty, menstruation and the menopause. Psychological factors which are involved in many cases are conflicts, frustrations and other situations that maintain tension with accumulative effect.

Depression

Depression is, of course, a natural response of normal individuals to personal failures and problems of all kinds. Usually these reactions are a temporary affair and seldom lead to the seeking of medical advice. When depression begins to dominate a person's life and has little or no relation to recent outside events, then it must be regarded as an illness. It is an illness that may often go unrecognized and untreated, one that may have the most serious of consequences in the form of suicide.

Depressive illnesses are usually classified into two main kinds. Reactive depression describes the illness when it occurs as a response to some outside cause, e.g. a bereavement or an unhappy love affair; the symptoms are, however, excessive in amount and persist for a long time. Sometimes no obvious precipitating cause can be discovered; here the illness is called an endogenous depression.

The features of depression have already been described under the heading of Manic-depressive psychosis. The important point which needs stressing is the risk of suicide. Threats of suicide or 'failed attempts' at suicide occupy a considerable number of medical beds in hospitals, and not only take up much of the time of medical staff but also strain the psychiatric resources of general hospitals. Although the official policy is that every case of attempted suicide should receive skilled psychiatric assessment, a number of cases (estimated to be as high as 20 per cent) are never in fact seen by a psychiatrist.

Psychosomatic illness

These illnesses are what one can describe as being physical expressions of emotions or mental disorders. 'Stress' of various sorts, particularly that resulting from loss of love or some relation, or aggression, often precipitate the appearance of these psychosomatic disorders. Some diseases that have a psychosomatic origin, diseases such as asthma, peptic ulcer and hypertension, also seem to have a strong constitutional element; these diseases occur more often among family members of patients with the disorders than among the families of patients with other diseases. The list of diseases in which psychological stress often plays a role is long and includes hypertension, peptic ulcer, bronchial asthma, ulcerative colitis, thyrotoxicosis, coronary artery disease, migraine, diabetes mellitus and rheumatoid arthritis.

The control of mental illnesses

General

From our brief survey of the kinds of mental illnesses, it is quite obvious that no single measure can prevent the bulk of these illnesses, and indeed the causes of most mental illness still lies in the realm of speculation. Genetic counselling and family planning have an important part to play in the control of those mental illnesses, including mental deficiency, in which there are clear genetic influences. These specific examples apart, this is one of the most difficult of all fields of preventative medicine. Whenever social, economic and cultural conditions change rapidly, there is usually an alarming increase in mental and behavioural disorders. This effect is by no means restricted to developed countries; the same results are seen in developing countries of the world. The urban environment is certainly a potentially unhealthy place in which to live. Crime, delinquency, alcoholism, drug addiction, prostitution, mental illness and suicide are all penalties of the urban way of life. An additional problem is the burden of the increasing proportion of old people in many populations; in industrialized societies there has been a considerable rise in the rates of admission of old people to mental hospitals in recent years. The aged, *par excellence*, pose the problem of loneliness—a major cause of ill health and unhappiness in societies (Figures 30.3, 30.4).

The unit requiring treatment—individuals, family or society?

The promotion of mental health involves attack at all levels of society and the cooperation of many individuals and organizations, each with their own special skills—central government, local authorities, town planners, architects, general practitioners, psychiatrists, teachers and all the diverse activities of welfare organizations, both voluntary and local authority. Emotional illness in the individual is increasingly recognized as a manifestation of a sick family, and control measures should be aimed at this larger group. The families' 'group mentality' is the target for assessment and treatment. Some of the advantages of this type of approach can be seen from the following example.

A boy of seventeen develops attacks of right-sided abdominal pain and diarrhoea. His mother takes him to see the local general practitioner. On their way out of the house father shouts to the mother 'while you are there, get yourself

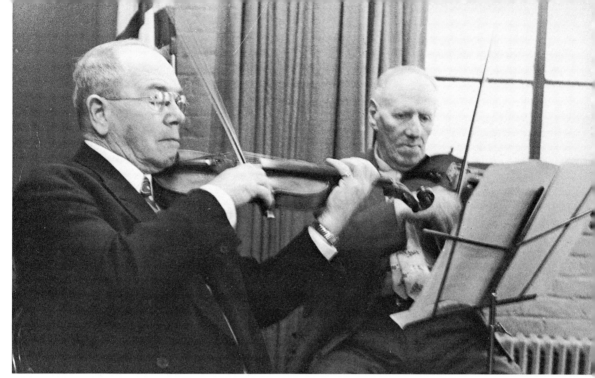

Figure 30.3 (above)   One million New Yorkers over 60 years of age are beset by loneliness. Problems of old age are accentuated by loneliness. These two men attend the Sirovich Day Centre, one of twenty-two old people's centres in the City run by private institutions with the support of the Health Department. (*WHO photo by Homer Page.*)

Figure 30.4 (below)   Everywhere in the world more people are living longer. Special health, welfare and occupational and recreational services and community centres can be provided for those who outlive their close friends and relatives. The photograph shows a new resident of a community development block for old people in Sweden proudly showing visitors the family portraits. (*WHO photo by Jan Dolden.*)

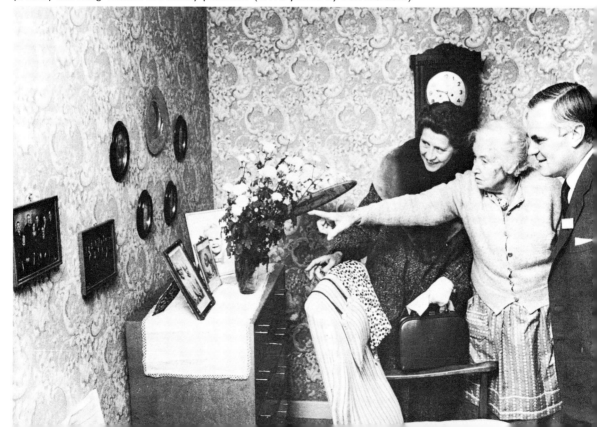

sorted out as well'. The mother has been depressed and frigid for some time and the father has been increasingly irritable and tense, which has done little for his 'nervous indigestion'.

At the G.P's the mother does not mention her depression and frigidity. The G.P. has the boy admitted to a surgical ward at a local hospital, where he had stayed two months previously under observation as a case of suspected appendicitis. On this occasion he is operated upon. Uncertain of the diagnosis, the surgeon makes a long incision to give him room to look around the abdominal contents. No abnormality is seen and a normal appendix is removed. The boy makes an uneventful recovery and is discharged home feeling well. Within weeks of his return home the abdominal symptoms reappear, now with frequent diarrhoea with slime in the stools. He is referred for further investigations. Barium enema and sigmoidoscopy are carried out with no abnormal findings. He has several interviews with a psychiatrist and is started on a course of 'tranquillizers' and a drug to reduce the activities of the bowel. He makes a dramatic improvement and the abdominal symptoms disappear.

The boy's improvement coincides with a deterioration in the relationships between his parents. Father's indigestion becomes more troublesome and a whole series of fruitless investigations are carried out. A G.P. locum with training and interest in psychiatry appears on the scene and mother and father are eventually interviewed together. It appears that the onset of the son's abdominal symptoms and the deterioration in the relationship between the parents coincided with the return home of a daughter on long vacation from the university. A brilliant young woman, all of her father's hopes and ambitions were pinned upon her. She began to mix with a 'hippie' set and spent several evenings away from home. Father felt unable to interfere with his daughter's way of life, in spite of the fact that he was very anxious about its possible effects upon her academic career. Mother refused to interfere, and indeed she had no hopes of an academic career for her daughter; all she wanted for her daughter was that she should stay at home, marry and live in the same locality.

The father then became increasingly irritable and spent his feelings on his son. The son was not academically bright and was receiving special coaching at a private school to try to get some 'O' levels. The persistent bickering between the two males made the mother depressed and frigid.

This then was the 'sick' family. Treatment of individual members of the family proved to be an extremely expensive and unsuccessful way of dealing with the problems. If, in this situation, one member is treated and so improved, the whole balance of the family becomes disturbed, triggering off emotional and psychosomatic illnesses in the other members. If, instead, the family is treated as a unit, all members are likely to benefit.

Day hospitals

This change in the unit being treated is one of the advances in psychiatric medicine that has emerged in recent years. We have already mentioned the trend away from 'institutionalization' of the mentally ill towards care within the community. Until fairly recently, mental hospitals were for the care of the various psychoses—

Figure 30.5 An example of what a dynamic, optimistic psychiatrist can do to help the mentally ill. Under his guidance a traditional insane asylum in the Philippines, housing 4300 patients instead of the 1000 for which it was built, is being transformed into a place for treatment and cure where anyone can go for advice and assistance. The iron bars and grills within the patio compound were removed; games and athletic contests were organized; music was heard for the first time in the hospital at daily concerts given by a band of talented patients; classes in painting, ceramics, handicrafts were started. Family participation in treatment is encouraged and group discussions with the families of out-patients are held regularly to foster understanding of the needs of the patient and the role that the family can play in bringing about a cure. From this hospital, also, teams go out to try to discover illness in its earliest stages. The photograph shows a schizophrenic in a violent outburst of anger being calmed by Dr Jose M. Clarin.

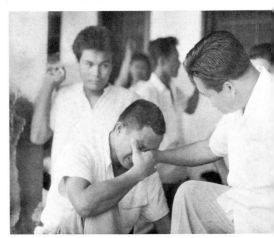

schizophrenia, the organic dementias and manic-depressives—and admission was usually by way of a certificate and with the attendance of a magistrate. These serious illnesses are relatively uncommon compared with the number of neuroses—anxiety, depression, psychosomatic disease and the like. When the ideas of psychiatrists such as Freud began to influence British medicine, the management of these neuroses also became part of psychiatry, although patients were usually treated in out-patient departments of general hospitals. A new kind of hospital has now emerged to bridge the gap between these two kinds of care of the mentally ill—i.e. the mental hospital for psychotics and the general hospital out-patient clinic for neurotics. This is the day hospital, which allows large numbers of people to be treated and supervized and supported without the need for admission. The introduction of a range of new and effective drugs in the 1950s which could control anxiety or depression (the psychotropic drugs, see page 368) gave impetus to this development. The pleasant appearance and informal running of these day hospitals is a far cry from the grim Victorian atmosphere of many existing mental hospitals. The function of these day hospitals overlaps somewhat with the 'day centres' which are run by local authorities, providing long-term occupational and social support for the physically and mentally handicapped (including the elderly). In most areas of the country these day centres, rather than day hospitals, care for the mentally subnormal.

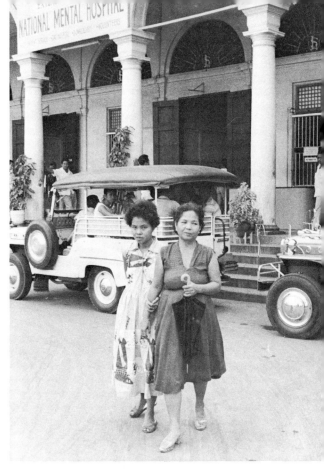

Figure 30.6   There is no barred door to this Manila hospital. Many who require expert help are well enough to stay with their families which prevents them from losing touch with reality. They visit the hospital at regular intervals as out-patients. This mother is taking her daughter home after treatment. (*WHO photo by Eric Schwab.*)

The range of the various treatments for mental disorders. Psycho-analysis

In considering the treatment of patients with mental illness a clear distinction has to be made between the major mental illnesses, the psychoses (e.g. schizophrenia and manic-depressive psychoses) and the neuroses (anxiety, depression and the psychosomatic diseases). The earliest form of treatment for neurotic illnesses was the technique of psycho-analysis—a prolonged relationship between doctor and patient in which the patient gained some insight into his problems. These techniques were developed in the mid-nineteenth century by workers such as Charcot, Freud, Adler and Jung. The basis of much of this work lies in the recognition that there are powerful mental processes that can and often do remain hidden from the conscious mind. At first the technique of hypnotism was used to tap these hidden mental processes. Freud discovered, however, that hypnotism was not necessary. By

getting his patients to relax on a couch in a dreamy condition, speaking freely about every kind of thought that fleeted through the mind, discussing dreams and feelings, he was able to obtain some image of the deep unconscious mental processes. Each facet that could be discovered in this way was slowly and painfully followed up, so taking the patient back along a devious and often painful route into his past life where it was hoped the source of the neurotic illness would be found.

From these studies Freud built up his own picture of the architecture and functioning of the mind and the disorders of mental processes that may lead to neurotic illness (see Sigmund Freud, *An Outline of Psycho-Analysis*, Hogarth Press, 1949). Freud laid great stress on the significance of a vast and complex unconscious mind, whose workings we do not appreciate as words or pictures but as emotions. We are only permitted certain glimpses of these processes if they are allowed to emerge into consciousness by the 'endopsychic censor'. Any force or idea that this censor disapproves of is driven back into the unconscious. Here it does not remain dormant, it has its own quota of life energy ('libido') and its activities may manifest themselves indirectly in the form of neurotic illness. Freud saw the 'endopsychic censor' as banishing many unpleasant and painful memories into the unconscious mind, so that the individual no longer remembers them. In the process of psycho-analysis the censor has to be persuaded to allow these memories to rise up into consciousness so that their pent-up energies can be released. The relationship between patient and psycho-analyst is of a very special nature. Freud asserted that the patient regarded the analyst 'as the return—the reincarnation—of some important figure out of his childhood or past, and consequently transfers on to him feelings and reactions that undoubtedly applied to this model. It soon became evident that this transfer is a factor of undreamt of importance—on the one hand an instrument of irreplaceable value and on the other a source of serious dangers.'

Thwarted sexual urges, with their associated guilt, were to Freud the commonest cause of neurotic illness. Some of the followers of Freud had other ideas about the kind of mental forces that were the source of neurosis. Their techniques of psycho-analysis, however, followed that of Freud, and all of them stressed the importance of conflicts in early development in the shaping of neurotic reactions later in life.

These psycho-analytical methods of treatment have made major contributions to our understanding of possible causes of mental illness and possible treatments. On the other hand, the limitations of classical psycho-analysis are profound. In the first place their use is limited to neurotic illnesses—anxieties, depression, phobias and the like. They have little or no place in the management of psychoses (schizophrenia, manic-depressive illnesses etc.) or of mental deficiencies. Secondly, psycho-analysis is a lengthy and costly treatment; the available resources are quite inadequate to treat the millions of neurotics in the world by psychoanalysis. Even the available physical methods of treatment for mental illness, such as electroconvulsive therapy (see below), are too expensive to deal with this problem. The only form of treatment that a single psychiatrist can administer to hundreds of patients simultaneously is in the form of psychotropic drugs (see page 368). Nowadays classical psycho-analysis has become divorced from the bulk of medicine and psychiatry in Great Britain at least, and it is an uncommon form of treatment of mental disorders.

Behaviour therapy

Behaviour therapy is the name given to methods of psychological treatment which arise from studies of the learning process; it aims to modify existing behaviour and to develop more desirable patterns of behaviour. This kind of treatment has its roots in experimental studies of animals and man himself—of which Pavlov's experiments with dogs are a classic. These latter experiments involved a study of the factors involved in the regulation of the secretion of digestive juices. Pavlov and his workers noticed that the flow of saliva in a dog's mouth was a reflex activity (a spontaneous and automatic action made in response to definite stimuli). Saliva was made when it was required. The taste of meat was seen to be the prime stimulus that caused the secretion of saliva, but this stimulus could be linked (associated) in the 'mind' of the dog with other stimuli—the smell of the feeder's hand, or the sound of feeding utensils—so that these other stimuli could also cause a flow of saliva, even in the absence of food. Pavlov found that it was possible to teach a dog when to respond to an 'associated' stimulus and when not to respond. If a dog was allowed to smell meat but not allowed to eat it then the response of the secretion of saliva to the stimulus of smell alone became weaker and weaker until the dog did not salivate when he smelt meat. If the dog was presented with meat and at the same time a bell was rung, the animal would eventually associate these two stimuli—i.e. meat and bell—so that the animal would salivate at the ringing of the bell alone. This reflex activity of salivation was thus 'conditioned' to the stimulus of a bell ringing. The mechanism of conditioning is useful to the animal in nature, for it helps it to 'forecast' what is going to happen and to take the appropriate action in readiness. The dog could start to salivate, for example, when he saw the keeper approaching from a distance at meal times. This kind of conditioning gives the appearance of intelligent behaviour.

Similar conditioning of responses can be produced experimentally in man. Watson, for example, produced automatic reactions of fear of rats in an eleven-month old boy by repeatedly presenting an unpleasant stimulus, a loud noise, whenever the boy approached a rat. In 1924 Jones successfully treated fears in children by the reverse of this process—by presenting the feared object when the child was engaged in a pleasurable activity—eating sweets. From these kinds of studies developed the idea that neurotic 'fears' may be in the nature of conditioned emotional responses. A variety of kinds of neurotic behaviour are now being treated by means of artificial learning situations in which conditioning plays a vital role. Thus alcoholics, drug addicts, compulsive gamblers or sexual perverts may be presented with their particular brand of pleasure—be it drink, a drug, pictures of race meetings, or photographs of abnormal sexual activity—and at the same time they receive an unpleasant stimulus such as an electric shock or an injection to produce vomiting. The aim of this activity is to encourage the individual to associate this particular activity with an unpleasant stimulus, i.e. to condition him. This particular kind of treatment is called 'aversion therapy'. Conditioning treatment may also have positive aspects. This involves re-inforcing *desirable* behaviour by praise, food, attention, cigarettes etc., while at the same time *undesirable* behaviour results in withholding of attention and the token rewards. This kind of treatment can be carried out in groups, such as wards of patients. Obviously this may be a very prolonged form of treatment and it may need much ingenuity to find the rewards and punishments that are most appropriate for a particular patient.

Physical methods of treatment

Convulsive therapy

As long ago as 1798 injections of camphor were used to produce convulsions in mental patients in the hope of improving their condition. In 1937 the technique was revived, using an electric shock passed through the front of the brain to produce the convulsion (E.C.T.—Electro-Convulsive Therapy). In the early days of this treatment accidents occurred because of the powerful muscular contractions that occurred during the convulsion; these contractions were often powerful enough to fracture a bone as strong as the femur. It became apparent, however, that the convulsion itself was not necessary to obtain benefit from the treatment, and patients are now anaesthetized and relaxed with a short acting, paralysing drug before the electric current is passed across the brain; the paralysing drug prevents the powerful muscle spasms. The way in which this treatment produces its beneficial effects are unknown, but certainly several types of mental patients are improved by it, e.g.

depressives, schizophrenics and manic-depressives. Disturbances of memory and concentration commonly follow this treatment, although modern refinements of the technique in which only one side of the front of the brain receives an electric current have reduced these effects.

Brain surgery—prefrontal leucotomy

Brain surgery is a drastic and irreversible form of treatment for mental illness, and it is resorted to only when all other treatments have been shown to be of no effect. The operation of prefrontal leucotomy was developed by Moniz, a professor of neurology in Lisbon. The frontal lobes of the brain seemed to be the logical point of surgical interference; these areas of the brain had no special physical function assigned to them —they seemed to be the seat of intellectual life. Experiments in apes had showed that extensive destruction of these frontal areas of the cerebral hemispheres improved their emotional stability with little effect on 'intellectual' functions. The operation, developed by Moniz, was designed to interrupt connections between the frontal areas of the brain and the deeper parts. The operation itself is not particularly dangerous or difficult. A fine knife or needle is inserted through a small opening into the skull and carefully directed to sever the fibres that carry the 'emotional impulses' from the deeper parts of the brain up to the frontal areas.

The results of this operation are complex. The individual experiences less emotional charge so that he feels and reacts less intensely; parallel with this there is less tendency to worry. There is also a release of some inhibitions so that there may be more impulsiveness. Intellectual changes of a subtle kind may appear, with a reduced tendency to think in abstract terms. The main indications for this operation are found in the chronically ill who are incapacitated by excess of emotion in the form of tension and anxiety. Modern refinements of the operation in which, instead of completely isolating the frontal lobe, only certain fibre connections are interrupted, have reduced the damaging effects on personality and intellect.

Drugs

Until the 1950s the use of drugs had a limited place in the treatment of mental illness. The drugs available—such as morphia, hyoscine, paraldehyde and the barbiturates—were used mainly to decrease restlessness and excitement or to promote sleep. Sometimes sedatives were used to produce continuous narcosis—'sleep treatment'—or to relax the patients to such a point that they were able to talk freely of their problems and release pent-up emotions. Since 1935 insulin was used to produce either a state of deep coma (in the treatment of schizophrenia) or to stimulate appetite in cases of mental illness where loss of appetite and weight were prominent features.

In 1951 a potent drug called chlorpromazine (Largactil) was introduced and it was soon found to be a powerful agent for the control of agitated and difficult schizophrenic patients. Chlorpromazine and its derivatives are now standard treatment for schizophrenia, and valuable long-acting derivatives (whose effects last for a month after injection) have made it possible to treat schizophrenics on an out-patient basis. It is estimated that in a ten year period, at least 20 million patients have received this drug and tens of thousands of publications have dealt with its actions. Chlorpromazine was followed by a whole host of 'psychotropic drugs', tranquillizing drugs for the management of anxiety and anti-depressants that act specifically on depressive symptoms.

These psychotropic drugs have revolutionized the treatment of mental illness of many kinds. They do not cure the illness but they are powerful suppressors of the symptoms of the illness. They are most effective when they are combined with other forms of treatment such as advice in solving emotional problems and social, occupational and physical rehabilitation. In addition to their specific effects on the various symptoms of mental illness, they can also so alter the mental and emotional state of a patient as to make him more receptive to these other forms of treatment. The use of these drugs has lessened the need for physical forms of treatment such as electro-convulsive therapy. Some patients may, however, still need E.C.T. if depression is severe or if they do not respond adequately to anti-depressive drugs.

Summary

In this chapter we have presented, in a very compressed form, the 'spectrum' of mental illnesses, their treatments and possible methods of prevention. We are still only on the threshold of understanding the causes of mental illness and the way in which the available methods of treatment produce their effects. Prevention lags even further behind; without a vast increase in the resources for the study of this aspect of mental health, the outlook is not very promising. It is perhaps inevitable that, with major physical illnesses still uncontrollable and with half the world suffering from poverty and malnutrition, the prevention and treatment of mental illness is still in its infancy.

Bibliography

This bibliography includes most of the books that we have found of value in the preparation of this book. It is by no means comprehensive but further reading lists may be found in these volumes. Wherever possible we have tried to include references for the non-specialist reader and these are marked by an asterisk.

Many World Health Organization Publications have been listed in the bibliography. In the U.K. these publications may be obtained from Her Majesty's Stationery Offices; all postal orders should be sent to P.O. Box 569, London, S.E.1. Orders may also be addressed to: World Health Organization, Distribution and Sales Unit, Geneva, Switzerland, from whom a catalogue of publications can be obtained.

Accidents

Accident Prevention and Life Saving. John H. Hunt. (Edinburgh: E. and S. Livingstone Ltd., 1965.)

Accidents in Childhood. Facts as a Basis for Prevention. (WHO Technical Report Series, No. 118, 1957.)

Domestic Accidents. E. Maurice Backett. (WHO Public Health Papers, No. 26, 1965.)

New Safety and First Aid. A. Ward Gardner and P. S. Royland. (London: Pan Books, 1970.)

Road Traffic Accidents: Epidemiology, Control and Prevention. L. G. Norman. (WHO Public Health Papers, No. 12, 1962.)

Bacteria

Bacteria. A. H. Dadd. (London: Hutchinson Educational Books, 1972.)

Biological Principles of Fermentation. J. G. Carr. (London: Heinemann Educational Books Ltd, 1968.)

Microbes and Man. John Postgate. (Harmondsworth: Penguin Books, 1969.)

Microbial Toxins. A Comprehensive Treatise. (Vols. I, II, and III) Bacterial Protein Toxins. Ed. Samuel J. Ajl *et al*. (London: Academic Press, 1970.)

The Biology of Fungi, Bacteria and Viruses. Greta B. Stevenson. (London: Edward Arnold, 1970.)

Cancer

Cancer Control. First Report of an Expert Committee (Geneva 1962). (WHO Technical Report Series, No. 251, 1963.)

Cancer Treatment. Report of an Expert Committee (Geneva 1965), (WHO Technical Report Series, No. 322, 1966.)

Epidemiology of Cancer of the Lung. Report of a Study Group (Geneva 1959). (WHO Technical Report Series, No. 192, 1960.)

Prevention of Cancer. Report of a WHO Expert Committee (Geneva 1963). (WHO Technical Report Series, No. 276, 1964.)

Domiciliary Care of the Patient with Cancer (The Marie Curie Memorial Foundation Symposium on The Prevention of Cancer). Ed. R. W. Raven. (London: W. Heinemann Medical Books, 1970.)

What We Know About Cancer. Ed. R. J. C. Harris. (London: Allen and Unwin, 1970.)

Communicable diseases

Aerobiology; Proceedings of the 3rd International Symposium. Ed. I. H. Silver. (London: Academic Press, 1970.)

Epidemic Diseases. A. H. Gale. (Harmondsworth: Pelican Books, 1959.)

Infectious Diseases. A. M. Ramsay and R. T. O. Emond. (London: W. Heinemann Medical Books, 1967.)

Natural History of Infectious Disease. Sir Macfarlane Burnet. (Cambridge University Press, 1953.)

Plague. R. Pollitzer. Monograph Series No. 22. (WHO, 1954.)

Poliomyelitis. R. Debré *et al*. (WHO Monograph Series No. 26, 1955.)

Streptococcal and Staphylococcal Infections. Report of a WHO Expert Committee. (WHO Technical Report Series, No. 394, 1968.)

The Birth of Penicillin and the Disarming of Microbes. R. Hare. (London: Allen and Unwin, 1970.)

Tuberculosis. 8th Report of a WHO Expert Committee (Geneva 1964). (WHO Technical Report Series, No. 290, 1964.)

Uses of Epidemiology. J. N. Morris. (Edinburgh: E. and S. Livingstone, 1964.)

Cardiovascular disease

Arterial Hypertension and Ischaemic Heart Disease: Preventative Aspects. Report of a WHO Expert Committee (Geneva 1961). (WHO Technical Report Series, No. 231, 1962.)

Cardiovascular Diseases Mortality, 1954–1956, 1958–1960. Epidemiological and Vital Statistics Report. (WHO, 1963, vol. 16, No. 2.)

'Coronary Disease'. *The Practitioner*, No. 1208, vol. 202, February 1969.

Hypertension and Coronary Heart Disease: Classification and Criteria for Epidemiological Studies. First report of the Expert Committee on Cardiovascular Diseases and Hypertension (Geneva 1958). (WHO Technical Report Series, No. 168, 1959.)

'Peripheral Vascular Disease'. *The Practitioner.* No. 1233, vol. 206, March 1971.

Study Group on Atherosclerosis and Ischaemic Heart Disease. Report (Geneva 1955). (WHO Technical Report Series, No. 117, 1957.)

Dental health

Adult Dental Health in England and Wales in 1968. (London: HMSO, 1970.)

Expert Committee on Water Fluoridation. First Report (Geneva 1957). (WHO Technical Report Series, No. 146, 1958.)

*Caring for Teeth. (London: Consumers Association, 1970.)

Periodontal Disease. Report of an Expert Committee on Dental Health (Geneva 1960). (WHO Technical Report Series, No. 207, 1961.)

Drugs and alcoholism

Alcohol and Alcoholism. Report of an Expert Committee (Geneva 1954). (WHO Technical Report Series, No. 94, 1955.)

Amphetamines, Barbiturates, LSD and Cannabis. Their Use and Misuse. (London: HMSO, 1970.)

*Drugs: Medical, Psychological and Social Facts. Peter Laurie. (Harmondsworth: Penguin Books, 1969.)

Drugs: The Parents' Dilemma. A. R. K. Mitchell. (Royston: Priory Press, 1969.)

Expert Committee on Addiction-Producing Drugs. 15th Report. (WHO Technical Report Series, No. 343, 1966.)

Services for The Prevention of Dependence on Alcohol and other Drugs. 14th Report of the WHO Expert Committee on Mental Health (Geneva 1966). (WHO Technical Report Series, No. 363, 1967.)

Teaching About Drugs. A Curriculum Guide K-12. (American School Health Association, 1971.)

'The Problem of Addiction', *The Practitioner.* No. 1196, vol. 200, February 1968.

Treatment and Care of Drug Addicts. Report of a Study Group (Geneva 1956). (WHO Technical Report Series, No. 131, 1957.)

*WHERE on Drugs—A Parents Handbook. (Cambridge: Advisory Centre for Education, 1970.)

Food hygiene and food-borne disease

Brucellosis. Fourth Report of the Joint FAO/WHO Expert Committee (Geneva 1963). (WHO Technical Report Series, No. 289, 1964.)

Food-borne Infections and Intoxications. Ed. Hans Riemann. (London: Academic Press, 1969.)

'Food Irradiation Stymied'. Edward Edelson. *New Scientist.* 30th May, 1968.

Food Poisoning and Food Hygiene. Betty C. Hobbs. (London: Edward Arnold, 1970.)

Hygiene in Milk Production, Processing and Distribution. M. Abdussalam *et al.* (WHO Monograph Series, No. 48, 1962.)

Meat Hygiene. V. E. Albertsen *et al.* (WHO Monograph Series, No. 33, 1957.)

Microbiological Aspects of Food Hygiene. Report of a WHO Expert Committee with the participation of FAO.

Milk Pasteurisation: Planning, Plant, Operation and Control. H. O. Kay *et al.* (WHO Monograph Series, No. 14, 1953.)

Pesticide Residues in Food. Report of the 1968 Joint FAO/WHO Meeting. (WHO Technical Report Series, No. 417.)

The Control of Tuberculosis. A Survey of Existing Legislation. Reprint from International Digest of Health Regulation. 1963, vol. 14, No. 4. (WHO Technical Report Series, No. 399, 1968.)

Fungi

Laboratory Methods in Microbiology. W. F. Harrigan and Margaret E. McCance. (London: Academic Press, 1966.)

Materials and Methods in Fermentation. G. L. Solomons. (London: Academic Press, 1969.)
The Impact of Fungi on Man. Willard A. Taber and Ruth Ann Taber. (London: John Murray, 1969.)
The Yeasts. A treatise in three volumes. (Vol. 1 Biology of Yeasts. Vol. 2 Physiology and Biochemistry of Yeasts. Vol. 3 Yeast Technology.) Ed. by A. H. Rose and J. S. Harrison. (London: Academic Press, 1970.)

General texts

A Biology of Man. Margaret E. Hogg. (London: Heinemann Educational Books, 1962.)
Environmental Health. Ed. P. Walton Purdom. (London: Academic Press, 1971.)
Health of Mankind. Ciba Foundation 100th Symposium. Ed. G. Wolstenholme and M. O'Connor. (London: J. and A. Churchill, 1967.)
Microbe Hunters. Paul de Kruif. (New York: Harcourt, Brace & Co., 1926.)
Pasteur and Modern Science. Rene Dubos. (London: Heinemann Educational Books, 1961.)
Physiology, Environment and Man. Ed. D. H. K. Lee and D. Minard. (London: Academic Press, 1970.)
Public and Community Health. W. S. Parker. (London: Staples Press, 1970.)
The Second Ten Years of the World Health Organization, 1958–1967. (WHO, 1968.)

Health education

A Handbook of Health Education. Department of Education and Science (HMSO 1968).
A Textbook of Health Education. D. Pirrie and A. J. D. Ward. (London: Tavistock Publications, 1962.)
Expert Committee on Health Education of the Public. 1st Report (Paris 1953). (WHO Technical Report Series, No. 89, 1954.)
Methods and Materials in Health Education. H. and N. Schneider. (London: W. B. Saunders, 1964.)
Teacher Preparation for Health Education. Report of the Joint WHO/UNESCO Committee (Geneva 1959). (WHO Technical Report Series, No. 193, 1960.)
Planning and Evaluation of Health Education Services. (WHO Technical Report Series, No. 409.)
UNESCO Source Book for Health Education. C. E. Turner. (Harlow: Longmans, 1971.)

Human genetics

An Introduction to Medical Genetics. J. A. Fraser Roberts. (Oxford University Press, 1967.)
Genetic Counselling. 3rd Report of the WHO Expert Committee on Human Genetics. (WHO Technical Report Series, No. 416, 1969.)
Genetic Counselling. W. Fuhrmann and F. Vogel. (Harlow: Longmans, 1969.)
Genetic Counselling. 3rd Report of the WHO Expert Committee on Human Genetics. (WHO Technical Report Series, No. 416.)
Human Genetics and Public Health. 2nd Report of the WHO Expert Committee on Human Genetics (Geneva 1963). (WHO Technical Report Series, No. 282, 1963.)
Human Heredity. C. O. Carter. (Harmondsworth: Penguin Books, 1962.)
Research on Genetics in Psychiatry. Report of a WHO Scientific Group (Geneva 1965). (WHO Technical Report Series, No. 346, 1966.)
The Science of Genetics. Charlotte Auerbach. (London: Hutchinson Educational Books, 1970.)
Screening for Inborn Errors of Metabolism. (WHO Technical Report Series, No. 401.)

Immunity and immunization

A History of Immunization. H. J. Parish. (Edinburgh: E. and S. Livingstone, 1965.)
Basic Immunology. E. R. Gold and D. B. Peacock. (Bristol: John Wright, 1970.)
Biological Defence Mechanisms. Ian Carr. (Oxford: Blackwell Scientific, 1971.)
Cell Mediated Immune Responses. (WHO Technical Report Series, No. 423.)
Cellular Immunology. Sir Macfarlane Burnet. (Cambridge University Press, 1969.)
Essential Immunology. I. M. Roitt. (Oxford: Blackwell Scientific, 1971.)
Genetics of the Immune Response. (WHO Technical Report Series, No. 402, 1968.)
'Immunization in General Practice'. *The Practitioner.* No. 1234, vol. 206, April 1971.
The Role of Immunization in Communicable Disease Control. (WHO Public Health Papers, No. 8, 1961.)
The Traveller's Health Guide. A. C. Turner. (London: Tom Stacey, 1971.)
The Use of Human Immunoglobulin. Report of a WHO Expert Committee (Geneva 1965). (WHO Technical Report Series, No. 327, 1966.)

Victory with Vaccines. H. J. Parish. (Edinburgh: E. and S. Livingstone, 1968.)

The Practice of Community Mental Health. Ed. H. Grunebaum. (London: J. and A. Churchill, 1970.)

Mental health and disease

Aspects of Depression. Ed. E. S. Schneidman. (London: J. and A. Churchill, 1970.)

Aspects of Family Mental Health in Europe. D. Buckle *et al.* (WHO Public Health Papers, No. 28, 1965.)

Behaviour Therapy: Appraisal and Status. C. M. Franks. (New York: McGraw-Hill, 1969.)

Changing Man's Behaviour. H. R. Beech. (Harmondsworth: Penguin Books, 1969.)

Diagnosis and Drug Treatment of Psychiatric Disorders. D. F. Klein and J. M. Davis. (Edinburgh: E. and S. Livingstone, 1969.)

Epidemiological Methods in the Study of Mental Disorders. D. D. Reid. (WHO Public Health Papers, No. 2, 1960.)

Expert Committee on Mental Health. Report on the 1st Session (Geneva 1949). (WHO Technical Report Series, No. 9, 1950.)

Report on the 2nd Session (Geneva 1950). (WHO Technical Report Series, No. 31, 1951.)

Maternal Care and Mental Health. J. Bowlby. (WHO Monograph Series, No. 2, 1952.)

Mental Health Problems of Ageing and the Aged. 6th Report of the Expert Committee on Mental Health (Geneva 1958). (WHO Technical Report Series, No. 171, 1959.)

Prevention of Suicide. (WHO Public Health Papers, No. 35.)

Psychiatry To-day. D. Stafford-Clark. (Harmondsworth: Penguin Books, 1971.)

'Psychology and Psychiatry in General Practice'. *The Practitioner.* No. 1227, vol. 205, September 1970.

Psychology in Relation to Medicine. R. M. Mowbray and T. F. Rodger. (Edinburgh: E. and S. Livingstone, 1970.)

Psychosomatic Disorders. 13th Report of the WHO Expert Committee on Mental Health (Geneva 1963). (WHO Technical Report Series, No. 275, 1964.)

Psychotherapy: A Dynamic Approach. P. A. Dewald. (Oxford: Blackwell Scientific, 1970.)

The Community Mental Hospital. 3rd Report of the Expert Committee on Mental Health (Geneva 1952). (WHO Technical Report Series, No. 73, 1953.)

The Development of the Infant and Young Child: Normal and Abnormal. R. S. Illingworth. (Edinburgh: E. and S. Livingstone, 1969.)

The Mentally Subnormal Child. (WHO Technical Report Series, No. 75, 1954.)

Parasites

Amoebiasis. Report of a WHO Expert Committee. (WHO Technical Report Series, No. 421.)

Animals Parasitic in Man. G. Lapage. (Harmondsworth: Pelican Books, 1957.)

Chemotherapy and Drug Resistance in Malaria. W. Peters. (London: Academic Press, 1970.)

Control of Ascariasis. Report of a WHO Expert Committee (Geneva 1967). (WHO Technical Report Series, No. 379, 1967.)

Epidemiology and Control of Schistosomiasis. Report of a WHO Expert Committee (Geneva 1966). (WHO Technical Report Series, No. 372, 1967.)

'Fascioliasis—A large outbreak'. E. W. Hardman *et al. British Medical Journal,* No. 5721, vol. 3, 1970.

Filariasis (Wuchereria and Brugia Infections). 2nd Report of a WHO Expert Committee (Geneva 1966). (WHO Technical Report Series, No. 359, 1967.)

Malaria. 13th Report of a WHO Expert Committee (Geneva 1966). (WHO Technical Report Series, No. 357, 1967.)

Parasitic Protozoa. A. Wiseman, J. R. Baker and B. J. Gould. (London: Hutchinson Educational Books, 1969.)

Soil—Transmitted Helminths. Report of a WHO Expert Committee on Helminthiasis (Rio de Janiero, 1963). (WHO Technical Report Series, No. 277.)

Onchoceriasis. 2nd Report of a WHO Expert Committee (Geneva 1965). (WHO Technical Report Series No. 335, 1966.)

Zoonoses. 3rd Report of a Joint FAO/WHO Expert Committee. (WHO Technical Report Series, No. 378, 1967.)

Populations and contraception

Basic and Clinical Aspects of Intra-Uterine Devices. Report of a WHO Scientific Group (Geneva 1966). (WHO Technical Report Series, No. 332, 1966.)

Biology of Fertility Control by Periodic Abstinence. Report of a WHO Scientific Group (Geneva 1966). (WHO Technical Report Series, No. 360, 1967.)

'Family Planning'. *The Practitioner.* No. 1225, vol. 205, July 1970.

Family Planning. J. F. Robinson. (Edinburgh: E. and S. Livingstone, 1968.)
Family Planning Today. Ed. Alan Rubin. (Oxford: Blackwell Scientific, 1970.)
Legal Abortion. The English Experience. A. Hordern. (London: Pergamon Press, 1971.)
Manual of Family Planning and Contraceptive Practice. Ed. M. S. Calderone. (Edinburgh: E. and S. Livingstone, 1970.)
Population and Food Supply. Essays on Human Needs and Agricultural Prospects. Ed. Sir Joseph Hutchinson. (Cambridge University Press, 1969.)
The Agonising Choice: Birth Control, Religion and the Law. N. St. John Stevas. (London: Eyre & Spottiswood, 1971.)
The Contraceptive Pill. J. F. Robinson. (Edinburgh: E. and S. Livingstone, 1965.)
World Population and Food Supply. J. H. Lowry. (London: Edward Arnold, 1970.)

Radiation and health

Atomic Radiation and Life. Peter Alexander. (Harmondsworth: Penguin Books, 1957.)
Ionizing Radiation and Health. Bo Lindell and R. Lowry Dobson. (WHO Public Health Papers. No. 6, 1961.)

Smoking

Commonsense about Smoking. C. M. Fletcher et al. (Harmondsworth: Penguin Books, 1965.)
Scientific Basis of Drug Dependence. Ed. Steinberg. (London: J. and A. Churchill, London, 1969.)
Smoking and Health Now. A Report of the Royal College of Physicians. (London: Pitman, 1971.)
Smoking, Health and Personality. H. J. Eysenck. (London: Weidenfeld and Nicolson, 1965.)
The Biochemistry of Bladder Cancer. E. Boyland. (Illinois: C. C. Thomas, 1963.)

Venereal diseases

Venereal Diseases. R. S. Morton. (Harmondsworth: Penguin Books, 1966.)
Venereal Diseases. Ambrose King and Claude Nicol. (London: Baillière Tindall & Cassell, 1969.)

Viruses

Arboviruses and Human Disease. (WHO Technical Report Series, No. 369, 1967.)
Mechanisms of Virus Infection. Ed. Wilson Smith. (London: Academic Press, 1963.)
Techniques in Experimental Virology. Ed. R. J. C. Harris. (London: Academic Press, 1964.)
The Biology of the Large RNA Viruses. Ed. R. D. Barry and B. W. J. Mahy. (London: Academic Press, 1970.)
Viruses and Man. F. M. Burnet. (Harmondsworth: Penguin Books, 1953.)
'Virus Diseases'. *The Practitioner.* No. 1193, vol. 199, November 1967.

Water and water-borne diseases

Cholera. R. Pollitzer. (WHO Monograph Series, No. 43, 1959.)
Cholera. 2nd Report of a WHO Expert Committee (Manila 1966). (WHO Technical Report Series, No. 352, 1967.)
Community Water Supply. Report of a WHO Expert Committee. (WHO Technical Report Series, No. 420.)
Research into Environmental Pollution. Report of Five WHO Scientific Groups. (WHO Technical Report Series, No. 406, 1968.)
Treatment and Disposal of Wastes. Report of a WHO Scientific Group. (WHO Technical Report Series, No. 367, 1967.)
Water Pollution Control in Developing Countries. (WHO Technical Report Series, No. 404.)

Zoonoses

'Allergy to Animals: A Zoological Hazard?' P. Hunter-Jones. *New Scientist*, 1966, 513–31, 615–16.
'Human viral and bacterial infections acquired from laboratory rats and mice'. R. G. Somerville. (Laboratory Animals Centre. Collected Papers 1961, 10, 21–32.)
Rabies. 5th Report of a WHO Expert Committee. (WHO Technical Report Series, No. 321, 1966.)
Zoonoses. 2nd Report of the Joint WHO/FAO Expert Committee (Stockholm 1958). (WHO Technical Report Series, No. 169, 1957.)
Zoonoses. Ed. J. Van Der Hoeden. (Barking, Essex: Elsevier, 1964.)

Addresses of organizations

The following organizations may be able to provide further information and also possibly visual aids and visiting speakers.

British Red Cross Society, Heald Road, Bowdon, Altrincham, Cheshire.

Central Council for Health Education, Tavistock House North, Tavistock Square, London W.C.1.

Chest and Heart Association, Tavistock House North, Tavistock Square, London, W.C.1.

Clean Air Association, Field House, Breams Buildings, London E.C.4.

Gas Council, 4/5 Grosvenor Place, London S.W.1.

General Dental Council, 37 Wimpole Street, London W.1.

Marriage Guidance Council, 58 Queen Anne Street, London W.1.

Ministry of Health, Public Relations Officer, 1 Alexander Fleming House, London S.E.1.

Oral Hygiene Service, Hesketh House, Portman Square, London W.1.

Royal Society for the Prevention of Accidents, Terminal House, 52 Grosvenor Gardens, London S.W.1.

National Association for Maternal and Child Welfare, Tavistock House North, Tavistock Square, London W.C.1.

National Dairy Council, Charing Cross Road, London W.1.

N.S.P.C.C., Victory House, Leicester Square, London W.C.2.

St. John Ambulance Brigade, 25A Farncombe Road, Worthing, Sussex.

National Association for Mental Health, 39 Queen Anne Street, London W.1.

U.K. Alliance, Alliance House, 12 Caxton Street, London S.W.1.

Films and filmstrips

Films and filmstrips on aspects of Health Education may be obtained from the following organizations:

Boulton Hawker Films Ltd., Hadleigh, Suffolk.

British Instructional Films, 2 Dean Street, London W.1.

Camera Talks, 31 North Row, London W.1.

Central Film Library, Government Buildings, Bromyard Avenue, London W.3.

Chest and Heart Association, Tavistock House North, Tavistock Square, London W.C.1.

Concord Films Council, Nacton, Ipswich, Suffolk.

Diana Wyllie Ltd., 3 Park Road, London N.W.1.

E.F.V.A. Foundation Film Library, Brooklands House, Weybridge, Surrey.

Encyclopaedia Britannica Ltd., Dorland House, 18–20 Lower Regent Street, London S.W.1.

Esther Films, c/o Macmillan & Co. Ltd., 4 Little Essex Street, London W.C.2.

Gas Council, 4/5 Grosvenor Place, London S.W.1.

Gateway Educational Films Ltd., 470–472 Green Lanes, London N.13.

General Dental Council, 37 Wimpole Street, London W.1.

Imperial Chemical Industries Ltd., I.C.I. House, Millbank, London S.W.1.

Medical Recording Service, Kitts Croft, Writtle, Chelmsford, Essex.

Petroleum Films, 4 Brook Street, London W.1.

Rank Film Library, 1 Aintree Road, Perivale, Greenford, Middx.

R.A.V. Ltd., P.O. Box 70, Great West Road, Brentford, Middx.

Ron Harris, Cinema Services Ltd., Glen Buck Studios, Surbiton, Surrey.

R.O.S.P.A., Terminal House, 62 Grosvenor Gardens, London S.W.1.

Sound Services Ltd., Wilton Crescent, London S.W.19.

The London Foundation for Marriage Education, 78 Duke Street, London W.1.

Unilever Films, Unilever House, Blackfriars, London E.C.4.

Visigraph Ltd., Rowberry Street, Bromyard, Herefordshire.

Walt Disney Productions, 83 Pall Mall, London S.W.1.

Index